ANTHONY J. ADAMS, O.D., Ph.D.
Dean and Professor of Optometry & Vision Science
School of Optometry
University of California
Berkeley, California 94720

Tony Adams.

9/1/93

ENVIRONMENTAL VISION

ENVIRONMENTAL VISION

Interactions of the Eye, Vision, and the Environment

Donald G. Pitts, O.D., Ph.D.

College of Optometry
University of Houston
Houston, Texas

Robert N. Kleinstein, O.D., M.P.H., Ph.D.

School of Optometry
University of Alabama at Birmingham
Birmingham, Alabama

Butterworth–Heinemann
Boston   London   Oxford   Singapore   Sydney   Toronto   Wellington

To the Memory of
Oscar W. Richards, Ph.D.
born January 5, 1902, died January 31, 1989

A pioneer scientist in the field of Environmental Vision
who inspired the writing of this book.

To our lovely wives, Laura and Roberta,
for the many years of love, understanding, assistance, and support
that made the many years of research and the writing of this book possible.
DGP/RNK

Every effort has been made to ensure that the drug dosage
schedules within this text are accurate and conform to
standards accepted at time of publication. However, as
treatment recommendations vary in the light of continuing
research and clinical experience, the reader is advised to verify
drug dosage schedules herein with information found on
product information sheets. This is especially true in cases of
new or infrequently used drugs.

Recognizing the importance of preserving what has been
written, it is the policy of Butterworth–Heinemann to have the
books it publishes printed on acid-free paper, and we exert our
best efforts to that end.

Library of Congress Cataloging-in-Publication Data
Environmental vision : interactions of the eye, vision, and the
    environment / [edited by] Donald G. Pitts, Robert N. Kleinstein.
        p.   cm.
    Includes bibliographical references and index.
    ISBN 0-7506-9051-8
    1. Industrial ophthalmology.   2. Vision disorders—
Environmental aspects.   I. Pitts, Donald G.
II. Kleinstein, Robert N.
RE825.E56   1993
617.7—dc20   93-1290
                                                   CIP

British Library Cataloguing-in-Publication Data
A catalogue record for this book is available from the British
Library.

Butterworth–Heinemann
80 Montvale Avenue
Stoneham, MA 02180

10 9 8 7 6 5 4 3 2 1

Printed in the United States of America

Contents

Contents

Section IV: Special Problems and Solutions
in Environmental Vision   359

CHAPTER FIFTEEN
Protecting the Eye from Welding   361
Donald G. Pitts, O.D., Ph.D.

CHAPTER SIXTEEN
Special Clinical Problems   373
Debra Bezan, M.Ed., O.D. and Donald G. Pitts,
O.D., Ph.D.

CHAPTER SEVENTEEN
Vision and Drugs   387
Marilyn E. Schneck, O.D., Ph.D. and Anthony J. Adams,
O.D., Ph.D.

Index   409

Contributing Authors

Anthony J. Adams, O.D., Ph.D.
School of Optometry
University of California, Berkeley
Berkeley, CA

Ian L. Bailey, O.D., Ph.D.
School of Optometry
University of California, Berkeley
Berkeley, CA

Debra Bezan, M.Ed., O.D.
College of Optometry
Northeastern State University
Tahlequah, OK

Anthony P. Cullen, O.D., Ph.D.
School of Optometry
University of Waterloo
Waterloo, Ontario, Canada

Jimmy Jackson, M.S., O.D.
Cataract and Refractive Surgical Center
Richmond, VA

Robert N. Kleinstein, O.D., M.P.H., Ph.D.
School of Optometry
University of Alabama at Birmingham
Birmingham, AL

Alan L. Lewis, O.D., Ph.D.
College of Optometry
Ferris State University
Big Rapids, MI

Donald G. Pitts, O.D., Ph.D.
College of Optometry
University of Houston
Houston, TX

Marilyn E. Schneck, O.D., Ph.D.
School of Optometry
University of California, Berkeley
Berkeley, CA

James E. Sheedy, O.D., Ph.D.
Allergan Humphrey
Research and Development
San Leandro, CA

Gregory L. Stephens, O.D., Ph.D.
College of Optometry
University of Houston
Houston, TX

Preface

Environmental Vision emphasizes concepts and methods for solving problems that occur through the interaction of the eyes and vision of people with their environment. There are many environmental problems that cannot be solved with traditional clinical procedures—problems such as prescribing protection treatments for occupational and radiation hazards, designing environmental lighting for optimal visual performance, diagnosing work-related disease, providing treatment and patient education in the optimal use of video display terminals, assessing the risk of ultraviolet radiation on the eye, and establishing eye and vision health programs. These and other environmental vision problems are increasingly being recognized as our knowledge of environmental hazards expands, as people become more aware of their environments, as vision becomes increasingly important in our information society, and as employers compete globally.

Environmental vision is an immense, complicated, and complex field. This book has been written to emphasize the most important areas in this field. By design, we have emphasized the workplace and occupational environments; however, the concepts and principles contained herein apply to all environments such as the home, sports, and recreation. Optometrists, other clinicians, health physicists, industrial hygienists, human factors engineers, and occupational physicians will be able to apply the material in the book to solving the environmental problems they encounter.

Optometry student clinicians need to assess their patient's visual tasks, visual environments, and visual performance needs in order to provide quality eye care. In recent years there has been an emphasis on disease diagnosis, treatment, and co-management. This emphasis is important but must not overlook the fact that people need to see and perform well in their many environments. In addition to ruling out or treating disease, student clinicians must assess their patients' many visual tasks, the variety of environments in which these tasks are accomplished, and how their patients' visual performance can be maximized. The importance of this assessment—making correct diagnoses of environmental problems and needs and determining appropriate treatments to maximize patients' visual performance in their environments—cannot be overemphasized. It is a key responsibility of all optometrists.

To provide the concepts and information needed to solve environmental vision problems, our book has been divided into four sections. Section I presents environmental optometry, recommended standards of care, occupational morbidity and mortality, costs of eye injuries, the occupational history, the clinical task analysis, the practice of occupational optometry, the design of eye-vision health care programs, and the identification of occupational disease.

Section II presents the basic concepts of radiant energy and how it interacts with matter; photometric principles; the effect of the sun as a source of radiant energy and ocular hazards; the principles for selecting light sources; the effect of contrast and glare on the visual task; the hazards of exposure to ultraviolet, visible, infrared, microwave, and ionizing radiation; and the principles and uses of lasers in industry and clinics.

Section III presents the principles for determining the need for eye protection, methods for calculating safe exposures, the spectral transmittance and selection of ophthalmic materials for eye protection, the principles for designing optimal sunglass lenses, and the use of contact lens materials in the workplace.

Section IV presents selected applications of environmental vision problems and their solutions. These problems include the use of video display terminals, the relationship between vision and driving, protection from radiant energy used in welding and tanning parlors, special problems involving eye hazards from clinical instruments, and the effect of common social drugs on vision.

Many portions of this book have been developed from lecture notes and research interests of the authors. The lack of a textbook in this field has been a serious handicap in its development. Because of the vastness of the field and the occasional uncertainty of sources for some information, we recognize that complete references may not have been given for some material in this textbook. If this oversight does occur, then let us know so that we may insert appropriate corrections and change future editions.

Environmental vision problems have existed for centuries. They began to receive wide recognition during the industrial revolution in the 19th century. The field of industrial vision evolved from the realization that workers performed better with sufficient light to the realization that eye protection would improve production. Other benefits such as fewer accidents and more contented workers were recognized later.

During the middle and latter half of the 20th century the benefits of eye protection began to be recognized in many occupations, sports activities, hobbies, and activities around the home. A signal event was the approval of legislation, the Occupational Safety and Health Act of 1970, which emphasized worker protection. Eye protection and eye safety have generally been recognized as important in most businesses and industries.

Unfortunately, there is little recognition that people need to have optimal vision to perform well on-the-job, at school, in sporting activities, and at home. Many industries, for example, that have well-designed programs for ensuring eye protection, do not recognize the importance of optimal vision designed for the visual tasks of their employees. Awareness and emphasis on optimizing visual performance is essential as our society and its technology change. The laser, space flight, deep-sea explora-

tion, the silicone chip, the widespread use of computers, and future technology all will require excellent visual performance.

Although this is the first textbook on environmental vision, we need to recognize some of the pioneers in this field. Tiffin (1942), Weston (1949), Kuhn (1950), Hofstetter (1956), Fletcher (1961) and many others contributed their expertise to the field and literature in industrial and occupational vision. It was Oscar W. Richards who most likely proposed the term *environmental vision* and convinced one of us (DGP) that a book in the field was needed. Although a topic outline was developed in 1979, along with plans for a coauthored book, Professor Richards was unable to pursue the task and asked DGP to "finish the job." Because of teaching, research, and other responsibilities, this task was delayed until 1988. Because of his interest and teaching in the field, RNK was independently beginning plans to write a similar book. Fortunately, we discovered our mutual interest in the field and the need for a textbook and were able to collaborate on *Environmental Vision*. Because of the scope of the field, we sought colleagues with special areas of expertise. We are indebted to them for their contributions and wish to thank them for their help. We believe that the team has produced an excellent textbook.

In addition to our contributors, we wish to personally thank everyone who assisted us in this enormous and time-consuming task. Ms. Hazel Davis and Ms. Alvenia Daniels conscientiously processed the many words, copies, and different versions for which we are truly grateful. Ms. Enita L. Torres spent long hours perfecting figures, and Ms. Kay Stroud assisted with her photographic expertise. Mr. Murry D. Getz helped with his excellent consultation regarding visual design. Ms. Becky Estrada and other librarians assisted in documentation, referencing, and making certain references were correct. Without all of this behind-the-scenes support, this task would have been much more difficult.

Not long before his death, Oscar telephoned me (DGP) and asked if the book would be written. My prompt answer was that it would be, and since it is now completed, Oscar, I hope you are happy with the result.

Donald G. Pitts, O.D., Ph.D.
Robert N. Kleinstein, O.D., M.P.H., Ph.D.

SECTION ONE

VISION AND THE ENVIRONMENT

Vision and the environment defines and emphasizes the importance of environmental and occupational optometry for the optometrist providing primary care. Every patient seen by the optometrist functions in a wide variety of environments. These may be the ordinary environments of a typical home or office, or unusual environments, such as unique industries, sports, or outerspace. The patient's environments need to be assessed in order to provide high quality care. The optometrist should provide treatments so the patient can maximize both visual performance and physical performance. The hazards in the environment also need to be assessed so that patients and especially their eyes and vision can be protected. Environmental and occupational vision assessments should become the common standard of comprehensive eye and vision care.

This section emphasizes occupational optometry, an important part of environmental optometry. Chapter 1 discusses the enormous, unseen, and unappreciated costs of eye injuries and vision disorders in the workplace. To improve the quality of patient care, optometrists need to use the basic survey occupational history and one of the practical occupational questionnaires in the chapter that can be easily modified for in-office use. Many important occupational services can be provided by most optometrists and used to expand the services they offer in their communities.

The application of occupational optometry in practice is emphasized in Chapter 2. Guidelines are presented for designing occupational eye and vision health care programs, providing vision screening, eye and vision protection, establishing procedures for emergencies, and for suspecting occupational diseases. The expectations of business and the optometrist who works with business and industry full- or part-time are discussed along with the economics related to providing occupational services. Several summary tables, key Appendices 1-1 to 1-5 will help the optometrist who provides occupational services in practice or in business and industrial settings.

1

CHAPTER ONE

Occupational Optometry and Primary Care

Robert N. Kleinstein, O.D., M.P.H., Ph.D.

All optometrists need to be actively involved in environmental optometry because of the large number of their patients in the work force,[1,2] the high incidence of eye injuries and prevalence of vision problems among working adults,[3-6] the importance of the workplace in the economic life of both individuals and families, and the aging of the work force. "A substantial amount of illness, injury and death is attributable to or affected by occupational and environmental conditions."[7] By focusing their expertise on their patient's work and workplace, optometrists can improve patients' visual performance and performance on the job, remove workplace hazards, prescribe and provide eye protection, and train workers. The success of individuals in the workplace ultimately determines the success of society as a whole.[6]

The vision and visual performance of an employee and applicant for work need to be assessed. Both the worker and the employer need to know whether the worker's eyes and vision have what it takes to get the job done. The efficiency with which employees see is directly related to how efficiently and safely they perform on the job.[8] "No other physical defect is so amenable to correction as is faulty vision, and hardly any other so affects job performance. . . . Vision, in two important ways, stands apart from other human factors related to job success. First, the quality of visual performance can be measured quickly, comprehensively and dependably. Second, when vision is below desirable levels it can be improved readily in a high percentage of cases and at relatively low cost to the individual.[8]

The workforce in the United States has 121,000,000 men and women in many occupations (Table 1-1).[1] Over 90% of employers and 80% of workers in business and industry work in organizations of fewer than 500 employees.[9] Organizations with fewer than 300 employees have 50% of the workers and comprise 75% of the business and industry in the United States.[10] Unfortunately, almost 50% of people in business and industry are in organizations with no health care plans or services.[7,11] In those organizations that provide health care services, it is unknown how many provide occupational optometry services or any eye and vision protection services. All workers need the services and expertise of occupational optometrists. Every organization would benefit by having its employees maximize their visual performance.

1.1 Environmental Optometry— An Essential Part of Primary Care

Definitions of Environmental and Occupational Optometry

Environmental optometry is the branch of optometry that broadly considers the relationship of people's eyes and vision to all aspects of their environments, including home, school, work, recreation, transportation, underwater, and outerspace. The breadth of services and problems considered in environmental optometry are considerable. The optometrist will analyze and solve problems that arise through the interaction of patients with their environments, will design optimal visual environments for the needs of patients, and will evaluate environments to improve visual performance.

Occupational optometry is the branch of environmental optometry that considers all aspects of the relationship between work and vision, visual performance, eye safety, and health. This complex relationship includes the worker's eyes and visual system, as well as the worker and the workplace environments. The emphasis of occupational optometry is high quality patient care with two major priorities: (1) prevention of work-related eye diseases, injuries, and vision disorders; and (2) enhanced performance of workers on the job.

A secondary but important concern of occupational optometrists is disease prevention and health promotion. "Occupational disease is one of the great 'unders' of American health care—under recognized, under reported, under compensated, under studied, and under prevented."[12] The optometrist has a significant role in disease prevention and health promotion.

Primary Care and Environmental Optometry

"Almost all adults spend a significant portion of their lives working in a variety of occupational settings. . . . There is considerable evidence that exposure to hazards in the workplace can cause or exacerbate illness. To the extent that [optometrists] care for persons of working age, all [optometrists] are engaged in the practice of occupational [optometry]."[13,14] The need for primary care optometrists to address the environmental and occupational eye and vision health care needs of their patients in the workplace is as crucial as the need for their management of other eye diseases and vision disorders. In providing high quality eye and vision care, optometrists need to know the environments of their patients, the type of work their patients do and how it may affect their eyes, vision, and health.

The primary care optometrist is the major resource for patients concerned about home, work, and other environmental eye and vision problems and hazards. The recognition, diagnosis, treatment, and prevention of occupational and environmental eye and vision problems are part of the obligation and responsibility that optometrists have to their patients.[7] Prevention must be addressed in all environments including work, home, and recreation.

Employment status and occupation	All Persons	Male	Female
	Population in thousands		
Total labor force	**111,770**	**62,581**	**49,189**
Currently employed	104,045	58,479	45,566
Executive, administrative, and managerial occupations	12,616	8,299	4,317
Professional specialty occupations	13,514	6,870	6,644
Technicians and related support occupations	3,259	1,656	1,603
Sales occupations	11,601	6,091	5,510
Administrative support occupations, including clerical	16,215	3,262	12,953
Private household occupations	836	50	786
Protective service occupations	1,595	1,363	232
Service occupations, except protective and household	10,353	3,519	6,834
Farming, forestry, and fishing occupations	3,218	2,719	499
Precision production, craft, and repair occupations	12,966	11,858	1,108
Machine operators, assemblers, and inspectors	7,881	4,633	3,249
Transportation and material moving occupations	4,522	4,152	370
Handlers, equipment cleaners, helpers, and laborers	3,659	3,011	647
Unknown occupation and military	1,811	997	814
Currently unemployed	7,725	4,102	3,623

From National Center for Health Statistics, Collins JG, Thornberry OT. Health characteristics of workers by occupation and sex: United States 1983–85. Advance data from Vital and Health Statistics, DHHS Pub. No. (PHS) 89–1250, No. 168. Hyattsville, Public Health Service, MD, 1989.

TABLE 1-1
Population Distribution of Persons 18 Years of Age and Over in the Labor Force by Employment Status, Occupation, and Sex: United States, 1983–1985

The primary care optometrist must be alert to potential occupational or environmental causes of patients' problems.[7] Patients have injuries, illnesses, and risk factors that are work-related. Optometrists need to identify and diagnose occupational and environmental problems, health risks, analyze patient's problems, decide how best to solve these problems, prescribe treatments to improve visual performance or restore function, manage eye injuries and diseases, and provide treatments including patient education for preventing risks to eyes and vision.[13]

Inadequate Occupational Optometry Education

"There is increasing concern that our highly sophisticated health care system is not well prepared to address problems related to occupational and environmental factors."[7] This concern occurs at the same time that workers and employers look to the health care system for information about health risks and exposures, for diagnosis and treatment of diseases caused and exacerbated by toxic environmental exposures, and for guidance about prevention.[7] Unfortunately, many primary providers of health care are not well trained in this area. In the estimated 50% of medical schools that require it, students receive about four hours on occupational health over four years.[7,13,15] Optometrists receive an estimated 20 to 80 hours of didactic and 5 to 10 hours of clinical occupational training during four years of school, although variability among programs is high. Although some occupational diseases are discussed, they are not consistently presented, and the occupational perspective is not usually emphasized.

Optometrists in practice are faced with the problem that their education has emphasized diseases and disorders but not occupational diseases, injuries, problems, and their solutions and their prevention. Practitioners do not observe environmental and occupational diseases and problems very frequently among their patients because of inadequate training and history taking. Therefore they consider them to be infrequent. This view ignores the prevalence of occupational diseases, injuries, hazards, and the importance of recognizing risk factors and treating environmental problems. Occupational risk factors are not low in frequency, nor are health problems that affect one's ability to work. Many clinicians fail to take a comprehensive view of the work relatedness of their patient's health problem.[7]

The average optometrist does not appear to consider occupational and environmental vision care to be part of the mainstream of clinical practice.[7] Inadequate education, the low frequency of reported occupational injuries and diseases, the lack of awareness and concern for occupational problems including their prevention, and the inadequate occupational histories taken by clinicians result in inadequate delivery of clinical preventive and occupational services.[7]

Goals of Primary Care and Occupational Optometry

The three major goals related to occupational optometry for optometrists in private practice are based on the definitions, priorities, and problems previously discussed, as well as on the basic fact that high quality patient care cannot be delivered to adults without assessing the patient's occupation and working environment. These goals are as follows:

1. To incorporate environmental optometry into private practice and assess the impact of vision disorders and eye diseases on the ability of patients to work.
2. To assess the impact of work and the work environment on the performance of the worker on the job, at home, and during recreation.
3. To understand the relationship between health and work and to recognize, diagnose, treat, and prevent work-related illnesses and injuries.[7,16]

Minimum Standard of Care

Based on these three major goals, the optometrist needs to meet several objectives to achieve a minimum standard of care:

1. Complete an occupational history on each adult patient, including an assessment and interpretation of it.
2. Identify and diagnose conditions that may be occupationally induced and make appropriate referrals if necessary.
3. Assess their patient's visual needs and provide treatment for maximizing their on-the-job performance.
4. Initiate preventive measures for patients and others with the same eye and vision risks.

To provide this minimum standard of care, optometrists need to:

1. Know the basic principles of occupational and environmental disease, including such concepts as latency, threshold dose, and multifactorial etiology.[7,17]
2. Take an appropriate survey or diagnostic occupational history in those clinical situations in which occupational or environmental disease is part of the differential diagnosis.[7]
3. Conduct a task analysis to maximize each patient's visual and work performance on the job.
4. "Be sensitive to the ethical, social, and legal implications in the diagnosis of and intervention for occupational and environmental disease" (see Appendix 1-1).[7]
5. "Be alert to the opportunities for the prevention of occupational and environmental illnesses and injuries in patients under their care."[7]
6. Appreciate and understand the work environments of their patients.
7. Understand their responsibilities within the workers' compensation system.
8. "Call known or suspected hazards to the attention of public health agencies or other entities as indicated by the history and information obtained."[7,18]
9. Be knowledgeable about reimbursement of patient care costs under third-party programs using ICD-9-CM codes such as unspecified contusion

of the eye, injury of eye not otherwise specified (NOS) (921.9), penetration of eyeball with non-magnetic foreign body (871.6), and superficial injury of cornea (918.1).[19]

Optometric clinicians practicing in the community have a very important role in occupational optometry because employee health services in business and industry cannot serve more than a small portion of the nation's workers. Millions of workers employed in organizations too scattered or too small to justify in-plant services will look to their primary care optometrist for guidance on what to do to avoid adverse health effects and to protect their eyes and vision. Optometrists must become knowledgeable about industries in their communities and fully understand and appreciate the work of their patients in order to meet their professional responsibilities.

1.2 Occupational Morbidity and Mortality

Business and industry have difficulty "seeing" safety problems. Reduced vision performance is not easily observed or even recognized as a potential problem. Eye injuries or injuries resulting from impaired vision are not usually seen because no single accounting figure is labeled "eye injury" or "impaired vision injury" costs. These costs are dispersed in training, insurance, legal, and other budget items. The cost of one serious disabling eye injury or eye loss or impaired vision injury would pay for many occupational optometry eye and vision health care programs (Tables 1-2 to 1-16).

An estimated 11,000 workers are killed annually in occupational accidents and 100,000 die annually from occupational diseases.[3,13,20,21] It is unknown how many of these are associated with poor vision. There are about 400,000 new cases of occupational diseases recognized each year.[2,16,21]

Cases of disease and eye injuries are underestimated because there is no reporting, national registry, or data collection system. A national registry was started in 1985, but only voluntary reports of penetrating eye injuries were included.[58] Underestimation also occurs because of the long latency between exposure and disease manifestation and the multifactorial causes of chronic diseases. There is generally a lack of recognition, diagnosis, and research related to occupational eye diseases.[7]

Eye Injuries and Vision Disorders: Prevalence, Incidence, Time Lost, Costs, Compensation

About 50% of adults in the United States have difficulty seeing clearly at distance and about 60% have difficulty seeing at near when no corrective lenses are worn.[6] With lenses, the prevalence of impaired distance vision is still over 30%, and the prevalence of impaired near vision is about 40%.[6] Because a significant percentage of the population has impaired vision, it is very likely that similar percentages of people in the workplace have impaired vision. Poor vision reduces the performance and productivity of workers on the job and increases their risk of having disabling accidents and injuring their co-workers.

Workplace injuries are difficult to estimate. The National Safety Council estimates that there are over nine million disabling injuries annually, including almost two million that occur on the job.[3] Days lost annually to occupational injury or illness average 49 per 100 full-time employees; these range from 14/100 in the communication industry to 247/100 in the trucking industry.[22] Among these on-the-job disabling injuries there are 4%, or 70,000, that are disabling eye injuries (Table 1-2).[3] The National Society for the Prevention of Blindness (NSPB) estimates that there are 300,000 disabling eye injuries in the workplace annually.[10] A disabling eye injury usually means that an eye injury is severe enough to cause a worker to miss at least one day of work or at least the subsequent shift. Disabling eye injuries significantly underestimate the actual number of eye injuries in the workplace.

Work injuries due to accidents, including eye injuries, caused over 35,000,000 work days to be lost in 1987.[3] The incidence rates for lost work days varies with the industry (Table 1-3). This time lost is a significant cost to business, and programs to reduce work injuries in the workplace are very important.[2]

Some states, such as California, maintain a supplemental data system to collect detailed work injury information from workers' compensation data. This is very useful in identifying work-related injuries by nature of injury, accident type, age and sex, body part, and source of injury. By determining injury rates, industries and patients with the highest risk of eye injuries can be identified (see Table 1-7).

There were many causes of eye injuries and illnesses reported by industry in California in 1989 for
Text continues on page 13.

Work Accidents					
Accidents by Part of Body Injured (% of Total Accidents)		Compensation by Part of Body Injured (% of Total Compensation)		Disabling Work Injuries (Number)	
Eyes	4%		1%	Eyes	70,000
Head (Except Eyes)	4%		3%	Head (Except Eyes)	70,000
Neck	2%		2%	Neck	40,000
Arms	10%		7%	Arms	180,000
Hands	5%		2%	Hands	90,000
Fingers	13%		5%	Fingers	230,000
Back	22%		32%	Back	400,000
Trunk	9%		9%	Trunk	160,000
Legs	13%		12%	Legs	230,000
Feet	4%		2%	Feet	70,000
Toes	2%		1%	Toes	40,000
Body Systems	2%		6%	Body Systems	20,000
Multiple	10%		18%	Multiple	180,000

Average Workers' Compensation Payments			
Part of Body Injured	Total Cases Closed (%)	Average Indemnity Compensation*	Average Medical Payment*
Total	**100.0%**	**$ 4,035**	**$2,012**
Head	5.1	3,312	1,874
Eye	1.1	2,502	1,164
Neck	1.7	5,303	2,453
Upper Extremities	25.6	2,234	1,382
Arm	4.2	3,024	1,591
Wrist	4.4	2,915	1,538
Hand	4.1	2,114	1,328
Finger	11.7	1,627	1,150
Trunk	37.0	4,583	2,224
Back	26.2	5,193	2,358
Lower extremities	20.0	2,848	1,734
Leg	9.5	3,704	2,356
Foot	3.6	2,129	1,118
Toe	1.8	1,209	791
Multiple	9.0	7,323	3,610
Body system	1.2	20,940	3,110
Nonclassifiable	0.3	7,219	2,202

Cases   Compensation ($)
*Average payments are based on 353,449 closed cases from nine states in 1985.
From Accident Facts. Chicago, National Safety Council, 1989, with permission.

TABLE 1-2
Work Accidents and Average Workers' Compensation Payments by Part of Body

Industry	SIC Code*	Incidence Rates per 100 Full-Time Employees§					
		Total Cases	Lost Workday Cases	Cases Involving Days Away From Work & Deaths	Nonfatal Cases Without Lost Workdays	Lost Workdays†	Days Away From Work
All Industries		**7.59**	**3.05**	**1.86**	**4.53**	**60**	**41**
Agriculture, forestry & fishing		**11.83**	**5.84**	**4.19**	**5.97**	**121**	**102**
Agricultural production crops	01	14.67	7.02	4.10	7.61	111	78
Forestry	08	4.05	1.84	1.84	2.21	58	56
Mining		**6.06**	**1.62**	**1.18**	**4.43**	**49**	**38**
Metal mining	10	11.25	2.46	1.96	8.76	87	68
Bituminous coal & lignite mining	12	11.32	2.71	2.52	8.61	120	90
Oil & gas extraction	13	3.30	1.07	0.63	2.22	20	15
Nonmetallic minerals, except fuels	14	5.99	1.81	1.25	4.17	56	46
Construction		**8.02**	**3.42**	**2.93**	**4.59**	**71**	**63**
General building contractors	15	8.64	3.22	2.71	5.40	89	80
Heavy construction contractors	16	7.59	3.33	2.82	4.25	65	57
Special trade contractors	17	14.83	6.11	6.07	8.69	127	123
Manufacturing		**8.05**	**3.00**	**1.59**	**5.05**	**58**	**37**
Durable goods		9.52	3.51	1.78	6.01	67	42
Lumber and wood products	24	10.11	5.14	4.18	4.95	120	98
Sawmills and planing mills	242	12.27	6.29	5.02	5.98	128	105
Millwork, plywood, and structural members	243	8.88	4.67	3.68	4.18	114	87
Furniture and fixtures	25	13.80	6.07	1.76	7.72	124	32
Household furniture	251	10.36	2.96	1.89	7.40	40	32
Stone, clay, and glass products	32	11.55	4.76	2.54	6.79	102	78
Cement, hydraulic	324	13.47	3.06	2.40	10.41	100	76
Concrete, gypsum, and plaster products	327	8.18	2.48	2.27	5.70	52	48
Miscellaneous nonmetallic mineral products	329	8.05	3.78	3.06	4.26	85	77
Primary metal industries	33	12.42	3.59	1.79	8.82	79	52
Blast furnace and basic steel products	331	10.90	3.00	2.22	7.89	90	77
Iron and steel foundries	332	20.45	5.06	1.66	15.38	90	46
Primary nonferrous metals	333	14.18	4.64	1.92	9.53	90	51
Nonferrous rolling and drawing	335	9.01	3.07	1.32	5.93	59	30
Fabricated metal products	34	11.15	3.87	1.89	7.28	68	40
Metal cans and shipping containers	341	12.23	3.51	1.32	8.71	56	30
Cutlery, hand tools, and hardware	342	10.71	3.16	2.56	7.55	81	54
Fabricated structural metal products	344	7.82	2.51	2.03	5.30	56	51

TABLE 1-3
Occupational Injury and Illness Incidence Rates by Industry, 1987

Industry	SIC Code*	Incidence Rates per 100 Full-Time Employees§					
		Total Cases	Lost Workday Cases	Cases Involving Days Away From Work & Deaths	Nonfatal Cases Without Lost Workdays	Lost Workdays†	Days Away From Work
Manufacturing *continued*							
Durable goods							
Metal forgings and stampings	346	21.82	7.32	1.66	14.49	103	30
Miscellaneous fabricated metal products	349	8.27	3.09	2.32	5.18	63	54
Machinery, except electrical	35	8.59	3.11	1.74	5.48	57	34
Farm and garden machinery	352	9.44	4.02	0.56	5.43	53	10
Construction and related machinery	353	9.59	3.33	2.09	6.26	72	46
Metalworking machinery	354	11.52	5.32	3.08	6.21	73	57
Special industry machinery	355	7.90	2.50	1.90	5.40	59	52
General industrial machinery	356	8.01	2.95	2.50	5.06	49	40
Office and computing machines	357	1.86	0.87	0.58	1.00	16	6
Refrigeration and service machinery	358	15.50	4.57	2.43	10.93	84	45
Miscellaneous machinery except electrical	359	11.21	4.43	0.86	6.78	98	35
Electric and electronic equipment	36	4.68	1.86	1.12	2.83	38	23
Electric distributing equipment	361	13.00	5.80	3.02	7.21	96	57
Electric industrial apparatus	362	6.92	2.67	1.43	4.24	60	37
Household appliances	363	8.75	2.52	2.05	6.23	55	46
Electric lighting and wiring equipment	364	8.07	3.77	1.67	4.29	79	36
Communication equipment	366	3.13	1.01	0.64	2.12	19	12
Electronic components and accessories	367	4.81	1.50	0.73	3.30	28	13
Miscellaneous electrical equipment and supplies	369	7.58	4.36	3.72	3.21	81	66
Transportation equipment	37	11.07	4.22	1.80	6.84	69	43
Motor vehicles and equipment	371	21.46	8.15	2.90	13.31	134	77
Aircraft and parts	372	5.47	1.78	1.42	3.70	29	24
Ship and boat building and repair	373	18.13	7.80	4.20	10.33	118	76
Railroad equipment	374	13.33	4.79	4.74	8.55	122	120
Guided missiles, space vehicles and parts	376	2.41	0.86	0.35	1.54	12	6
Instruments and related products	38	4.36	1.49	0.94	2.87	30	22
Measuring and controlling devices	382	6.85	2.59	1.97	4.27	46	37
Medical instruments and supplies	384	4.40	1.68	0.96	2.70	39	28
Miscellaneous manufacturing industries	39	9.12	4.90	3.92	4.21	104	82

TABLE 1-3

Occupational Injury and Illness Incidence Rates by Industry, 1987, continued

Industry	SIC Code*	Incidence Rates per 100 Full-Time Employees§					
		Total Cases	Lost Workday Cases	Cases Involving Days Away From Work & Deaths	Nonfatal Cases Without Lost Workdays	Lost Workdays†	Days Away From Work
Manufacturing *continued*							
Nondurable goods		6.64	2.50	1.40	4.13	50	32
Food and kindred products	20	11.18	4.54	3.10	6.64	91	66
Meat products	201	25.01	9.21	4.18	15.80	158	84
Dairy products	202	7.12	2.89	2.17	4.23	59	44
Preserved fruits and vegetables	203	11.10	3.72	2.13	7.38	83	52
Grain mill products	204	9.39	2.66	2.48	6.72	50	42
Bakery products	205	8.15	4.90	4.66	3.25	115	110
Beverages	208	7.31	2.75	2.17	4.55	62	45
Miscellaneous foods and kindred products	209	7.93	3.15	2.37	4.78	80	68
Textile mill products	22	5.56	1.52	0.48	4.04	27	14
Weaving mills, cotton	221	6.57	1.69	0.44	4.87	28	16
Knitting mills	225	8.19	1.87	0.81	6.32	38	24
Apparel and other textile products	23	6.76	3.17	0.95	3.59	52	28
Miscellaneous fabricated textile products	239	6.97	2.48	1.20	4.49	55	36
Paper and allied products	26	9.38	3.10	2.20	6.28	75	58
Paper mills, except building paper	262	9.88	2.83	1.93	7.04	73	58
Miscellaneous converted paper products	264	6.74	2.89	1.94	3.84	58	42
Paperboard containers and boxes	265	11.05	5.11	4.00	5.92	119	97
Printing and publishing	27	6.78	3.37	2.21	3.41	60	38
Newspapers	271	6.90	3.76	3.53	3.13	68	61
Commercial printing	275	9.13	3.73	2.00	5.40	53	28
Chemicals and allied products	28	4.12	1.58	0.62	2.54	29	14
Industrial inorganic chemicals	281	5.50	1.98	1.07	3.51	39	28
Plastic materials and synthetics	282	3.87	1.42	0.43	2.45	25	12
Drugs	283	3.10	1.36	0.71	1.74	23	12
Soap, cleaners and toilet goods	284	3.98	1.90	1.23	2.08	32	23
Paints and allied products	285	5.86	2.49	0.66	3.36	39	15
Industrial organic chemicals	286	3.97	1.45	0.44	2.51	26	10
Agricultural chemicals	287	4.75	1.48	0.70	3.27	33	17
Miscellaneous chemical products	289	4.61	2.05	0.91	2.56	40	23
Petroleum and coal products	29	6.50	2.49	1.27	4.01	49	30
Petroleum refining	291	6.64	2.57	1.12	4.06	49	27
Paving and roofing materials	295	6.51	2.52	2.25	3.99	58	51
Rubber and miscellaneous plastics products	30	6.60	3.05	1.77	3.55	66	41
Miscellaneous plastics products	307	7.47	3.34	2.02	4.13	78	51
Leather and leather products	31	9.72	4.23	2.29	5.49	68	40

TABLE 1-3
Occupational Injury and Illness Incidence Rates by Industry, 1987, continued

Industry	SIC Code*	Total Cases	Lost Workday Cases	Cases Involving Days Away From Work & Deaths	Nonfatal Cases Without Lost Workdays	Lost Workdays[†]	Days Away From Work
				Incidence Rates per 100 Full-Time Employees[§]			
Transportation & public utilities		**6.28**	**3.46**	**2.45**	**2.81**	**67**	**48**
Railroad transportation	40	7.47	5.45	3.56	2.01	157	113
Local and interurban passenger transit	41	15.28	8.37	8.35	6.91	259	258
Local and suburban transportation	411	15.60	8.94	8.93	6.66	145	145
Trucking and warehousing	42	20.76	15.94	15.60	4.82	226	220
Trucking, local and long distance	421	22.30	17.57	17.55	4.73	247	246
Water transportation	44	6.56	3.66	3.47	2.88	100	91
Transportation by air	45	4.94	2.75	2.21	2.19	33	27
Pipelines, except natural gas	46	4.28	1.31	1.14	2.97	26	21
Communication	48	2.11	0.80	0.72	1.32	17	13
Electric, gas, and sanitary services	49	5.39	2.63	1.52	2.75	51	31
Electric services	491	4.49	2.08	1.07	2.41	43	24
Gas production and distribution	492	6.94	3.51	2.58	3.43	63	45
Water supply	494	13.07	6.20	5.94	6.86	119	109
Wholesale & retail trade		**5.38**	**2.45**	**1.85**	**2.93**	**51**	**38**
Wholesale trade—durable goods	50	8.77	3.79	2.76	4.98	80	57
Wholesale trade— nondurable goods	51	2.82	1.64	1.52	1.17	26	24
Retail trade		**3.66**	**1.57**	**1.07**	**2.09**	**39**	**28**
Automotive dealers and service stations	55	3.66	1.51	1.08	2.14	35	30
Services		**5.09**	**2.19**	**2.03**	**2.90**	**35**	**28**
Business services	73	1.32	0.58	0.46	0.74	9	7
Amusement and recreation services	79	13.92	5.83	4.53	8.09	114	102
Hospitals	806	9.06	3.97	3.75	5.09	60	50
Educational services	82	4.13	2.30	2.30	1.82	37	35
Public administration (government)		**13.81**	**4.35**	**3.83**	**9.46**	**103**	**89**
Executive legislative and general	91	16.33	4.72	4.26	11.61	125	113
Police protection	9221	8.90	2.51	2.37	6.37	32	31
Fire protection	9224	14.59	6.61	5.36	7.98	63	56
State departments of transportation		9.37	4.30	4.30	5.06	57	57
Offices		2.23	0.96	0.43	1.27	15	12
Research and development or laboratory		2.43	0.77	0.40	1.65	14	7

*SIC codes are from the Standard Industrial Classification Manual, 1972 Edition.
[†]Lost workdays include both days away from work and restricted workdays.
[§]Incidence rates use 200,000 employee hours as the equivalent of 100 full-time employees.
Table based on reports of National Safety Council members participating in the Occupational Safety/Health Award Program and may not be representative of all industries listed.
From Accident Facts. Chicago National Safety Council, 1989, with permission.

TABLE 1-3
Occupational Injury and Illness Incidence Rates by Industry, 1987, continued

workers' compensation benefits. The major causes were scratches and abrasions (66.8%). Other causes were diseases of the eye (13.6%), burns and scalds (7.0%), cuts, lacerations and punctures (5.1%), radiation effects (5.0%), infective or parasitic diseases (1.6%), and other (0.9%).[23]

Unlike the widespread awareness of medical costs in industry, the high workplace costs associated with untreated vision disorders are unrecognized and not easily quantifiable. These costs are found in reduced productivity of workers and unnecessary high rates of spoiled or second-class products. These costs also include the costs of accidents and co-worker injuries that could have been prevented if vision disorders had been treated. No business or industry accounts for the costs of untreated vision disorders, and therefore they are not recognized as a significant problem.

The costs associated with some eye and some vision injuries can be estimated because of the need for treatment[57] and workers' compensation costs, both of which are "visible." Within a specific workplace, the amount paid for eye injuries can be significant, especially if an eye is lost. The direct costs of a single employee losing one eye ranges from about $40,000 to $115,000.[20,24] Workers' compensation laws have the loss of one eye as a scheduled benefit ranging from $5,699 to $157,685, depending on the state.[24] These are minimal costs because they do not include the indirect costs associated with eye loss (Tables 1-2, and 1-4).

A national insurance company evaluated its workers' compensation costs in 1985. They found the direct cost for an eye lost by a single employee was $80,000. In addition, the indirect costs were very conservatively estimated to be four times the direct costs or $320,000, including training, lost time, investigation and other costs.[25] Indirect costs include many items, for example, work-stoppage time or slowed production, costs of finding and training replacement workers, damaged equipment repair, accident investigation and reporting time, first aid provision, legal fees, and judgments.

The overall total costs for eye injuries are high. NSPB estimates that 300,000 disabling eye injuries in 1982 cost business and industry $330 million in lost production time, medical bills, and compensation.[10] In one state, the average direct cost of a lost time eye injury was $3,000, with an average loss of 10.5 work days.[10] These costs included only eye in-

Type of industry	Percent
Printing/publishing	46.8
Stone, clay, glass and concrete	44.5
Transportation equipment	44.1
Apparel and leather products	42.9
Electronic and electrical products	40.8
Fabricated metal products	40.1
Miscellaneous	40.0
Primary metal industries	39.1
Textile mill products	38.1
Furniture and fixtures	38.0
Unclassified	37.9
Rubber products	36.3
Industrial/commercial machinery	35.8
Measuring/analyzing/controlling inst.	33.3
Food and kindred products	30.6
Chemical products	28.5
Nonmanufacturing	28.4
Lumber and wood products	28.4
Paper products	27.3
All types	37.2

From National Association of Manufacturers, Medical Benefits 6(12):1, June 30, 1989, with permission.

TABLE 1-4
Medical Costs as a Percentage of Net Profit (1988) from Selected Industries

juries, not indirect costs or costs associated with vision disorders.

The same average direct cost of a single lost time eye injury of about $3,000 has been reported by a national insurance company[25] and by a 3-year study conducted by the National Council on Compensation Insurance.[26] Using data from seven states, these sources estimated the average direct cost of each disabling eye injury in 1985 was $3,057. When they included indirect costs, conservatively estimated at four times the direct costs, the total cost for each disabling eye injury was $15,285.[26] These direct costs are consistent with data from the Bureau of Labor Statistics (BLS) (Table 1-2).

There are indications that the NSPB estimates are of the correct magnitude. The state of Ohio reported 6,457 work-related eye accidents in 1980, and the average direct costs, including health care and compensation costs, were $20,000,000. This report did not include indirect costs, which were estimated to be 4 to 10 times the direct costs. Assuming a conservative six times multiplier for indirect costs, the total costs for these eye accidents in Ohio would have been $140,000,000.[20]

In 1980, Ohio had 1/20th of the total U.S. workforce with fewer blue collar workers than exist nationally on a percentage basis. Extrapolating from Ohio to the United States, the total U.S. costs in 1980 for eye injuries would have been $2.8 billion.[20] Others have estimated the total U.S. costs for eye injuries to be $0.5 to $2.1 billion.[3] Although the actual costs are unknown because there is no national reporting system, eye injuries are a major cost that could be significantly reduced.

Using all these studies, one can estimate the total cost of an eye loss at about $160,000 to $320,000, and $460,000 if a federal employee is involved. (Federal employees receive higher direct compensation for eye loss than other employees.) The total cost of a disabling eye injury is about $15,000. These costs are high, have a negative impact on small business and industry, and usually can be prevented.

Prevention of Eye Injuries

The NSPB estimates that 90% of eye injuries are preventable.[10] BLS conducts an annual survey to define injury and illness experience in the United States. They also have a supplementary data system for detailed studies of specific problems. Their last investigation of eye injuries used voluntary reports of injuries that were required to be reported by state workers' compensation laws (Table 1-5). Cases were excluded from their survey if the injury resulted in a fatality or the loss of vision in both eyes or if more than 90 days had elapsed between the time of the injury and the beginning of the survey. About 50% of workers surveyed responded to the questionnaire.[27]

The criteria for workers' compensation vary by state. Some states require that all workers' compensation cases be reported regardless of time lost from work, but other states limit reporting to cases involving 1 to 8 days lost time from work. These criteria result in a definite underreporting of eye injuries, because an eye injury that resulted in

"only" a week lost from work would not be reported in some states.[27] There were other limitations to this survey.

The optometrist has a key role in preventing eye injuries and visually related injuries to co-workers. The most apparent role is to prescribe eye protection designed for the specific job, usually in the form of safety spectacles. The less apparent role is to make certain that a person has good visual skills for his or her job.[28] ". . . Data . . . from numerous studies indicate conclusively that vision is related to accident experience and that workers whose visual skills are adequate for their jobs are less likely to experience industrial accidents."[29] Because the need for good visual skills is not obvious, the optometrist will often need to educate management about this need and its importance in productivity and accident prevention.

At the time of the accident, about 60% (3 out of 5) workers in the BLS eye injury survey who experienced impact or chemical burn injuries to the eye were not wearing eye protection (Table 1-5).[27] Most injured workers were on the job doing their normal activities and received many different types of eye injuries (Table 1-6). Of the objects striking the eye, almost 60% were less than 0.5 mm, which is smaller than a pinhead, and 20% were about 1 mm in diameter. Two thirds of the objects were traveling faster than a hand-thrown object. Chemical contact was responsible for 20% of the injuries (Table 1-6).[27]

Of the remaining 40% of the workers who had eye injuries, all were wearing some form of eyeglasses or eye protection when the accident occurred. The most common eyeglasses used had no side shields. Over 70% of these injured workers thought they had safety glasses; however, almost 40% reported there were no special markings on their lenses, and another 40% did not know if their lenses were marked. Therefore, 40% to 80% of the workers with eyeglasses were not wearing safety glasses.[27]

The most frequent explanations given by the unprotected workers who were injured was that eye protection was not normally used in their work or was not needed for the task they were performing. Three fifths of the workers reported that they had received safety information regarding eye protection, including where to use it and what kind to wear.[27]

These BLS data strongly indicate that the occupational optometrist has a definite and significant role in providing primary preventive vision health

Industry division	All workers		Workers wearing eye protection	
	Number	Percent	Number	Percent
Total	**1,052**	**100**	**435**	**100**
Agriculture, forestry, and fishing	32	3	3	1
Mining	8	1	6	1
Construction	228	22	69	16
Manufacturing	506	48	283	65
Transportation and public utilities	32	3	9	2
Wholesale trade	65	6	17	4
Retail trade	72	7	16	4
Finance, insurance, and real estate	7	1	–	–
Services	91	9	30	7
Public sector	9	1	1	<0.5
Industry unspecified	2	<0.5	1	<0.5

Type of eye protection	Number	Percent

Indicate what type of eye or face protection, if any, you were wearing when the accident occurred.

Total	**1,048**	**100**
Not wearing any eye or face protection	613	58
Glasses—no side shields	181	17
Glasses—full-cup side shields	94	9
Glasses—flat-fold side shields	57	5
Welding goggles	2	<0.5
Soft-side goggles	21	2
Cup type goggles	3	<0.5
Face shield	68	6
Welding helmet	9	1

If you were wearing glasses, what kind were they?

Total	**347**	**100**
Industrial safety glasses	250	72
Regular glasses	90	26
Don't know	7	2

Did the glasses have any special marking on the lens such as manufacturing trademark, etc?

Total	**330**	**100**
No	125	38
Yes	61	18
Don't know	144	44

Dashes indicate that no data were reported from state workers' compensation reports. Percentages may not add to 100 due to rounding. This survey data included 750 cases and was based on the injury report prepared for workers' compensation. All usable data in incomplete questionnaires was used. The cases were based on the voluntary participation of 19 state agencies, which reviewed 188,000 injury reports, of which 2,118 were within the scope of the survey.
From the U.S. Department of Labor, Bureau of Labor Statistics: Accidents Involving Eye Injuries. Report 597. April 1980.

TABLE 1-5
Eye Injuries by Industry Division and Type of Eye Protection, Selected States, July–August 1979

Type of accident	All workers		Workers wearing eye protection	
	Number	Percent	Number	Percent
How did the accident occur?				
Total	**1,052**	**100**	**435**	**100**
Flying or falling object struck you	727	69	355	82
Struck non-moving object	21	2	5	1
Liquid or chemical injured you	216	21	59	14
Occurred in another way	88	8	16	4

Nature of injury	All workers		Workers wearing eye protection	
	Number	Percent	Number	Percent
Total	**1,052**	**100**	**435**	**100**
Amputation or enucleation	1	<0.5	1	<0.5
Burn (chemical)	212	20	57	13
Contusion, crushing, bruise	37	4	4	1
Cut, laceration, puncture	192	18	80	18
Scratches, abrasions	558	53	280	64
Multiple injuries	5	<0.5	1	<0.5
Eye, other diseases of the eye	3	<0.5	1	<0.5
Other injury, not elsewhere classified	3	<0.5	1	<0.5
Nonclassifiable	41	4	10	2

Survey data for this table is described in Table 1-9.
From the U.S. Department of Labor, Bureau of Labor Statistics: Accidents Involving Eye Injuries. Report 597. April 1980.

TABLE 1-6
Eye Injuries by Type of Accident and Nature of Injury, Selected States, July–August 1979

care and education for workers and patients. Sixty percent of workers in this survey were not wearing eye protection; almost half or more of the 40% who did wear eyeglasses were not using safety materials. These data support the very high eye injury costs previously discussed.

The optometrist must be involved in preventing these eye injuries and reducing injury costs. By providing high quality environmental and occupational care, optometrists will help reduce and prevent the pain and suffering experienced by their patients at their workplace. Accidents occur too quickly to be avoided and therefore must be prevented. For example, a woodchip from a table saw travels at 103 miles/hour or 2 feet in 0.013 seconds and can penetrate the eye.[29] The best prevention approach combines the skills and expertise of the optometrist with

the support of management in requiring the assessment of visual skills and the wearing of protective equipment (Tables 1-6 and 1-7).

Trends Affecting Optometrists

Occupational optometry has become very important because of many societal changes in the past several decades, including the following:

1. A growing awareness that exposures to hazardous substances in the workplace, home, and general environment may cause or contribute to the origins of disease and influence its natural history.[7,13,30]

2. An increasing awareness of the effects of the visual environment (lighting, contrast, glare, and

Industry	Eye Injuries		All Injuries	
	Number	Rate	Number	Rate
Total	**19,556**	**15.5**	**430,408**	**340.9**
Agriculture[†]	1,394	31.9	21,036	480.7
Mining	82	19.7	1,448	348.1
Construction	4,096	63.6	53,616	833.1
Manufacturing	4,906	22.7	74,612	345.7
Transportation[§]	836	14.9	27,726	493.9
Wholesale Trade	938	12.2	25,588	333.5
Retail Trade	2,264	10.3	73,498	333.9
Finance[††]	302	3.6	10,226	122.3
Service	2,928	8.8	76,494	229.4
Government[**]	1,810	11.0	66,164	402.2

*Disabling cases are those that cause absence from work for at least a full day or shift beyond the day of occurrence
[†]Agriculture includes forestry and fishing
[§]Transportation includes communication and utilities
[††]Finance includes insurance and real estate
[**]Government includes state and local government
From California Work Injuries and Illnesses—1989, and from unpublished data—San Francisco, California Department of Industrial Relations, Division of Labor Statistics and Research; with permission.

TABLE 1-7
Number and Rate (per 10,000 employees) of Eye and Total Work-Related Disabling* Nonfatal Injuries Under Workers' Compensation by Industry in California, 1989

exposure to ultraviolet, infrared, ionizing, and microwave radiation) on vision, vision performance, and perception.

3. An increasing concern regarding the economic and social costs of premature mortality and preventable disability and injuries.[30]

4. A continuing increase in the costs of health care and the benefits of reducing costs through preventing diseases and injuries by early detection and effective management.[30]

5. An expansion of legislation, regulation, case law, and labor-management agreements that increase responsibility of employers for the physical and mental health of their workers.[31]

6. An increasing number of women in the work force and concerns for the future reproductive health of both women and men.

An increase in international competition with need for increased worker productivity and flexibility.

7. A transformation of the United States from an industrial to an information-based economy and the increasing complexity of the workplace.

8. An aging of the work force.

9. An increasing insistence of workers to be informed and to participate in all areas that affect their personal welfare.[7,31]

10. An increasing interest by employers, insurance carriers and the public in health promotion and disease prevention.[7]

With these changes, vision and visual performance are becoming even more important. This importance includes the unappreciated use of vision changes as sentinel events in the recognition of environment and workplace hazards.

One result of these changes and the high prevalence and incidence of vision disorders and eye injuries in the workplace is the beginning recognition of the importance and need for the optometrist who is knowledgeable or specializes in environmental optometry. Excellent vision is essential for workers to be productive and to avoid potentially injurious situations. Environmental optometric care is a vital and necessary part of the health care services that primary care optometrists provide. Because of the number of small businesses or work units that are too small to justify a full-time optometrist, environmental vision services for most workers will be provided by the optometrist practicing in the community.[20,30]

Within their community, optometrists need to provide high quality care, regardless of their patients' field of employment. Optimal patient management requires taking occupational case histories that assess work-related tasks, including vision requirements, and determining the need for vision and eye protection and the best method for providing it. In addition, the optometrist must assess risks from environmental hazards and the impact of current eye diseases and vision disorders on job performance, as well as diagnose work-related occupational diseases.

Many practicing optometrists will have the opportunity to become professionally involved with business and industry in their local communities. Sections in this chapter are written for optometrists who are interested in this area and who are employed part-time or full-time in business and industry or who serve as consultants to them. Clinicians in private practice and those working in industry need to understand how to establish occupational optometric eye and vision health care programs, how to establish vision standards, the distinction between impairment and disability, the role of regulatory agencies, and the evaluation of potential hazards. With this information, optometrists can provide significant services that will economically benefit business and industry, improve the quality of eye and vision care for their patients, and improve the visual performance of their patients on the job. Most importantly, they will prevent pain, suffering, and permanent visual impairment in their patients.

1.3 Occupational History

Work-Related Problems and Risk Factors

Persons who have vision problems impairing their work performance or who are at risk for eye injuries and other work-related hazards enter optometrists' offices every day. Unfortunately, most optometrists, like other primary care providers, rarely consider work-related causes in their differential diagnosis of patient problems or in an assessment of preventive treatments. Because of this, they may miss the opportunity to make diagnoses that could have an early impact on an existing disease or prevent other diseases, for example, by stopping exposure to environmental hazards.[13]

The occupational history is an essential part of the patient interview and history. ". . . Clinicians who would never omit the family history from a thorough interview, or disregard the patient's current medication in the evaluation of a new or unexplained problem, will ignore or disregard that part of the patient's history dealing with one-third of the patient's life. Often, mention of the patient's current occupation will be omitted entirely from the record or will be confined to billing information."[36] The omission of the occupational history is a serious clinical problem.

The problem of not assessing occupational disease and risk factors is not new. In the 1990 health objectives for the nation, the Department of Health and Human Services (DHHS) identified the clinical setting as an important site for achieving its goals to prevent occupational illness and injury.[7] A key objective stated that by 1990, over 70% of all primary health care providers should be routinely eliciting occupational health information as part of each patient history.[7] In addition, every primary provider should know how to interpret the information and present it to patients in an understandable manner. Unfortunately, the 1986 midcourse review concluded that this objective was unlikely to be met by 1990 and no recent information indicates that it has been met.[7] Some occupational diseases are required to be reported.[32]

In 1700, Bernardino Ramazzini recommended that the teachings of Hippocrates be appended. He asked that one more question be added: "What occupation does he follow?"[21] As indicated by the 1990 objective just mentioned, no more attention or time appears to be allocated to the patient's occupation today than nearly three centuries earlier.[33,34] Today the occupational history remains one of the major clinical tools that the optometrist needs to use to recognize, diagnose, and manage eye and vision problems in the workplace.[13]

OCCUPATIONAL HEALTH HISTORY
"The occupational health history is fundamental to the assessment of the work-relatedness of health problems and should become a routine component of any comprehensive health history." This history requires much more than a superficial question about the patient's job title.[16] Like other parts of the patient history, the occupational history can be adopted and modified to meet the needs of each patient. For most primary care problems, the occupational history has two components: (1) the survey or basic occupational history, and, if needed, the diagnostic occupational history; and (2) the task analysis.

SURVEY (BASIC) OCCUPATIONAL HISTORY
The survey occupational history can easily be incorporated into the optometrist's traditional patient interview and history.[13,16,21] The key points to include are a description of current and past jobs and occupations; employment status (including unemployed, retired); exposure to hazards; and an assessment of the work-relatedness of the chief complaint or diagnosis. Questions that can be modified to address these key points follow:[13,16]

1. Describe your current and longest-held former jobs, including duties, materials used, and existing potential hazards including eye and vision hazards.
2. Are you now or have you ever been exposed to high intensity light, radiation, noise, chemicals, fumes, dusts, or biologic agents? Include a brief assessment of types, intensity, and duration.
3. Do you believe that any of your problems (signs or symptoms) are related to your work (or activities or hobbies at home)?
4. Did any change in your normal work tasks (procedures or processes) occur before you noticed your recent problem?
5. Do any of your co-workers have problems similar to yours?

Using these questions, the optometrist can determine if there is a relationship between the chief complaint or diagnosis and work-related or home-related activities or exposures, either present or past. Attention should also be given to other factors that may contribute to the problem such as cigarette smoking, medications, or drug or alcohol use.[16] For example, a complaint of poor night vision (dark adaptation) could be caused by exposure to carbon monoxide from cigarette smoke or engine exhaust.[35] The occupational survey history is not burdensome. It can readily be abbreviated, expanded, or focused and, like all other parts of the history, it should never be eliminated.[36]

These survey questions may help to establish the diagnosis of occupational or environmental problems.[13] The finding of a temporal relationship between the symptoms and the performance of tasks or exposures at work is very important information. An occupational cause should be suspected when symptoms decrease when the patient is away from work, such as during weekends or vacations, and reappear with return to work.[13] A symptom such as a headache that occurs at work and disappears when the patient is away from work very likely has a work-related cause. Other symptoms may mimic systemic diseases.

The second key question regarding exposure to environmental hazards helps assess the patient's current or past exposures to energy or agents that could be harmful.[17,18] Hazards can affect the patient's physical or mental health status and even result in death. The history of exposures may be the

determinant of the diagnosis. Hazards that could impact the eye or visual system are commonly classified as physical (e.g., radiation, noise, temperature extremes, heavy lifting and repetitive motion); chemical (e.g., lead, mercury, dust, gases, fumes, solvents, acids, caustics); biologic (e.g., viruses, bacteria, parasites, fungi); psychologic (e.g., boredom, work shift fatigue, risk of falling, repetition),[37] and ergonomic (e.g., improper tool or work area design, unnecessary lifting, poor vision conditions).

Diagnostic Occupational History

The diagnostic history is used when the survey occupational history increases the optometrist's suspicion that the patient's signs or symptoms are related to work or the environment.[13] This expansion of the basic occupational history collects more information about the patient and the work environment. Additional questions are asked to identify and diagnose specific occupational associations and hazards.

There are four key steps in taking the diagnostic history. They can be completed efficiently beginning with the use of a self-administered history form.[16] The key information to collect and assess is the following:

1. A listing of all jobs.
2. Identification of all places of employment and products manufactured, where appropriate.
3. Description of all operations performed on the job.
4. Assessment of illnesses in other workers similar to those of the patient.

The patient should include a detailed description of the work performed. Often it is useful to have the patient describe a typical day at work and to identify the work environment and the common tasks performed.[16] Unusual work procedures should also be assessed, such as end-of-the-month maintenance with hazardous substances or other occasional exposures to hazardous substances. The job title, nature of the job, and the products manufactured should be obtained for all past jobs (Tables 1-8 to 1-12; Fig. 1-1).

The optometrist needs to listen and be sensitive to potential hazards during the occupational interview

Your Company
Is there an occupational health program?
Does the company give physical examinations?
What is the industrial hygiene policy?
Is there a safety program?
Are you informed of the results of examinations or of workroom air samplings?

Your Job
What exactly were you doing when you became ill?
Were you working your regular shift?
What material(s) do you work with?
If it is liquid, does it give off vapor ("fumes") which can be breathed?
Does it ever spill on your skin?
Does it ever soak your clothing?
If you used protective devices, are these maintained by the company?
Do you exchange your respirator when it gets dirty or when you smell the chemical through the mask?
Does the company ever hold information meetings to tell you about the material you work with?
Is any chemical being used near you by other employees?
Do you become ill during the week at work and then get better over the weekend?
Do you get sick when you return to work? After a weekend off? After your vacation?
Has any new substance been introduced that you work with?
Has the brand of any material been changed?
Has there ever been a spill at your work station?
Has the equipment ever broken down?
Has anything interrupted the usual work process?
Have you ever changed jobs because of your health?
Has there ever been an OSHA inspection of your workplace?

If so, what was found and what action was taken?
Is there an exhaust ventilation system used at your work station?
Does anyone ever take air samples where you work?

Your Fellow Workers
Have any of your fellow workers been ill in the same way you are? When?
Have any complained of being unable to have children or having children born with defects?

Your Hobbies and Habits
What do you work with at home? Glue? Pesticides? Your car? Furniture refinishers? Photographic chemicals?
Do you smoke? What, where, and how much? How old when you started? How old when you quit?
Do you drink? What and how much?
Do you use firearms?
Do you play rock music? How long per day?
Do you drive heavy farm machinery?
Where do you have your work clothes washed?
Do you have any pets at home?
Do you take any medicines?

Your Feelings About Your Job
Do you like your job?
Are you still good at your job?
Have you had trouble holding a job?
Do you get frustrated at work?
Do you like (odd) shift work?
Is your job more than you can handle?
How do you feel about your foreman?
Is there much stress in your job?
Do you look forward to retirement?

From Felton JS: The occupational history: A neglected area in the clinical history. J Fam Pract 11:38, 1980; with permission.

TABLE 1-8
Occupational History Questions

with the patient. Hazards may exist that are not obvious from job titles. It is useful to ask the patient directly about potential hazards because workers are often well-informed about their workplace exposures. Workers who are not informed will require additional follow-up. People who should be approached if more information is needed are the plant manager, safety engineer, or appropriate employee representatives (Tables 1-13 to 1-16).

When hazardous exposures are assessed, it is useful to estimate the exposure dose. The dose is a function of how frequently the patient performs common tasks in a hazardous environment during a typical day and the duration of the exposure. The frequency, duration, and intensity of exposure all summate when dose is estimated. When chemical hazards are suspected, the optometrist can ask the worker or manufacturer for a Material Safety Data Sheet (MSDS) (Table 1-17) that lists ingredients and environmental information.[18] Other clues to exposure doses are the use of personal protective equipment and clothing. Clinicians can use a standard approach for evaluating work-related diseases (Table 1-18).

1. Name _____ Date _____
2. Current position (job) _____
   Type of business _____
   Description of work activities _____

3. Are you exposed to or do you work with any chemicals, dusts, or fumes? Yes ___ No ___ Don't know ___
4. Do any co-workers have medical complaints similar to yours? Yes ___ No ___ Don't know ___
5. Do you think you have a medical problem related to or aggravated by your work? Yes ___ No ___ Don't know ___
6. Have you ever worked with any of the following materials?

Asbestos	_____	Plastics	_____
Solvents	_____	Radiation	_____
Petroleum products	_____	Lead	_____
Vehicle or engine exhaust	_____	Mercury	_____
Degreasers	_____	Other metals	_____
Paints	_____	Welding, brazing, soldering	_____
Glues	_____	Insulation	_____
Grease and oil	_____	Other dusts	_____
Pesticides	_____	Other gases	_____
Silica	_____	Noise	_____

7. Have you ever done any of the following types of work?

Plumbing or pipefitting	_____	Mining	
Shipyard work	_____	Forge or foundry work	_____
Building construction	_____	Chemical plant work	_____

8. Have you worked in any other environments or with any other materials about which you are concerned? Yes ___ No ___
   If yes, describe: _____

9. Do you have any hobby activities that involve use of or exposure to dusts, chemicals, or fumes?
   Yes _____ No _____
   If yes, describe: _____

Starting with your first job, list your complete occupational history. Include summer jobs and part-time jobs.
Dates (month/yr.)
From   To   Employer   Job   Exposures

From McCunney RJ: Handbook of Occupational Medicine. Boston, Little, Brown and Company, 1988; with permission.

TABLE 1-9
Sample Occupational History Form

An expanded OSHA regulation (OSHA Hazard Communication Standard 1910.122), referred to as the employee right-to-know law, became effective in 1988. This applies to any employer, including optometrists, who uses flammable, corrosive, reactive, or toxic materials that can cause injury to people. Employers are required to inform employees about any hazardous materials in their working area, label hazardous chemicals, provide protective clothing and eyewear, provide training in safety procedures, and make MSDS available to employees for all hazardous chemicals (Table 1-17).

Any determination of work or work exposures should include the possibility of nonoccupational exposures or of exposures occurring in the home. These nonoccupational exposures may potentiate or contribute to the effect of hazardous exposures at the workplace. In addition to hazardous materials used within the home, there may also be neighborhood pollution produced by nearby businesses and

I. Work and Exposure History

A. Current Employment
Questions 1–7 refer to your current or most recent job.

1. Job title _____

2. Type of industry _____

3. Name of employer _____

4. Year job began _____
   Still working? _____
   Yes _____ No _____ If no, year job ended _____

5. Briefly describe this job, noting any part that you feel may be hazardous to your health. _____
_____

6. Do you wear protective equipment on this job?
   Yes _____ No _____ If yes, check equipment used:
   Gloves _____ Air supply respirator _____
   Mask respirator _____ Coveralls or aprons _____
   Hearing protection _____ Safety glasses _____

7. In this job, are you exposed to any of the following?
   If yes, mark those to which you are exposed:
   Fumes and dusts _____ Elements and metals _____
   Solvents _____ Other chemicals _____ Noise _____
   Vibration _____ Excess heat/cold _____
   Emotional stress _____ Other _____

B. Employment History
It is important that we know all the jobs you have had. Job #1 is your current or most recent job. Beginning with the job before this one—Job #2—please fill in as much of the information requested as you can remember, and continue to do so until all previous jobs have been listed. Include any military service you have had. If you need additional space, use the back of this form.

	YEARS From—To	JOB TITLE	EXPOSURES
Job #2	_____	_____	_____
Job #3	_____	_____	_____
Job #4	_____	_____	_____
Job #5	_____	_____	_____

	YEARS From—To	JOB TITLE	EXPOSURES
Job #6	_____	_____	_____
Job #7	_____	_____	_____
Job #8	_____	_____	_____
	_____	_____	_____

C. Other Exposures

1. Does anyone in your household work at a job that you suspect involves exposures that may be brought home from work (e.g., asbestos fibers on clothes)?
   Yes _____ No _____

2. Are there any industries in the area in which you live that may pollute your environment?
   Yes _____ No _____

3. Do you have any hobbies that expose you to chemicals, metals, or other substances?
   Yes _____ No _____

4. Have you ever smoked cigarettes? ("No" means less than 20 packs of cigarettes in your entire life.)
   Yes _____ No _____
   If yes, please answer the following:
   a. Do you now smoke cigarettes (that is, as of 1 month ago)? Yes _____ No _____
   b. How many years have you smoked? _____
   c. Of the entire time you have smoked, about how many cigarettes per day do or did you smoke on the average?
   _____

II. General Health History

1. Is there any particular hazard or part of your job that you think relates to your problems? Yes _____ No

2. Do any of your coworkers have problems or complaints similar to yours? Yes _____ No _____

From Rosenstock L: Clinical Occupational Medicine. Philadelphia, WB Saunders, 1986; with permission.

TABLE 1-10
Sample Occupational History Form

This questionnaire has been developed to assist us in designing the types of glasses that will best suit your lifestyle and offer fashion and protection, as well as comfort and affordability.

Name _____ Employer _____

Type of Work _____

Address _____

City _____ State _____ Zip _____ Phone _____

1. Do you currently use more than one pair of glasses?
   yes ___ no ___
2. If so, is your second pair for a special application such as:
   office ___, dresswear ___, occupational safety wear ___,
   active sports ___, home safety wear ___, other ___?
3. Are safety or protective eye glasses required for your work?
   yes ___ no ___
4. If so, are safety glasses provided by your company?
   yes ___ no ___
5. If you do precision work on the job, is your prescription written for the correct distance from your eyes to your tools?
   (close range is 14") yes ___ no ___
6. If you use a computer on the job or at home, do you experience visual fatigue, frequent headaches, blurred vision or difficulty in focusing after extended work on a VDT?
   yes ___ no ___
7. For either precision work or computer use, approximately what different ranges of vision must your eyes accommodate? close (14") ___, intermediate (26") ___, greater than 36" ___?
8. Do your hobbies and leisure time activities include:
   ___ Gardening/yard work ___ Basketball/racquetball
   ___ Tennis/golf/hiking   ___ Auto mechanics
   ___ Hunting/fishing   ___ Home repair with power tools
   ___ Active sports such as soccer, softball
   Other _____

9. Are your eyes sensitive to sunlight? yes___ no ___
10. Do you spend a substantial amount of time driving?
    yes ___ no ___
11. Do you spend a substantial amount of time outdoors, on the job or off? yes ___ no ___
12. What is potentially the most hazardous activity you participate in regularly in terms of your vision?
    _____
13. When was the last time you broke your glasses and what was the cause? Frame stress ___, impact to lenses ___, other ___
14. If you had a comfortable and attractive pair of glasses for special applications such as: the computer, active sports, or home workshop, would you wear them:
    1) consistently ___, 2) sometimes ___, 3) rarely ___.
15. How important is the cost factor in buying a secondary pair of special application or protective eyewear?
    1) primary consideration ___, 2) reasonably important ___, 3) not a major factor ___.
16. If your children wear glasses, do they wear industrial strength protective eyewear everyday? yes ___ no ___
17. Do your children have specially constructed and approved sports glasses for participation in sports?
    yes ___ no ___

Modified from Titmus Optical, Protective Products Division, Petersburg, Virginia; with permission.

TABLE 1-11
Lifestyle Protection Patient Questionnaire

industries. Personal habits may also contribute to environmental exposures that interact or add to occupational exposures (Table 1-14).[13,16]

Task Analysis

The second component of the occupational history is the task analysis. This analysis is a detailed assessment of the patient's work-related tasks. The assessment is done to maximize vision perfor- mance and minimize or eliminate eye and vision hazards. This is very important because different jobs will make different visual demands upon the worker and require different visual skills.[28] "How well we see and what we see are determining factors in how efficiently and safely we perform at our occupations."[8] A patient questionnaire is often helpful (Table 1-19). The task analysis requires the training and skills of the occupational optometrist or the primary care optometrist experienced in this area.

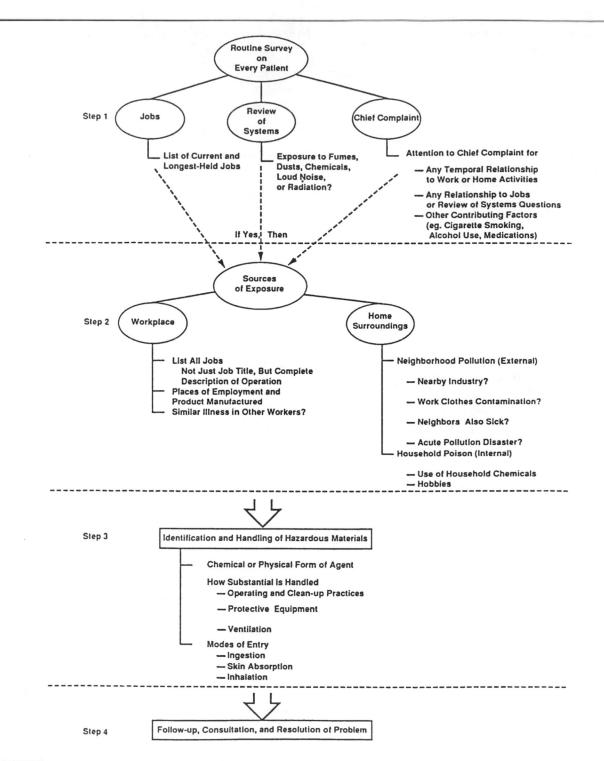

Step 1

Routine Survey on Every Patient

Jobs
List of Current and Longest-Held Jobs

Review of Systems
Exposure to Fumes, Dusts, Chemicals, Loud Noise, or Radiation?

Chief Complaint
Attention to Chief Complaint for
— Any Temporal Relationship to Work or Home Activities
— Any Relationship to Jobs or Review of Systems Questions
— Other Contributing Factors (eg. Cigarette Smoking, Alcohol Use, Medications)

If Yes, Then

Sources of Exposure

Step 2

Workplace
List All Jobs
  Not Just Job Title, But Complete Description of Operation
Places of Employment and Product Manufactured
Similar Illness in Other Workers?

Home Surroundings
Neighborhood Pollution (External)
— Nearby Industry?
— Work Clothes Contamination?
— Neighbors Also Sick?
— Acute Pollution Disaster?
Household Poison (Internal)
— Use of Household Chemicals
— Hobbies

Step 3

Identification and Handling of Hazardous Materials
Chemical or Physical Form of Agent
How Substantial Is Handled
— Operating and Clean-up Practices
— Protective Equipment
— Ventilation
Modes of Entry
— Ingestion
— Skin Absorption
— Inhalation

Step 4

Follow-up, Consultation, and Resolution of Problem

From Goldman RH, Peters JM: The occupational and environmental health history, JAMA 246:2831, 1981.© American Medical Association; with permission.

TABLE 1-12
Algorithmic Approach to History Taking and Diagnosis of Occupational Problems

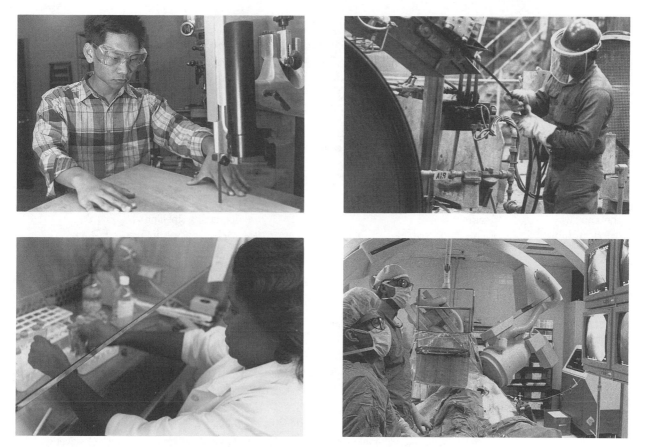

FIGURE 1-1
People in a wide variety of occupations. The diversity of occupations and tasks within occupations require the optometrist to take an occupational history for all patients.

The optometrist does the task analysis using a broad primary care and visual science perspective with an extensive knowledge of visual and ophthalmic optics, binocular vision and oculomotor control, psychophysical principles, photopic and scotopic illuminance requirements, color contrast, contrast, glare, ergonomic performance, static and dynamic acuity, stereopsis, radiant exposure thresholds, environmental assessment and analysis skills, and many other factors. The specific application of this extensive knowledge to the worker's visual performance and eye safety will enable the worker to perform safely and maximize on-the-job performance. The older or disabled worker may have special needs that need to be addressed. Unfortunately, many employers, employees, and some clinicians make a serious mistake by assuming that the treatment of a worker's

distance refractive error is all that is needed for eye and vision safety and performance.

It is important for the optometrist, patient, and employer to recognize that eye care improves job performance. "Visual skills and visual deficiencies can often be improved by professional eye care and treatment. Many employees in industry have a pattern of visual skills that is not adapted to their jobs. Often such employees are unaware of the visual handicaps under which they are working. The ophthalmic professions—ophthalmology and optometry—are able to rehabilitate . . . a large majority of employees whose vision is not adapted to their jobs."[28] Workers with good vision are more productive (quantity and quality); have fewer accidents, including lost time accidents; and are more likely to remain on the job (less turnover).[28]

	Agent	Potential Exposures
Immediate or Short-term Effects		
Dermatoses (allergic or irritant)	Metals (chromium, nickel), fibrous glass, epoxy resins, cutting oils, solvents, caustic alkali, soaps	Electroplating, metal cleaning, plastics, machining, leather tanning, housekeeping
Headache	Carbon monoxide, solvents	Firefighting, automobile exhaust, foundry, wood finishing, dry cleaning
Acute psychoses	Lead (especially organic) mercury, carbon disulfide	Handling gasoline, seed handling, fungicide, wood preserving, viscose rayon industry
Asthma or dry cough	Formaldehyde, toluene diisocyanate, animal dander	Textiles, plastics, polyurethane kits, lacquer use, animal handler
Pulmonary edema, pneumonitis	Nitrogen oxides, phosgene, halogen gases, cadmium	Welding, farming ("silo filler's disease"), chemical operations, smelting
Cardiac arrhythmias	Solvents, fluorocarbons	Metal cleaning, solvent use, refrigerator maintenance
Angina	Carbon monoxide	Car repair, traffic exhaust, foundry, wood finishing
Abdominal pain	Lead	Battery making, enameling, smelting, painting, welding, ceramics, plumbing
Hepatitis (may become a long-term effect)	Halogenated hydrocarbons, e.g. carbon tetrachloride, virus	Solvent use, lacquer use, hospital workers
Latent or Long-term Effects		
Chronic dyspnea Pulmonary fibrosis	Asbestos, silica, beryllium, coal, aluminum	Mining, insulation, pipefitting, sandblasting, quarrying, metal alloy work, aircraft or electrical parts
Chronic bronchitis emphysema	Cotton dust, cadmium, coal dust, organic solvents, cigarettes	Textile industry, battery production, soldering, mining, solvent use
Lung cancer	Asbestos, arsenic, nickel, uranium, coke-oven emissions	Insulation, pipefitting, smelting, coke ovens, shipyard workers, nickel refining, uranium mining
Bladder cancer	β-Naphthylamine, benzidine dyes	Dye industry, leather, rubber-working, chemists
Peripheral neuropathy	Lead, arsenic, n-hexane, methyl butyl ketone, acrylamide	Battery production, plumbing, smelting, painting, shoemaking, solvent use, insecticides
Behavioral changes	Lead, carbon disulfide, solvents, mercury, manganese	Battery makers, smelting, viscose rayon industry, degreasing, mfg/repair of scientific instruments, dental amalgam workers
Extrapyramidal syndrome	Carbon disulfide, manganese	Viscose rayon industry, steel production, battery production, foundry
Aplastic anemia, leukemia	Benzene, ionizing radiation	Chemists, furniture refinishing, cleaning, degreasing, radiation workers

From Goldman RH, Peters JM: The occupational and environmental health history. JAMA 246:2831, 1981. © American Medical Association; with permission.

TABLE 1-13
Examples of Environmental Causes of Medical Problems

Common Dangerous Products

Product	Potentially Hazardous Agents
Disinfectants	Cresol, phenol, hexachlorophene
Cleaning agents and solvents	
Bleaches	Sodium hypochlorite (Clorox)
Window cleaner	Ammonia
Carpet cleaner	Ammonia, turpentine, naphthalene, 1,1,1-trichloroethane
Oven and drain cleaners	Potassium hydroxide, sodium hydroxide
Dry-cleaning fluids, spot removers	1,1,1-Trichloroethane, perchloroethylene, petroleum distillates
Paint and varnish solvents	Turpentine, xylene, toluene, methanol, methylene, chloride, acetone
Pesticides	Malathion, dichlorvos, carbaryl, methoxychlor
Emissions from heating or cooling devices	
Gas stove pilot light	Nitrogen oxides
Indoor use of charcoal grill	Carbon monoxide
Leaks from refrigerator or air conditioner cooling systems	Freon
Microwave ovens	Microwave radiation
Sun lamps	Ultraviolet radiation

Common Hazards in Hobbies

Activity	Potential Hazard
Painting	Toxic pigments, eg. arsenic (emerald green), cadmium, chromium, lead, mercury; acrylic emulsions, solvents
Ceramics	
Raw materials	Colors and glazes containing barium carbonate; lead, chromium, uranium, cadmium
Firing	Fumes of fluoride, chlorine, sulfur dioxide
Gas-fired kilns	Carbon monoxide
Sculpture and Casting	
Grinding silica-containing stone	Silica (silicon dioxide)
Serpentine rock with asbestos	Asbestos
Woodworking	Wood dust
Metal casting	Metal fume, sand (silica) from molding, binders of phenol formaldehyde or urea formaldehyde
Welding	Metal fume, ultraviolet light exposure, welding fumes, carbon dioxide, carbon monoxide, nitrogen dioxide, ozone or phosgene (if solvents nearby)
Plastics	Monomers released during heating (polyvinyl chloride), methyl methacrylate, acrylic glues, polyurethanes (toluene 2,4-diisocyanate), polystyrene (methyl chloride release), fiberglass, polyester of epoxy resins
Woodworking	Solvents, especially methylene chloride
Photography	
Developer	Hydroquinone, metal
Stop bath	Weak acetic acid
Stop hardener	Potassium chrome alum (chromium)
Fixer	Sodium sulfite, acetic acid-sulfur dioxide
Hardeners and stabilizers	Formaldehyde

From Goldman RH, Peters JM: The occupational and environmental health history, JAMA 246:2831, 1981. © American Medical Association; with permission.

TABLE 1-14
Examples of Common Dangerous Products and Hazards in Hobbies

Occupation or Activity	Exposures*	Selected Potentially Hazardous Exposures	

Agriculture, farming, and pest control	A,B,F,K	A. Aerosols, Vapors, Gases
		  Carbon monoxide
			H. Metals, Metal Fumes
			  Aluminum

Automobile, aircraft manufacturing and repair	A,C,E,H,K,M	Formaldehyde Hydrogen sulfide	Arsenic Cadmium
Bakers, food handlers	B,L,M	Ethylene oxide	Chromium
Boiler operations and cleaning	A,C,E,K	Nitrogen dioxide	Cobalt
Ceramics and masonry	E,H	Ozone	Iron
Carpentry, woodworking, and lumber industry	B,I,J,K,N	Phosgene Smoke	Lead Mercury
Chemical industry and users	A–N	Sewer gas	Nickel

Construction work, demolition, road work, maintenance, and plastering	C,D,E,K,J,N	Sulfur dioxide
		Inert gases
		Welding fumes
			I. Organic Dust
			  Cotton dust
			  Wood dust

Dry cleaning, and laundry	J,M,N	B. Biological Inhalants	Poison oak
Electric, electronics	C,E,H,J,M	Bacteria	J. Petrochemicals
Foundry work	A,C,E,H,K	Fungi	Asphalt and tar
Health care, laboratory work, and dental work	A,B,C,D,E,G,K,L,M,N	Molds Spores	Creosote Coal tar

Machinery, grinding, and metal work	A,C,H,K,M,N	C. Corrosive Substances
		  Acids
			PBB (polybrominated
			  biphenyls) and PCB

Mining	A,E,G,K	Alkalis	(polychlorinated
Oil industry, petrochemical	A,C,J,K,N	Ammonia	biphenyls)
Paper industry	E,N	Chlorine	Petroleum distillates
Plastic manufacturing	E,J,L	Phenol	K. Physical Agents
Plumbing, pipefitting, and shipfitting	A,C,E,H,K	D. Dyes, Stains Aniline dyes	Heavy lifting Noise
Printing, lithography	D,I,K,N	Azo dyes	Thermal stress
Sandblasting, spray painting	A,E,H,K,N	Benzidine	Vibration

Shipyard, dock work, and transportation	A,C,E,H,J,K,N	E. Inorganic Dusts, Powders
		  Asbestos
			L. Plastics
			  Vinyl chloride

Textile industry	A,D,E,I,N	Beryllium	Epoxy resins
Welding	A,E,H,M	Coal dust	Acrylonitrile
X-ray occupations	G	Fiberglass Nickel Silica Talc	Styrene Methyl ethyl ketone peroxide M. Sensitizing Agents

		F. Insecticides, Herbicides
		  Carbamates
			Methane diisocyanate,
			  toluene diisocyanate

		Hallogenated hydrocarbons	Nickel Platinum
		Organophosphates Phenoxyherbicides	Proteolytic (detergent) enzymes
		G. Electromagnetic Radiation	Aliphatic amines
		Radioactive materials	N. Solvents
		Ultraviolet	Benzene
		X-ray	Carbon disulfide
		Yellowcake	Carbon tetrachloride
		Microwaves	Chloroform Methanol Trichloroethylene Xylene Glycol ethers (cellusolves)

From The Occupational and Environmental Health Committee of the American Lung Association of San Diego and Imperial Counties, California: Taking the occupational history. Ann Intern Med 99:641–651, 1983, with permission.

TABLE 1-15
Inventory of Occupations and Major Hazardous Exposures

1. Occupational lung diseases: asbestos, byssinosis, silicosis, coal workers' pneumoconiosis, lung cancer, occupational asthma
2. Musculoskeletal injuries: disorders of the back, trunk, upper extremity, neck, lower extremity; traumatically induced Raynaud's phenomenon
3. Occupational cancers (other than lung): leukemia, mesothelioma; cancers of the bladder, nose, and liver
4. Amputations, fractures, eye loss, lacerations, traumatic deaths
5. Cardiovascular diseases: hypertension, coronary artery disease, acute myocardial infarction
6. Disorders of reproduction: infertility, spontaneous abortion, teratogenesis
7. Neurotoxic disorders: peripheral neuropathy, toxic encephalitis, psychoses, extreme personality changes (exposure-related)
8. Noise-induced loss of hearing
9. Dermatologic conditions: dermatoses, burns (scaldings), chemical burns, contusions (abrasions)
10. Psychologic disorders: neuroses, personality disorders, alcoholism, drug dependency

NOTE: The conditions listed under each category are to be viewed as *selected examples,* not comprehensive definitions of the category.

From the Centers for Disease Control: Leading work-related diseases and injuries—United States. MMWR 32(2):24–26,32; 32(14):189–191, 1983.

TABLE 1-16
The 10 Leading Work-Related Diseases and Injuries in the United States, 1982

The occupational optometrist begins the task analysis with an assessment of the visual requirements of the job. Although a complex process, the task analysis requires the assessment of the following data:[38-43]

1. Job description, including all the different tasks and procedures done during the usual work day, indoors or outdoors. Infrequent tasks should also be described, along with their frequency and duration. Working positions should be assessed including standing, sitting, walking, and driving.
2. Distance from the worker's eyes to the work areas, accommodative and convergence demands.
3. Work movement: fixed or changing, slow or rapid, constant or intermittent, vertical, horizontal, or rotary.

4. Work area size, centrally and peripherally.
5. Visual attention requirements: fixed or changing, casual or concentrated, detailed or gross, constant or intermittent duration.
6. Work and surround area illumination: quantity, quality, and direction of lumination; reflectance; disability or minimal glare; brightness ratios; and contrast.
7. Color discrimination requirements: gross, fine, none.[44]
8. Stereoacuity requirements: detailed, gross, none.
9. Position of work surface: at, below, or above eye level; angle of work with respect to straight-ahead position, to left, or to right.
10. Eye and vision hazards: metal or nonmetal particles, dust, fumes, chemicals (splash), moving machinery, radiation from ultraviolet (UV), infrared (IR), radio frequency (Rf), microwave, and laser sources.
11. Size of task details: fine, medium, gross. Visibility.
12. Peripheral vision requirements.

This information is used to determine the visual requirements for each job and the type of eye and vision protection required. Task analysis is used to determine not only visual requirements but also to maximize the worker's visual performance on the job.[45] Assessment of visual requirements ensures that the task can be performed properly and safely with high productivity. The optometrist uses complex judgments in determining these requirements and treatments (see Tables 1-20 to 1-22).

Several corporations have developed educational materials for clinicians and the public about the importance of occupational eyecare. One example is the lifestyle guide describing selected occupations, their common visual tasks, and recommendations based on visual factors developed by Vision-Ease (Fig. 1-2).[42]

1.4 Occupational Optometry Services

The overall goals of occupational optometry are the prevention of eye and vision injuries and the enhancement of performance on the job through maximizing vision performance. Prevention has the

Material Safety Data Sheet May be used to comply with OSHA's Hazard Communication Standard, 29 CFR 1910.1200. Standard must be consulted for specific requirements.	**U.S. Department of Labor** Occupational Safety and Health Administration (Non-Mandatory Form) Form Approved OMB No. 1218-0072
IDENTITY *(As Used on Label and List)*	*Note: Blank spaces are not permitted. If any item is not applicable,* *or no information is available, the space must be marked to* *indicate that.*

Section I

Manufacturer's Name	Emergency Telephone Number
Address *(Number, Street, City, State, and Zip Code)*	Telephone Number for Information
	Date Prepared
	Signature of Preparer *(optional)*

Section II—Hazardous Ingredients/Identity Information

Hazardous Components (Specific Chemicals Identity: Common Name[s])	OSHA PEL	ACGIH TLV	Other Limits Recommended	% (optional)

Section III—Physical/Chemical Characteristics

Boiling Point	Specific Gravity ($H_2O = 1$)
Vapor Pressure (mmHg.)	Melting Point
Vapor Density (AIR = 1)	Evaporation Rate (Butyl Acetate = 1)
Solubility in Water	
Appearance and Odor	

TABLE 1-17
Material Safety Data Sheet

Section IV—Fire and Explosion Hazard Data

Flash Point (Method Used)		Flammable Limits	LEL	UEL

Extinguishing Media

Special Fire Fighting Procedures

Unusual Fire and Explosion Hazards

Section V—Reactivity Data

Stability	Unstable	Conditions to Avoid
	Stable	

Incompatibility *(Materials to Avoid)*

Hazardous Decomposition or Byproducts

Hazardous Polymerization	May Occur	Conditions to Avoid
	Will Not Occur	

Section VI—Health Hazard Data

Route(s) of Entry:	Inhalation?	Skin?	Ingestion?

Health Hazards *(Acute and Chronic)*

Carcinogenicity:	NTP?	IARC Monographs?	OSHA Regulated?

Signs and Symptoms of Exposure

Medical Conditions
Generally Aggravated by Exposure

Emergency and First Aid Procedures

TABLE 1-17
Material Safety Data Sheet, continued

Section VII—Precautions for Safe Handling and Use

Steps to Be Taken in Case Material is Released or Spilled

Waste Disposal Method

Precautions to Be Taken in Handling and Storing

Other Precautions

Section VIII—Control Measures

Respiratory Protection *(Specify Type)*

Ventilation	Local Exhaust		Special
	Mechanical *(General)*		Other

Protective Gloves   Eye Protection

Other Protective Clothing or Equipment

Work/Hygienic Practices

(Reproduce locally)   OSHA 174 Sept 1985

Reprinted from the U.S. Department of Labor, Occupational Safety and Health Administration, 1985.

TABLE 1-17
Material Safety Data Sheet, continued

higher priority because of the tragic and costly consequences of serious eye and vision injuries and loss. All optometric services provided are related to these goals (Table 1-23).

Occupational optometry services may be provided in individual or group private practices, multispecialty group clinics, and in business or industry plants.[45] One exception to this may be the evaluation of environmental hazards. However, hazard evaluation can be done in the private practice setting by an experienced optometrist familiar with the businesses or industries in the community and with patients who are knowledgeable about their jobs and environments.

The provision of occupational optometric services is determined by the nature of the business or industry, the number of employees, the enlightenment of management regarding preventing eye injuries and maximizing worker performance, and the types of workplace hazards and injuries. These services include pre-employment and preplacement evaluations; vision screenings; periodic examinations,

1. Determine the diagnosis accurately:
   a. Uniformity of diagnosis among cases
   b. Standard diagnostic practices or clearly defined case definition
2. Describe working conditions (occupational history)
3. Review toxicity of materials (literature review)
4. Evaluate information on dose and response:
   a. Consider dose-response relationships from epidemiologic studies
   b. Consider factors that modify exposure
   c. Consider exposure to analogous substances
5. Consider plausible alternative explanations
6. Review aggregate data related to the hypothesis that materials at work caused the illness:
   a. Features that substantiate the proposed relationship
   b. Alternative explanations and their likelihood
   c. Type of cause considered to be present (e.g., de novo, aggravation, predisposition)

From McCunney, RJ: Handbook of Occupational Medicine. Boston, Little, Brown and Company, 1988; with permission.

TABLE 1-18
Summary of the Evaluation of Work-Related Diseases

including diagnosis and management of work-related eye and vision problems; rehabilitation and postinjury care; pre-termination and pre-retirement vision assessments; health assessments; evaluation of potential hazards and environmental surveys; standards determination; eye and vision policy establishment; health education and safety seminars for individual workers and groups of workers; determination of regulatory compliance or adherence; and administrative services, including the operation of occupational eye and vision health programs and specialized material billings.

Pre-Employment and Preplacement Evaluations

Pre-employment evaluations are conducted to determine if a worker's eyes and vision will satisfy the anticipated on-the-job visual demands. These evaluations document pre-existing eye and vision conditions and are important when assessing subsequent environmental exposures. Preplacement evaluations are similar to pre-employment evaluations;

however, they are conducted after a worker has been hired to determine the positions for which a person is visually qualified.

Vision Screening

Vision screenings are conducted to determine if workers have the minimum vision needed for a specific job and to screen workers for eye and vision problems or diseases. For example, in many states, periodic vision screenings are done to be certain people have the minimum vision needed for driving. The screening does not replace an eye examination. In any screening, there will be a percentage of false positive and false negative results depending on the prevalence of the condition, the nature of the tests, and the screening criteria used. The selection of tests and criteria for passing are an important service provided by the occupational optometrist.

Periodic Examinations

There are three different types of periodic examinations. The first is an occupational vision examination to assess occupational vision demands.[46] This examination emphasizes an analysis of the visual demands of the job, work hazards, and the work environment. It also includes an assessment of external and internal eye health, refraction if appropriate, and assessment of work-related oculomotor, accommodative, and binocular functions.

The second type of periodic examinations is a supplemental occupational vision examination limited to a task analysis.[39,42] This examination includes an analysis of the visual demands of the job and may include a review of work hazards and the job environment. It also includes a review of the eye examination results provided by the employee's optometrist for relevance to job demands. Additional procedures may be done when judged to be significant to the employee's job requirements and work safety.

The third type is the comprehensive optometric eye and vision examination. This examination is done at regular intervals to assess eye and vision problems, to rule out suspected diseases or disorders, and to provide early identification of risk factors and health problems such as hypertension and diabetes.

Employee _____

Employer _____

The O.V.S. panel member doctor needs the following information for the analysis of your occupational vision needs and for the design of appropriate occupational/protective eyewear.

Brief job description _____

Please check each item related to your job:

Work is performed while:

☐ Standing	☐ Sitting	☐ Walking	☐ Driving
☐ Indoors	☐ Outdoors	☐ Viewing a video screen*	☐ Other

*Persons doing frequent, prolonged tasks may complete a VIDEO SCREEN OCCUPATIONAL VISION REQUIREMENTS form.

Seeing directions and distances:

☐ Eye level   Viewing distance is _____ inches/feet.

☐ Below eye level   Viewing distance is _____ inches/feet.

☐ Above eye level   Viewing distance is _____ inches/feet.

☐ Other directions and distances *(please describe)*

Viewing area (field of view) at:

Far distance is	☐ Large	☐ Medium	☐ Small
Intermediate distance is	☐ Large	☐ Medium	☐ Small
Near distance is	☐ Large	☐ Medium	☐ Small

Size of tasks at:

Far distances	☐ Large	☐ Medium	☐ Small	☐ Very Small
Intermediate distances	☐ Large	☐ Medium	☐ Small	☐ Very Small
Near distances	☐ Large	☐ Medium	☐ Small	☐ Very Small

Work Environment:

Temperature:	☐ Hot	☐ Cold	☐ Average
Lighting:	☐ Bright	☐ Dark	☐ Average
Humidity:	☐ High	☐ Low	☐ Air conditioned

Other *(please describe)* _____

Eye hazards:

☐ Metal particles	☐ Non-metal particles	☐ Dust	
☐ Fumes	☐ Chemical splash	☐ Moving machinery	
☐ Infrared	☐ Ultraviolet	☐ Glare	☐ Radiation

Other *(please describe)* _____

Special vision requirements:

☐ Depth perception _____

☐ Color discrimination _____

☐ Other *(please describe)* _____

TABLE 1-19
Patient Questionnaire—Occupational Vision Requirements

- Job description
- Visual working distance. Accommodative convergence/demand
- Work movement
- Work area size
- Visual attention requirements
- Illumination of work and surround
- Color discrimination requirements
- Stereoacuity needs
- Work position and orientation
- Eye and vision hazards
- Task size
- Peripheral vision requirements

TABLE 1-20
Task Analysis—Diagnosing Occupational Vision Needs

Rehabilitation and Post-Injury Care

Rehabilitation services may be required depending on the results of the periodic screenings or examinations. If needed, these are usually provided by the patient's optometrist. Specialized services may be provided by the occupational optometrist for unique job tasks, when these are not available in the community. Post-injury follow-up care will usually be provided by the patient's optometrist but may be coordinated with the occupational optometrist.

Pre-Termination and Pre-Retirement Eye and Vision Assessment

Although rarely done, there should be an eye and vision assessment of all employees leaving a business or industry, either voluntarily or involuntarily. This reduces the risk of future claims for work-related eye diseases and vision impairments.

Health Assessment

Health assessments are done to identify the presence or rule out the existence of systemic diseases, including those that may affect the eye and visual system.

These assessments include a detailed health history including exposures to environmental hazards. Physical assessment of the eye, internally and externally, and systemic screening tests such as measurement of blood pressure, screening for cholesterol, and the ordering of blood tests are commonly done. The assessment may include consultation with an occupational physician if needed. These assessments are especially important for workers who rarely have general physical examinations or for those who have had an acute or chronic exposure to environmental hazards.

Evaluation of Potential Hazards

Evaluation of potential hazards can be done during an initial environmental survey, for example, when the optometrist first establishes a relationship with a business or industry as a consultant. This survey should be repeated periodically to determine whether new hazards have developed. For example, it should be repeated with a change in a manufacturing process or an environmental change that could cause glare or poor contrast. An evaluation of hazards should also be done in response to a specific problem area or in response to any eye or vision accident.

The determination of hazards and their assessment and remediation requires the application of the environmental optometrist's knowledge in the areas of industrial hygiene, toxicology, epidemiology and biostatistics, optometric surveillance, risk assessment and OSHA requirements. These areas are important in the recognition, evaluation, and control of eye and vision hazards and injury prevention. Because of the complexity of the workplace, the occupational optometrist usually interacts with other workplace professionals. These professionals may include the safety engineer, the occupational nurse or physician, the industrial hygienist, the plant manager, the chairman of the safety committee, union safety personnel, and others.

Standards Determination

Determination of standards and their assessment are very important during the implementation of an

Desirable

Accountant	Illuminating engineer
Anaesthetist	Interior decorator/designer/planner
Architect	
Artist—graphic, commercial, advertising	Jeweller
Auctioneer	
	Librarian
Bartender	Lighting director (stage, film, TV)
Bacteriologist	
Baker	Manicurist
Beautician	Metallurgist
Botanist	Milliner
Brewer	Miner
Butcher	
Builder/bricklayer	Nurse
Buyer—textiles, yarn, tobacco, food, e.g., fruit, cocoa; timber	
	Optometrist/ophthalmologist
Carpenter	Osteopath
Carpet/lino fitter/planner	
Chiropodist	Painter
Clothes designer	Pharmacist assistant (counter service)
Cook or chef	Physician
Coroner	Physical Therapist
Confectioner	Post Office counter assistant
Cosmetics director (stage, film, TV)	Potter
Dental surgeon and technician	Sales person (fabrics, drapery, yarns, wool, carpets)
Draughtsman	garments/footwear
Dressmaker	china and glass
Driving Instructor	linen
Driver in public services, e.g., bus	cosmetics/toiletries
	jewellery
Engineer (various)	confectioner
	stationer
Farmer	storekeeper
Florist	Shoe repairer
Forester	Surgeon
Furrier	
	Tanner
Gardener and landscape gardener	Tailor
Geologist	Telephone switchboard operator
Gemologist, e.g., setting stones, diamond grader	Theatre/stage props manager
Grocer	
	Veterinary surgeon
Hairdresser	
Horticulturist	Waiter
	Window dresser
	Zoologist

Essential

Armed forces	Electrical work—electrician
	electronics technician
Civil aviation, military aviation	color TV mechanic
Color matcher in dyeing, textiles, paints, inks,	motor mechanic
colored paper, ceramics, cosmetics	telephone installer
Carpet darner/inspector, spinner, weaver,	Police—Certain grades
bobbin winder	Navigation—pilot, fisherman, railways

From Voke J: Industrial and occupational consequences of defective color vision. Optician, February 1, 1980; with permission.

TABLE 1-21
Careers and Occupations in which Good Color Vision Is Desirable and Essential

Visual Skills	Typical		Occupational/Job Related							How Determined[1]
	Driving (far)	Reading (near)	Computer Operator	Clerical & Admin.	Inspection & Close Work	Operators of Mobile Equip.	Machine Operators	Mechanics & Skilled Techs.	Unskilled Laborers	
Locating, Scanning, Tracking	✓		✓	✓	✓	✓	✓	✓	✓	? • *
Peripheral (side) Vision	✓		✓	✓	✓	✓	✓	✓	✓	? • † *
Depth Perception	✓				✓	✓	✓	✓	✓	† *
Color Discrimination	✓		?		✓	✓	✓	✓		† *
Glare Recovery	✓		✓		✓	✓	✓	✓		*
Eye Hand Coordination	✓		✓	?	✓	✓	✓	✓		*
Focusing Range & Speed	✓		✓	✓	✓	✓	✓	✓		? • *
FAR (distance) Central Vision (clarity)	✓		✓	✓	✓	✓	✓	✓	✓	• † *
Equal Focus	✓					✓	~	~		• *
Sustaining Focus	✓					✓	~	~		• ? *
Ease of Single Vision	✓					✓	~	~		• † *
Sustaining Single Vision	✓				✓	✓	~	~		• ? *
NEAR (close vision) Central Vision (clarity)	✓	✓	✓	✓	✓	~	✓	✓	~	• † *
Equal Focus		✓	✓	✓	✓	~	✓	✓		• *
Sustaining Focus		✓	✓	✓	✓	~	✓	✓		• ? † *
Ease of Single Vision		✓	✓	✓	✓	~	✓	✓		• *
Sustaining Single Vision	✓	✓	✓	✓	✓	~	✓	✓		? • *

[1] How visual skills are determined:
• Typical examination for eyeglasses
† Vision screening on the job site
* Vision examination related to job demands
Copyright © 1986, Occupational Vision Services, Inc., Burbank, California.

TABLE 1-22
Visual Skills Needed for Various Activities

- Pre-employment/preplacement evaluation
- Vision screening
- Periodic examinations
    Occupational vision examination
    Supplemental occupational examination
    Comprehensive eye and vision examination
- Rehabilitation and postinjury care
- Pre-termination and pre-retirement eye and vision assessment
- Health assessment
- Hazard evaluation
- Standards determination
- Policy establishment
- Health education–health promotion, injury/disease prevention
- Regulatory compliance
- Administrative services

TABLE 1-23
Occupational Optometry Services

occupational program. Most jobs do not have existing vision standards, and these must be established. Standards may apply to entire job classes or to individual positions, depending on their importance and hazardous nature (Appendices 1-2 and 1-3 and Chapter 2). Standards are not intended to exclude workers from positions but to serve as a guide for worker placement. Some workers may need supplemental vision devices to meet specific job vision standards. Visually demanding tasks may require the use of supplemental vision devices, for example, the use of a microscopic device for inspection or supplemental lighting for assessing fine details.

Jobs or tasks that are extremely hazardous or have high risk of injury must have established vision standards that are enforced. For example, the vision of an overhead crane operator must be consistent with a high regard for safety. If an experienced crane operator suffered a gradual reduction in vision due to the development of age-related macular degeneration, for example, the worker would eventually need to be placed in another job or have the present job modified.

Federal and state agencies have regulations that apply to most businesses and industries.[49] Fields such as construction and specific occupations such as welders have additional regulatory requirements.

Occupational optometrists should be familiar with the regulations that apply to the businesses or industries with which they or their patients work.

All optometrists need to be familiar with the Occupational Safety and Health Act (OSH Act) of 1970 (Appendices 1-2–1-5).[48,50,51] This act was passed by Congress to promote the health and safety of the work force and involves the setting of workplace standards by the Occupational Safety and Health Administration of the U.S. Department of Labor. It specifically identified and recognized the American National Standards Institute Z.87.1[50] standards for safety eyewear, which are reviewed in Chapter 2.

The Americans with Disabilities Act of 1990, Public Law 101-336, is another example of federal laws with which the occupational optometrist needs to be familiar. The purpose of this law is to protect disabled Americans and integrate them into society. In brief, the law (1) establishes standards for "program accessibility," (2) requires entities to evaluate whether their services and facilities discriminate against people with disabilities, and (3) establishes procedures for complaints.[59] According to this law a disabled person is one who "has a physical or mental impairment that substantially limits a 'major life activity,' or has a record of such an impairment, or is regarded as having such an impairment."[59] Visual impairments are included in this definition. Examples of factors with which occupational optometrists need to be familiar include signage, visual alarms, building design, and medical care facilities.[60]

Establishing Policies

Few businesses and industries have established written eye and vision policies. The occupational optometrist commonly assists in establishing these policies. Major points that need to be addressed are which job classifications must use ocular personal protective devices, what penalties will occur if they are not used, and who will pay for occupational eye examinations.[30,46] Other policy issues are discussed in Chapter 2.

Eye and Vision Health Education

Health education is an essential service of optometrists concerned with occupational eye care. It can be delivered within the private practice to individual patients, to small groups of workers at safety meetings, to safety personnel, or to large employee groups. The message of eye and vision health education needs to be consistent with the overall goals of occupational optometry: prevention and performance. Workers need to know how to manage eye and vision injuries prior to movement of an injured worker, how to recognize hazardous practices and environments, how to work safely, and how to report hazards needing change. Workers using personal protective equipment (PPE) should learn how to recognize when their own equipment needs replacement. Workers need to understand the necessity of using PPE, the risks of not using it, and their responsibility for helping protect co-workers and visitors from accidents and hazards. PPE use is enhanced with understanding, comfort, availability, and appearance. The occupational optometrist needs to be familiar with basic principles of health education, including determining the needs of the patient, setting goals, selecting and implementing educational techniques, and evaluating outcomes. Most educational programs will include definitions of the knowledge, behavior, and motivation needed to achieve specific education goals.

Regulatory Compliance

Businesses and industries need to be in compliance with many government and other regulations. These may be mandatory or voluntary. The occupational optometrist advises management regarding the adequacy or inadequacy of its compliance with regulations affecting workers' eyes, vision, exposure to hazards, and meeting good manufacturing practices.

Administrative Services

Many small and medium-sized businesses and industries do not have occupational health programs. They may not have any full-time occupational optometrists, other clinicians or safety professionals. The occupational optometrist may provide some administrative services for these organizations, such as the operation of their occupational eye and vision health care programs, and do specialized billing.

1.5 Occupational Health Care

The history of occupational health care is long and fascinating.[34] The relationship between work and acute hazardous exposures has been recognized since the early 1500s.[9,16] Chronic effects were not recognized until the late 19th century.[51] The early 20th century saw the formation of the Industrial Medical Association, and the specialty of occupational medicine developed in the 1960s.[50] Unfortunately the development of health insurance plans and specialized medical training caused occupational health care and concerns to be minimized. In recent years, the concern for occupational health has been increasing.

With the passage of the OSH Act in 1970, a national law was written "to assure safe and healthful working conditions for working men and women . . ." (see Appendices 1-4 and 1-5).[48] In spite of this federal mandate and societal concern for occupational health, there exist today only about 1000 out of 600,000 physicians who are board-certified in occupational medicine.[7] With these very limited numbers, compared to the 121,000,000 workers in the population, it is apparent that workers with occupational injuries and illnesses will receive care from optometrists and other primary care providers who do not specialize in occupational services.

Occupational safety and health has developed in four stages in the 20th century:[52]

Stage 1: Emphasis on treatment of traumatic injuries and minimal accident prevention
Stage 2: Emphasis on diagnosis and development of diagnostic tests, including tests for vision screening. Expansion of workers' compensation programs in the 1930s
Stage 3: Emphasis on worker conservation during World War II with its worker shortages
Stage 4: Emphasis on regulation and management responsibilities in the 1970s

1.6 History of Occupational Optometry

Optometry developed during the early 20th century to provide the eye and vision care needed by individuals and workers. Eye protection dates back thousands of years with the use of face shields with eye holes by a variety of people, including Eskimos, who used various materials with eye slits for protection from the ultraviolet radiation in sunlight.[53,54] The first protective spectacles for foundry workers were made in 1870 and known as "melter's glasses."[54] Protective eyewear today ranges from plano safety spectacles to gold-coated sun shields used by the astronauts. In the 1940s and 1950s, the specialty of industrial optometry developed with major emphasis on eye safety and injury prevention and minimal attention to improving performance on the job.

Interest in the specialty practice of both industrial optometry and industrial medicine was highest following World War II. Following World War II, there was a long period when there was little interest in this area. Recently, the interest in occupational optometry appears to be increasing. Hopefully, it will be rejuvenated as occupational medicine has been. "The clinical discipline of occupational medicine which was largely unstudied, untaught, and unpracticed in major medical centers as recently as a decade ago, underwent unprecedented rejuvenation in the 1980s. Spurred by national regulatory programs and requirements, widespread litigation concerning toxic injury, and altered perception of environmental risks, the demand for the services of occupational medicine has risen sharply, especially outside the workplace."[17]

Optometry has matured from a profession with concern about spectacles to one with a broad concern about the patient's health and well-being. As providers of primary care, optometrists have progressed from limited concerns about vision in industry to broad concerns about occupational and environmental eye and vision care. Yesterday's industrial optometrist is today's environmental optometrist.

Occupational optometry will continue its evolution into a significant part of the health care system. With the transformation of society into the information age, the aging of the work force, the increasing complexity of the workplace, and the need for higher productivity to meet international competition, vision and visual performance will need to be maximized. All primary care optometrists will be required to meet this need.

References

1. U.S. Dept. of Commerce, Bureau of the Census. Statistical Abstract of the United States: 1990. Washington, D.C., Bureau of the Census, 1990.

2. National Center for Health Statistics, Collins JG, Thornberry OT. Health Characteristics by Occupation and Industry of Employment: United States, 1983–85. Advance Data from Vital and Health Statistics, No. 168. DHHS Pub. No. (PHS) 89-1250. Hyattsville, MD, Public Health Service, 1989.

3. National Safety Council. Accident Facts. Chicago, National Safety Council, 1989.

4. National Center for Health Statistics. Monocular Visual Acuity of Persons 4–47 years, United States, 1971–72. DHEW Pub. No. (HRA) 78-1654, Series 11, No. 206. Rockville, MD, U.S. Department of Health, Education, and Welfare, 1978.

5. National Center for Health Statistics. Characteristics of Persons with Corrective Lenses, United States, 1971. DHEW Pub. No. (HRA) 75-1520, Series 101, No. 93. Rockville, MD, U.S. Department of Health, Education and Welfare, 1974.

6. Rubenstein RS, Lohr KN, Brook RH, Goldberg GA. Conceptualization and Measurement of Physiologic Health for Adults, Vol 12: Vision Impairment, 1982. Santa Monica, CA, Rand, 1982.

7. Institute of Medicine, Division of Health Promotion and Disease Prevention. Role of the Primary Care Physician in Occupational and Environmental Medicine. Washington, D.C., National Academy Press, 1988, pp. 1–4, 16, 17, 22, 23, 29, 55, 72, 87.

8. Sherman RA. Eyes for the job. Ind Med Surg 1970; 39:60–63.

9. Shepard WP. The Physician in Industry. New York, McGraw-Hill, 1961.

10. National Society for the Prevention of Blindness. A Guide for Controlling Eye Injuries in Industry. Chicago, NSPB, 1982.

11. Ibid 1, Table 678, p 413.

12. National Safe Workplace Institute. Beyond Neglect. Chicago, National Safe Workpklace Institute, 1990.

13. McCunney RJ (ed). Handbook of Occupational Medicine. Boston, Little, Brown and Co, 1988.

14. American College of Physicians. The role of internist in occupational medicine: A position paper of the American College of Physicians. Am J Ind Med 1985; 8:95–99.

15. Levy, BS. The teaching of occupational health in U.S. medical schools: 5 year follow up on an initial survey. Am J Pub Health 1985; 75:79–80.

16. Rosenstock L, Cullen MR. Clinical Occupational Medicine. Philadelphia, WB Saunders, 1986.

17. Cullen MR, Cherninck MG, Rosenstock L. Occupational Medicine. N Engl J Med 1990; 322:594–601.

18. Grant WM. Toxicology of the Eye (3rd ed). Springfield, IL, Charles C. Thomas, 1986.

19. National Center for Health Statistics. The International Classification of Diseases, 9th revision, Clinical Modification (2nd ed). DHHS Pub. No. (PHS) 80-1260. Washington, DC, U.S. Department of Health and Human Services, 1980.

20. Thackray J. The high cost of workplace eye trauma. Sight-saving 1982; 51(1):19–22.

21. Felton JS. The occupational history: A neglected area in the clinical history. J Fam Pract 1980; 11:33–39.

22. U.S. News & World Report, July 19, 1982.

23. Division of Labor Statistics and Research. California Work Injuries and Illnesses. San Francisco, California Department of Industrial Relations, 1989.

24. U.S. Chamber of Commerce. Analysis of Workers' Compensation Laws. Washington, DC, U.S. Chamber of Commerce, 1989.

25. Hall E. Protective Eyewear, proper care helps stop injuries, blindness at work. Occup Health Saf 1987;70–71, 80.

26. Bromberg J, Hirschfelder D. Workplace eye injuries: The problem and the solution. Prof Safety 1984; 6:15–20.

27. U.S. Department of Labor. Accidents Involving Eye Injuries. Report 597. Washington, DC, Bureau of Labor Statistics, 1980.

28. U.S. Army. Occupational and Environmental Health—Occupational Vision. Technical Bulletin TB Med 506. Headquarters, Dept of the Army, December 1981.

29. Vinger PF. Eye Safety. Fine Woodworking 1988; 70–72.

30. Alderman MH, Hanley MJ. Clinical Medicine for the Occupational Physician. New York, Marcel Dekker, Inc, 1982.

31. U.S. Department of Health and Human Services. Healthy People 2000: National Health Promotion and Disease Prevention Objectives, Conference Edition. Washington, DC, U.S. DHHS, 1990.

32. Centers for Disease Control. Mandatory reporting of infectious diseases by clinicians, and mandatory reporting of occupational diseases by clinicians. MMWR 1990; 39 (No. RR-9): 1–17.

33. Feinstein AR. Clinical Judgment. Baltimore, Williams and Wilkins, 1967, p 299.

34. Felton JS. Two hundred years of occupational medicine in the U.S. J Occup Med 1976; 18:809–817.

35. von Restorff W, Hevisch S. Dark adaptation of the eye during carbon monoxide exposure in smokers and nonsmokers. Aviat Space Environ Med 1988; 59:928–931.

36. Guidotti TL. Taking the occupational history. Ann Intern Med 1983; 99:641.

37. Dobson VN, Lindesmith LA, Horvath EP, Zeng C, Blumenthal MS. Diagnosing occupationally induced diseases. Wis Med J 1981; 80:19.

38. Koven AL. Right eyes for the right job. Trans Am Acad Ophthalmol Otolaryngol 1947; 50:46.

39. Fox SL. Industrial and Occupational Ophthalmology. Springfield, IL, Charles C. Thomas, 1973.

40. Environmental/Occupational Vision Committee. How to Become an Occupational Vision Consultant. St. Louis, American Optometric Association, 1988.

41. Tiffin J, Wirt SE. Determining visual standards for industrial jobs by statistical methods. Trans Am Acad Ophthalmol Otolaryngol 1945; 50:72.

42. Vision-Ease Lens Dial. St. Cloud, MN.

43. Committee on Occupational Vision. Optometrist's Manual on Environmental Vision. St. Louis, American Optometric Association, 1969.

44. Steward JM, Cole BL. What do color vision defectives say about everyday tasks? Optom Vis Sci 1989; 66:288–295.

45. Gunning JN, Jr, Soles EM, Miller SC. Guidelines for an occupational vision program. J Am Optom Assoc 1979; 50:935–938.

46. Occupational Vision Services. OVS Panel Member Manual. Burbank, CA, OVS, 1990.

47. Mahlman HE. Handbook of Federal Vision Requirements and Information (2nd ed). Chicago, Professional Press, 1982.

48. Williams-Steiger Occupational Safety and Health Act of 1970 (Public Law 91–596), December 29, 1970 (84 Stat 1590).

49. A.M. Best Company. Best's Safety Directory. Oldwick, NJ, A.M. Best, 1989.

50. American National Standards Institute, American National Standard Practice for Occupational and Educational Eye and Face Protection. ANSI Z87.1, 1968, 1979, 1989. Des Plaines, IL, American Society of Safety Engineers, 1989.

51. Zenz G. Occupational Medicine (2nd ed). Chicago, Year Book Medical Publishers, 1988.

52. Cowles SR. Occupational health. In Ladou J (ed): Introduction to Occupational Health and Safety. Chicago, National Safety Council, 1986.

53. Guidelines for special eyewear. National Safety News 1978; 117:43.

54. Technical Staff, Wilson Safety Products. Designing an eye protection program with insight. Occup Health Saf 1982; 11:20–26.

55. Paton D, Goldberg MF. Injuries of the Eye, the Lids and the Orbit. Philadelphia, WB Saunders, 1968.

56. Stein AV. Hazardous Materials Training Programs.

57. Klopfer J, Tielsch JM, Vitale S, See L-C, Canner JK. Ocular trauma in the United States: eye injuries resulting in hospitalization 1984–1987. Arch Ophthalmol 1992; 110:838–842.

58. Dannenberg AL, Parver LM, Brechner RJ, Khoo L. Penetrating eye injuries in the workplace; the national eye trauma system registry. Arch Ophthalmol 1992; 843–848.

59. Levitan D, Pfeiffer D. The Americans with Disabilities Act of 1990: A compliance overview. National Civic Review, Spring–Summer 1992; 81:143–154.

60. Federal Register, vol. 56, No. 144, Friday July 26, 1991, rules and regulations; Part III, Department of Justice 28 CFR Part 36, Nondiscrimination on the basis of disability by public accommodations and in commercial facilities; final rule.

Appendix 1-1

Code of Ethical Conduct for Physicians Providing Occupational Medical Services, Adopted July 23, 1976 by the American College of Occupational Medicine with Permission

"These principles are intended to aid physicians in maintaining ethical conduct in providing occupational medical service. They are standards to guide physicians in their relationships with the individuals they serve, with employers and workers' representatives, with colleagues in the health professions, and with the public.

Physicians should:

1. accord highest priority to the health and safety of the individual in the workplace;
2. practice on a scientific basis with objectivity and integrity;
3. make or endorse only statements which reflect their observations or honest opinion;
4. actively oppose and strive to correct unethical conduct in relation to occupational health service;
5. avoid allowing their medical judgment to be influenced by any conflict of interest;
6. strive conscientiously to become familiar with the medical fitness requirements, the environment and the hazards of the work done by those they serve, and with the health and safety aspects of the products and operations involved;
7. treat as confidential whatever is learned about individuals served, releasing information only when required by law or by over-riding public health considerations, or to other physicians at the request of the individual according to traditional medical ethical practice; and should recognize that employers are entitled to counsel about the medical fitness of individuals in rela-

tion to work, but are not entitled to diagnoses or details of a specific nature.

8. strive continually to improve medical knowledge, and should communicate information about health hazards in timely and effective fashion to individuals or groups potentially affected, and make appropriate reports to the scientific community;
9. communicate understandably to those they serve any significant observations about their health, recommending further study, counsel or treatment when indicated;
10. seek consultation concerning the individual or the workplace whenever indicated;
11. cooperate with governmental health personnel and agencies, and foster and maintain sound ethical relationships with other members of the health professions; and
12. avoid solicitation of the use of their services by making claims, offering testimonials, or implying results which may not be achieved, but they may appropriately advise colleagues and others of services available."

Appendix 1-2

OSHA Self-Inspection Checklist for Eye and Face Protection[49]

"This checklist covers most of the important eye & face protection requirements of the OSHA regulations and standards. It is intended to serve as a general reference tool, not a comprehensive review. It may be necessary to make changes to cover specific hazards in your own industry or plant.

To use the checklist, locate the subject(s) which apply to your situation, review the specific requirements, and indicate whether or not your workplace is in compliance."

Subject	Yes	No	Requirements	Action/ Comment
General			Equipment provided against potential hazards: flying objects, glare, liquids, injurious radiation Equipment is durable, comfortable & appropriate for hazard Equipment can be sanitized and cleaned Employees wearing protective glasses have appropriate equipment Equipment marked with name of manufacturer Manufacturer's limitations made known & enforced Equipment meets ANSI Standard Z87.1—1968	
Abrasive Blasting			Operators have appropriate eye & face protection	
Abrasive Wheels & Tools			Employees wear eye protection Eye shield attached to bench or floor stand	
Bakeries			Goggles or face shields worn near open kettles of hot fat	
Battery Rooms & Battery Charging			Face shields worn when handling acids or batteries Eye drenching facilities within 25 ft. of work	
Bolting, Riveting Fitting-Up & Plumbing-Up			Eye protection worn as needed for hazards	
Caissons & Cofferdams			Protective equipment worn as needed	
Chemical, Paint & Preservative Removers			Goggles or face shields worn for handling & application	
Compressed Air			Protective equipment worn as needed	
Construction			Equipment meets all general eye & face protection requirements Protection against radiant energy meets ANSI standard Proper laser safety goggles worn by employees exposed to laser beams Goggles labeled with: laser wavelengths for which use is intended, optical density of those wavelengths, & visible light transmission	
Excavating Trenching & Shoring			Protective equipment worn as needed	
Forging Machines			Goggles worn by those using lead in forge/die shops	
Helicopters			Employees receiving load are provided with & use complete eye protection	
Laser Beams			Proper laser safety goggles worn by employees Goggles labeled with: laser wavelengths for which use is intended, optical density of those wavelengths, & visible light transmission	
Longshoring Operations			Longshoremen do not work where exposed to light rays, hot metal or sparks from welding or cutting operations	

Subject	Yes	No	Requirements	Action/ Comment
Maritime			Equipment meets all general eye & face protection requirements—ANSI Z2.1. Suitable face shield or goggles worn to protect against flying particles, molten metal or liquid chemical in chipping, caulking, drilling, etc. operations Proper filter lenses worn to protect against radiant energy Cargo handlers around flying particles & heavy dust wear appropriate protection—ANSI Z87.1—1968	
Painting			Eye and face protection worn when handling highly volatile toxic & flammable solvents	
Mechanical Paint Removers			Operators wear goggles or face shields	

Pulp, Paper & Paperboard Mills			Equipment meets all general ANSI eye & face protection requirements
			Emergency showers & bubblers located where caustic soda burns might occur and in lime slaking operations
			Rotary tenders, smelter operators & smelt spout cleaners have filter lenses for harmful rays
			Protective equipment worn:
			  in pulpwood crane & stacker operations
			  in pulp chip handling
			  in handling alum, clay, soda ash, lime, bleach powder, sulfur, chlorine & liquid acid or alkali
			  in opening rag bales
			  in barker feed operation
			  by splitter block operator
			  by knot cleaner operators
			  in inspection, repair or maintenance of acid towers
			  in lime slaking operations
			  for removing hand plate of digester
			  in mechanical pulp processing when exposed to falling materials
			  in acid handling
			  in banding of skids, cartons, etc.
			  in unloading railcars or trucks with steel bands or wires	

Pulpwood Logging			Eye or face protection meets ANSI Z87.1—1968 standard for chips, saw-dust and flying particles	
Sawmills			Eye protection worn in handling chemicals	
Tanks—Open Surface			Workers wear tight chemical goggles or face shields & have eye wash facilities available	
Telecommunications			Side & frontal eye protection worn for working with storage batteries Suitable eye protection wherever flying objects are a hazard Insure employees do not look into energized source of microwave radiation	
Textiles			Large supply of fresh, clean water where acids or caustics used Eye or face protectors worn when handling acids or caustics in bulk, repairing pipes, etc.	

Subject	Yes	No	Requirements	Action/ Comment
Tools, Portable Powered			Operators & assistants of explosive actuated fastening tools have appropriate protection	
Toxic Cleaning Solvents			Suitable equipment worn around these substances	
Tunnels & Shafts			Protective equipment worn as needed	

Welding, Cutting & Brazing			Goggles, helmets & hand shields used in arc welding & cutting operations, excluding submerged arc welding
			Goggles used during gas welding or oxygen cutting operations
			Transparent face shields or goggles worn in resistance brazing & welding operations
			Helmets & hand shields:
			    are made of material that insulates against heat & electricity
			    are not readily flammable
			    can be sterilized
			    protect from direct radiant energy from arc
			    are provided with easily removable filter plates & cover plates
			    will not readily corrode or discolor skin
			    are ventilated to prevent fogging
			    lens glass is tempered & free from striae, air bubbles, waves, etc.
			    lenses have permanent marking of source & shade
			    all filter lenses & plates meet ANSI test for transmission of radiant energy, Z87.1—1968
			Welding booth or noncombustible screens provided wherever work permits
			Workers & others adjacent to welding areas are protected by screens or shields & wear appropriate goggles	

Appendix 1-3

Where to Find OSHA Personal Protective Equipment Requirements[49]

Appendix 1.1 and 1.3. OSHA standards are currently being revised. For the latest standards and section numbers OSHA should be consulted to determine if any changes have occurred.
From Best's Safety Directory. Copyright © 1989, A.M. Best Company, Oldwick, New Jersey.

In addition to the general personal protective equipment requirements in Subpart I, which apply to all employers, requirements scattered throughout the standards specify certain equipment in specific industries. Some standards briefly refer to one type of equipment; others go into more detail on many different types . . . to see all the different types of equipment required under one standard, find that standard in the list below (standards are in numerical order).

General Industry Standards	Eye and Face	Head	Respiratory	Hand & Arm	Body & Leg	Foot
Section						
Ventilation (abrasive blasting, spray finishing, open surface tanks) (1910.94)	X		X	X	X	X
Storage & Handling of Andrydrous Ammonia (1910.111)			X			
Sanitation (wet processes) (1910.141)						X
Helicopters (1910.183)	X	X		X	X	
Forging Machines (1910.218)	X			X	X	
Mechanical Power Transmission Apparatus (1910.219)					X	
Guarding of Portable Powered Tools (explosive actuated fastening tools) (1910.243)	X	X				
Welding, Cutting, & Brazing (1910.252)	X	X	X	X	X	
Pulp, Paper, & Paperboard Mills (1910.261)	X	X	X	X	X	X
Textiles (1910.262)	X	X	X	X	X	
Sawmills (1910.265)	X		X	X	X	X
Pulpwood Logging (1910.266)	X	X	X	X		X
Telecommunications (1910.268)	X	X		X	X	
Procedures During Dive (1910.422)				X		
Equipment (for Diving) (1910.430)			X		X	

Construction Standards	Eye and Face	Head	Respiratory	Hand & Arm	Body & Leg	Foot
Section						
Gases, Vapors, Fumes, Dusts, & Mists (1926.55)					X	
Working Over or Near Water (1926.106)					X	
Signaling (1926.201)					X	
General Requirements (tools—hand & power) (1926.300)	X					
Abrasive Wheels & Tools (1926.303)	X					
Ventilation & Protection in Welding, Cutting, & Heating (1926.353)	X				X	
Welding, Cutting & Heating in way of Preservative Coatings (1926.354)			X			
General Requirements (electrical) (1926.400)			X	X		
Battery Rooms & Battery Charging (1926.403)	X			X	X	
Helicopters (1926.551)	X	X			X	
Marine Operations & Equipment (1926.605)					X	
General Protection Requirements (excavations, trenching, & shoring) (1926.650)	X	X	X	X	X	X

Construction Standards	Eye and Face	Head	Respiratory	Hand & Arm	Body & Leg	Foot
Tunnels & Shafts (1926.800)	X		X	X		
General Requirements (power transmission & distribution) (1926.950)				X		
Tools & Protective Equipment (power transmission & distribution) (1926.951)		X		X		

Maritime Standards	Eye and Face	Head	Respiratory	Hand & Arm	Body & Leg	Foot
Section						
Precautions before Entering (1915.2)			X			
Toxic Cleaning Solvents (1915.32)	X		X	X	X	
Chemical Paint & Preservative Removers (1915.33)	X		X	X	X	
Mechanical Paint Removers (1915.34)	X		X	X	X	
Painting (1915.35)	X		X	X	X	X
Ventilation & Protection in Welding, Cutting & Heating (1915.51)	X	X	X		X	
Welding, Cutting & Heating in Way of Preservative Coatings (1915.53)			X			
Guarding of Deck Openings & Edges (1915.73)					X	
Working Surfaces (1915.77)					X	
Health & Sanitation (1915.97)	X					
Abrasive Wheels (1915.134)	X					
Powder Actuated Fastening Tools (1915.135)	X					
Lifesaving Equipment (1915.154)					X	
Hazardous Cargo (1917.22)					X	
Hazardous Atmospheres & Substances (1917.23)			X			
Fumigants, Pesticides, Insecticides & Hazardous Preservatives (1917.25)			X			
Terminals Handling Intermodal Containers or Roll-on Roll-off Operations (1917.71)					X	
Terminals Handling Menhaden & Similar Species of Fish (1917.73)			X			
Welding, Cutting & Heating (Hot Work) (1917.152)	X		X		X	
Hazardous Cargo (1918.86)					X	
Ventilation & Atmospheric Conditions (1918.93)			X			
Longshoring Operations in the Vicinity of Repair & Maintenance Work (1918.95)	X					
First Aid & Life Saving Equipment (1918.96)					X	
Protection Against Drowning (1918.106)					X	

Appendix 1-4

Public Law 91-596, The Occupational Safety and Health Act of 1970: Congressional Findings and Purpose[3,48]

An Act

To assure safe and healthful working conditions for working men and women: by authorizing enforcement of the standards developed under the Act; by assisting and encouraging the States in their efforts to assure safe and healthful working conditions; by providing for research, information, education, and training in the field of occupational safety and health: and for other purposes.

Be it enacted by the Senate and House of Representatives of the United States of America in Congress assembled, That this Act may be cited as the "Occupational Safety and Health Act of 1970".

Congressional Findings and Purpose

Sec. (2) The Congress finds that personal injuries and illnesses arising out of work situations impose a substantial burden upon, and are a hindrance to, interstate commerce in terms of lost production, wage loss, medical expenses, and disability compensation payments.

(b) The Congress declares it to be its purpose and policy, through the exercise of its powers to regulate commerce among the several States and with foreign nations and to provide for the general welfare, to assure so far as possible every working man and woman in the Nation safe and healthful working conditions and to preserve our human resources—

1. by encouraging employers and employees in their efforts to reduce the number of occupational safety and health hazards at their places of employment, and to stimulate employers and employees to institute new and to perfect existing programs for providing safe and healthful working conditions;

2. by providing that employers and employees have separate but dependent responsibilities and rights with respect to achieving safe and healthful working conditions;

3. by authorizing the Secretary of Labor to set mandatory occupational safety and health standards applicable to businesses affecting interstate commerce, and by creating an Occupational Safety and Health Review Commission for carrying out adjudicatory functions under the Act;

4. by building upon advances already made through employer and employee initiative for providing safe and healthful working conditions;

5. by providing for research in the field of occupational safety and health, including the psychological factors involved, and by developing innovative methods, techniques, and approaches for dealing with occupational safety and health problems;

6. by exploring ways to discover latent diseases, establishing causal connections between diseases and work in environmental conditions, and conducting other research relating to health problems, in recognition of the fact that occupational health standards present problems often different from those involved in occupational safety;

7. by providing medical criteria which will assure insofar as practicable that no employee will suffer diminished health, functional capacity, or life expectancy as a result of his work experience;

8. by providing for training programs to increase the number and competence of personnel engaged in the field of occupational safety and health;

9. by providing for the development and promulgation of occupational safety and health standards;

10. by providing an effective enforcement program which shall include a prohibition against giving advance notice of any inspection and sanctions for any individual violating this prohibition;

11. by encouraging the States to assume the fullest responsibility for the administration and enforcement of their occupational safety and health laws by providing grants to the States to assist in identifying their needs and responsibilities in the area of occupational safety and health, to develop plans in accordance with the provisions of this Act, to improve the administration and enforcement of State occupational safety and health laws, and to conduct experimental and demonstration projects in connection therewith;

1.2. From the Williams-Steiger Occupational Safety and Health Act of 1970 (Public Law 91-596) December 29, 1970 (84 Stat 1590).

12. by providing for appropriate reporting procedures with respect to occupational safety and health which procedures will help achieve the objectives of this Act and accurately describe the nature of the occupational safety and health problem;

13. by encouraging joint labor-management efforts to reduce injuries and disease arising out of employment.

Appendix 1-5

Public Law 91-596, The Occupational Safety and Health Act of 1970: Selected Sections

Purpose

The purpose of the OSH Act is "to assure safe and healthful working conditions for working men and women; by authorizing enforcement of the standards developed under the Act; by assisting and encouraging the states in their efforts to assure safe and healthful working conditions; by providing for research, information, education, and training in the field of occupational safety and health; and for other purposes."[49]

Section 5(a), THE GENERAL DUTY CLAUSE

Specific Sections Relevant to Optometrist Responsibilities

Each employer (1) shall furnish to each of his employees employment and a place of employment which are free from recognized hazards that are causing or are likely to cause death or serious physical harm to his employees; (2) shall comply with Occupational Safety and Health Standards promulgated under this Act. Under the General Duty Clause, employee responsibilities are that: "each employee shall comply with Occupational Safety and Health Standards and all rules, regulations, and others pursuant to this Act which are applicable to his own actions and conduct."[30]

This clause requires employers to meet a standard of performance that is consistent with their industry. The phrase "recognized hazard" is not limited to hazards that are visible but include hazards that are not obviously visible, e.g., toxic products.

Protective Equipment

"The OSHA standards dealing with personal protective equipment consists of three types of requirements. Section 1910.132 is a set of general requirements covering all types of equipment and all situations where it is needed; the other sections of Subpart I Personal Protective Equipment give requirements for one particular type of equipment; and certain paragraphs in standards not primarily concerned with personal protection call for protective equipment to be used under the working conditions regulated by the section.

For certain hazards all three provisions may be applicable. If no specific conditions cover the conditions, the general requirements in section 1910.132 shall apply. If eye and face or head or specific types of protection are used for hazard protection, then this equipment must conform to the requirements in specific sections such as 1910.133, Eye and Face Protection.[49]

General Requirements (1910.132)

(a) Provide, require the use of, and maintain in a sanitary and reliable condition, all protective equipment which is necessary to protect employees from any hazard which could cause injury or illness.

(b) Assure adequacy of employee-owned equipment, including proper maintenance and sanitation.

(c) Check adequacy of equipment design and construction for the intended purpose.[49]

General requirements (tools—hand and power) (1926.300), abrasive wheels and tools (1926.303), ventilation and protection in welding, cutting, and heating (1926.353), battery rooms and battery charging (1926.403), helicopters (1926.551), general protection requirements (excavations, trenching, and shoring) (1926.650), tunnels and shafts (1926.800).

Maritime Standards

Toxic cleaning solvents (1915.32), chemical paint and preservative removers (1915.33), mechanical paint removers (1915.34), painting (1915.35), ventilation and protection in welding, cutting and heating (1915.51), abrasive wheels (1915.134).

Eye and Face Protection (1910.133)[48,49] General Requirements

All eye and face protective equipment used by employees must meet the requirements of (1910.133) which covers the employer's general responsibility and refers to ANSI standard Z87.1-196 as the source of guidance in the selection of eyewear for specific hazards. Such equipment may also be specified in a standard not primarily concerned with protective equipment if the working conditions regulated by the standard may require eye and face protection. . . . If no other standard specifies protection for the working conditions at hand the requirements of (1910.133) still apply.[49]

General Requirements

(1) Employers must make available and require employees to use suitable eye and face protective equipment where eye injuries may otherwise occur such as where hazard of flying objects, glare, liquids, and injurious radiations exist.

(2) Protective equipment must: (i) provide protection against the hazards it is designed for; (ii) be reasonably comfortable under the conditions of use; (iii) fit snugly and not interfere with the wearer's movement; (iv) be durable; (v) be capable of being disinfected; (vi) be easily cleanable; (vii) be kept clean and in good repair.

(3) Protective equipment for people who wear corrective glasses must be one of the following: (i) spectacles with protective lenses which also provide optical correction; (ii) goggles to be worn over spectacles without disturbing their adjustment; (iii) goggles with corrective lenses behind the protective lenses.

(4) Protective equipment must be marked to identify the manufacturer.

(5) The employer must inform the user of the limitations and precautions indicated by the manufacturer and see that such information is strictly observed.

(6) Design, construction, testing, and use of eye and face protective devices must be in accordance with the ANSI standard for Occupational and Educational Eye and Face Protection Z87.1-1968. The ANSI standard has been revised in 1979 and in 1989. Although the OSHA requirements have not been changed, these newer revisions should be consulted where appropriate.

CHAPTER TWO

Occupational Optometry in Practice

Robert N. Kleinstein, O.D., M.P.H., Ph.D.

2.1 Practice of Occupational Optometry

Preparation and Concepts

Before approaching business and industry to establish a consultative arrangement or an occupational optometric eye and vision program, the primary care optometrist must be prepared. This preparation includes knowing details about the business or industry such as the manufacturing process, the different types of jobs and their visual performance demands, eye safety hazards, the related Occupational Safety and Health Administration (OSHA) requirements, the potential suppliers of personal protective equipment (PPE), the number of employees and their approximate age distributions, and the special language associated with each industry. For example, in the construction industry, the optometrist should understand the terms *foundations, framing, trusses, rough plumbing, drywall, glazing, air hammers*, and *chipping*. In the steel industry, such terms as *slabs, galvanized sheets*, and *continuous casting* are used and should be understood.

The optometrist needs to determine the motivation of (or may need to motivate) local business or industry in starting a new occupational vision and eye safety program or in establishing a consultative arrangement. Unless the business or industry is motivated, no new programs will be initiated. There are many benefits of these programs including such things as solving a specific worker's eye and vision problem, preventing eye and vision injuries or accidents, preventing injuries to co-workers, decreasing accidents resulting in permanent disability, meeting OSHA regulations, lowering insurance costs, eliminating the potential future cost to the company and poor publicity from a worker losing an eye, matching employee abilities to the vision demands of the job to improve efficiency,[1] improving competitiveness and increased productivity from improved worker visual performance, reducing spoilage and defective products, and improving morale through increased concern by the company for its employees. Other program benefits are preventing accidents to co-workers and subsequent lawsuits, and the proper placement of employees, which saves unnecessary training costs, replacement costs, and inefficient workers. This sampling of reasons can be used by the optometrist or by organizations to justify the use of optometric occupational services.

There are several practical concepts that the optometrist must not overlook. The primary purpose of business and industry is to make a profit. Without a profit, the business or industry cannot afford to provide occupational optometric services. These services should be consistent with the economic mission of the organization and improve the long-term profitability of the organization, either directly or indirectly.[2]

We have seen that business and industry benefit from establishing occupational eye and vision health programs by reducing or eliminating both the direct and indirect costs associated with an injured worker. Maximizing the visual performance of workers for the visual demands of the job reduces the production of poor quality materials, reduces accidents, and improves the efficiency and quantity of production in both blue- and white-collar occupations. The loss of one eye of one worker can often more than pay for the entire annual costs associated with an occupational eye and vision program. Addressing workers' vision needs may also eliminate potential regulations and reduce long-term liability. For example, providing eye care for users of video display terminals may prevent new government regulation in this area.

Expectations of Business and Industry

Business wants competent, objective optometric services from professionals who understand the workplace and the ethical obligations associated with providing their services.[3,4] Attention to the unique aspects of occupational health, coupled with quality optometric care, enables optometrists to have a major role in reducing occupational injury and illness as they work as part of the health care team employed by the industry. With the optometrist's excellent interpersonal skills and understanding of human psychology, the adjustment to the occupational team is not difficult. Unlike private practice patients, most workers are in good health and are usually within one location.

Expectations of the Optometrist Providing Occupational Optometry Services

In a parallel manner, the occupational optometrist has expectations from business and industry that are as important as the profit motive is to business.[3]

Unless occupational services can be provided with few limitations or restrictions, the optometrist will probably not be satisfied, regardless of remuneration or status. The organization that significantly restricts the optometrist will not attract the best person with concerns about providing the highest quality of occupational services. The optometrist must place the interests of the worker above all and not be either business- or labor-oriented.[4]

The occupational optometrist should have an appropriate status in the organization. The optometrist should have direct access to the people or groups who make and implement policy decisions because the optometrist's observations and recommendations are important to the safety and optimal operation of the workplace. The optometrist must be an effective member of the team, whether a part- or full-time relationship exists, while understanding that final policy decisions are always the responsibility of management.

Staff support for the optometrist is necessary for a wide range of important tasks including the maintenance of records for worker information, the identification of workplace hazards and the recommendations for their remediation, the occurrence of injuries and their treatment, and the implementation of eye and vision protection policies approved by management. Support will be necessary for ensuring compliance with federal OSHA and state workplace requirements, correspondence with community professionals, follow-up of referred workers, completion of workers' compensation and other insurance reports, and preparation of annual reports and budget requests. The extent of staff support will depend on the relationship of the occupational optometrist with business and industry, the size of the organization, and the scope of occupational services provided.

The occupational optometrist should expect to receive adequate remuneration for the services and time provided. This includes direct services and meetings with management and staff. Usually, both business and the optometrist will benefit from a contractual relationship with stated expectations including responsibilities (consultant, part-time or full-time employee), and remuneration (fee for service, consulting fee, or retainer). Like many other services, inexpensive services usually result in inadequate results.

Delivering Occupational Optometry Services

Optometrists should visit the local plant or business to improve their ability to communicate with workers and to understand the manufacturing or business process and its environmental hazards. "In order to understand the jobs at a given organization, it is necessary to observe the work actually being done—on site."[4] These visits enable optometrists to adapt their services to the specific needs of each business and industry.

The occupational optometrist must have a high sense of optometric ethics and must not use business and industrial relationships to take advantage of fellow optometrists. Existing good relationships between workers and their optometrists must be respected and preserved. The optometrist must be able to interact with other professional colleagues. The occupational optometrist can prevent misunderstandings by strengthening relationships with business, industry, and the local optometric community.

A statewide model exists for providing occupational vision services. Occupational Vision Services, Inc. (O.V.S.) is a nonprofit, mutual benefit corporation organized under California law which now has about 1000 panel members.[5] The corporation was established to meet the occupational vision and protective eyewear needs of business and industry. O.V.S. offers a wide range of services including consulting, job site analysis, visual ability screening, occupational vision examinations, and other occupational/protective professional services, such as designing personal protective equipment (PPE), ordering PPE, providing quality control, and dispensing and educating workers to use PPE in the workplace. Quality protective safety eyewear and PPE are provided economically through volume purchases, and costs are directly billed to clients with minimal administrative fees. The administrative services of O.V.S. include selecting appropriate panel member doctors for client location(s), establishing panel member peer review and mediation to assure quality care, controlling orders for quality assurance and compliance with specifications and ANSI standards, placing orders, shipping and handling, and computerized accounting and billing. All services and PPE are coordinated to provide an effective, quality-oriented occupational protective eyewear program.[5] Many of the components of the O.V.S. model are also found in the optometric occupational vision care and eye protection program developed by the Alberta Optometric Association.[6]

2.2 Designing an Occupational Eye/Vision Health Care Program

The design of the occupational eye and vision health care program may be relatively simple for small organizations or complex for large organizations. However, there are common elements to all programs, such as assuring that workers possess adequate vision to meet the demands of their jobs, protecting workers' eyes and vision against hazards, and ensuring health care for workers sustaining eye injuries or diseases affecting the visual system.[7,8] If employees and applicants are not having their vision tested, then neither the employee nor the employer know if the employee has the vision and visual skills to do the job and achieve the results that management will expect.[9]

Health care costs are a major concern of business and industry, as discussed in Chapter 1. The proposal of a new *health care* program (occupational eye and vision health care program) may be met with strong resistance because of the suggestion of increased health care costs. In fact, the well-designed occupational eye and vision program should reduce costs, as previously described. If business or industry management has strong concerns about health care costs and may not listen to a proposal for a new health care program, then the occupational optometrist should use another title for the program. Possible program titles are: occupational eye health and vision care program, occupational eye and vision program, or occupational eye injury prevention and vision performance program.

Program Components

Each eye and vision health care program needs to have clearly stated goals and objectives. The occupational optometrist by training and experience is well equipped to develop these goals and objectives. The process for establishing the program must have the support and commitment of management from the chief executive officer to the line supervisors.[8] Successful programs must be both well-designed and effectively implemented.[9,12]

The eye and vision health care program has five general components: (1) Establishing objectives and communicating them to all employees, (2) collecting baseline data, (3) developing the health care plan, (4) implementing the plan, and (5) evaluating the plan and modifying it where necessary. These steps apply to small and large organizations (Tables 2-1–2-3).

General Objectives

According to Alderman and Hanley,[2] there are seven basic overall objectives for the occupational health care program which can be modified to establish a similar set of objectives for most organizations:

1. To protect employees against health and safety hazards in their work environment.
2. To protect the general environment of the community, insofar as practical and feasible.
3. To facilitate placement of workers.
4. To assure adequate (optometric) care and rehabilitation of the occupationally ill and injured.
5. To provide health education and encourage personal health maintenance.
6. To expand the scope of (optometric) services for employees and their families, as appropriate for local circumstances, beyond strictly work-related injuries and illnesses.
7. To provide surveillance and examination and implement other practices and procedures to achieve compliance with all regulations (e.g., OSHA regulations) affecting the company's operations.[2]

Specific Objectives

The objectives for the health care program should be explicit and address major problems of occupational eye and vision health.[5,9,18] The overall rationale should be stated. For most programs the rationale is to prevent eye and vision injuries, enhance vision performance, and improve productivity.

Objectives vary by type of business or industry and with the occupational problems and environment that are present. There are a wide range of

- Environmental survey of the work place: formal or informal, preliminary or detailed
- Task analysis: vision requirements of job, matching worker to job
- Vision screening: test battery, periodic testing
- Vision standards: minimum requirements, safety and performance
- Hazard evaluation: recognition, evaluation, control
- Applicant and preplacement eye and vision examinations: match visual abilities and job requirements, confidentiality of records
- Safety and health education and training: specific prevention programs, supervisors and workers
- Periodic surveys: safety and health inspections, identification of new hazards
- Accident investigation: vision contribution, impact on eyes and vision
- Protection of eyes and vision: engineering, administrative and personal protective equipment; lens cleaning program
- Provision of personal protective equipment: maintenance and replacement
- Program policies: direct communication between the occupational optometrist and management, compliance with use of protective equipment as a condition of employment
- Program administration: organization responsibilities, optometrist responsibilities
- Program monitoring: periodic evaluation, program successful or needs changing
- Occupational health and safety requirements: OSHA, state
- Eye injury management: emergency procedures, treatment and followup
- Assistance with personal health maintenance
- Risk assessment: relative, absolute

TABLE 2-1
Elements of Occupational Eye and Vision Health Care Programs

specific objectives that may be developed (Table 2-4). Many objectives will be unique and designed for a specific business or industry.

All specific objectives should relate to the goals and overall objectives for the eye and vision health care program. Each objective needs to be stated simply and contain clear, measurable, and attainable outcomes that are easily understood. The success in

meeting these objectives should be assessed annually and the results communicated to everyone within the organization.

Data Collection and Plan Development

Collection of basic information is needed for the development of the occupational eye and vision program (Tables 2-1–2-3). Because almost all programs include elements targeted to identify and solve problems, there are four areas in which data need to be gathered: products and processes, work force, laws, and additional information.

- Determination of degree of eye hazard for each job or work area
- Analysis of job classes to determine the required visual skills for optimal job performance
- Development of a guide listing vision standards and eye-protection requirements for each job title or job classification
- Vision screening to determine whether workers possess the required visual skills indicated by the job analysis:
    Annual job-related vision screening examinations of personnel in highly hazardous areas and jobs
    Preplacement and biennial vision screening for other workers with any potentially eye-hazardous occupations
    Elective periodic vision screening for employees in non–eye-hazardous occupations
- Referral of employees not possessing the desired visual skills for a complete professional vision examination and recommended therapy
- Supervision of eye protection and eye hygiene
- First aid and immediate care, plus follow-up care of occupational eye injury and disease
- Worker health protection with respect to proper eye protection and the benefits of an occupational vision program
- Periodic surveys of work area to
    Promote adequate illumination
    Evaluate other aspects to ensure safe, comfortable, and efficient visual performance

From US Army Technical Bulletin TB Med 506, Occupational and Environmental Health, Occupational Vision, December, 1981.

TABLE 2-2
Components of an Occupational Vision Program

- Providing professional staff
- Surveying eye hazards in the workplace
- Utilizing engineering controls to remove, attenuate, and control damaging energy at its source
- Promoting a vision screening program
- Providing visual analysis services
- Initiating a fitting/dispensing program
- Starting a verification/inspection program
- Instituting a sight conservation education program
- Furnishing an inspection/replacement program
- Recommending an enforcement program supported by management

---

From Nakagawara, VB: Functional model of an eye protection program: Guide for the clinical optometrist. J Am Optom Assoc 59:12, 925–928, 1988; with permission.

TABLE 2-3
Model of an Eye Protection Program

PRODUCT AND PROCESSES

Data need to be gathered that describe the products, processes, and operations of the organization.[2] The data can be collected from on-site surveys and existing publications. This data is needed for both blue- and white-collar organizations, including those in which the primary function is information processing.

The data have two important uses: First, it is useful in facilitating placement of employees. Placement is improved when there is a clear understanding of the work and the visual tasks to be performed. This is very important when individuals have handicaps and for compliance with the American Disability Act. Accommodations can usually be made to enable the handicapped worker to perform satisfactorily on the job.[2] Second, this information helps to identify any existing or potential hazards in the business or industry. These may result from the working conditions, procedures, materials, or processes. Hazards can also result from how materials are used, handled, stored, distributed, and the nature of the processes to which the materials are subjected. Data are usually available from industrial hygiene surveys, toxicity testing, scientific literature, previous concerns or complaints from former and current workers, customer problems, suppliers and industry pub-

lications. After identifying hazards, the optometrist can design the occupational program to prevent or limit them.[2]

WORK FORCE

The age, sex, length of service, employee classifications, and stability of the workforce are important considerations in developing the occupational eye and vision program. The occurrence and severity of accidents and diseases should be reviewed. If possible, an estimate of "near accidents" should be made. This should be done even if the accident rate is low. The areas or job categories in which accidents occur provide important insights for program design.

- Eye and vision injuries will be reduced to no more than one injury per 100 workers per year. Some organizations may establish an objective of zero injuries per year.
- All workers will wear personal protective eye protection in identified eye hazard areas.
- Every hazardous operation will be reviewed annually by the occupational optometrist, industrial hygienist, and safety engineer to determine whether eye and vision protection needs to be improved.
- Each worker will have an annual occupational vision screening to determine if the worker's vision remains adequate for the tasks being performed.
- Eye safety and emergency procedures will be reviewed annually during mandatory safety meetings for all workers.
- All new employees will receive a preplacement eye and vision evaluation to determine if any job restrictions will be necessary because of impaired or reduced vision.
- All new employees will be given a 3-hour safety orientation with at least 45 minutes for discussing eye and vision safety and emergency first-aid procedures.
- An environmental survey will be performed annually to identify eye and vision hazards; written recommendations for their remediation will be presented to management within 30 days of the survey.
- All eye injuries and accidents will be reviewed by the occupational optometrist to determine the cause of the injury or accident and what needs to be done to prevent future occurrences. A program to identify and investigate near misses will be established to prevent injuries.

TABLE 2-4
Examples of Specific Objectives for Occupational Health Plans

Other useful workforce information is the company's cost for workers' compensation insurance compared to similar companies. If the costs are above average, there may be existing hazards or operations that can be modified to reduce injuries and insurance costs. It is important to determine the reasons for above- or below-average costs.

LAWS

Most businesses and industries must comply with an increasing number of federal and state regulations. The Occupational Safety and Health Act of 1970, Public Law 91-596, which established OSHA, is the major federal law affecting working conditions in business organization.[10] The occupational health care program will enable the company to comply with many of the OSHA requirements regarding industrial surveys, use of protective equipment, recordkeeping and training and education of employees.[2]

ADDITIONAL INFORMATION

One of the early steps in developing the occupational eye and vision program is to identify additional data needs. The need for data must be weighed against the additional costs of collecting the data. In many instances, population data can be used for an organization, especially when direct business or industry data are not available. For example, the predicted need for vision corrections can be estimated from the need occurring in the general population. In the United States about 50% of all adults have vision problems that are not treated (see Chapter 1). This suggests that vision screening would be appropriate in any business or industry. These data also suggest that most business and industry productivity could be improved through better vision performance in the workplace.

There are a number of functions or services that can be components of an occupational eye and vision program. Not every plan will include all of these elements or components, but all should be considered in the development of every occupational program (Tables 2-1–2-3).

After the plan elements are selected and prioritized, the resources required to implement the plan must be determined. These resources will include personnel, space, equipment, administrative support, funding and education. The costs of the program should be compared to the anticipated benefits. The organization's management will usually want to know this information before approving the occupational eye and vision care program. The costs for the different elements in the program can usually be accurately estimated using data collected, as described above, personnel salary information, PPE costs, optometric occupational part-time, consulting, or in-office service costs, and other factors.

The benefits of the occupational health care program are not as easy to estimate as are costs. Many benefits are long term with potential savings and others are intangible, such as improved employee morale. In addition, few organizations are willing to do research before and after an occupational program is implemented to quantitate improvements in productivity, reductions in defective production, and decreased injury costs. Nonetheless, it is important to attempt to demonstrate these benefits.

Benefits can be classified as either direct or indirect. Benefits from occupational programs are many, such as fewer workers with eye and vision injuries, resulting in less time lost from work; fewer clinical costs; a decreased downtime of production processes; reduced administrative costs associated with accident reporting and investigation and decreased training and replacement costs for the worker off the job; reduced workers' compensation insurance premiums; increased worker productivity when the occupational program includes assessment and improvement of vision performance with subsequent improved worker performance; decreased number of rejected products or poor production performance; reduction in nonproductive time resulting from asthenopia, eyestrain, and headaches associated with vision problems and premature daily eye fatigue; and improved morale resulting from organizational support and concern for workers' problems and welfare.

Implementation of the Occupational Eye and Vision Health Program

Implementation of the occupational eye and vision health program will follow the objectives and elements that are approved by management. The resources and budget for the plan will be the determining and limiting factor in the focus and scope of the occupational program. The implementation phase of the program should be straightforward, if everyone has communicated well and all program elements are well understood.

As the occupational program is implemented, delays or increased costs may be encountered. Depending on the organization's economic performance and the impact of external environmental strategic factors, the budget for the program may be adjusted up or down. If circumstances change, the occupational optometrist will need to take into account resource changes when implementing the program. This needs to be done within the framework of the program. Alternative sources of supply or modified services may need to be considered if resources are reduced. If basic changes in the occupational program are needed, it is important to keep management informed. Excellent records and documentation must be maintained so that the program can be evaluated.

There are several key points in implementing an occupational health program. Management must support the program, from the president or CEO to the line supervisors. Program design is difficult and requires the skills and knowledge of the occupational optometrist, whose background includes education in occupational and environmental optometry, applied optics, psychophysics, eye injury and disease diagnosis and management, health care, communication, epidemiology, and practice-patient interaction. Development of the program requires the interaction and efforts of many people including management, safety personnel, workers, and industrial hygienists. The program will likely contain many but not all of the elements described, and these will vary with each business and industry. However, there are several essential elements such as the vision screening, the environmental survey, and the task analysis.

Evaluation of the Program

There are many approaches for evaluating the occupational program. For example, one approach would be to compare accident rates before and after implementation of the program. Another approach would be to compare productivity or worker morale before and after implementation. Unfortunately, most organizations do not collect the data needed for such comparisons.

Two other approaches to evaluation can be used: efficiency and effectiveness. Efficiency can be evaluated by reviewing resource costs, number of functions and number of services that were in the program and determining if they could be reduced while keeping the quality, scope and effectiveness of ther program the same.[2] After this comparison, sources of cost variance can also be investigated. The feedback provided from this comparison will strengthen the occupational program.

Effectiveness is another evaluation approach that can be used, although it is difficult because the monetary value of many outcomes cannot be assigned easily. Effectiveness can be assessed by comparing the problems identified during the data collection phase and the extent to which the occupational program has solved them.[2]

2.3 Vision Screening

Purpose

Vision screening is an important element in the occupational health program that has objectives to identify eye and vision problems that decrease productivity and to identify eye diseases at an early stage when interventions can save an employee's vision. Screening also establishes baseline data for future comparisons to rule out eye disease or vision conditions that may be considered work-related. It is important in assessing vision for job placement. Vision screening is designed to meet the specific needs of industry and business.

Principles

All screenings tests must be selective and emphasize the working population at risk. Screening is based on a number of principles:

1. The problem must be important. Vision disorders and selected age-specific or industry-specific eye diseases are important problems.

2. The problems need to have reasonable prevalence in order to be screened for efficiently.

3. The eye and vision disorders, problems or diseases should be identified in their latent stage before symptoms appear; in the workplace this principle

may not always be followed because the early symptomatic worker may be screened before being referred for care.

4. The tests should be both valid and reliable. When the costs of false negative and false positive results are evaluated, it is usually less expensive to have the occupational optometrist do at least the initial screening and follow-up screening at periodic intervals. During interim periods, other nonprofessional methods of vision screening may successfully be employed under the optometrist's direction.

5. The tests need to be acceptable to the workers or they will resist being screened.

6. The test should be cost-effective with benefits (direct and indirect) outweighing the costs. If feasible, tests should be noninvasive.

7. Treatment should be acceptable, available, and effective.

8. Adequate follow-up should be done to ensure that workers receive the necessary treatment.

9. Vision screenings must include appropriate and adequate tests; a casual testing of distance acuity with a Snellen chart is not sufficient.

The tests used for vision and eye screening need to meet all of these criteria (Table 2-5).[11]

Location

Vision screenings should be provided in the plant or on site at the business or industry. When many previously screened workers are receiving a periodic screening and no serious problems are suspected, then screening on the job site is preferred because time off the job can be minimized and workers returned to work rapidly. Screening in an office setting is advantageous if unique equipment is needed to perform special tests or if very few workers are screened. For example, when threshold perimetry is needed following an accident, an office visit for the injured worker is useful and cost-effective.

Types and Frequency of Screening

Vision screening can be used for many purposes. The first purpose is for pre-employment testing to determine if a potential employee has the visual abilities to perform the job so training is not wasted on someone unable visually to perform a job. For example, workers hired to operate looms in textile mills need excellent stereopsis and ability to discriminate colors. When a thread breaks, the loom operator needs to replace it with a thread of identical color or the material is downgraded and has reduced value.

A second major purpose of screening is for surveillance of the experienced worker's vision (Table 2-6). The early identification of workers who are developing vision problems enables treatment to be provided before these problems interfere with productivity or contribute to accidents. For example, a forklift operator who develops an increase in myopia has impaired ability to judge distances. When stacking pallets, the myopic operator will likely misjudge their position due to uncorrected blur. Pallets improperly positioned could fall and injure another worker or damage finished materials.

Workers between the ages of 20 and 38 years should be screened biannually. Those performing critical tasks or tasks requiring excellent visual abilities should be screened annually. Workers over age 38 years should be screened annually, especially for near vision performance. Other easily and rapidly administered screening tests should be considered depending on the size and age of the workforce, such as screening for elevated intraocular pressure. Periodic screening is important because visual function and visual performance change with age.

A third purpose of screening is for exit screening. Exit screenings should be done to document the vision abilities of the worker who is ending employment. Exit screenings document and protect the

- Important problems (diseases or disorders)
- Appropriate prevalence of problems
- Asymptomatic problems
- Validity and reliability of tests
- Acceptable and appropriate tests
- Cost-effective tests
- Treatment available, effective and acceptable
- Treatment available
- Adequate follow-up available

TABLE 2-5
Eye and Vision Screening Principles

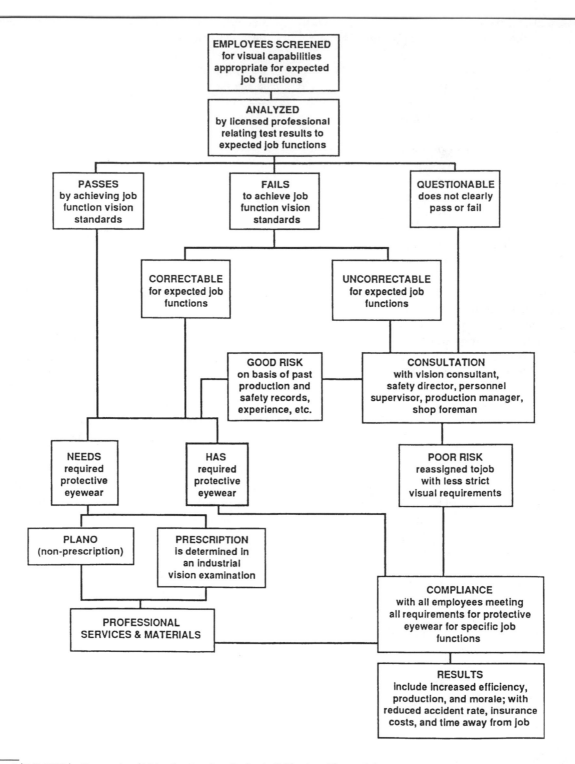

TABLE 2-6
Vision Screening Flow Chart

organization against subsequent claims for work-related disability related to vision impairment.

Screening Tests

There are two types of eye and vision screening tests that should be used in business and industry: general tests, used to assess the basic visual abilities and functions needed by all workers, and specialized tests, used to test specific abilities needed by workers with demanding vision or job requirements, such as airline pilots, crane operators, and inspectors. The general tests usually include visual acuity measured at both distance and near, preferably aided, with the near distance being the job working distance; peripheral vision to rule out major peripheral vision defects; heterophorias at distance and near; ophthalmoscopy; and color vision. These screening tests enable the optometrist to determine whether workers can see adequately to perform their tasks, need corrective lenses at distance and near, have adequate peripheral vision for avoiding accidents and operating motor vehicles, possess adequate binocular vision to perform tasks safely and comfortably, can avoid fatigue with frequent near vision tasks, have healthy eyes and have normal color vision.

Specialized tests are necessary for selected workers, depending on the tasks they perform. For some jobs, glare recovery, threshold visual fields, and dark adaptation need to be tested. Detailed color vision tests, such as the Farnsworth-Munsell test, are needed when tasks require excellent color discrimination.

Baseline color vision tests are useful for workers potentially exposed to environmental hazards that may first be detected by changes in color vision, such as exposure to certain solvents and other chemicals. Baseline threshold visual field tests are useful for workers whose visual field can become impaired after exposure to environmental hazards. Specialized stereoscopic vision testing is needed for workers who have tasks that require above average stereoacuity. Accommodative-convergence testing, including near point of convergence, accommodative facility, and other binocular tests, may be needed for the prepresbyopic worker doing specialized near tasks.

One form of testing not commonly used is the questionnaire. All potential or newly hired workers should be screened by a questionnaire in addition to

the vision screening. A questionnaire is useful in identifying worker's eye and vision symptoms on or off the job, which may suggest potential problems needing early remediation. Workers must be assured that honest answers will not result in the loss of their job, will be used only by the occupational optometrist, and will be kept confidential. Early identification of problems helps organizations because early treatment costs less than later treatment and early treatment of eye and vision problems in experienced workers saves retraining and replacement costs.

Vision Standards

Screening tests do not take the place of a comprehensive eye examination. Workers who do not pass a screening test should be rescreened before referral. Optometrists need to be sure that test memorization is not used during rescreening by selecting a different chart or approach to testing. Workers who do not pass the second test or to whom a second test is not given should be referred to community optometrists who are knowledgeable and experienced in occupational optometry for a definitive examination (Table 2-7). If additional information is needed, the occupational optometrist can be consulted.

Periodically, the screening false-negative rate should be determined. This can be done by rescreening a sample of workers who initially screened negative. The number who test positive during the rescreening were previously falsely identified as negative. This information is helpful for maximizing screening validity.

The criteria for each vision screening test may vary with the job or task to be performed and the needs of the individual business and industry.[12-15] The need for establishing vision standards has long been recognized, and there are general criteria that can be used for most organizations. These criteria were developed by Tiffin and his co-workers at the occupational research center at Purdue University.[12,16] These results are still widely accepted because no other studies have superseded them. For the many thousands of new jobs that have developed since their research was completed, the optometrist will need to modify the Purdue standards or develop new ones. Examples of businesses and technology which did not exist at the time the prior research was

---

Name _____ Age _____
Job Classification _____
Company _____
Currently Wearing Glasses or Contact Lenses   Yes _____   No _____
_____

Eye Screening Program—Examining Doctor's Report

1. Visual acuity—distance   Uncorrected _____
                                                             Corrected _____

2. Visual acuity—Near (_____")   Uncorrected _____
                                                             Corrected _____

3. Indications of refractive error _____
4. Heterophoria—heterotropia   Distance _____
                                                             Near _____

5. Ocular motility   Restricted _____
                                                             Unrestricted _____

6. Near point of convergence _____
7. Eye disease   External _____
                                                             Internal _____

8. Degree of binocularity _____
9. Color vision   Normal _____
                                                             Weakness _____

10. Further tests recommended
11. Doctor's comments and recommendations

Modified from Auerbach HH, Renyo JD: Report on a comprehensive in-plant industrial eye screening program. NJ J Optom, Jan–Mar 1972; with permission.

TABLE 2-7
Sample Vision Screening Report Form

done include: video display terminals, the entire electronics and semiconductor industry, the widespread use of private and commercial aircraft, the expansion of the research and development industry within universities and industry, and the automation and expansion of the textile industry.

Tiffin et al studied several million workers in thousands of different jobs.[12,16] They compared visual aptitudes in workers doing the same or similar jobs. The visual attributes that correlated to success on the job were identified. The visual characteristics that were found in a majority of good workers and absent in a majority of poor workers were studied to determine their value and relative importance. Using this information, specific visual requirements were developed for different job classifications. They categorized jobs into six classifications or families (Tables 2-8 and 2-9.)[12,16]

Some jobs may have eye and vision standards that are state or federally mandated.[17] Examples of these include operators of commercial vehicles such as interstate trucks, buses or commercial aircraft, as well as military positions. The occupational optometrist should consult appropriate references to determine these standards.

The Purdue job classification standards assume that each worker has binocular vision.[12,16] Binocular vision is necessary for work requiring stereoacuity, binocular peripheral vision, and wide assessment of fields of view such as in some rapid production inspection tasks. Workers with monocular vision or workers with good vision in only one eye, whether monocular or not, should not be automatically excluded from most jobs. However they should not be placed in jobs requiring good depth perception such as operators of most cranes, mobile equipment, and power machinery.

Workers with monocular vision must wear and use personal protective equipment at all times.[18,19] Their PPE should include safety spectacles with

Class I	Clerical and administrative personnel These workers primarily prepare and analyze data and figures and use accounting, typing, or other business machines, or do general office and administrative work.
Class II	Inspection personnel These workers primarily do visual inspection for small defects, or of small parts, operate small machines, and assemble or fabricate parts at distances close to the eyes.
Class III	Mobile equipment operators These workers operate trucks, fork lifts, cranes, boats and ships, tow motors, power shovels, graders, and high lift equipment.
Class IV	Machine operators These workers use machines such as lathes, drill presses, shapers, power saws, mills, or others where the actual operation is at or within arm's reach. If the machine requires the observation of work beyond arm's reach, more stringent requirements should be set up for the distance visual acuity.
Class V	Unskilled laborers These workers include janitors, guards, porters, hand truckers, longshoremen, loaders, and others.
Class VI	Mechanics and skilled tradesmen These workers do nonrepetitive jobs, e.g., carpenters, electricians, servicemen, setup men, plumbers, masons, painters, auto mechanics, welders, riveters, and others.

From Fox SL: Industrial and Occupational Ophthalmology, Springfield, IL: Charles C. Thomas, 1973; with permission.

TABLE 2-8
Job Classifications—Purdue Study

safety frames, safety lenses made from polycarbonate plastic and sideshields of solid plastic or mesh. In some cases, it may be best to recommend to management that some monocular workers change jobs in order to minimize or eliminate the risk to their single, remaining eye. For example, consider an experienced worker in a steel plant who handles tinplate strips and who loses one eye due to injury or to diabetic retinopathy. This worker should be reassigned to a position where there is no risk of metal strips getting under safety glasses and penetrating the remaining eye.

2.4 Occupational Eye and Vision Protection

All workers are exposed to occupational hazards or risks because a zero risk environment or workplace does not exist. Hazards may range from asthenopia associated with the use of video display terminals and falls resulting from poor vision to chemical burns of the cornea and macular burns from class IV lasers. The occupational optometrist must identify hazards and risks for existing work-related tasks and environments.[1] Priorities must be established with the most hazardous workplaces receiving first attention. After the most serious hazards and risks are managed successfully, others with lower priorities need to be managed. A risk assessment should be conducted for any new procedures or processes that are being considered or introduced into a business or industry.

Approaches to Protection

There are four major approaches for reducing or minimizing eye and vision hazards in industry and business—engineering, administrative, personal protective equipment, and redesign. These approaches include all the elements in the organization: tasks, environments, machinery, workers.[20,21] The engineering approach is usually the best because it builds into the task or process safety materials or devices that protect the worker from hazards or eliminates them. A simple example is the use of thermoplastic (Plexiglas) shields in front of machine tools, grinding equipment, and other metal forming tools. Another example is confining laser radiation to the inside of the laser housing.

Class	Far Vision		Near Vision		Stereo-Depth Perception	Max. Permissible Distance Phoria		Max. Permissible Near Phoria	Normal Color Vision
	Each Eye	Binoc-ular	Each Eye	Binoc-ular		Vertical	Lateral	Lateral	
I	20/30	20/25	20/25	20/20	Required	0.5^{Δ}	4^{Δ} Eso. 5^{Δ} Exo.	6^{Δ} Eso. 7.5^{Δ} Exo.	Usually Required
II	20/35	20/30	20/25	20/20	Required	0.5^{Δ}	4^{Δ} Eso. 5^{Δ} Exo.	6^{Δ} Eso. 7.5^{Δ} Exo.	Usually Required
III	20/25	20/20	20/35	20/30	Required	0.5^{Δ}	4^{Δ} Eso. 5^{Δ} Exo.	6^{Δ} Eso. 7.5^{Δ} Exo.	Required
IV	20/30	20/25	20/30	20/25	Required	0.5^{Δ}	4^{Δ} Eso. 5^{Δ} Exo.	6^{Δ} Eso. 7.5^{Δ} Exo.	Usually Required
V	20/30	20/25	20/35	20/30	Not Required	1.0^{Δ}	No Limitations	No Limitations	Not Required
VI	20/30	20/25	20/25	20/20	Required	0.5^{Δ}	4^{Δ} Eso. 5^{Δ} Exo.	6^{Δ} Eso. 7.5^{Δ} Exo.	Usually Required

From Fox SL: Industrial and Occupational Ophthalmology. IL: Charles C. Thomas, Springfield; 1973, and Tiffin.[54]

TABLE 2-9
Summary of Visual Requirements for Each Job Classification

Administrative or task-oriented approaches to reducing hazards are based on limiting exposure; they also involve training, safe work practices, housekeeping, and similar practices. Workers doing tasks in hazardous areas can have their risk reduced by reducing their total exposure. Proper scheduling with enforcement of maximum exposure durations can reduce workers' risks. For example, workers exposed to low level radiation in a nuclear power plant can be scheduled or rotated so that their exposure, even within protective clothing, is minimized.

Personal protective equipment is the most common approach to reducing hazardous exposures because it is cost-effective. It does not require engineering costs or the increased number of employees that the administrative approach may require. PPE varies widely from eye and vision protection to respirators, sound-reducing ear plugs or muffs and whole body protection. PPE is frequently used when there are no alternative solutions. For example, workers who perform ground tasks around commercial air-planes need hearing protection. There are at present no alternative engineering or administrative approaches that are more practical. Another example is the welding supervisor who needs PPE to minimize or eliminate the risk from exposure to welding arcs. Protection cannot be provided by engineering or administrative approach because of the supervisor's mobility and the nature of the job. There are guidelines for selecting many types of PPE (Table 2-10).

The redesign or environment-oriented approach for reducing hazards or risks is expensive because it requires the redesign of the manufacturing process or the substitution of alternative procedures in order to eliminate or reduce risks and hazards. However, during the initial design of a new plant, office or process, factoring safety into the design can be very useful and cost-efficient. Consultation with the occupational optometrist during the design process can eliminate or reduce hazardous eye and vision conditions and maximize visual performance. For example, inadequate lighting frequently contributes to hazardous environments, accidents, and reduced

	Selection Chart			Protector Guidelines		
	Tasks	Hazards	Protector Type	Protectors	Limitations	Not Recommended
I M P A C T	Chipping, grinding, machining, masonry work, riveting, and sanding.	Flying fragments, objects, large chips, particles, sand, dirt, etc.	B,C,D, E,F,G, H,I,J, K,L,N	Spectacles, goggles, faceshields SEE NOTES (1) (3) (5) (6) (10) For severe exposure add N	Protective devices do not provide unlimited protection. SEE NOTE (7)	Protectors that do not provide protection from side exposure. SEE NOTE (10) Filter or tinted lenses that restrict light transmittance, unless it is determined that a glare hazard exists. Refer to OPTICAL RADIATION.
H E A T	Furnace operations, pouring, casting, hot dipping, gas cutting, and welding.	Hot sparks	B,C,D, E,F,G, H,I,J, K,L,*N	Faceshields, goggles, spectacles *For severe exposure add N SEE NOTE (2) (3)	Spectacles, cup and cover type goggles do not provide unlimited facial protection. SEE NOTE (2)	Protectors that do not provide protection from side exposure.
		Splash from molten metals	*N	*Faceshields worn over goggles H,K SEE NOTE (2) (3)		
		High temperature exposure	N	Screen faceshields. Reflective faceshields. SEE NOTE (2) (3)	SEE NOTE 3	
C H E M I C A L	Acid and chemicals handling, degreasing, plating	Splash	G,H,K *N	Goggles, eye cup and cover types. For severe exposure, add N	Ventilation should be adequate but well protected from splash entry	Spectacles, welding helmets, handshields
		Irritating mists	G	Special purpose goggles	SEE NOTE (3)	
D U S T	Woodworking, buffing, general dusty conditions	Nuisance dust	G,H,K	Goggles, eyecup and cover types	Atmospheric conditions and the restricted ventilation of the protector can cause lenses to fog. Frequent cleaning may be required.	
O P T I C A L R A D I A T I O N	WELDING: Electric Arc		O,P,Q	TYPICAL FILTER LENS SHADE / PRO-TECTORS SEE NOTE (9) 10-14 / Welding Helmets or Welding Shields	Protection from optical radiation is directly related to filter lens density. SEE NOTE (4). Select the darkest shade that allows adequate task performance.	Protectors that do not provide protection from optical radiation. SEE NOTE (4)
	WELDING: Gas		J,K,L, M,N,O P,Q	SEE NOTE (9) 4-8 / Welding Goggles or Welding Faceshields		
	CUTTING			3-6		
	TORCH BRAZING			3-4	SEE NOTE (3)	
	TORCH SOLDERING		B,C,D, E,F,N	1.5-3 / Spectacles or Welding Faceshield		
	GLARE		A,B	Spectacle SEE NOTE (9) (10)	Shaded or Special Purpose lenses, as suitable. SEE NOTE (8)	

TABLE 2-10

Selection Chart for Determining Types of Protection for Hazards Caused by Impact, Heat, Chemical, Dust, and Optical Radiation Hazards Not Including Lasers

PROTECTIVE DEVICES

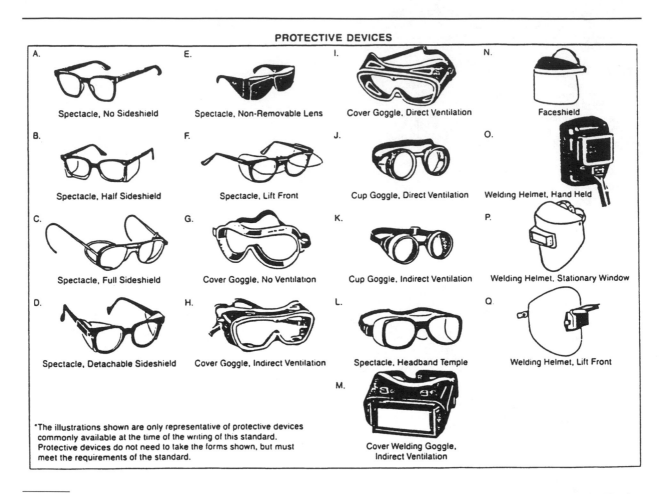

A. Spectacle, No Sideshield
B. Spectacle, Half Sideshield
C. Spectacle, Full Sideshield
D. Spectacle, Detachable Sideshield
E. Spectacle, Non-Removable Lens
F. Spectacle, Lift Front
G. Cover Goggle, No Ventilation
H. Cover Goggle, Indirect Ventilation
I. Cover Goggle, Direct Ventilation
J. Cup Goggle, Direct Ventilation
K. Cup Goggle, Indirect Ventilation
L. Spectacle, Headband Temple
M. Cover Welding Goggle, Indirect Ventilation
N. Faceshield
O. Welding Helmet, Hand Held
P. Welding Helmet, Stationary Window
Q. Welding Helmet, Lift Front

*The illustrations shown are only representative of protective devices commonly available at the time of the writing of this standard. Protective devices do not need to take the forms shown, but must meet the requirements of the standard.

From American National Standards Practice for Occupational and Educational, Eye and Face Protection, ANSI Z87.1-1989, approved by the American National Standards Institute on February 2, 1989 and published by the American Society of Safety Engineers.

NOTES:

(1) Care shall be taken to recognize the possibility of multiple and simultaneous exposure to a variety of hazards. Adequate protection against the highest level of each of the hazards must be provided.

(2) Operations involving heat may also involve optical radiation. Protection from both hazards shall be provided.

(3) Faceshields shall only be worn over primary eye protection.

(4) Filter lenses shall meet the appropriate standard (see Chapter 15).

(5) Persons whose vision requires the use of prescription (Rx) lenses shall wear either protective devices fitted with prescription (Rx) lenses or protective devices designed to be worn over regular prescription (Rx) eyewear.

(6) Wearers of contact lenses shall also be required to wear appropriate covering eye and face protection devices in a hazardous environment. It should be recognized that dusty and/or chemical environments may represent an additional hazard to contact lens wearers.

(7) Caution should be exercised in the use of metal frame protective devices in electrical hazard areas.

(8) Refer to standard on Special Purpose Lenses.

(9) Welding helmets or handshields shall be used only over primary eye protection.

(10) Non-sideshield spectacles are available for frontal protection only.

TABLE 2-10
Selection Chart for Determining Types of Protection for Hazards Caused by Impact, Heat, Chemical, Dust, and Optical Radiation Hazards, Not Including Lasers, continued

productivity. Retrofitting a workplace with new lighting fixtures can be costly, whereas the inclusion of appropriate fixtures during the design development phase of a new project is easy and requires minimal, if any, additional costs.

Personal Protective Equipment for Eyes and Vision

The use of personal protective equipment for eye and vision protection is task specific and begins with the identification of eye and vision hazards in the workplace. This identification usually involves the occupational optometrist and may also involve the industrial hygienist, safety engineer, and management. The assessment of hazards is one of the roles of the occupational optometrist. This assessment evaluates the relative risk of hazards to workers, the hazard's risk of causing permanent eye and vision impairment, and the frequency of eye and vision injuries in the workplace.

Management and workers need to clearly understand their responsibilities in the provision and use of personal protective equipment. This includes the consequences of nonuse as stated in safety policies, such as worker responsibility for work-time lost when injured while not using required PPE. Some organizations with very dangerous hazards make the consequences of nonuse of PPE the immediate loss of the job.

It is important that PPE including prescription safety lenses be designed for the worker's task. The occupational optometrist, or the primary care optometrist with knowledge about industry and business, must design the PPE and safety spectacles. The selection of proper ophthalmic materials for occupational needs and tasks are discussed in Chapter 10. The design of filters and sunglasses for eye protection against harmful radiation is discussed in Chapters 9 and 11. Safety standards for eye and vision protection are established by the American National Standards Institute. The current standards for industry are the ANSI Z87.1-1989 standards,[22] which are discussed in Chapter 9. Photochromic lenses and contact lenses in the work environment are presented in Chapters 9 and 12. The technical aspects and clinical uses of lasers are covered in Chapters 7 and 8.

Lighting in Industry

Another major role of the occupational optometrist is the assessment of lighting in industry. Environmental lighting is important in maximizing worker performance and productivity. Too much illumination causes glare and visual fatigue, whereas inadequate illumination causes asthenopia, increases the risk of accidents, and reduces productivity. These problems are discussed in Chapter 5.

2.5 Evaluating Potential Hazards

Industrial Hygiene

The primary care optometrist needs to have a working knowledge of many related disciplines, such as epidemiology, industrial hygiene, and toxicology, in order to provide high quality occupational optometry services. Industrial hygienists in particular can help assess health risks and the need for examinations of workers who are exposed to environmental hazards, including those hazards impacting on the visual system and eyes. The efforts of the industrial hygienist and optometrist are complementary.[4,7,23]

Hazards

The hazards found in the workplace can be divided into five types: gases/vapors, liquids (including splash hazards), dusts/fumes/mists, physical agents, and biologic agents (Table 2-11).[24] Another hazard classification is chemical, physical, biologic, psychologic, and ergonomic (Survey History, Chapter 1).[7] An understanding of these hazards is important because they can have an effect on the eyes and visual system. Each hazard can have different routes of entry and may require different approaches for prevention and control.

Vapors are the gaseous states of substances that are normally in the liquid state at room temperature. *Dusts* may be nuisance, toxic, or pneumoconiosis-producing dusts. Respirable-sized dust particles are commonly 10 μm or smaller. *Fumes* are solids that have been vaporized and subsequently condense. A *mist* is a liquid that is dispersed into the air as fine

Pollutant	Source	Diameter	Common Example(s)
Dust	Solid: given off by a mechanical process	100+ μm	Coal, ash, cement
Fumes	Solid: formed by vapor condensation through a sublimination, distillation, calcination, or chemical reaction	0.03–0.3 μm	Zinc oxide, lead oxide
Mist	Liquid: formed by vapor condensation (and a possible chemical reaction)	0.5–3.0 μm	Sulfuric acid mist
Smoke	Solid: particles resulting from incomplete combustion of carbon material	0.05–1.0 μm	Cigarette smoke
Spray	Liquid: formed by atomization of a parent liquid	10+ μm	Water

From Klopfer J: Effects of Environmental Air Pollution on the Eye. J Am Optom Assoc 60:773–778, 1989; with permission.

TABLE 2-11
Classification of Particulate Pollutants

droplets. *Physical agents* include ionizing and nonionizing radiation, coherent radiation from lasers, noise, heat, cold, and vibration. *Biologic agents* include bacteria, insects, molds, viruses, and fungi.

The industrial hygienist can sample and monitor work environments for most of these hazards. For many of these agents there are recognized exposure guidelines, such as the American Conference of Government Industrial Hygienists (ACGIH) Threshold Limit Values (TLV),[23,25] the National Institute for Occupational Safety and Health (NIOSH) Recommended Exposure Limits,[20] and OSHA Permissible Exposure Limits. With the exception of lasers, ultraviolet (UV), visible infrared (IR), microwave (MW), and ionizing radiation, there are almost no threshold limit values for hazards affecting the eye and vision. The occupational optometrist needs to work with the industrial hygienist to establish eye and vision hazard guidelines for the work environment and processes and products at the individual work site. Conservative values, based on the scientific literature, should be established where none currently exist. Values can also be established by extrapolating from exposures in other work environments.

Most industries use a safety color code to identify some hazards. Some industries such as air, sea, railroad, and highway transportation have their own unique color codes. In general, yellow designates caution and is used to mark physical hazards where a worker could strike something, stumble, fall, trip, or get caught between objects. Orange designates dangerous machine parts where a worker could be cut,

crushed, shocked, or exposed to moving gears, belts, and similar equipment. Purple designates radiation hazards. Black and/or white designates traffic markings and housekeeping identification. In addition to these codes, red designates fire protection equipment, danger, and stop, such as stop buttons on machinery. Green designates safety and first-aid equipment.[26]

Toxicology

The effects of toxic substances on the eye have been recognized as an important occupational health problem.[33] There are serious or potentially serious effects on the eye and visual system from over 50% of the chemicals listed as being hazardous. Therefore, a high priority of the occupational health specialist must be to set and maintain occupational hygiene standards for chemical eye protection.[7,20,28,29]

Toxicology is the study of the actions and adverse effects of chemical agents in living organisms. These effects may or may not be reversible and may injure individual cells, organs, or the entire person. Toxicology's major objective is to identify the damage that is produced by chemical substances and the doses at which this damage is produced.[23,25] With this information, acceptable levels of exposure can be predicted for humans who are exposed to chemical substances during their manufacture, use, and disposal.[4,27] Toxicity ranges from extremely toxic (a lethal dose being taste or a few drops) to relatively harmless (a lethal dose being a quart).[27,30]

Exposure to Toxic Agents

The major routes of contact for toxic agents are inhalation through the lungs, absorption through the skin, ingestion through the gastrointestinal tract, and parenteral administration of blood. Toxicity is determined by the level and frequency of exposure and the dose. As the frequency and dose increase, the toxicity increases; this is described as the *dose-response relationship.* The duration of the exposure is also important. Two smaller doses are sometimes less toxic than one large dose. Different effects may be observed within 24 hours of acute exposure compared to chronic exposure exceeding 24 hours.[4]

The optometrist needs to become familiar with the potentially toxic agents with which workers become exposed. This process begins with the identification of the agents, their potential for exposure and their methods of absorption, distribution, metabolism, and excretion. This information can be found through the OSHA Hazard Communication Standard, which requires that information regarding materials used or handled be made available to employees. For many products with trade names or for products that contain several constituents, the Material Safety Data Sheet (MSDS) provides important information. Literature can be found for many toxic materials by searching computerized databases such as MEDLINE, TOXLINE, and NIOSH/TIC.

Epidemiology

Epidemiology is the study of the determinants and distribution of diseases and disorders in populations.[11] Epidemiologic studies in occupational settings are used for investigating the causes of diseases including eye diseases and vision disorders, health risks associated with occupational exposures, the natural history or development of diseases and disorders, and new methods of diagnosing or preventing occupational problems. It can be useful to collaborate with an occupational epidemiologist in the design of in-house or in-plant studies of workers and their environment and to use epidemiologic studies in quantifying risk of eye and vision hazards.

2.6 Emergency Procedures

The eye is always at risk for injuries and trauma from workplace hazards. In spite of the best hazard assessment and risk identification and control program, there will be unforeseen events or combinations of circumstances that result in injury to the eye. Because of this, the occupational optometrist needs to include an emergency response plan within the occupational eye and vision program.

The eye is at risk for injuries from thermal or chemical burns, flash injuries from welding, abrasions, and lacerations from many physical agents. All injuries must be considered as emergencies until proven otherwise.

Ocular Emergencies and Urgencies

The first step in the development of an emergency response plan is to develop procedures, medical support, supervisor and worker training programs and to identify those events that are true emergencies, urgencies, and less urgent conditions. True emergencies are those events that require an immediate response—ideally within seconds or within minutes at worst. Urgencies are those events that may require some immediate first aid and will require treatment within 1 to 2 hours. Less urgent conditions are those that require treatment within several days to 1 to 2 weeks (Table 2-12).[8]

The second step is to identify the most hazardous areas within the industry or plant and to place emergency eyewash or eyecare stations in each area. After doing this, monthly inspection of these eyewash or eyecare stations, including test operation, must be instituted to prevent the stations from becoming inoperative and unusable in an emergency. Appropriate signs must be in place with the eyewash fountain well marked to allow quick identification of the station. A portable eyewash system should be placed next to the permanent fountain to allow irrigation to be continued while the worker is transported.[31,32] All eyewash fountains should meet the ANSI Z358.1-1981 standard.

The single most important treatment of chemical burns of the eye and adnexa is copious irrigation within seconds of the injury. Any immediately available nontoxic liquid should be used. Fingers will be needed to keep the eyelids wide open. The injured

- **True emergencies (therapy should be instituted within minutes):**
    Chemical burns of the cornea
    Central retinal artery occlusion
- **Urgent situations (therapy should be instituted within 1 to several hours):**
    Penetrating injuries of the globe
    Acute narrow-angle glaucoma
    Pupillary block glaucoma (lens or vitreous incarcerated in pupil); lens in anterior chamber
    Orbital cellulitis/cavernous venous thrombosis
    Corneal ulcer
    Gonococcal conjunctivitis
    Corneal foreign body
    Corneal abrasion
    Acute iritis and formation of synechiae
    Giant cell arteritis with acute ischemia of optic nerve
    Acute retinal tear with hemorrhage
    Acute retinal detachment
    Descemetocele
    Hyphema
    Lid laceration
- **Semiurgent situations (therapy should be instituted within days whenever possible or sometimes weeks):**
    Optic neuritis
    Ocular tumors
    Exophthalmos
    Previous undiagnosed chronic simple glaucoma
    Old retinal detachment
    Strabismic or other remediable amblyopias
    Blowout fracture of the orbit

From Deutsch & Feller: Paton and Goldberg's Management of Ocular Injuries, 2nd ed., Philadelphia, WB Saunders, 1985; with permission.

TABLE 2-12
Ocular Conditions Defined As True Emergencies, Urgent Situations, and Semiurgent Situations

person should roll the eyeball as much as possible to expose all of the anterior surface to irrigation. Irrigation should continue for a minimum of 30 minutes, depending on the chemical.

The third step is the training of supervisory personnel in the identification of and response to ocular emergency injuries. This should be followed by education of workers in all hazardous areas. The use of hands-on training or drills with actual workers is valuable. This training should be provided to all new workers and periodically updated for experienced workers.

The fourth step is the preparation of posted and stated procedures for the immediate management of the worker with an eye injury. Designing these procedures usually will involve consultation with the occupational optometrist or the community primary care optometrist.

The fifth step in the plan development is the development of an accident reporting process. This involves establishing procedures for thoroughly recording the history of the injury, including when, where, how, and why it occurred.[18] This information should be included in the employee's record and a copy sent to the consulting clinician.

Chemical injuries can also occur outside the workplace. For example, there are many common household chemicals including sodium hydroxide (drain cleaner), sodium hypochlorite (swimming pool chlorine), ammonium hydroxide (household ammonia), sulfuric acid (battery acid), and acetic acid (vinegar) that can cause eye injuries.[33]

Mechanisms of Ocular Response to Injury

Although there are a large number of oculotoxic substances, the eye generally responds to injury with a primary response at the site of injury, a later more generalized ocular inflammatory response, and a specific and characteristic ocular response to systemically active substances.[8] Not every response is the same because the eye is composed of a series of complex interrelated structures. The response of the eye to insults from different chemicals and the biphasic ocular inflammatory response should be understood.[8]

2.7 Occupationally Related Illnesses and Diseases

Principles

Optometrists need to understand the principles of occupational disease in order to provide the best care for their patients. Frequently the optometrist is the only clinician regularly consulted by the worker and therefore has the responsibility for identifying occupational diseases or illnesses and for arranging treatment for the worker.[4]

There are certain principles that apply to all work-induced disorders:

1. "The clinical and pathologic expression of most occupational diseases are indistinguishable from those of nonoccupational diseases."[34] Although there are exceptions, most occupational illnesses are not easily distinguishable from common disorders of nonoccupational origin.

2. "For many occupational diseases, there is a latent interval between the onset of exposure and the first expression of the disease."[34] The optometrist must be aware that conditions of recent onset may be derived by exposure to occupational toxins from many years past.

3. "Many occupational factors act in concert with nonoccupational factors to cause disease."[34] There are often multiple causes of work-related problems and diseases. Thus several risk factors may synergistically enhance their contribution to the risk of developing certain conditions. For example, smoking by workers exposed to a low-risk aerosal carcinogen on the job may enhance their risk of lung cancer.

4. "Occupational factors of importance may be difficult to ascertain by the clinician and may have as yet unestablished biologic significance."[34] This is true because there are over 20,000 toxic substances widely used, and many toxins occur in mixtures or as contaminants of other products.[34] Unfortunately toxologic data of both old and new substances are limited for many potential hazards.

5. "The clinical effects of toxic exposures are related to exposure."[34] The effect of any substance is related to its toxicity, the amount that the body absorbs, its effect (direct-acting, carcinogenic, allergic), and how it is eliminated.[34] There is often a threshold dose.

Suspecting Occupational Disease

Persons suffering from work-related illnesses enter optometrists' offices every day. It is important to consider work-related causation as part of the differential diagnosis. By doing this, diagnoses can be made that will influence the course of a disease and prevent impairment.[4] There are many environmental causes of health problems, including commonly used chemicals, household products, and materials used in hobbies (Tables 1-13–1-15). They illustrate the importance of the occupational history and identifying different exposures that can cause diseases and illnesses. Neurologic presentations including ataxia, headaches, encephalopathy, visual field loss, peripheral neuropathy, and tremors can also occur with exposures to neurotoxic substances.[4,35,36]

If occupational disease is suspected, the following steps should be taken:

1. Use the diagnostic occupational history
2. Define sources of potential exposure
3. Identify and describe the hazards
4. Resolve the problem and follow-up

2.8 Economics of Occupational Optometry

Remuneration

Optometrists who provide occupational eye and vision services to business and industry may be compensated in different ways depending on the relationship the optometrist has with the organization. The optometrist may be a part-time employee, a consultant under contract, or receive fee-for-service payments under a retainer that covers agreed-upon services. Optometrists may also have an informal relationship whereby services are provided on a fee-for-service basis within limits set by the health care program. Other arrangements are possible, including full-time employment. Capitated arrangements should generally be avoided unless the optometrist chooses rates that are protective in the event 100% utilization occurs.

Fees are determined after assessing many factors in addition to the organizational relationship: the services the organization needs or requests (concerning which the occupational optometrist may need to educate management); the size of the organization; the number of specialized jobs; the hazards in the workplace; and the duration of the optometrist-business relationship. The complexity of the organization and the number of specialized work positions that will require specialized knowledge and services also must be considered.

The optometrist will need to determine the potential income lost by being away from a successful practice and not being available to patients and the costs involved in keeping the practice open to meet patients' needs for services. Once these costs are known, the optometrist will have a baseline for determining fees for services associated with the provision of occupational services out of the office. These fees can be adjusted when a contractual or long-term relationship is established.

For primary care optometrists who provide services within their private practices the establishment of fees is simpler. For the occupational vision examination, supplemental examination and in-office screening, the optometrist can use existing fee schedules and adjust them for the specialized services and time required for providing them. Separate fees are usually established for each service provided. For a long-term commitment or contract for in-office services, the fees can be appropriately modified.

In determining compensation, the optometrist needs to consider both the direct and indirect benefits of working with business and industry. The direct benefits are receiving direct compensation for services, whereas the indirect benefits are becoming known to a large group of workers and subsequently providing services for their families and friends. Another indirect benefit is providing noncovered services to workers for care that is not related to the workplace. For example, workers may need services for off-the-job injuries or need services and materials associated with sporting activities. Because these indirect benefits are difficult to determine and may be provided by other optometrists, it is best not to emphasize them when establishing realistic fees for services.

Practice Building

Frequently the well-established optometrist is approached and asked to become involved with business or industry. After initial consultations or part-time involvement, the busy optometrist realizes that there may be an economic loss associated with being out of the office. At this point, many optometrists end their relationship with business and industry. A better approach and one that serves to expand the scope of the practice and the overall gross practice income is to hire an optometric associate. The associate will not have the patient following of the established optometrist, and with the guidance of the established optometrist can successfully provide the specialized services needed by industry and help ex-

pand the practice. With time and the success of the new optometrist, this process can be repeated and additional optometrists added to the practice.

Common Primary Care Occupational Services

Within the private practice setting there are five areas of occupational service that can be provided in addition to services commonly offered:[5]

1. Occupational vision examinations
2. Supplemental occupational vision examinations
3. Professional services related to PPE and safety eyewear
4. Industrial vision screenings
5. Preplacement examinations

The occupational vision examination is the most comprehensive of these services. This service is usually provided to workers who have specific job requirements or to determine if workers' vision meets job requirements. It is also useful for workers changing, transferring, or being considered for promotion to new positions that will have different vision requirements. This examination usually includes an occupational history, task analysis, external and internal eye health assessment, binocular vision assessment, and other tests necessary for the employee's job requirements and work safety. Depending on the local community and business or industry, several of the additional procedures may be regularly included and fees adjusted accordingly.

The supplemental occupational vision examination essentially provides an analysis of the job's visual demands, work hazards, and the worker's environment. It also includes a review of the eye examination results provided by the worker's optometrist or nonoptometrist eye care provider. Occasionally, additional procedures may be provided for assessing a specific job requirement or safety need of the worker.

Professional services related to PPE and safety eyewear are an important service provided by the occupational optometrist. These services are usually considered to be relatively trivial by business and industry and, as a result, they usually provide little remuneration for them. Management needs to be educated about the importance of professional services related to PPE and safety eyewear for both protection and performance.

There are three major services that need to be provided for safety eyewear to be successfully prescribed, including the appropriate selection of the safety eyewear (assessing eye position, symmetry, vertex distances, field of view, refractive error, and peripheral vision requirements); the occupational design of the safety lenses if prescription vision correction is necessary or if occupational prescriptions enhance performance (material, base curve, position of major reference point, design and position of multifocal segments or progressive addition lenses, coatings, tints); and the training of the worker in the use of the safety eyewear, including education regarding its nonuse. When all three of these services are professionally provided and the safety eyewear used on the job, workers will be protected from hazards. For some jobs additional PPE will be needed in addition to safety eyewear.

When inappropriate eyewear is selected, employees eyes and vision will not be protected. An electrician prescribed a metal frame that subsequently comes into contact with an open circuit and causes traumatic electrical insult to the eyes and face would not have been adequately protected, despite the wearing of a safety frame. A worker prescribed safety glasses but not prescribed safety sideshields who subsequently receives a penetrating injury from the side and loses vision would not have been adequately protected. Most workers in different job classifications also need eyewear that enhances their vision performance while protecting their eyes according to the requirements and exposures of the job.

The third service needed for PPE and safety eyewear to be used successfully is the training of the worker in its use. All of the efforts in PPE, eyewear and lens design are useless without the worker's understanding of the use and limitations of the safety eyewear. Workers must understand, for example, that no materials are completely unbreakable, that damaged safety materials need to be replaced immediately, that frames out of adjustment will interfere with their visual performance and must be corrected, that certain areas of their lenses provide the best vision and under which environmental conditions lens aberrations will become a handicap. With safety eyewear, it is crucial that the order be verified for accuracy and that the eyewear meets ANSI ophthalmic and safety standards. Industrial vision screenings and preplacement examinations are discussed earlier in this chapter.

2.9 Visual Impairment and Visual Disability

Definitions of Impairment and Disability

Work-related diseases and injuries to the eye and visual system can cause visual impairment and disability. The occupational optometrist needs to be able to assess workers to determine and document their visual impairments. Based on this determination of impairment, the worker may or may not be assessed as being disabled. *Impairment* refers to the loss of bodily function. The objective loss of the function of the eye or visual system pathway is a loss compared to the function that previously existed. Impairment is independent of the patient's profession, work, or other factors, whereas disability is not.

Disability refers to the impact of the impairment on work or social functioning. Determination of disability is a function of the person's age, sex, education, economic factors, and social environment, as well as the impairment. Disability may be short-term or temporary—usually less than 6 months' duration, or long-term, which includes permanent disability. Disability may also be partial or total and work-connected or work-aggravated.[34] Permanent total disability means that the person will never be able to work regularly at any available job for which the person is physically or educationally suited.[34]

Work-related or work-connected refers to illness or injury that resulted from some exposure at work. The cause of work-related impairment is often difficult to establish. The legal standard of cause is used, and this refers to a greater than 50% likelihood that the exposure was responsible for the impairment. Legal causes can be any established risk factor that substantially increases the risk of disease, or a factor that is suspected but cannot be proved to be responsible.[34]

Evaluation of Disability

The evaluation of a worker for determination of disability requires a detailed comprehensive occupational history; a comprehensive eye and vision examination that results in diagnostic results; and an assessment of the probable cause of the disease or illness. Evaluation requires a professional assessment to determine whether the condition is or is not impairing, whether it is progressive or stable, and whether there is any limit on returning to work. The standard guide for assessing visual impairment is the American Medical Association (AMA) Guide to Evaluation of Permanent Impairment, The Visual System.[37] Disability may be categorized by duration, type, and severity.

In assessing impairment and disability, it is important to know that the same impairment may cause different disabilities in different individuals. A laborer with a reduction in visual acuity to 20/50 may not be disabled, whereas an engineer with the same acuity doing drafting may be disabled. Adaptation to disability also differs with the individual and is a function of the person's age, education, occupational skills, work attitudes, and motivation.

Disability may be long-term, extended, short-term, or temporary. Disability can also be classified along a continuum of different degrees of severity. Total or severe refers to a degree of disabililty that precludes work. Partial impairment refers to those workers who are unable to return to the same work that they did before becoming impaired or to those who can work full-time at the same job but with some limitations.

Programs for Disabled Workers

The United States has had an uneven response to the impairment and resulting disability suffered by workers from work-related diseases, risk factors, and injuries. This is unfortunate, given the magnitude of the problems that occur. At present, there are many disparate and uncoordinated public and private programs to provide income through cash payments or services. There are different definitions of disability such as occupational or nonoccupational, different benefit amounts and periods, and different financing approaches. Many programs are limited to specific groups or occupations, such as veterans or railroad workers, or only cover specific diseases, such as black lung disease. All of these programs use measurement of impairment as indicators and criteria for disability. For eye and visual system impairment, visual acuity and visual field measurements are most often used. Following is a brief discussion of the most common programs.

Social Security Disability Insurance (SSDI) is the broadest program and includes everyone except federal civilian workers and one fourth of all state and local government employees. It pays benefits to disabled workers under age 65 years, to disabled dependent widows of insured workers, and others. The SSDI is designed to pay only those who are totally disabled, their dependents, and disabled dependents. Beneficiaries must be unable to engage in any substantial gainful activity (regardless of location or job availability) because of a physical or mental impairment that is expected to last at least 12 months or result in death. This definition is the most restrictive of any program.[34]

Blindness in the Social Security program means visual acuity of 20/200 or less in the better eye with the use of a correcting lens or visual fields of 20° or less. The worker must also have completed a 5-month waiting period, have a history of substantial and recent work, have contributed to the Social Security system for 5 of the 10 years before becoming disabled, and meet other requirements. At present, there are about 3 million disabled workers and 2 million dependents receiving SSDI benefits.

Workers' compensation programs are no-fault insurance programs provided through state law and disability is defined by each state.[2,34] These programs vary greatly in their coverage and benefits provided. Farm workers and small groups have usually been excluded, but coverage for most other workers is mandatory for almost all states. Most programs provide prompt and reasonable income and health care benefits for people injured at work or with a work-related illness regardless of fault; encourage employers to maximize interest in safety and rehabilitation through experience-rating their insurance premiums; and eliminate payment for fees associated with legal actions.

Workers are eligible if they have an occupational injury or disease leading to inability to work or death. Benefits are paid for temporary or permanent and partial or total disability. An eligible worker receives benefits to cover loss of income and other expenses such as health care. Case benefits are calculated as a percentage of earnings at the time of injury or death. Benefits may also be paid for loss of an eye or other organs even if no loss of wages occurs.

Optometrists need to be familiar with details of their state's workers' compensation program and with the general principles of workers' compensation, as noted by Rosenstock and Cullen:[34]

1. Illness must be deemed work-related or work-aggravated on a more-probable-than-not basis in order for the patient to qualify.
2. If an illness is determined to be work-related, the physician must so inform the patient and assist in taking appropriate steps to file a worker's compensation claim.
3. Benefits for work-related illness, compared to injuries, are frequently contested.
4. Third-party law suits are outside the worker's compensation system in general.
5. Because it is a no-fault system, the worker cannot sue an employer. One can sue a supplier or other third party because of dangerous or defective equipment, but this is covered under liability laws.[34]

Health insurance will usually not reimburse health care costs for work-related problems. If any worker is impaired from a work-related accident or disease, the occupational optometrist needs to determine which program may provide benefits by consulting with state officials, OSHA personnel, and others as needed.

2.10 Occupational Safety and Health Legislation

The Williams-Steiger Occupational Safety and Health Act of 1970 (OSH Act), Public law 91-596, was signed on December 29, 1973, and became effective April 28, 1971.[10] The purpose of this legislation is "to assure safe and healthful working conditions for working men and women" (Appendix 1-4 in Chapter 1). This legislation has had a positive and dramatic impact on the health and safety of the American workforce. The law provided enabling legislation that authorized administrative interpretations of the act, which serves as the basis for the promulgation of regulations.[2]

The law established two agencies: OSHA and NIOSH. OSHA is mandated to protect workers from work site hazards by establishing health and safety standards, enforcing standards by work site inspections, and assisting employers in solving work site problems through consultations with federal or state OSHA agencies.[10] NIOSH was established to conduct research about workplace hazards at the work site and through other methods such as reviews of the scientific literature. Based on this research, NIOSH produces criteria documents, which then serve as the basis for OSHA standards. NIOSH also can conduct health hazard evaluations (HHE) at the request of the employer, employee, or others. These evaluations use industrial hygienists and others as appropriate. NIOSH in 1973 was assigned to the Center for Disease Control for administrative purposes. The results of NIOSH studies are presented as recommendations to OSHA. Generally, the Department of Labor establishes standards that affect workers.

This legislation covers all workers or employees and employers except those who are self-employed, work on farms where only the immediate family members are employed, or are covered by other agencies or legislation such as miners, railroad workers, truck drivers, and federal employees.

The OSH Act has four categories of standards: general industry,[38] maritime, construction and agriculture. If OSHA has not passed a specific standard for an industry, then the employer must follow the act's general duty clause, which states that each employer shall establish a place of employment that is free from recognized hazards that are considered or likely to cause death or serious physical harm to employees.[2]

All occupational optometrists need to review the OSHA laws and become familiar with them because they apply to the businesses and industries with which they are engaged.[38,45] The OSH Act provides for workplace inspections, the priorities for such inspections, workers' rights, record-keeping requirements, and employee education and training. It also has specific requirements for protective equipment and requires that eye and face protection meet the American National Standard for Occupational and Educational Eye and Face Protection, ANSI Z87.1 (Appendices 1-2 and 1-3 in Chapter 1).[22]

2.11 Program Policies

A major responsibility of the occupational optometrist is to recommend and help develop occupational eye and vision program policies. These policies should be compiled and made available to all employees. Some examples of policy questions follow:

1. Program Scope and Design[43]
   a. Who [person(s) or group] will be responsible for designing the program?
   b. Will the program include all employees or only those in selected job categories?
   c. What will be the key components of the program?
2. Program Implementation
   a. Who will be responsible for implementing the program?
   b. Will the program be implemented at one time or phased in?
   c. Who will review and approve the program?
   d. Who will educate employees about the program and promote it?
3. Pre-employment and Preplacement Evaluations
   a. Will all potential employees have their visual skills evaluated?
   b. Will experienced employees have their visual skills evaluated periodically?
   c. Who will determine the minimum skills needed for employees to work safety and efficiently?
4. Record-keeping
   a. What information needs to be kept and for how long?
   b. Who is responsible for maintaining the records?
   c. Who has access to the records and how is confidentiality maintained?
5. Wearing and Using Personal Protective Equipment
   a. Will 100% enforcement of PPE use be required?
   b. Will visitors, subcontractors, and management be required to wear PPE?
   c. Who is responsible for maintaining and replacing PPE?
6. Selection and Costs of Personal Protection Equipment
   a. Who pays for occupational and other eye examinations?
   b. Will freedom of choice by the employee be allowed for this service?
   c. Who will design, order, and dispense PPE?
   d. What PPE and safety frames, safety lenses, tints, and antireflection or antiscratch coatings will be allowed?
   e. Who will pay for damaged PPE replacement?

7. Compliance-Adherence
   a. What mandatory disciplinary action will be used for those who do not comply with the program?
   b. What safety incentives will be offered?
   c. What safety and PPE signs will be posted?
   d. What PPE education will be provided?
8. Eyewashes and Eye Safety Stations
   a. How many are needed, where will they be located, and who will maintain them?
   b. How will they be identified?
   c. Who will educate workers on their use?
   d. Who will be responsible for maintaining them?
9. Emergency Procedures
   a. What anticipated hazards will require emergency procedures?
   b. Who will establish emergency procedures?
   c. Who will educate employees about established safety procedures?
   d. Who will be responsible for supervising emergency procedures?
10. Safety and Health Education
    a. How frequently will education programs be provided?
    b. Who will be responsible for designing and delivering this education?
    c. What education responsibilities will employees have for their education?
11. Vision Screening
    a. Who will design the general and specific screening tests?
    b. What applicants and employees will be screened? How frequently?
    c. Who will pay for subsequent eye care if employees do not pass the screening?
12. Hazards Evaluation
    a. Who will be responsible for periodic hazard evaluations?
    b. What evaluation procedures will be used after a worker is injured on the job?
    c. How will changes in the workplace, production processes, or materials be evaluated for new hazards before they are implemented?
13. Program Monitoring and Evaluation
    a. Will the program be monitored and evaluated?
    b. How will the monitoring and evaluating be done and by whom?
    c. Who will be responsible for the program evaluation?

The development of policies for the occupational eye and vision health care program are important. These policies help establish the specific details of the program and affect how it will be implemented. The knowledge and expertise of the occupational optometrist is essential when business and industry establish these policies.

References

1. Gates AG. Vision Conservation: Job Performance and Eye Safety. Dangerous Properties of Industrial Materials Report 1987; 7(4):2–6.
2. Alderman MH, Hanley MJ. Clinical Medicine for the Occupational Physician. New York, Marcel Dekker, Inc, 1982.
3. Shepard WP. The Physician in Industry. New York, McGraw-Hill, 1961.
4. McCunney RJ (ed). Handbook of Occupational Medicine. Boston, Little, Brown and Co, 1988.
5. Occupational Vision Services. OVS Panel Member Manual. Burbank, CA, OVS, 1990.
6. McQueen JC. An occupational vision care program that works. Can J Optom 1983; 45:155–157.
7. Zenz G. Occupational Medicine, 2nd ed. Chicago, Year Book Medical Publisher, 1988.
8. Deutsch TH and Feller DB: Paton and Goldberg's Management of Ocular Injuries 2nd ed. Philadelphia, WB Saunders, 1985.
9. Nakagawara VB. Functional model of an eye protection program: Guide for the clinical optometrist. J Am Optom Assoc 1988; 59:925–928.
10. Williams-Steiger Occupational Safety and Health Act of 1970 (Public Law 91-596), December 29, 1970 (84 State 1590).
11. Mausner JS, Kramer S. Epidemiology—an Introductory Text. Philadelphia, WB Saunder, 1985.
12. Tiffin J. Industrial Psychology (3rd ed). New York, Prentice-Hall, 1952.
13. Sheedy JE. Fire fighter vision standards. J Am Optom Assoc 1884; 55:365–375.
14. Sheedy JE, Keller JT, Pitts D et al: Recommended vision standards for police officers. J Am Optom Assoc 1983; 10:925–928.
15. DeHaan WV. The Optometrist's and Ophthalmologist's Guide to Pilots Vision. Boulder, CO, American Trend, 1982.
16. Kuhn HS. Eyes and Industry (2nd ed). St. Louis, Mosby, 1950.
17. Mahlman HE. Handbook of Federal Vision Requirements and Information (2nd ed). Chicago, Professional Press, 1982.
18. Fox SL. Industrial and Occupational Ophthalmology. Springfield, IL, Charles C. Thomas, 1973.
19. Leggo C. A second look at one-eyed applicants and employees. Ind Med 1955; 21:473–476.
20. National Institute for Occupational Safety and Health. Strategies for the Prevention of Leading Work-Related Diseases and Injuries, Part 1. Washington, DC, Association of Schools of Public Health, 1986.
21. Guidelines for special eyewear. National Safety News 1978; 117:43.
22. American National Standards Institute. American National Standard Practice for Occupational and Educational Eye and Face Protection. ANSI Z87.1, 1968, 1979, 1989. Des Plaines, IL, American Society of Safety Engineers, 1989.
23. Olishifski JB (ed). Fundamentals of Industrial Hygiene (2nd ed). Chicago, National Safety Council, 1979.
24. Klopfer J. Effects of environmental air pollution on the eye. J Am Optom Assoc 60 1989; 773–778.
25. Plog BA (ed). Fundamentals of Industrial Hygiene (3rd ed). Chicago, National Safety Council, 1988.
26. Hofstetter HW. Industrial Vision. Philadelphia, Chilton, 1956.
27. Srivastava AK, Gupta BN. Oculotoxins: Effects, implications, and importance in occupational health. Am J Ind Med 1989; 16:723–726.
28. Grant WM. Toxicology of the Eye (3rd ed). Springfield, IL, Charles C Thomas, 1986.
29. Ctein A, Veritas. Hazardous materials training programs, Photomethods 1990; 33:14–15.
30. LaDou J. Introduction to Occupational Health and Safety. Chicago, National Safety Council, 1986.
31. Ziegler TJ. Interested in saving face? Emergency eyewashes may be the answer. Occup Health Saf 1989; 58:26–27, 29.
32. Cox WR. Eyewash stations provide first aid for chemical contamination. Occup Health Saf, 1986; 155:50–60.
33. Nelson JD, Kopietz LA. Chemical injuries to the eyes: Emergency, intermediate and long-term care. Postgrad Med 1987; 81:62–75.
34. Rosenstock L, Cullen MR. Clinical Occupational Medicine. Philadelphia, WB Saunders, 1986.
35. Harrington DO. The Visual Fields (3rd & 6th eds). St. Louis, Mosby, 1964, 1990.
36. Fengsheng H. Occupational toxic neuropathies—An update. Scand J Work Environ Health 1985; 11:321–330.
37. Committee on Rating of Mental and Physical Impairment. Guides to the Evaluation of Permanent Impairment, Chapter VII, The Visual System. Chicago, American Medical Association, 1971.

38. Occupational Safety and Health Administration. General Industry Safety and Health Standards. OSHA 2206 (29 CFR 1910). Washington, DC, U.S. Department of Labor, 1976.

39. Klopfer J. OSHA and the optometrist. J Am Optom Assoc 1987; 64:540–542.

40. Felton JS. 200 Years of Occupational Medicine in the U.S. Journal of Occupational 1976; 18:809.

41. Cowles SR. Occupational Health. In Introduction to Occupational Health and Safety. Chicago, National Safety Council, 1986.

42. Cullen MR, Cherninck MG, Rosenstock L. Occupational medicine. N Engl J Med 1990; 322:594–601.

43. Gunning JN, Jr, Soles EM, Miller SC. Guidelines for an Occupational Vision Program. J Am Optom Assoc 1979; 50:935–938.

CHAPTER THREE

Ophthalmic Standards

James E. Sheedy, O.D., Ph.D.

3.1 Functions of Standards

Ophthalmic standards are established: (1) To provide a standard nomenclature, definitions and terminology so that various segments of an industry can work together more effectively and efficiently; (2) to provide quality control; and (3) to provide protection for the public. For example, it is important that a common definition of the Diopter be accepted by lens manufacturers, equipment manufacturers, and optometrists. If different segments of the industry used a different wavelength to specify the refractive power of a lens, the industry would be seriously handicapped. For this reason, an international definition of the Diopter has been established by the International Standards Organization (ISO).

Definitions of base curve, curvature, and standard methods for specifying and measuring ophthalmic lenses are necessary for clinicians, laboratories, and lens manufacturers to communicate. Ophthalmic frame parameters and measurement systems are standardized so that clinicians, laboratories, and frame and lens manufacturers can communicate effectively for business. Contact lens standards on water content assist in defining the boundaries between rigid and soft contact lenses. Standards on low vision aids provide methods for specifying the magnification of various devices so that manufacturers and clinicians can communicate for the benefit of the patient.

The American National Standards Institute (ANSI) Z80.1 standards for ophthalmic lens tolerances establishes the lens quality criteria for optical laboratories, optometrists and others. Standards for semifinished lens blanks establish the quality expectation between ophthalmic lens manufacturers and the optical laboratory. The values of these latter tolerances take into account the abilities and technologies of manufacturers and laboratories to enable the laboratories to meet the ANSI Z80.1 standards. ANSI standards for hard and soft contact lenses establish the quality control expectations between the contact lens manufacturers and clinicians. ISO standards for ophthalmic instruments establish quality control tolerances for manufacturers such as the horizontal and vertical alignment for viewing telescopes, on the lens powers in the ophthalmoscope, and measuring accuracy for lensometers. The standard for automated refractors establishes a calibration procedure.

ANSI Z87.1 is the standard for occupational and industrial eye and face protection that specifies the properties of eye protective materials. The impact resistance portion of ANSI Z80.1 specifies the minimum protective properties of dress ophthalmic lenses. The ANSI Z80.3 standard on nonprescription sunglasses specifies the minimum UV protective properties of over-the-counter sunglasses.

3.2 Effectiveness of Standards

Most standards-setting bodies in the United States are voluntary, nongovernmental groups. Because the standards that they develop usually have an effect upon trade, commerce, and the public good, any group that can be affected by the establishment of a standard can participate in the development of that standard. For example, ANSI procedures state, "Any person (organization, company, government agency, individual, and the like) with a direct and material interest has the right to participate by (1) expressing a position and its basis, (2) having that position considered, and (3) appealing if adversely affected."

Standards organizations require that a consensus of those participating in the standard agree upon the standard before it is adopted. Consensus can be interpreted in many ways. For example, the ANSI procedures state, "Consensus is established when . . . substantial agreement has been reached by directly and materially interested categories. Substantial agreement means much more than a simple majority, but not necessarily unanimity. Consensus requires that all views and objections be considered, and that a concerted effort be made towards their resolution."

Since standards-setting bodies are voluntary organizations, the standards, by themselves, do not establish governmental policy or law and are therefore unenforceable. However, since all interested parties participate in the development of the standard, and consensus is required for the adoption of a standard, general voluntary adherence to the standard usually occurs. A manufacturer who does not use the terminology, measurement methods, and tolerances of the

standard will generally be placed in a disadvantageous position in the marketplace. For example, an optical laboratory that does not meet or use the ANSI Z80.1 tolerances would develop a reputation for providing poor quality lenses.

In some cases, standards that have been adopted by a voluntary standards organization become mandatory when they are adopted by a governmental agency. This occurred when the Food and Drug Administration (FDA) adopted the impact-resistant testing of ophthalmic lenses as described in ANSI Z80.1. When this became FDA policy, all dress ophthalmic lenses dispensed in this country had to meet this standard. Similarly, since the Occupational Safety and Health Administration (OSHA) adopted ANSI Z87.1 as government policy, all industrial safety eyewear must meet that standard.

International standards are also developed by voluntary standards setting organizations such as ISO. Such an organization, by itself, has no jurisdiction; however, many standards adopted by the ISO and other international groups have the force of international law because of the General Agreement on Tariffs and Trade (GATT). Member nations of the United Nations have signed the GATT and are thereby bound by its provisions. The GATT standards code requires governments to use international standards, where they exist, in national technical rules and regulations concerning international trade. The purpose of this is to eliminate technical barriers to trade that may be caused by differences in national laws, regulations, and standards. Therefore, the GATT treaty effectively gives ISO standards the force of international law.

3.3 American National Standards Institute

ANSI has played the dominant role in the domestic area of ophthalmic products, although it supports standards in many different areas. Previously, the institute was named the American Standards Association (ASA); most people are familiar with the ASA rating of photographic film, a product that still carries the old name.

ANSI is a nonprofit institute that accredits and approves committees, each of which is configured to develop standards for a particular segment of products. No employees of ANSI participate in the work of the committees. The committees are composed of professional societies, trade associations, other organizations, and individuals. Each committee must meet the requirements established by ANSI in order to be accredited. Standards developed by each committee must be shown to have met a consensus (as defined earlier); they also must be held open by ANSI for public comment before the standards are adopted.

Many ANSI standards committees are formed to develop a single standard, whereas others develop many standards in a particular area depending on the needs of the industry. In the area of ophthalmics, the primary committee is ANSI Z80, the committee on ophthalmic standards. The voluntary groups that participate in the standards development activities of ANSI Z80 are shown in Table 3-1. This is a broad-based group of manufacturers, optometrists, ophthalmologists, opticians, laboratories, federal agencies, and public and general interest groups.

Table 3-2 lists the ANSI standards that are related to ophthalmic products and those with a Z80 designation have been developed by the ANSI Z80 Committee. Subcommittees within Z80 develop these standards, which are then presented to ANSI Z80 for approval and to ANSI for adoption. All ANSI standards must be revised, reaffirmed, or withdrawn every 5 years. For this reason, the work of standards committees is ongoing just to maintain standards. Ophthalmic standards that have been developed by committees other than ANSI Z80 are also shown in Table 3-2. These standards relate to industrial safety, safe use of lasers, sports protective eyewear, and the design of video display work stations. Each area is developed by a separate committee comprising different voluntary groups that have expertise in each of the particular areas.

3.4 Other Domestic Standards Organizations

Numerous other organizations within this country establish standards; however, none of these standards organizations have impacted the field of ophthalmics as greatly as has ANSI. The American Society for Testing and Materials (ASTM) is a standards-setting organization that has numerous committees that work on standards in particular areas of industry. It has been particularly active in setting standards for the testing and quality of materials used in industry. ASTM has developed some standards for sports eye protective equipment (Table 3-2) that have subsequently been adopted by ANSI. The Illuminating Engineering Society (IES) sets standards for lighting including those related to the quality and quantity of light in various occupational, recreational, and home environments (see Chapter 5). A more complete list of vision–related standards and standards organizations is available from the American Optometric Association.[1] The names and

American Academy of Ophthalmology
American Academy of Optometry
American Ceramic Society
American Optometric Association
Association of Schools and Colleges of Optometry
Contact Lens Institute
Contact Lens Manufacturers Association
Contact Lens Society of America
Food and Drug Administration
Industrial Equipment Association
National Association of Manufacturing Opticians
National Academy of Opticianry
National Association of Opticians and Optometrists

National Bureau of Standards
National Institutes of Health
National Society to Prevent Blindness
Opticians Association of America
Optical Laboratories Association
Optical Manufacturers Association
Optical Society of America
Sunglass Association of America
United States Army
United States Air Force
United States Navy
Veterans Administration

TABLE 3-1
Organizational Members of ANSI Z80

Standard	Description
Z80.1	Prescription Ophthalmic Lenses
Z80.2	First–Quality Rigid Contact Lenses
Z80.3	Nonprescription Sunglasses and Fashion Eyewear
Z80.4	Contact Lens Accessory Solutions for Conventional Contact Lenses
Z80.5	Dress Ophthalmic Frames
Z80.6	Physicochemical Properties of Contact Lenses
Z80.7	Intraocular Lenses
Z80.8	First Quality Soft Contact Lenses
Z80.9	Low Vision Aids
Z87.1	Occupational and Education Eye and Face Protection
Z136.1	For the Safe Use of Lasers
ANSI/ASTM	Specification for Eye and Face Protective Equipment for Hockey Players
F513-85 ANSI/ASTM	Specification for Eye Protectors for Use in Racquet Sports
F803-85 ANSI/ASTM	Specifications for Ski Goggles
ANSI/HFS 100	Human Factors Engineering of Video Display Terminal Work Stations

TABLE 3-2
ANSI Standards on Ophthalmic Products

American National Standards Institute
1430 Broadway
New York, NY 10018
(212) 642–4900

American Society for Testing and Materials
1916 Race Street
Philadelphia, PA 19103
(215) 299–5400

Illuminating Engineering Society
345 East 47th Street
New York, NY 10017
(212) 705–7916

TABLE 3-3
Selected Domestic Standards Organizations

addresses of the domestic organizations discussed here are presented in Table 3-3.

3.5 Standards–Setting Organizations in Other Countries

Many other industrial nations have a standards–setting organization. These include the British Standard Institute, Standards Association of Australia,

Canadian Standards Association, Afnor (France), DIN (West Germany), and Japan's Standards Association which are the standards organizations in each of these countries. These organizations usually are more dominant than ANSI is in the United States. In most countries, the national standards organizations are branches of the government or receive governmental support—very much unlike ANSI, which is entirely voluntary and receives no government support. With the growing importance of international trade and international standards, the greater organization and support of the foreign standards–setting organizations often places the U.S. committees in a trailing position in the development of international standards. Currently, some U.S. governmental agencies are considering providing support to the U.S. standards organizations.

The International Standards Organization

The ISO has the largest influence on ophthalmic standards. ISO standards cover all technical fields except electro-technical standards, which are covered by the International Electro-technical Commission (IEC). The ISO was established in 1946 by the national standards associations from 25 countries.

ANSI was the founding member organization from the United States and continues as a member today. A list of the ophthalmic–related standards that have been adopted by the ISO or are in development by ISO/TC 172 are presented in Table 3-4. Information about ISO standards is available from ANSI.

The ISO work is carried out by 164 Technical Committees (TCs). The TC of greatest interest to the field of ophthalmics is ISO/TC 172, the Technical Committee on Optics and Optical Instruments. TC 172 is divided into subcommittees, each of which has several working groups to develop the specific standards documents. Experts from the various countries participate in the working groups and subcommittees. Within the working groups, individual experts agree on the recommended drafts for the standards. These drafts are then presented to the subcommittee, where a vote is made at the meeting according to participating nations (one vote for each nation). This vote determines whether the draft document should be submitted to the TC. If it is approved to be submitted to the TC, then the TC will send the draft document for mail ballot to the participating country member standards organizations. Several levels of voting and approval are necessary before a document is adopted as an ISO standard.

The participating nations in the work of ISO/TC 172 are presently Australia, Austria, Canada, France, Germany, Italy, Japan, United Kingdom, United States, and the former Soviet Union. Twelve other nations have observer status.

International standards have the potential for strong influence on international trade products through the GATT. Member countries of the United Nations have agreed that products traded internationally will meet international standards if such standards exist. This is enforced only if countries choose to require compliance with the ISO standard before a product can be imported into that country. Presently no countries are limiting imports on the basis of meeting the standards. However, the first ISO/TC 172 standards have only recently been adopted and some countries may begin using them to limit imports.

The European Economic Communities (EEC), which was formed in 1992, is one of the organizations that will use the ISO standards. The EEC has established a greater European standards organization called the European Committee for Standardization (CEN). The purpose of CEN is to establish European standards for goods that will travel across EEC borders to prevent goods of an inferior quality

Chart Projectors	Measuring System for Spectacle Frames
Contact Lenses	Objective Refractometers
Contact Lenses: Biocompatibility—Rabbits	Ophthalmometers (Keratometers)
Contact Lenses: Determination of Chemical Purity	Refractor Heads
Contact Lenses: Determination of Curvature	Retinoscopes
Contact Lenses: Determination of Refractive Index	Rigid Contact Lens Specifications
Contact Lenses: Determination of Thickness	Screws, Nuts, and Rivets
Contact Lenses: Determination of Vertex Power	Slit-Lamp Biomicroscopes
Contact Lenses: Determination of Water Content	Specifications for Multifocal Lenses
Contact Lenses: Inclusion and Imperfections	Specifications for Progressive Lenses
Contact Lenses: Oxygen Transmission and Permeability	Specifications for SV Lenses
Contact Lenses: Solvent Extractions	Spectacle Frames
Contact Lenses: Spectral Transmittance	Synoptoscopes
Contact Lenses: Standard Solutions	Terms for Boxing System and Formers
Finished SV Lenses, General Requirements	Test Lenses for Focimeters
Focimeters	Tonometers
Formers	Trial Case Lenses
Fundus Cameras	Trial Frames
Indirect and Direct Ophthalmoscopes	Visual Acuity: Optytype Correlation
Laser Photocoagulators	Visual Acuity: Standard Optotype
Marking of Spectacle Frames	

TABLE 3-4
Ophthalmic Standards Adopted Or Under Development by the ISO

from one country from being shipped into another and sold to the detriment of domestically produced goods. The CEN is largely adopting the ISO standards for ophthalmic products or other appropriate national standards if ISO standards do not exist. It appears likely that these standards and some form of product certification will be used to screen imports into the EEC and it is also likely that other countries will do the same. Manufacturers of export products must be aware of the ISO standards and manufacture products accordingly.

Another international standards organization is the Commission Internationale de l'Eclairage (CIE), the International Commission on Illumination. The CIE develops international lighting standards but also develops and adopts various scientific documents that address issues in lighting applications.

3.6 Clinical Standards

The standards established by ANSI, ISO, and the other standards setting organizations are generally related to products or industrial applications. These groups, however, are not the appropriate bodies to establish clinical testing standards. It is necessary that any clinical testing standards be established by clinicians because the manufacturing groups do not have clinical expertise nor should they be directly involved in the relationship between doctor and patient.

A good example involves the standardization of visual acuity testing. It is necessary to standardize visual acuity testing so that measurements can be repeatable and comparable. Clinical testing standards for visual acuity established by the National Academy of Sciences Committee on Vision[2] and adopted by the Consilium Ophthalmologicum Universale[3] were developed by a group of clinicians who understand the issues of clinical care. ISO, however, has adopted standards for the measurement of visual acuity for daylight certification purposes only that specifically exclude clinical testing, as well as standards for the design of visual acuity chart projectors. These standards do not address the method of measurement of visual acuity.

References

1. Sheedy JE, Chioran GM. Vision Standards Bibliography. St. Louis, 1981. American Optometric Association, 1981.
2. National Academy of Sciences–National Research Council: Recommended standard procedures for the clinical measurement and specification of visual acuity: Report of Working Group 39. Adv Ophthalmol 1980; 41:103–148.
3. Visual Functions Committee, Concilium Ophthalmologicum Universale: Visual Acuity Measurement Standard. San Francisco, International Council of Ophthalmology, 1984.

SECTION TWO

RADIATION, LIGHTING, AND VISION

Radiation, lighting, and vision describes the electromagnetic spectrum and the measurement of the optical spectrum in both radiometric and photometric terms. The theoretical concept of the blackbody or full radiator and the physical laws that govern its radiant emittance are important basic concepts in understanding ocular damage from radiation and the clinical application of eye protection. In addition, the radiation of commonly used sources is provided to aid in the evaluation of the visual environment, its effects on the eye, and the need for protection of the eye against damage.

The relationship of the sun and its radiation to the environment is discussed with emphasis on ocular damage from sunlight. The effects of reduced or increased amounts of ozone on the environment is introduced. It is hoped that the information on this vital topic will stimulate a desire in the reader to seek additional information.

The International System of Units (SI) is used for both the base units and derived units. Tables and explanations of the SI units are provided at the end of Chapter 4 in Appendix 4-1.

CHAPTER FOUR

The Electromagnetic Spectrum

Donald G. Pitts, O.D., Ph.D.

4.1 Basic Principles

The Electromagnetic Spectrum

The electromagnetic spectrum (EMS) has no precise lower or upper limit and represents the radiation that extends from the secondary cosmic rays with a wavelength of 10^{-14} m to long AC circuits with a wavelength of 10^8 m. The EMS is usually divided into cosmic radiation, X-radiation (X-rays), ultraviolet radiation (UVR), visible spectrum (VIS) radiation, infrared (IR) radiation, microwave (MW) radiation, and radio frequency (RF) radiation (Fig. 4-1).

The boundaries between the different divisions of the EMS are somewhat arbitrary, and each of the regions tends to overlap.

The distance between two points in a light wave having the same phase defines the wavelength λ. The unit of measure of the wavelength is the nanometer (nm), which is equal to 10^{-9} m. Units such as the Angstrom (Å), micron (μm), and millimicron (mμ), which have been used in the past to designate wavelength will be converted to nanometers. For conversion purposes, 10 Å equals 1 nm, 1 mm equals 10^3 nm, and 1 micron (μm) equals 1 nm $\times$ 10^3.

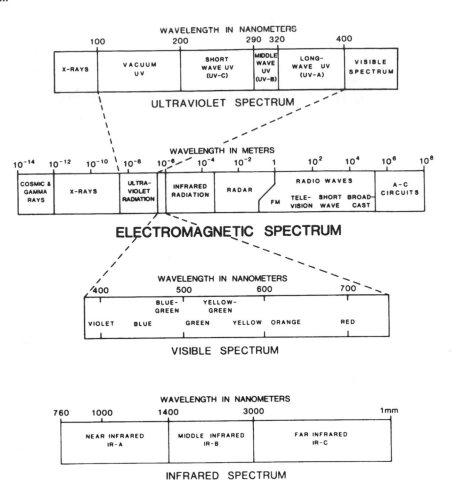

FIGURE 4-1
The electromagnetic spectrum. The integers above the EMS represent the wavelength in meters (m). The widths for each part of the EMS are proportional to their wavebands. The optical spectrum consisting of the UV, VIS, and IR spectra are expanded to present more detail.

Frequency (ν) and wavenumber (ν') are also used to designate certain portions of the EMS, and it may be convenient to relate them to the wavelength. The wavelength λ is equal to the velocity of radiant energy in a vacuum c divided by the frequency ν, or $\lambda = c/\nu$. Therefore, the frequency may be calculated when the wavelength and velocity of the radiation are known. The wave number ν' is the frequency divided by the velocity of radiant energy in a vacuum, or $\nu' = \nu/c$, and its unit is the reciprocal centimeter (cm^{-1}).

Cosmic radiation includes the wavelength range from 10^{-14} to 10^{-12} m. Cosmic radiation is encountered in space, and this region of the EMS will be considered briefly in the chapter on ionizing radiation. X-rays extend from 10^{-8} to about 10^{-9} m, and the discussion covering X-rays will emphasize their effects on the retina and lens.

Ultraviolet radiation (UVR) (100–380 nm), visible radiation (VIS) (380–760 nm), and infrared radiation (IR) (760–10^6 nm) constitute the optical spectrum. UVR between 315 and 380 nm is known as UVA or the near UV, UVR that lies between 290 nm and 315 nm is called UVB or middle wave UV, whereas UVC or the far UV lies between 290 nm and 200 nm. UVR possessing wavelengths shorter than 190 nm exists only in a vacuum and is not naturally found on Earth; in fact, 288 nm is the lower limit of UVR that reaches Earth.

The division of the UV portion of the optical spectrum is based roughly on its photobiologic action. The radiations in the UVC and UVB regions are most effective in producing photokeratitis. UVB produces corneal damage to the epithelium, stroma, and endothelium but, more importantly, this waveband is involved in the production of lenticular opacities (cataracts) after moderate acute and chronic exposures. The UVA waveband requires massive radiant exposures to produce damage to the cornea and lens of the eye, but can easily damage the retina. The process by which UVR damages biologic tissue is primarily photochemical, but there is some evidence that UVR at 350 nm and above produces thermal damage.

The VIS spectrum is commonly referred to as light and extends from about 380 to 760 nm. The VIS spectrum is efficient in exciting the visual pigments in the photoreceptors and is responsible for initiating vision. When sufficiently intense, the VIS spectrum can result in retinal damage. The process of ocular damage from the VIS spectrum was thought to be thermal in nature but has been shown to be partially photochemical.

The IR portion of the spectrum begins at about 760 nm and extends to 10^6 nm or 1 mm. The IR spectrum has been divided by the Commission Internationale de l'Eclairage (CIE) into IRA (760–1400 nm); IRB (1400 nm [1.4 μm] to 3000 nm [3 μm]); and IRC (3000 nm [3 μm] to 1,000,000 nm [1 μm]). The MW and RF portions of the EMS are described by their frequency instead of their wavelength. The overall RF and MW band is divided into six bands:

Frequency Band	Wavelength	Frequency Designation
Radio Frequency (RF)		
300–3000 KHz	1 km–100 m	Medium frequency (MF)
3–30 MHz	100 m–10 m	High frequency (HF)
30–300 MHz	10 m–1 m	Very high frequency (VHF)
Microwave Frequency (MW)		
300–3000 MHz	1 m–10 cm	Ultra-high frequency (UHF)
3–30 GHz	10 cm–1 cm	Super-high frequency (SHF)
30–300 GHz	1 cm–1 mm	Extremely-high frequency (EHF)

In industry, many operations use 6- to 38-MHz frequencies for plastic sealers and 18- to 31-MHz frequencies for dielectric sealers and heaters. Ultrasound in the 3- to 20-MHz frequency range is used clinically to measure the optical constants such as the axial length to localize intraocular foreign bodies, and to diagnose different pathologic conditions such

as ocular and orbital tumors. MW and RF damage biologic tissue by the process of heat.

As the frequency of the EMS increases from the long wavelength radio waves to the short wavelength cosmic rays, the energy associated with each photon or quantum particle increases. A photon or quantum of cosmic radiation possesses more energy than a quantum of the long radio waves. A quantum of UVR possesses more energy than a quantum of the VIS or IR spectra. The frequency of the EMS varies from 10^{22} Hz in the cosmic rays to 1.5×10^4 Hz in the long radio waves. There is a relationship between the wavelength λ, the velocity c, and the frequency ν of the EMS and, interestingly, these quantities can be measured. The quantities are related by the formula

$$c = \nu\lambda \text{ and } \nu = \frac{c}{\lambda} \qquad (4\text{-}1)$$

where c is the velocity of light (2.989×10^8 m/s), ν the frequency of light (Hz), and λ the wavelength of light (nm). The quantum energy of a photon may be calculated by $\varepsilon = h\nu$ and $\varepsilon = hc/\lambda$, where ε is the quantum, h the Planck's constant (6.547×10^{-34} J/s), and c the velocity of light. As energy from the optical radiations is incident on and is absorbed by solid materials, including biologic cells, changes occur at the molecular or atomic level.

Molecular and Ocular Damage

Radiation is essential for vision. However, too much radiation, or radiant energy, can damage the cornea, lens, and retina. To understand how radiation can damage the eye certain basic physical principles need to be reviewed including Einstein's relation, the Grotthus-Draper law, and power density. The atomic theory of Bohr and Einstein's relation can be used to explain these phenomena. Einstein's relation mathematically describes the energy necessary to cause an electron to be displaced:

$$E_k = h\nu - E_o \qquad (4\text{-}2)$$

where E_k is the kinetic energy possessed by an electron that leaves the material and E_o is the work function or energy required to free an electron from a solid material. The electron volt (eV) is the energy acquired by an electron when it is accelerated by a potential difference of 1V, and the eV = 1.602×10^{-12} J. When $E_o = eV$ and if λ is in nanometers then

$$E = \frac{1240}{\lambda[nm]} \text{ [eV]}$$

$$\text{and } E_o = eV \cdot 1.602 \times 10^{-19} \text{ J} \qquad (4\text{-}3)$$

$$\text{or } \lambda \text{ [nm]} = \frac{1240}{E[eV]}$$

The importance of Einstein's relation is that the energy of eV can be calculated when the wavelength of the absorbed radiation is known (Table 4-1).

Radiation must be absorbed by a molecule before a biologic effect may be observed (Grotthus-Draper law), and the absorption spectrum and photochemical properties are specific for a given molecule. The capture of a photon is required for the activation of a photochemical reaction, but not all absorptions result in a photochemical change because a number of mechanisms are available to the molecule to dissipate the energy from the excited electronic state back to the ground or preabsorption state. These mechanisms include fluorescence, phosphorescence, and nonradiative de-excitation.

Photochemical changes ordinarily result from the molecular absorption of a single quantum or photon of radiant energy. The photochemical change results from excitation when the absorbed energy achieves the required activation energy, which ranges from a few kilocalories (Kcal) to more than 100 Kcal. The

UV and VIS spectra are in the photon energy range that produces photochemical reactions. The absorption of UVR may inactivate enzymes or produce alterations in proteins in numerous biologic systems, but especially in the eye. Deoxyribonucleic acid (DNA) may be photochemically altered, and its repair process may be either normal or abnormal. Abnormal repair usually results in abnormal replication patterns in certain cells.

As an illustration of the precise nature of the photochemical reaction consider the following. When a molecule is exposed to energies in the 0.01- to 1-eV range, rotational and vibrational changes are induced in the molecule, causing a thermal effect. Absorption of photons with an energy level from 1 to 4 eV, found in the UV and VIS spectra of solar radiation, induces changes in the electrons of the molecule, i.e., results in a photochemical reaction. At 3.1 eV, the carbon-nitrogen bond is broken, whereas at 4.3 eV there is a disruption of the carbon-hydrogen double bond. The double carbon-carbon bond requires 6.3 eV for breakage, and the carbon-oxygen double bond requires 7.6 eV. These data demonstrate that there is a very precise cellular response to the absorption of radiant energy, and Table 4-1 allows determination of the approximate wavelength required to achieve the necessary eV levels. By understanding how molecular damage occurs, the clinician can appreciate and better explain the need for eye protection.

Absorption of energy results in the excitation of the electrons in the outer rings from a lower energy state to a higher energy state. The *singlet state* is achieved when a molecule that has an even number of electrons in its outer ring has the electrons all arranged in pairs with opposite spins. The *triplet state* describes a molecule that has an even number of electron pairs in its outer ring in which one pair has parallel spin. A molecule that has an odd number of electrons in the outer ring and, consequently, at least one electron with an unpaired spin is called a *radical*. If a molecule were excited to the singlet state, it retains its original electron spin and may return to the ground state. This reaction occurs in 10^{-9} s and the return to ground state is usually through fluorescence but may be through de-excitation. The electron spin may reach an excited metastable state (the triple state), which lasts as long as 10^{-4} to 10^{-1}s and results in phosphorescence when it returns to the ground state. These types of responses take place

Wavelength (nm)	Energy (eV)	Wavelength (nm)	Energy (eV)
100	12.40	700	1.77
200	6.2	800	1.55
300	4.1	1000	1.24
400	3.1	1400	0.88
500	2.48	1500	0.82
600	2.06	3000	0.41

See text for the levels of eV required to result in changes of biologic tissue.

TABLE 4-1
The eV and Kcal/mole Energy levels for Selected Wavelengths in the Optical Radiation Portion of the EMS

in the eye from exposure to the UVR contained in sunlight and may cause retinal damage, cataracts, and corneal damage.

The radiation from the EMS consists of waves of electric and magnetic fields oscillating in phase that are perpendicular to each other and to their direction of propagation. The symbol for the electric field is $[\overline{E}]$, and its unit is volt/meter [V/m], whereas the magnetic field symbol is $[\overline{H}]$, and its unit is the ampere/meter [A/m]. The $\overline{E}$ and $\overline{H}$ fields are vectors specified by both their magnitude and their direction of propagation. The electromagnetic waves travel in air at the velocity c or at a speed of 2.989×10^8 m/s, and the waves carry energy through space perpendicular to the direction of propagation. The power density of this energy is a vector product of $\overline{E}$ and $\overline{H}$: $P_d = \overline{EH}$ in [mW/cm^2] or W/m^2. One W/m^2 is equivalent to 1 mW/cm^2.

The power density P_d varies with the electric and magnetic properties of the medium through which it passes. The dielectric properties of a biologic system are very complicated and change at each interface between the different tissues. In spite of these difficulties, general guidelines can be established that describe the interaction of the EMS with the eye, other biologic systems, and matter:

1. *High Energy Photons* including frequencies greater than 10^{15} Hz that correspond to the gamma rays, X-rays, and UVR are called ionizing because they create ions by removing one or more orbital electrons from the atom or molecule. The negatively charged electron and positively charged ion may damage nearby molecules such as DNA, ribonucleic acid (RNA), and essential enzymes.

2. *Medium Energy Photons* include the VIS spectrum and IR. They add energy to the rotational and vibrational motion of the molecules and may cause small changes in the shapes of molecules. An example is that light strikes the rhodopsin molecule and causes a rotational change of the visual pigment, which initiates the visual stimulus.

3. *Low Energy Photons*, which include RF and MW, do not disrupt the electron structure of atoms, and many photons must be absorbed in order to produce an observable effect. These effects are usually expressed as an increase in temperature due to the vibrational motion induced by the absorption of energy.

The interactions of the EMS with matter are described by the measurement of the electric $\overline{E}$ and magnetic $\overline{H}$ fields, which are then empirically related to their effects on matter. The $\overline{E}$ field can free an ion or induce an asymmetric charge distribution on a molecule, which may be transient or permanent. The magnetic field $\overline{H}$ is defined in terms of its effect in rotating a permanent magnet dipole or in moving a charge that is perpendicular to the motion of the magnetic wave. The effects of the magnetic field $\overline{H}$ have been shown recently to have some effect on biologic systems, but the data are scanty.

Radiation Sources

There are a number of radiation sources that are used for medical, industrial, or lighting applications. Table 4-2 provides a listing of typical sources by frequency range, wavelength range, photon energy range, and the type of radiation.[1] The spectral irradiance of commercially available light sources for wavebands extending from the UV to the IR is presented in Table 4-3. To understand the theoretic as well as the practical aspects of radiation sources, it is necessary to understand the blackbody radiators and the laws that govern this theoretic constructs as well as the nonfull greybody radiators. (The various commonly used light sources will be described in Chapter 5, Basic Concepts in Environmental Lighting.) A more detailed look at the sun will provide a better appreciation of sunlight and allow the use of solar spectral irradiance in the evaluation of the danger of exposures to the eye. Finally, the radiometric measurement of radiant energy shall be incorporated into the realm of vision and photometry. The reader should then be able to manipulate radiometric measurements of various sources to determine their hazard and the protection necessary for our most precious sense, vision.

THEORETIC SOURCES
BLACKBODY RADIATORS. The distribution of energy in the EMS emitted by a hot body depends on the nature of the body. One may consider a theoretic body for which the radiation is only a function of temperature T and certain constants that are independent of the material from which the theoretic

TYPE OF RADIATION*	Frequency (Hz)	Wavelength Range	Photon Energy Range	Typical Sources
IONIZING	3×10^{21} to 3×10^{15}	10^{-4} nm to 100 nm	12.4 eV $\times 10^6$ to 12.4 eV	Linear accelerators, nuclear power plants, sun, radium, uranium, roentgen tubes.
ULTRAVIOLET [UV]				
UV-C	3×10^{15} to 1.03×10^{15}	100 nm to 290 nm	12.4 eV to 4.3 eV	Sunlight, electric arc welding, lasers, high pressure lamps, electron phosphor tubes
UV-B	1.03×10^{15} to 9.4×10^{14}	290 nm to 320 nm	4.3 eV to 3.9 eV	
UV-A	9.4×10^{14} to 7.5×10^{14}	320 nm to 400 nm	3.9 eV to 3.1 eV	
VISIBLE [VIS]	7.5×10^{14} to 3.9×10^{14}	400 nm to 760 nm	3.1 eV to 1.8 eV	Sunlight, tungsten lamps, fluorescent lamps, arc welding, gas welding, electron-phosphor tubes
INFRARED [IR]				
IR-A	3.9×10^{14} to 2.1×10^{14}	760 nm to 1400 nm	1.8 eV to 0.88 eV	Welding, hot bodies, thermal lamps, steel processing, furnaces, high pressure arc lamps
IR-B	2.1×10^{10} to 1.0×10^{14}	1400 nm to 3000 nm	0.88 eV to 0.41 eV	
IR-C	1.0×10^{14} to 3×10^{11}	3000 nm to 1 mm	0.41 eV to 1.2 meV	
MICROWAVES [MW]	3×10^{11} to 3×10^{8}	1 mm to 1 m	1.2 meV to 1.2 µeV	Klystron and magnetron tubes
RADIOFREQUENCIES [RF]	3×10^{8} to 3×10^{5}	1 m to 1 km	1.2 µeV to 1.2 neV	Radio transmissions, tuned circuits

*The divisions for the types of radiation are somewhat arbitrary but attempt to follow the CIE recommendations. For example, the UV divisions are based on the response of the eye to exposure but closely correspond to the CIE System.
(Adapted from Moss CH, Ellis RJ, Parr WH, Murray WE. Biological Effects of Infrared Radiation. DHHS (NIOSH) Publication No. 82–109. Washington, DC, Department of Health & Human Services, 1982.)

TABLE 4-2
Sources and Characteristics of Electromagnetic Radiations

TABLE 4-3
Spectral Irradiance [W/cm²] of Various Light Sources for Different Wavebands of the Electromagnetic Spectrum

LAMP Ordering Abbreviation		Color Temp	Initial Lumens	UV-C 200–240	UV-C 240–260	UV-C 260–280	UV-C TOTAL WATTS	UV-B 280–290	UV-B 290–300	UV-B 300–310	UV-B 310–320	UV-B TOTAL WATTS	UV-A 320–340	UV-A 340–360	UV-A 360–380	UV-A 380–400	UV-A TOTAL WATTS	Visible 400–500	Visible 500–600	Visible 600–700	Visible TOTAL WATTS
Filament																					
656	120V	2400°K	44	–	–	–	–	–	–	–	–	–	–	–	–	–	–	.014	.048	.120	.18
25A	120V	2560°K	256	–	–	–	–	–	–	.001	.002	.003	.001	.002	.003	.006	.012	.100	.330	.634	1.10
60A	120V	2820°K	855	–	–	–	–	–	–	.001	.004	.005	.006	.011	.017	.028	.062	.389	1.090	1.970	3.40
100A	120V	2900°K	1,750	–	–	–	–	–	.001	.003	.004	.008	.014	.025	.041	.062	.132	.843	2.240	3.860	6.90
500	120V	3000°K	10,500	–	–	–	–	–	.010	.024	.033	.067	.106	.180	.284	.424	.994	5.450	13.500	22.300	41.30
1500	120V	3050°K	33,000	–	–	–	–	–	.034	.084	.116	.234	.367	.615	.963	1.480	3.360	17.800	42.700	68.800	129.00
5MC64/7	120V	3200°K	141,000	–	–	–	–	–	.210	.501	.693	1.400	2.080	3.340	5.050	7.220	17.700	83.500	184.000	280.000	547.00
5MC64/3	120V	3350°K	165,000	–	–	–	–	–	.340	.797	1.060	2.190	3.120	4.760	7.080	9.930	24.900	106.000	217.000	313.000	636.00
Q6.6T4/1CL	200W	3050°K	4,450	–	.002	.006	.008	.005	.008	.011	.015	.039	.048	.082	.126	.187	.443	2.370	5.670	9.180	17.20
Q500T3/Cl	120V	3000°K	10,500	–	.004	.012	.016	.011	.016	.024	.033	.084	.105	.184	.288	.404	.981	5.480	13.500	22.900	41.90
Q1000T3/CL	240V	3200°K	20,850	–	.018	.054	.072	.048	.069	.096	.130	.343	.396	.639	.967	1.380	3.380	16.000	35.200	53.500	105.00
250A21/60	120V	3100°K	.070	–	–	–	–	–	–	.002	.007	.009	.039	.096	.160	.187	.482	.164	.000	2.620	2.80
Fluorescent																					
F40CW			3,200	–	–	–	–	–	–	–	.058	.058	.006	.019	.167	.128	.320	2.710	4.510	1.950	9.21
F40CWX			2,230	–	–	–	–	–	–	–	.038	.038	.007	.011	.127	.036	.180	2.010	3.030	2.800	7.83
F40WW			3,250	–	–	–	–	–	–	–	.058	.058	.010	.010	.150	.062	.232	1.690	4.480	2.570	8.74
F40WWX			2,180	–	–	–	–	–	–	.002	.028	.030	.011	.013	.116	.059	.199	1.200	2.810	3.410	7.42
F40D			2,660	–	–	–	–	–	–	.002	.048	.050	.011	.024	.186	.210	.431	3.820	3.860	1.390	9.06
F40SW/N			2,200	–	–	–	–	–	–	.002	.060	.062	.008	.015	.124	.085	.232	1.860	2.760	2.940	7.55
F40SGN			2,450	–	–	–	–	–	–	–	.059	.059	.007	.020	.154	.127	.308	2.810	3.420	2.190	8.42
F40DB			450	–	–	–	–	–	–	–	–	–	.002	.005	.050	.113	.170	1.500	.726	.106	2.33
F40B			1,160	–	–	–	–	–	–	–	.008	.008	.005	.071	.278	.436	.790	4.480	1.740	.246	6.47
F40C			4,350	–	–	–	–	–	–	–	.032	.032	.014	–	.081	–	.095	.792	7.920	.207	8.92
F40CC			2,850	–	–	–	–	–	–	–	.020	.020	.002	.001	.033	.054	.090	2.800	4.060	.990	7.85
F40VG			2,500	–	–	–	–	–	–	.028	.028	.028	.008	.010	.112	.045	.175	.740	3.640	2.800	7.18
F40GO			2,400	–	–	–	–	–	–	–	–	–	–	–	–	–	–	–	3.220	2.050	5.27
F40PK			1,160	–	–	–	–	–	–	–	.034	.034	.005	.002	.066	.005	.078	.535	1.150	3.070	4.77
F40R			200	–	–	–	–	–	–	–	–	–	–	–	–	–	–	–	.002	1.660	1.67
F40BL				–	–	–	–	–	–	.090	.235	.325	1.410	1.910	2.310	1.680	7.310	2.300	.340	–	2.64
F40BLB				–	–	–	–	–	–	.010	.095	.105	1.180	2.790	1.800	.420	6.190	.158	–	–	.16

	LAMP			UV-C Nanometers				UV-B Nanometers					UV-A Nanometers					Visible Nanometers			
Ordering Abbreviation	Color Temp	Initial Lumens	200–240	240–260	260–280	TOTAL WATTS	280–290	290–300	300–310	310–320	TOTAL WATTS	320–340	340–360	360–380	380–400	TOTAL WATTS	400–500	500–600	600–700	TOTAL WATTS
High Intensity Arcs																				
H85A3/UV		3,000	.204	.708	1.250	2.170	.126	.378	.405	1.080	1.990	.420	.195	2.150	.141	2.910	4.190	4.510	.564	9.26
H85A3		3,000	–	–	–	–	–	–	.006	.057	.063	.117	.120	1.760	.126	2.120	3.950	4.500	.537	8.99
MV400*		31,500	–	–	–	–	–	–	*	*	*	*	*	*	*	*	26.200	50.300	12.100	88.70
LU400*		42,000	–	–	–	–	–	–	*	*	*	*	*	*	*	*	10.300	55.300	39.600	105.00
H400A33-1		20,500	–	–	–	–	–	–	.350	1.190	1.540	2.070	1.190	16.300	.880	20.500	22.200	31.600	1.780	55.70
H400C33-1		20,000	–	–	–	–	–	–	–	.140	.140	.300	.360	6.560	.360	7.580	11.600	28.400	18.300	58.40
H400DX33-1		21,000	–	–	–	–	–	–	–	–	–	–	–	–	–	–	16.300	26.100	14.700	57.00
H400W33-1		22,000	–	–	–	–	–	–	.176	.880	1.060	1.120	.814	10.400	.770	13.100	17.200	33.600	8.270	59.00
H400R33-1		18,000	–	–	–	–	–	–	.018	.072	.090	.648	.666	9.140	.810	11.300	16.000	27.600	3.080	46.70
H400RC33-1		20,500	–	–	–	–	–	–	–	.184	.184	.676	.697	8.140	.144	9.660	14.000	29.500	18.900	62.50
H400RW33-1		22,000	–	–	–	–	–	.040	.440	2.020	2.460	2.110	.946	11.200	.616	14.900	16.900	32.700	7.810	57.50
H400Y33-1		12,000	–	–	–	–	–	–	–	–	–	–	–	.080	–	.080	.720	15.700	19.400	35.80
H1000A36-15		44,450	–	–	–	–	–	–	1.400	10.060	11.500	8.290	4.030	51.600	2.070	66.000	59.800	84.700	6.720	151.00
H1000C36-15		54,000	–	–	–	–	–	–	.030	.419	.450	.975	1.170	19.600	1.690	23.400	31.500	78.400	53.800	164.00
H1000W36-15		60,500	–	–	–	–	–	–	.400	2.350	2.790	4.920	4.550	36.100	2.900	48.500	46.600	91.300	24.600	163.00
H1000RC36-15		55,000	–	–	–	–	–	–	.165	.935	1.100	3.140	3.030	21.700	2.480	30.400	44.500	81.600	32.000	158.00
H1000RW36-15		58,000	–	–	–	–	–	–	.406	2.610	3.020	4.230	2.900	22.700	1.680	31.600	44.400	88.700	20.100	153.00
BH6		60,000	2.710	10.800	13.300	26.800	13.200	16.300	14.300	18.600	62.400	24.700	15.300	45.700	15.300	101.000	109.000	89.400	19.100	218.00
Germicidal																				
G30T6		220	–	13.110	.020	13.100	.020	.050	.030	.200	.300	.020	.020	.200	.010	.250	.600	.340	–	.94
G30T8		230	–	8.340	.010	8.350	.020	.030	.020	.160	.230	.010	.010	.170	.010	.200	.660	.330	–	.99
Sunlamp																				
RS		2,500	–	–	.004	.004	.050	.130	.340	.880	1.400	.230	.140	2.570	.130	3.070	2.440	4.160	.430	7.03
Photochemical																				
250UA-2		6,800	1.000	4.200	2.360	7.560	1.820	1.280	2.460	4.430	9.990	.890	.370	7.250	.280	8.790	6.640	10.600	.470	17.70
360UA-3		9,000	1.630	5.460	3.270	10.400	1.840	1.760	3.260	6.860	13.700	.970	.470	10.000	.750	12.200	10.500	13.800	.390	24.70
1200UA-11		49,600	8.080	41.100	22.400	71.600	16.700	12.700	24.100	46.800	100.000	8.250	3.440	68.600	2.660	83.000	49.900	76.900	2.440	129.00
1200UA-11B		45,500	–	.720	.910	1.630	2.630	4.030	9.320	22.800	38.800	5.540	2.570	54.600	2.670	65.300	49.400	77.300	2.850	130.00
3000UA-37		129,000	33.600	141.000	77.800	252.000	43.300	39.400	67.000	129.000	279.000	28.000	12.900	203.000	6.760	252.000	140.000	200.000	7.700	347
3000UA-9		120,000	–	–	–	–	–	.090	.370	1.660	2.120	2.010	2.140	73.900	3.950	82.000	130.000	187.000	6.990	323.00
H12T3		30,000	–	9.300	5.700	15.000	8.400	6.900	13.200	24.900	53.400	4.500	1.800	36.300	1.800	44.400	33.600	48.300	–	81.90
XE5000		275,000	–	19.500	25.000	44.600	13.800	16.500	18.200	20.000	68.500	43.700	49.000	56.700	65.500	215.000	408.000	337.000	320.000	1070.00

There is a 10 nm wavelength interval for the UVB, a 20 nm wavelength interval for the UVC and UVA and a 100 nm wavelength interval for the VIS spectrum. * UV data not available at this time.
From General Electric Corporation, Nela Park, Cleveland, Ohio, with permission.

TABLE 4-3
Spectral Irradiance [W/cm²] of Various Light Sources for Different Wavebands of the Electromagnetic Spectrum, continued

body is constructed. Such a theoretic body is available and is known as a blackbody radiator (it is also called a full radiator, Plankerian radiator, or cavity radiator). These terms describe a large body that completely encloses a hollow cavity. The cavity possesses a channel with a small opening to the exterior through which radiation is emitted. The smaller the opening compared to the size of the blackbody radiator, the more closely will be the radiator's approximation to a *true* blackbody. The full radiator is an important source of radiant energy because it obeys the laws of thermodynamics.

Planck demonstrated that the spectral radiant emittance $M_{e\lambda}$ of a full radiator should obey the following equation:

$$M_{e\lambda} = \frac{C_1{}^{\lambda-5}}{[e^{C_2/\lambda T}]} - 1 \qquad (4\text{-}4)$$

where $M_{e\lambda}$ is the spectral radiant emittance [W/cm^2-μm·sr], T the temperature [K], e the natural log, C_1 the constant 37,400 calculated from C1 = $2\pi C^2 h$, C_2 the constant 14,380 (International, 1948), and h Planck's constant (6.547×10^{-34} J/s).

When the wavelength is measured in micrometers, the spectral radiant emittance $M_{e\lambda}$ becomes W/cm^2-μm, and Planck's equation agrees remarkably well with experimental results. Figure 4-2 illustrates that the spectral radiant emittance $M_{e\lambda}$ of a full radiator increases as the absolute temperature increases.[2]

Stefan, using the laws of thermodynamics, reported that the total radiant emittance M_e per unit area of the blackbody was proportional to the fourth power of the absolute temperature. This concept has become known as the Stefan-Boltzmann law and is expressed mathematically:

$$M_e = \int_0^\infty M_{e\lambda}\Delta\lambda = \sigma T^4 [\text{W/cm}^2] \qquad (4\text{-}5)$$

where M_e is the total radiance emittance [W/cm^2], $M_{e\lambda}$ the spectral radiant emittance [W/cm$^2 \cdot$ μm], and T the absolute temperature; σ is calculated from $(C_1/15) (\pi/C_2)_4 = 5.68 \times 10^{12}$ W/cm2, with C_1 = 37,400 and C_2 = 14,380. The Stefan-Boltzmann Law indicates that each square centimeter of a blackbody at 1000 [K] radiates 5.68 W/cm^2.

As the temperature of a blackbody is raised, there is a shift or displacement of the wavelength (Fig. 4-2), at which the maximum emittance of the spectral energy occurs. Wien's Displacement Law states that

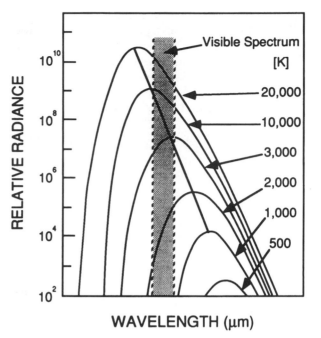

FIGURE 4-2
The effect of absolute temperature on the relative radiance and wavelength of a blackbody. There is an increase in total radiance, peak radiance, and peak of the wavelength as the temperture increases. The λmax, which is represented by the straight line drawn through the peaks, illustrates the shift from long wavelength to shorter wavelengths as the temperature increases. Vision and Visual Perception. From Riggs LA: Light as a stimulus for vision. In Graham CH (ed): 1966; with permission.

maximum spectral energy of a blackbody occurs at a wavelength (λ_{max}) that varies inversely as the absolute temperature of the blackbody:

$$\lambda_{max} = \frac{C_2}{T \cdot 4.9651} \qquad (4\text{-}6)$$

or

$$\lambda_{max} = 2898/T \qquad (4\text{-}7)$$

when λ max is in micrometers (μm) and the constant C_2 is 14,380. Figure 4-2 also illustrates that as the absolute temperature of the blackbody increases there is a shift in source radiant emittance to the shorter wavelengths. The λ_{max} wavelength does not occur in the VIS spectrum until the temperature of the body reaches 4000 [K].

The intensity of radiation per unit solid angle reflected from a diffusing surface varies with the cosine θ of the angle of incidence, measured from the normal to the surface and has been called Lambert's Cosine Law. It is also known that radiation varies as the square of the distance from the source—the inverse square law. Combining the two mathematically

$$E = \frac{I \cos \theta}{d^2} \qquad (4\text{-}8)$$

where E is the irradiance or illuminance of the source, I the radiant or luminous intensity of the source, θ the angle of incidence of the beam measured from the normal to the surface, and d the distance from the source. Actually, Lambert's law applies only to perfect emitters and perfect diffusers where the spectral emittance is independent of the direction of view. The full radiator or blackbody that emits the same radiance or luminance in all directions for each wavelength of the spectrum is said to be a Lambertian surface.

The Planckian radiator is a special case of a nonselective radiator that possesses a spectral radiation factor or a spectral emissivity factor of α = 1 for all wavelengths. Spectral radiance L_e is given by

$$L_{e\lambda} = \frac{1}{\pi} M_{e\lambda} \qquad (4\text{-}9)$$

where $L_{e\lambda}$ is the spectral radiance and $M_{e\lambda}$ is the spectral radiant emittance.

NONFULL RADIATORS (GREYBODY RADIATORS). Nonfull radiators are radiators with an emissivity factor α less than unity. The spectral radiance $L'_{e\lambda}$ of an actual greybody (e.g., tungsten) emitting only thermal radiation is always lower than the spectral radiance $L_{e\lambda}$ of a full radiator (Fig. 4-3) by the spectral emissivity factor α_λ:

$$L'_{e\lambda} = \alpha_\lambda L_{e\lambda} \qquad (4\text{-}10)$$

The spectral emissivity α_λ is a function of wavelength λ, temperature T, the direction of view θ, and is always less than unity. For a diffuse reflector, a portion of the incident radiation is absorbed and transformed into heat while the rest of the radiation is emitted diffusely according to Lambert's law. Lambert's law states that radiance L_e is independent of θ when the body is a perfect diffuser or blackbody radiator. The symbol ρ is called the diffuse reflection

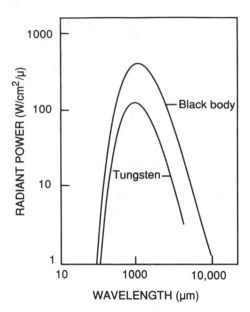

FIGURE 4-3
Comparison of the radiant power of a blackbody source and a greybody tungsten source. From Riggs LA: Light as a stimulus for vision. In Graham CH (2d): Vision and Visual Perception. New York, John Wiley and Sons.

factor and $\rho_\lambda = 1 - \alpha_\lambda$. For the full radiator, α = 1 and ρ = 0; i.e., the spectral emissivity of all wavelengths is equal, making the body a perfect radiator. For the perfect diffuser, α = 0 and ρ = 1 because all wavelengths are reflected and the thermal radiation of a perfect diffuser is zero.

It should now be clear why a blackbody made of any substance and having a small opening on its surface is a full radiator. The radiance of the hole is partly due to the radiation emitted by the element of the surface that is seen through the hole, while the diffusely reflected radiance is added to this element from other parts of the cavity.

If radiance $L_{e\lambda}$ from a single reflection = $\rho^1_\lambda L_{e\lambda}$, two reflections = $\rho^2_\lambda L_{e\lambda}$, three reflections = ρ^3_λ $L_{e\lambda}$, and for n reflections $\rho^n_\lambda L_{e\lambda}$, the total spectral radiance of the body would be

$$L'_{e\lambda} (1 + \rho_\lambda + \rho^2_\lambda + \rho^3_\lambda + \rho^n_\lambda) =$$
$$\frac{L'_{e\lambda}}{1-\rho_\lambda} = \frac{L'_{e\lambda}}{\alpha_\lambda} = L'_{e\lambda} \qquad (4\text{-}11)$$

which is the spectral radiance of the blackbody because $\alpha_\lambda = 1$. The laws of radiation for the greybody are the same as for the full radiator except that all energies are reduced by α_λ, the spectral emissivity factor. Based on this theory, we may now have a better understanding of manmade and natural sources.

STANDARD SOURCES

The ability to measure accurately the quantity of a physical or visual unit implies that the measurement is based on absolute standards or secondary standards traceable to the absolute standard. Because the performance of blackbody radiators can be predicted from fundamental physical properties of temperature and length (wavelength), the blackbody has become the standard source for radiant power or radiant flux. The blackbody can be duplicated in any desired location and is used to ensure that scientists are maintaining accurate procedures in measurement. Greybody sources can be compared with blackbodies in regions of spectral overlap and become an easily transportable secondary standard source. A second method of maintaining accuracy in measurements is to calibrate a detector against the blackbody radiator and to use it as a "standard detector" in measuring other sources.

In the United States, the National Bureau of Standards (NBS) develops standard sources, calibrates sources to be used as the comparison standard in the laboratory, and performs intercomparison measurements between standard sources and detectors. The NBS uses the two approaches just mentioned in maintaining primary radiometric standards. The NBS uses a blackbody source of accurately known temperature that obeys Planck's law for a primary standard. In addition, the NBS uses a self-calibrating or absolute receiver with nonselective spectral characteristics and with an absorptivity as close to unity as possible for measurements.

The NBS maintains several standard blackbody sources for purchase and use by scientists in optical radiation measurements:

- Standard of Thermal Radiation—a carbon filament lamp operated within 0.2% to 0.3% of a known voltage or amperage.
- Standard of Spectral Radiance—a tungsten ribbon-filament lamp that is calibrated for spectral irradiance over the region of 0.25 to 2.6 μm (250 to 2600 nm) with an accuracy of 8% at the shortest and 3% at the longest wavelengths.

- New Standard of Spectral Irradiance—a 200 W, quartz-iodine, coiled-coil tungsten filament operated at about 3000 [K]. Calibration curves for 250 to 2600 nm are provided with the same accuracy as above. More recently, the 200-W source has been extended to 1000 W. Higher radiant emittance allows closer calibration tolerances in the 225- to 2600-nm wavelength range.[3]
- Standard Deuterium Lamp—operates in 200- to 350-nm spectral region.[4]

Standard lamps are in a constant state of development and improvement. For example, the NBS Optical Radiation Section recently announced the availability of a new diagnostic standard for the UVB region (280 to 320 nm) of the spectrum. It is a special 20-W, 24-inch fluorescent lamp termed the B2-fluorescent lamp. Spectral irradiance values are provided in 1-nm wavelength intervals from 275 to 350 nm for a 1 cm^2 area of the lamp, with the measurement being made 50 cm from the lamp. In addition, a high irradiance, stable UVB source based on an argon maxi-arc lamp with irradiances of 8.9 W/cm^2-nm at 280 nm, 10 W/cm^2-nm at 300 nm, and 11 W/cm^2-nm at 320 nm measured in a region of the source 5 cm in diameter at a distance of 50 cm from the light source is available for use in the research laboratory.[5]

MACBETH LAMP

It is often desirable to be able to use readily available materials to approximate the spectral output of natural sunlight, and the MacBeth lamp is a source that accomplishes this goal. The MacBeth lamp is composed of a 500-W coiled tungsten filament lamp filtered by a CS1-62 Corning glass filter and a diffusing glass plate. The correlated color temperatures range from approximately 6800 [K] to 7500 [K] and may be varied by using a rheostat. A correlated color temperature is the chromaticity match of a selective radiator nearest to the chromaticity of a blackbody radiator. The MacBeth lamp is necessary for use in nearly all clinical and industrial chart-type color vision tests, including the pseudoisochromatic plates, and the D-15 and F-100 tests. MacBeth lamps are also excellent sources for industrial inspection processes that require acute color differentiation. A 500-W tungsten source filtered by the Corning CS1-62 filter makes an excellent source for color vision testing and other daylight requirements.

INCANDESCENT FILAMENT LAMPS

The most common form of filament lamp is the tungsten filament lamp, which is a greybody in spectral output with a radiant exitance of less than unity but approximately constant over the VIS spectrum. The light output is very close to the fourth power of the applied voltage (E^4) or to the eighth power of the applied amperage (I^8); therefore, varying the voltage to a tungsten source will change its spectral output.

The form of the filament is governed by its intended use and can be round wire, flat strip, round coil, flat coil, or coil-coiled. The lamp filaments slowly evaporate and condense on the cooler portions of the bulb envelope, causing the envelope to progressively blacken with a subsequent reduction in light output. More recently, iodine or other halogens (Cl, Fl, Br) have been placed inside the envelope, which causes the tungsten evaporated from the filament to migrate back to the filament instead of blackening the envelope. The theory is that the halogen vapor combines with the atoms of the evaporated tungsten to form tungsten halide. Tungsten halide is carried back to the filament where the higher temperature separates the tungsten and halide. The tungsten combines with the filament, and the halogen is set free to repeat the cycle. The advantages are that the envelope can be operated at higher temperatures and the lamp becomes more efficient while maintaining a higher output throughout its life. Halogen regenerative cycle lamps are more compact and usually have twice the life of an ordinary lamp with the same output rating.[6] Their small physical size allows an output that is more uniformly distributed. The higher operating temperature shifts the spectral output to the shorter wavelengths. These characteristics have been used to improve clinical diagnostic instruments, such as ophthalmoscopes and biomicroscopes.

The envelopes of incandescent lamps are usually made from lime glass. When greater resistance to thermal shock is required and the UV portion of the spectrum is desired, quartz is the material choice. The envelopes are filled with argon, nitrogen, or krypton gases. Most lamps use argon because of its low heat conductivity, which in turn results in a lower rate of tungsten evaporation. Often trace parts of nitrogen are used to prevent arcing between the lead-in wires. Krypton gas is heavier than nitrogen or argon and would provide better heat-conducting characteristics, but is too expensive for wide application.

Another characteristic of tungsten lamps is that their performance differs when an AC or DC power source is used. DC power results in a faster than normal migration of the filament to the envelope. This fast evaporation of the filament can be negated by reversing the polarity of the power once or twice a day during use. AC power produces a reduction in the rate of metal migration, but under certain conditions the eye can detect an AC ripple superimposed on the light output.

A special application of the tungsten filament lamp is its use as an IR heat source in the aerospace industry for heat testing, in the automotive and other industries for drying paints, in thermal process photocopy machines, and in radiant heating in certain areas for the comfort of people. IR lamps are tubular in shape, which allows their radiation to be controlled by optical systems, reflectors, prisms, and electrical control systems. The radiant heat is transferred directly from the tungsten source to the product without conduction or convection; consequently, IR lamps have an 87% efficiency when operated at their rated voltage.

FLUORESCENT LAMPS

A fluorescent lamp consists of a tubular, circular, or U-shaped evacuated envelope. The interior of the envelope is coated with a phosphor and contains a small amount of mercury and an inert, low pressure gas of either argon, krypton, or neon. The ends of the envelope contain an electrode, and passage of an electric current between the electrodes results in heat and the release of electrons that travel at high speeds between the electrodes. This causes an electric discharge through the mercury vapor and collisions of the electrode-generated, fast-moving electrons with the mercury atoms and the displacement of electrons of the mercury atoms from their orbits. The electrons of the mercury atom return to their original orbits and release the energy they have absorbed in the form of UVR at 254 nm. The UVR is absorbed by the phosphor and is re-radiated at longer wavelengths in the VIS spectrum that the eye sees as light.

The color of the light depends on the chemical composition of the phosphor material. The spectral output varies with the phosphor and the pressure of the lamp but results in a spectrum of about 2% UV, 23% VIS, 36% IR, and 39% convected and conducted heat (Table 4-3).[6,7]

A special application of the fluorescent concept is the cathode ray tube (CRT) that is used in oscilloscopes, radar, television, and the visual display terminals (VDT) for computer systems. The CRT consists of an evacuated glass envelope with the phosphor coating inside the front surface. The phosphor is activated by a narrow beam of electrons originating from the rear of the CRT. The electron beam activates the phosphor coating, which re-emits various intensities of light. The electron beam can be precisely controlled in position and intensity and can be modulated to produce the myriads of visual patterns that we have become accustomed to in television.

ARC LAMPS

Arc lamps differ from the tungsten and fluorescent lamps in their method of operation. The radiation of the arc lamp is emitted when an electrical discharge passes through air or a pressurized gas. There are three basic types of processes for arc lamps. In the first type, the source of radiation is derived from the crater of the hotter of the two electrodes; an example is the carbon arc lamp. The second type produces radiation essentially from the plasma ball of the ionized high pressure or low pressure gas that is located between the electrode. The last type of arc lamp uses a high frequency oscillatory field to produce radiation from the gas. The modes of operation of arc lamps do not differ materially because an electrical current must pass through the plasma of the gas.

A number of different gases are used, but argon, neon, sodium, mercury, xenon, and metal iodides are most commonly found. The radiant emittance differs spectrally according to the type of gas used in the lamp and the pressure under which the gas is maintained. Mercury produces a continuous spectrum covering the entire optical radiation spectrum but is very rich in UV and has the spectral emission lines of mercury superimposed on the spectral irradiance. Xenon produces a continuous optical spectrum that is richer in IR and is superimposed with xenon emission lines. The emission lines are narrow wavebands that possess a highly peaked, high intensity output. When mercury and xenon are combined, a continuous optical spectrum is obtained with an increased output in the UV waveband and a further increased output in the IR portion of the EMS.

ARC CRATER LAMPS

CARBON ARC.   The carbon arc is normally operated in air, and the arc is located between the two electrodes. The positive carbon electrode burns hotter and provides the main source of radiation. It is difficult to maintain a steady radiant emittance from the plasma ball generated between the two carbon rods because the carbon electrodes are consumed in the process, and care must be taken to maintain a constant distance in the separation of the rods. The radiation produced approximates that of a full radiator at 3800[K] and provides a spectrum containing UV, VIS, and IR radiation.

ARC DISCHARGE LAMPS

The arc discharge lamp falls into four categories: flame arc, low pressure arc, high pressure arc (HID), and electrodeless lamp. The flame arc is an extension of the carbon arc in which different substances in the core of the electrode are evaporated and create additional ions. The flame arc provides the highest luminance of any light source other than the sun. The term *low pressure arc* connotes that the pressure of the gaseous content of the lamp is below atmospheric pressure. The low pressure requires a high RF starting voltage to initially vaporize the gas inside the lamp. The emission of the lamp varies with the gas used in the envelope but consists mainly of spectral emission lines. Consequently, the output is essentially a group of narrow spectral lines that are used in calibrating optical instruments such as monochromators, spectrometers, and so on.

HID lamps are usually compact arc sources with arc lengths from 0.3 to 10 mm in length and with the gas under pressures up to 50 atm. Their output provides a high intensity continuous white spectrum with the lines of the gas superimposed on the spectrum. These HID lamps usually operate from a 30-W to 40-kW DC power supply and require a RF power supply to initiate the ionization of the gas to ignite the source.

A special type of HID lamp source is the metal arc lamp. It is claimed to be the most efficient source of white light in the modern lighting industry. The lamp consists of a central arc tube made from a quartz envelope that contains argon gas, mercury plus thorium iodide, sodium iodide, and scandium iodide. The gases and iodides are responsible for the efficiency and spectral distribution of the lamp. At the ends of the arc tube are the starting electrode and the main thoriated tungsten electrodes. A boro-silicate glass bulb protects the central arc tube and absorbs the UVR. The output varies from 14,000 to 155,000 lumens.

NATURAL SOURCES

THE SUN AS A RADIATION SOURCE.   The sun is such a common experience for each of us that we sometimes fail to appreciate its contribution to our lives and its importance to our environment. Professionals need to understand the characteristics of the sun because all humans are exposed to the sun as a source of radiant energy and the sun remains the most common source of UVR available for human exposure.

As an example of the importance of the sun, the recent changes in the ozone layer and its effect on the UV portion of the solar spectrum have been studied carefully over the past decade. Is this issue a scientific fad or does it have real meaning in our lives? Just as important is the prediction that as the air pollutants, particularly carbon dioxide, drift to the stratosphere, they act as a large lens and an insulator to produce the "greenhouse effect" that is manifest as a warming of the Earth. It has been predicted that during the 1990s, half of the summers would be as hot as the warmest summers of the 1951 to 1980 period. However, atmospheric dust from the eruptions of the volcanoes may alter this prediction.

Let's look at some of the facts regarding the sun. The sun is essentially a sphere of gas around which the Earth and other planets revolve. It is heated by the nuclear reaction derived from its center and provides heat, light, and energy for the entire solar system. The sun has a diameter of 13.84×10^5 km (865,000 miles), a mass of 1.91×10^{27} metric tons (2.1×10^{27} tons), and an average distance from the Earth of about 14.9×10^8 km (93 million miles). Since its axis of rotation is inclined about 7° to the pole of the Earth's orbit, the entire face of the sun can be seen during one rotational period. The period of rotation is a function of latitude, being 26 days at the Earth's equator and 34 days at the Earth's pole, while 27 days is usually taken as the rotational period for predicting effects on Earth.

The equinox is defined by the sun crossing the equator making night and day equal in the length of time. For the northern hemisphere, the spring equinox occurs on March 21 and the fall equinox occurs on September 22–23 each year. The solstice is the

point on the sun's orbit at which it is farthest north or farthest south of the equator. The limit of the northern boundary of the sun is called the Tropic of Cancer, which is located at latitude 23°27′ north of the equator, whereas the limit of the southern journey is the Tropic of Capricorn located at the latitude of 23°27′ south of the equator. These two celestial circles are parallel to the equator and define the region or zone around the Earth known as the Torrid Zone.

There are some interesting relationships between the sun and the eye. The sun subtends an angle of 0.00931 radians (0.53°) or 6.8×10^{-1} steradians at the surface of the Earth. The sun has an irradiance of 726.6 W/m^2 on Earth. The diameter of the sun on the human retina is approximately 159 μm. If we use an integrated ocular transmittance τ of 0.726 for the 300 to 1400-nm wavelength range, the retinal solar irradiance E_{er} is equal to 0.788 W/cm^2.

SOLAR CONSTANT.   The solar constant is defined as the total radiant energy in watts per meter squared received from the sun per unit time, per unit area, normal to the solar disk, at the mean Earth-sun distance in the absence of the Earth's atmosphere, i.e., in space. The value of the solar constant varies approximately 3.5% because of the Earth's elliptic orbit around the sun, and to reduce this variation the calculations are usually related to the mean Earth-sun distance. There are also small variations in the solar constant due to cyclic and sporadic changes in the sun that have not yet been determined. The value of the solar constant varies from 1353 W/m^2 to 1369 W/m^2, with a mean value of 1367 W/m^2 (0.1367 W/cm^2).[8-15] The variability of solar radiation and its use in determining the solar constant over the period of 1969 to 1980 was a low of 1365 W/m^2 with a high of 1369 W/m^2 and a mean of 1367 $W/m^2 \pm 2$ W/m^2, which is equivalent to 1.960 g cal/cm^2 min $\pm$ 0.003.[14,15] A recent report on the variation of the total solar irradiance from 1874 to 1988 suggests that solar irradiance has steadily increased since 1945, but the total temperature increase was only 0.02°C.[16] The NASA/ASTM standard solar constant value of 1353 $\pm$ 2 W/m^2 (1.940 g cal/cm2 min $\pm$ 0.03) was adopted in 1971 and 1974.[17,18] The uncertainty of measurements of the solar constant is on the order of 0.5%; however, it is 1.5% for the NASA/ASTM data. The NASA/ASTM total solar irradiance and spectral irradiance values will be used because they have been established as the standard in the

United States.[13,18] Annual UVR increases dramatically as the equator is approached, and because most of the world's population lives between the 40° to 50° latitudes, the increase becomes important when considering exposure (Fig. 4-4).[19,20] The highest levels of solar UVR fall on Earth during the summer solstice and autumn equinox (Fig. 4-4). People living in the far northern latitudes believe that they do not receive UVR, but the data show about 1.8 sunburn units (SBUs) or nearly 5×10^{-2} J/cm$^2 \cdot$ h of effective UVR in the summer months. Approximately 60% of effective UVR falls on the Earth between the hours of 10:00 a.m. and 2:00 p.m. (Fig. 4-4), and cities in the northern and southern hemispheres receive about the same effective annual UVB exposure when their latitudes do not differ greatly (compare Oakland, California, with Melbourne, Australia) (Table 4-4). The effect of altitude is not fully demonstrated in Table 4-4, because Bismarck, North Dakota at 0.51 km receives slightly more UVB than Davos, Switzerland at 1.58 km. However, Davos experiences many days of cloudiness, whereas Bismarck is located on the sunny plains. El Paso, Texas at 1.14 km and Fort Worth, Texas at 0.25 km clearly show the effect of altitude on the average annual effective radiant exposure at higher altitudes.[21] Of course, when latitude and altitude are combined, the average effective UVB per year at Moana Loa, Hawaii is almost double any other city. It is unfortunate, but the sunny areas of the high desert plateau in the southwestern United States were not included in the survey.

TOTAL SOLAR IRRADIANCE. The *total or global solar* irradiance received on the Earth's surface includes measurements made directly from the solar disk and indirectly from the solar radiation scattered by the atmosphere. The solar irradiance received on Earth by a surface normal to the center of the solar disk is called the *direct solar irradiance*. The solar radiation that reaches the earth and is then scattered by the atmosphere is termed *indirect or diffuse solar irradiance*. Most spectral irradiance values presented in tabular or graphic form are direct solar radiation measurement data for the different air masses of concern.

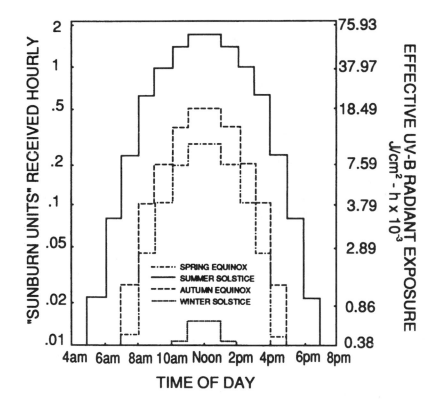

FIGURE 4-4
The effectiveness of sunlight at different times of day incident on a horizontal surface on Earth for the spring and autumn equinox and the summer and winter solstice of the four seasons of the year in northern latitudes. Sunburn units have been converted to effective UVB radiant exposures in J/cm^2-hr using 2500 minimal erythemal doses (MED) per year as the equivalent to 95 J/cm^2-yr. From Diffey BL. Environmental exposure to UV-B radiation. Revue on Environmental Health IV:317–337, 1984; with permission from Freund Publishing House, Ltd.

Location	Average Sunburn Units			Per Day	Per Hour	Annual Effective Radiant Exposure J/cm^2 = yr
	Latitude	Altitude (km)	Per Year			
Mauna Loa, HW	19.5N	3.38	7078	19.4	1.6	268.9
Tallahassee, FL	30.4N	<0.10	3825	10.5	0.9	145.4
El Paso, TX	31.8N	1.14	4889	13.4	1.1	185.8
Fort Worth, TX	32.8N	0.25	3583	9.0	0.8	136.2
Albuquerque, NM	35.0N	1.51	4511	12.4	1.0	171.4
Oakland, CA	37.7N	<0.10	3426	9.4	0.8	130.2
Melbourne, Aus	38.0 S	<0.10	3388	9.3	0.8	128.7
Philadelphia, PA	40.0	<0.10	2441	6.7	0.6	92.8
Honey Brook, PA	40.1N	0.21	2566	7.0	0.6	97.5
Des Moines, IA	41.5N	0.29	2759	7.6	0.5	104.8
Minneapolis, MN	44.9N	0.25	2403	6.6	0.6	91.3
Bismarck, ND	46.8N	0.51	2609	7.1	0.9	99.1
Davos, Switz	46.8N	1.58	2436	6.7	0.6	92.6
Belsk-Duzy, PO	51.8N	<0.10	1521	4.2	0.4	57.8

*Data were converted to radiant exposure in J/cm^2 using data from Scotto et al giving 2500 minimal erythemal doses (MED) per year as the equivalent to 95 J/cm^2 – yr. A MED and a sunburn unit are equivalent. From Diffey, BL: Environmental exposure to UV-B radiation. Revue on Environmental Health IV: 317–337, 1984; with permission from Freund Publishing House, Ltd.

TABLE 4-4
The Average Annual Effective Sunburn Units (SBUs) Received at Different Locations, Latitudes and Altitudes Around the World

It is necessary to know the attenuation of the atmosphere as solar radiation passes through it in order to compute the solar spectral irradiance falling on Earth. Air mass is an optical concept that is determined by the slant path from the sun to Earth. *Air mass* is defined as the ratio of the path length of solar radiation passing through the atmosphere at any specified angle to the path length when the sun is at zenith. Air mass is usually expressed as the secant of the solar angle to the zenith except for zenith angles of 62° or greater. When the sun is directly overhead, it is said to be at its *zenith*, and the angle between the center of the solar disk and the zenith is termed the *zenith angle*. The variations in solar luminance, correlated color temperature, irradiance for different zenith angles, and air masses for the solar disk are shown in Figure 4-5. The illuminance of the direct sunlight, the sky light, and the total sunlight falling on a horizontal surface on Earth for different altitudes above the Earth and for different air masses is

given in Table 4-5.[22] The data show that visible light decreases as the air mass increases and as the sun approaches the horizon.

Atmospheric attenuation increases with contamination such as water vapor, dust, and aerosol particles. Mercherikunnel and Richmond[23] have represented atmospheric attenuation as being due to Rayleigh scattering, turbidity, and the optical depth of ozone. Rayleigh scattering is found when the wavelength is short in comparison to the size of the particles in the atmosphere and causes the blue color of the sky. The optical thickness of Rayleigh scatter varies as λ^4 and has a value of 1.222 at 300 nm and 0.069 at 600 nm. *Turbidity* is the term used to describe the attenuation of solar radiation by atmospheric aerosols. The angstrom turbidity coefficients α and θ are wavelength-dependent and are related to the size distribution and density of the aerosols. The turbidity coefficient θ represents the small particle aerosols and varies in value from 0.02 for a very

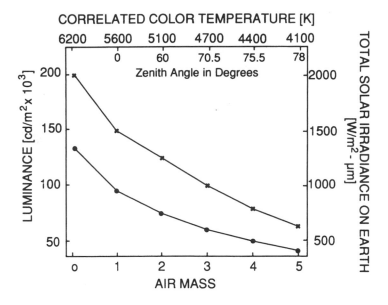

FIGURE 4-5
Relationship between the luminance of the solar disk, air mass, and zenith angle (χ). Changes in the total solar irradiance on Earth normal to the sun's rays (¢) with the change in air mass. Modified from Condron TP, Toolin RB, Stakutis VJ. Visibility, Chap 14. In Campen CF, Jr, Cole AE, Condron TP et al (eds): Handbook of Geophysics for Air Force Designers. Geophysics Res Direct, A.F. Cambridge Research Center, Air Research & Development Command, USAF, 1957.

clear atmosphere to 0.17 for a very turbid atmosphere; thus, higher θ values represent higher turbidity. The α coefficient is a wavelength exponent that is related to large particle aerosols. Its values vary from 0.5 to 2.5, with the larger value representing a smaller than average proportion of large particulate aerosols. The θ turbidity coefficient increases as the turbidity of the atmosphere increases, which should mean that small aerosols are responsible for high turbidity.

Turbidity is often related to air mass because as the air mass increases there is a concomitant increase in turbidity. There is also a greater absorption of UVR and the blue end of the visible spectrum. The larger zenith angle and the subsequent increase in air mass and turbidity at sundown results in the solar disk becoming orange or reddish-orange in appearance. This daily event should serve as a constant reminder that the atmospheric absorption of solar radiation is important in maintaining a balance in the ecology of the environment.

SOLAR SPECTRAL IRRADIANCE.   The solar spectral irradiance is the distribution of the solar constant radiant power as a function of wavelength in the absence of the Earth's atmosphere. The solar spectral irradiance for a solar constant of 1367 W/m^2 has over 96% of the solar spectral irradiance contained in the wavelength range from 270 to 2600 nm, while 49.6% lies in the 400- to 760-nm waveband.[23-27] It is re-

markable that half of the solar radiation is in the wavelength range that serves the human eye for vision, but what happens to the solar radiation as it passes through the atmosphere to Earth?

Absorption in the spectral region below 85 nm is due chiefly to molecular oxygen (O_2), O^-, N_2, and N_3. Between 85 nm and 200 nm, the absorption is principally by atomic oxygen O^-. At an altitude of 100,000 to 30,000 km and below, ozone absorbs all of the remaining solar UVR in the 200- to 288-nm wavelength range. Thus, practically all of the UVR to 288 nm is absorbed by the Earth's atmosphere.[28-31] Small changes in stratospheric O^-, O_2, N, N_2, and ozone (O_3), may result in a very small increase in the total solar energy but a disproportionate increase in the UVR below 340 nm would greatly increase the hazards of UVR.[32] Such an increase would be very dangerous to animal and plant life including humans; e.g., a 1% increase in UVR will result in a 2% increase in skin cancer.[33]

The standard NASA/ASTM solar irradiance for air mass = 0 (outside the Earth's atmosphere), air mass 1, and air mass 2, with their spectral irradiance values on Earth, are presented in Appendix Table 4-6 at the end of this chapter.[18] These data are the solar spectral irradiance measured at the average sun to Earth distance normal to the sun's rays.[23] The data for the 200- to 295-nm waveband in Appendix Table 4-6 were modified from Green et al.[34] The solar

SOLAR ALTITUDE	AIR MASS	DIRECT SUNLIGHT $lm\ m^{-2}*$		SKY LIGHT $lm\ m^{-2}*$		TOTAL $lm\ m^{-2}*$	
H [Km]	M	Evhd	Evpd	Evhs	Evps	Evht	Evpt
3	15.36	210	4026	2756	6318	2982	10344
5	10.39	1076	12378	3498	8030	4575	20452
7	7.77	2712	22066	4252	9128	6964	31216
10	5.60	6351	36059	5285	10258	11625	46285
15	3.82	14100	52851	6770	11517	20882	64369
20	2.90	22927	63077	8073	12271	31000	75348
25	2.36	32077	68788	9214	12702	41334	81483
30	2.00	41118	71258	10172	13024	51237	84282
35	1.74	50053	71473	10979	13132	61032	84605
40	1.55	58556	69858	11733	13132	70289	82990
45	1.41	66414	66414	12486	13132	78900	79546
50	1.30	73733	61893	13024	12917	86758	74810
55	1.22	80912	56188	13670	12702	93862	68890
60	1.15	86112	49730	14100	12379	100213	62108
65	1.10	91171	42518	14531	11733	105702	54250
70	1.06	95369	34678	14962	10979	110331	45747
75	1.04	98598	26372	15285	10010	113883	36382
80	1.02	100966	17761	15500	8977	116466	26695
85	1.01	102365	8966	15715	7836	118081	16792
90	1.00	103011	0	15931	6620	118942	662

*The illuminance units are lm/m², but the conversion to ft-cd can be made using the expression 1 lm/m² equals ft-cd × 10.764.
(Modified from Condron TP, Toolin RB, Stakutis VJ. Visibility, Chap 14. In Campen CF, Jr, Cole AE, Condron TP et al (eds): Handbook of Geophysics for Air Force Designers, 1st ed. Geophysics Res Direct., A.F. Cambridge Research Center, Air Research and Development, Command USAF, 1957.

TABLE 4-5
Illuminance from Direct Sunlight, Sky Light or Indirect Sunlight and Total or Global Illuminance on a Horizontal Surface (h) or a Vertical Plane (p) at the Earth's Surface for Different Altitudes H and Air masses M

spectral irradiance for air mass 1 incident on the Earth is plotted in Figure 4-6. The air mass 1 and 2 values were calculated using the U.S. standard atmospheric values for water vapor, O_3, and atmospheric turbidity, which are 20 mm of precipitable water vapor, 0.34 cm of O3, and an atmosphere with the turbidity parameters $\alpha = 1.3$ and $\theta = 0.04$.[34] To calculate the spectral irradiance Eeλ in W/m²-nm must be multiplied by the wavelength interval $\Delta\lambda$ in nm and summated over the waveband of concern:

$$E_e = \sum_{\lambda_1}^{\lambda_n} E_{e\lambda}\ \Delta\lambda \qquad (4\text{-}12)$$

The wavelength of the NASA/ASTM data has arbitrarily been set from 200 to 3005 nm because this waveband contains 99.03% of the sun's energy. Data on global and direct UVR have recently been published in the 280- to 340-nm wavelength range for radiation falling on a horizontal surface at different degrees of solar elevations and a variety of conditions (see Appendix Tables 4-7, 4-8, and 4-9 at the end of this chapter).[34-41] This wavelength range lies primarily in the actinic UVB range that is so very active in ocular and skin damage. These data will be used in subsequent calculations to establish ocular protection criteria against UVR exposure.

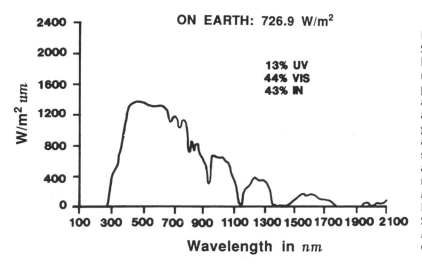

ON EARTH: 726.9 W/m²

13% UV
44% VIS
43% IN

Wavelength in *nm*

FIGURE 4-6
Spectral irradiance of the solar disk on Earth after undergoing absorption by nitrogen, oxygen, and ozone as it passes through the atmosphere. In addition, there is absorption by aerosols, water vapor, dust, and mixed gases. Finally, Rayleigh scattering, aerosol scattering, and multiple scattering by these components of the atmosphere produces the diffuse solar radiation component we call sky light. Modified from Mercherikunnel AT, Richard AT. Spectral Distribution of Solar Radiation. NASA Technical Memorandum 82021. Greenbilt, Goddard Space Flight Center 1980.

Unlike solar UVR, solar IR does not interact with O_3, O_2, or N during its propagation to Earth. However, IR is absorbed by atmospheric moisture, dust, carbon dioxide (CO_2) and other impurities, greatly reducing its total energy before it reaches Earth. IR interactions result in the absorption bands seen in the IR wavelengths of solar radiation. Incidentally, sunlight consists of approximately 13% UV, 44% VIS, and 43% IR.

The basic principles of the absorption and transmittance of solar radiation as it travels to Earth explain why it is easy to obtain a sunburn on a cloudy day. IR causes the skin to "feel" hot during sunbathing, but it is UVR that is responsible for the photochemical response called the suntan or sunburn. The skin does not "feel" UVR because its mechanism is photochemical. On a cloudy or overcast day, a greater portion of IR is absorbed by the moisture in the clouds; consequently, the sun does not feel as "hot" as on a normal sunny day, UVR is readily transmitted by the clouds and permitted to do its harm. Because the normal warning signs are absent, the sunbather is exposed to the UVR in sunshine longer during a cloudy day, which results in an unusually severe sunburn.

THE OZONE STORY.   Ozone (O_3) is produced in the stratosphere by the photolysis of O_2:

$$O + O_2 \Rightarrow O_3$$
$$O_2 + h\nu \Rightarrow 2O$$
$$2O + O_2 \Rightarrow O_3$$

where $h\nu$ represents the absorbed solar energy. The development of the supersonic transport in the United States created a concern that the pollutants from the jet engines would produce a degradation of the environment in the stratosphere. The result has been a series of studies and reports beginning in 1974 that were designed to analyze the impacts of the propulsion effluents of aircraft engines on the stratosphere and the impacts of the climatic changes on the biologic systems on Earth.[32,42,43] These studies concluded that climatic changes would result in an increase in solar UVR due to partial loss of O_3. Changes in temperature and precipitation associated with the decrease in O_3 and the increases in pollutants such as aerosol sulfates and water vapor were also forecast.

In reality the situation is not as clear as it appears in the introductory paragraph. Chlorofluorocarbons (CFCs), also called chlorofluoromethanes (CFMs), could potentially harm the stratosphere by interacting with O_3 to produce O_2 and result in a net increase in the UVR reaching Earth. The irony was that a mathematic model[45] based on a fixed amount of O_3 had predicted a significant decrease in UVR and VIS spectrum radiation on the Earth.

Part of the difficulty in understanding the release of atomic chlorine from the CFCs by UV photolysis was that all such compounds were simply referred to as fluorocarbons when, in reality, they consisted of four common compounds: trichlorofluoromethane, CFC = 11 (CCl_3); dichlorodifluoromethane, CFC = 12 (CCl_2F_2); trichlorotriflouroethane, CFC = 113 (CCl_2

· FCCL · F_2); and chlorodifluoromethane, CFC = 22 ($CHClF_2$), which are distinguished as chlorofluorocarbons, hydrofluorocarbons, and hydrochlorofluorocarbons. These compounds are used as refrigerants, propellants in aerosol cans, cleaning solvents for electronic parts, and as foaming agents for such plastics as styrofoam. They are released into the atmosphere and concentrate at from 25 to 40 km above the Earth.[46] It is the O_3 layer that protects humans, animals and plants on Earth while also preventing the CFCs from disassociation and robbing the stratosphere of O_3. The chemical reaction is described thusly:[47,48]

$$Cl + O_3 \Rightarrow ClO + O_2$$
$$ClO + O \Rightarrow Cl + O_2$$

Note that it is a two-chain reaction in which the Cl atom is not destroyed in the first reaction but reappears as a product of the second reaction to initiate the cycle repeatedly.[48] The Cl atoms ultimately return to Earth as hydrochloric acid (HCl) in rainfall but are not eliminated before destroying about 100,000 molecules of O_3. The initiator of the two-chain reaction is solar UVR shorter than 230 nm that does not get to Earth but is absorbed in the stratosphere by either O_2 or O_3 found in the stratosphere.

Using the effluent production of nitrogen oxide (N_{ox}) from the supersonic transport, we can predict an annual 12% depletion of the stratospheric O_3 in the northern hemisphere and 8% depletion in the southern hemisphere.[49] The hypothesis that CFCs should harm the O_3 in the stratosphere[44] had become accepted by 1979 because additional studies had established O_3 depletion rates of 7.5%, 10.8%, and 16.5% if the release of CFCs were continued at the 1977 rate.[50,51] More recently, a 12% reduction in stratospheric O_3 over an 11-year solar cycle or a 1.09% reduction per year has been reported.[52]

The intensive program to re-evaluate O_3 measurements shows rather conclusively that the stratospheric O_3 level has decreased over the past 17 years. An unexpected result was that there were larger than expected decreases in O_3 in the colder climates and higher latitudes.[53,54] This finding suggests that the process may be mediated by ice-chemistry phenomena. The Antarctic hole suffered a reported loss of 50% of the total O_3 in the hole and a 95% loss in the lower stratosphere in October 1987. In addition, there were record losses of O_3 outside the O_3 hole,

the hole lasted longer, the hole was colder than other years, and there was a total decrease in O_3 latitude 60° and farther south the entire year. In October 1988, however, the Antarctic O_3 level showed a recovery; that year the hole did not become as large and the loss of O_3 was not as great.[53]

Atmospheric scientists have searched for a reduction in O_3 in the Arctic similar to that found in the Antarctic but were unsuccessful until the winter of 1987–1988 when signs were found indicating a global O_3 loss.[55-58] Increased levels of CFCs destroy O_3 when stratospheric temperatures reach −80° to −85°C.[59] The temperatures are important because −77°C is required to form nitric acid clouds,[60] whereas −85°C or less is required to form water ice particles. Scientists do not feel that an O_3 hole will form in the Arctic like the one in the Antarctic because the weather patterns are different.[53] The International Ozone Trends panel reported an O_3 decrease from 1.7% to 3.0% for the period between 1969 and 1986.[61] Thus, a decrease in O_3 in the northern hemisphere and the chemistry of the Arctic stratosphere has been shown to possess the essential ingredients for the loss of O_3.[62,63] The trends are disturbing for the large populations that are located in the northern hemisphere.[60] The weight of evidence is that the CFCs are responsible for the observed changes in stratospheric O_3 in both the Antarctic and Arctic areas.[64]

The importance of the O_3 story to us is that the lower wavelength and the intensity of the UVR falling on the Earth depends on the integrity of the O_3 layer and the air mass of the atmosphere. The global, direct, and diffuse solar UVR reaching the ground has been calculated by incrementing the O_3 layer thickness in 25% steps, beginning at 0.16 atm-cm and extending to 0.40 atm-cm (see Fig. 4-9).[30-34] These data were used to calculate the percent increment or decrement in UVR and are plotted in Figure 4-7. The increases in UVR due to changes in the O_3 layer occur below 340 nm. As the O_3 layer reduces its thickness equivalency, there is a relatively larger increase in the short UV wavelengths that reach the Earth. Thus, there is a significant increase in the level of UVB irradiance and, at the same time, a shift to higher energy photons in the shorter wavelength UVB.

Evidence now being collected indicates that the plant and animal life of the Antarctic is being affected, but the definitive answer to the O_3 depletion

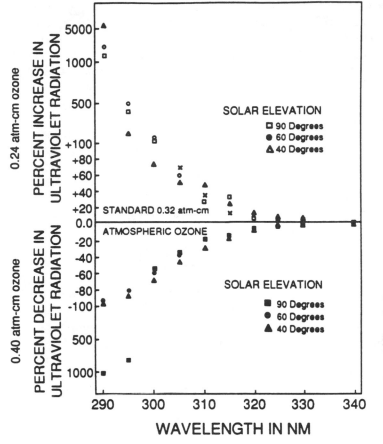

FIGURE 4-7
Calculated percentage of global UVR received on Earth for the 280- to 340-nm waveband at 40°, 60°, and 90° solar elevation for atmospheric O_3 concentrations of 0.24 and 0.40 atm-cm. These O_3 levels represent a $\pm$ 25% from the standard O_3 concentration of 0.32 atm-cm at the level of the stratosphere. Note that the curves asymtote at 340 nm indicating that all UVR changes take place at shorter wavelengths (Calculated from the data of Shettle and Green, 30, 34).

question is not complete.[60] There is predicted to be a 1% increase in skin cancer for each 2% of increase in UVR.[65] Taylor et al predict a 1% increase in the prevalence of UVR-induced senile cortical cataracts with each year of exposure to sunlight.[66] These events will be explored more fully in Section III, in which the effects of exposure of the eye to optical radiation are treated. The recognition by the United States, Europe, Canada, and other countries of the seriousness of the loss of the O_3 layer to the safety of plants and animals has led to several favorable actions. In September 1987, an ozone treaty was endorsed by more than 40 countries at a landmark meeting in Montreal.[67] The United States agreed to limit production of CFCs by 50% by June 1989.[64] Although the Treaty of Montreal is a proper move, it is recognized that limiting production of CFCs more severely to 20% of the 1986 level may not be adequate to stem the loss of O_3. The already progressive

loss of O_3 globally[56] has finally been recognized in Europe, and the EEC has banned all uses of CFCs by the end of the century.[68] Whether the atmosphere and stratosphere can recover from the years of CFC neglect remains to be answered.

4.2 Radiation and Vision

Radiometry and Photometry

The electromagnetic radiation (EMR) emitted by the previously discussed sources can be measured using physical methodology to establish its energy. *Radiometry* is the physical measurement of radiant energy or power flowing in beams of EMR including noncoherent, UV, VIS, and IR radiation. It constitutes the field of the measurement of the optical radiations in the 200- to 20,000-nm wavelength range. *Photometry* is concerned with the measurement of that portion of the EMS that is capable of stimulating the eye, resulting in the phenomena known as vision. The VIS spectrum has a waveband that begins at 380 nm and extends to 760 nm. There are other concepts that apply to both the radiometric and photometric systems that need to be understood. Table 4-6 defines some of the terms used to express these concepts.

Historically, the approach in explaining EMR has been accomplished by using three optical models. Geometric optics has treated EMR as rays that form images at the focal point of the lens. Physical optics considers EMR as a wavefront with interference and diffraction phenomena contributing to the image formation. Quantum optics establishes the discrete photon energies of the radiation and includes the concept of coherence.

The quantities, symbols, name, and units of radiometric and photometric terms are defined in Table 4-7 and Figures 4-8 and 4-9. The descriptions should assist in understanding the basic definitions, units, and symbols of the radiometric and photometric systems.

The ability of a light source such as a spotlight to illuminate a given surface from a distance uses the terms candle-power and intensity to define the source. Candle-power and intensity have been used interchangeably, but they have different meanings. The word *candle-power* should be applied to the light source; e.g., a bulb or lamp possesses so many candle-power. The word *intensity* should be used to describe the light that is produced by the source. Thus, a lamp possesses a certain candle-power but it produces light of a certain intensity. It is interesting that the concept of the luminance of a surface has always been interpreted as the illuminating capacity of each unit area of the surface of an extended source and not the source itself.

The derived International System of Units (SI) quantities, units, symbols, and definitions for radiometry and photometry are given in Table 4-7. The subscripts e and v should be used to indicate radiometric and photometric units, respectively. The symbols He or Hv designate radiant or luminous exposure and are often spectrally defined for research purposes. Spectral or wavelength quantities may be defined by adding the λ subscript to the symbol. Throughout the text, subscripts will be used to designate the portion of the eye that has received a

Radiometric Concepts	Photometric Concepts
Radiant Power (ϕ_e), also called radiant flux, is the time rate of flow of radiant energy. It is expressed in joules/second or watts.	*Luminous power* (ϕ_v) is light energy flow per unit time. It is also called luminous flux and is expressed in the basic unit of photometry, the lumen.
Irradiance (E_e) is the density of radiant power incident on a surface. It is generally measured in watts/square meter.	*Illuminance* (E_v), formerly called illumination, is the density of luminous power incident upon a surface. One lumen per square foot equals one foot-candle.
Radiant exitance (M_e) is the density of radiant power emitted from, transmitted through, or reflected from a surface. It was formerly known as radiant emittance and is measured in watts/square meter.	*Luminous exitance* (M_v) is the luminous power leaving a unit area of surface. It is measured in lumens/square meter. It was formerly called luminous emittance.
Radiant intensity (I_e) is the radiant power unit solid angle, traveling in a given direction. It is measured in watts/steradian.	*Luminous intensity* (L_v) is the luminous power per unit solid angle, traveling in a given direction. One lumen of power per steradian is one candela of intensity.
Radiance (L_e) is the radiant intensity per unit area leaving, passing through, or arriving at a surface in a given direction.	*Luminance* (L_v) is the luminous intensity per unit area leaving, passing through, or arriving at a surface in a given direction.

Used with permission of Dr. P. Pease.

TABLE 4-6
Definitions of Similar Terms Used in Radiometry and Photometry for the Most Commonly Used Units

Quantity	Symbol	Radiometric		Photometric	
		Name	Unit	Name	Unit
Energy	Q	Radiant energy	Joule [J]	Luminous energy	[1m s]
Energy per unit time	ϕ	Radiant power or flux	Watt [W][Js^{-1}]	Luminous power or flux	[cd sr][1m]
Power per unit area	E	Irradiance	[W m^{-2}]	Illuminance	[lx][1m m^{-2}]
Power per unit solid angle	I	Radiant intensity	[W sr^{-1}]	Luminous intensity	[cd][1m sr^{-1}]
Power per unit area and steradian	L	Radiance	[W m^{-2} sr]	Luminance	[cd m^{-2}][1m m^{-2} sr^{-1}]
Exposure per unit area	H	Radiant exposure	[J m^{-2}][W sm^{-2}]	Luminous exposure	[cd m^{-2}][1m s m^{-2}]

From Kostkowski HG, Saunders RD, Wand JF et al: Measurement of solar terrestrial spectral irradiance in the ozone cut-off region. *In* Chap 1, Self-Study Manual on Optical Radiation Measurements: Part III, Applications. NBC Technical Note 910-5. Washington, DC, US Government Printing Office, 1982.

TABLE 4-7
Comparison of the More Commonly Used SI Units for the Radiometric and Photometric Systems

threshold radiant exposure. Therefore, the symbols H_c, H_l and H_r will represent the threshold radiant exposure for the cornea, lens, and retina, respectively.

The SI units, symbols, and quantities for photometry in Table 4-7 need further amplification. The photometric units listed first in the table represent the accepted SI system using the candela, while the second set of units presents the photometric system in terms of the lumen. Adopting the lumen allows parallel concepts between the photometric and the radiometric systems because the lumen is equivalent to the watt, and the watt per second is equivalent to the lumen per second. When world standards organizations adopt the lumen for photometric definitions, both systems should become completely compatible both conceptually and mathematically.

The evolution of the photometric system has suffered from a plethora of different terms, definitions, and formulas used to express photometric units. The result is that photometric units that have been in common usage in different countries in the past must now be related to SI units. A chart of the units of luminance and their conversion factors is provided in Table 4-8. The units of illuminance and

their conversion factors are given in Table 4-9. In each instance, the SI standard unit is the first unit. The SI equivalent permits the earlier literature to be related to the present SI terminology. Care will be taken to present photometric data in SI units. However, it may be necessary to retain the original units for historical purposes and to include the SI conversions in the legend.

RELATIONSHIP BETWEEN RADIOMETRY
AND PHOTOMETRY
Historically, the candle has been used as the unit of luminous intensity and was the fundamental unit for all photometric quantities. The candle has been defined in terms of standard sperm candle, the Hepner lamp, the pentane lamp, the melting point of platinum, and other sources. Since the candle is based on visual comparison, photometric quantities cannot be defined on the basis of spectroradiometric curve measurements because photometric concepts would then be based on two different systems. The first is a psychophysical quantity based on visual comparison, whereas the second is a physical quantity based on physical measurements. What alternatives are available? The old definition based on the visual

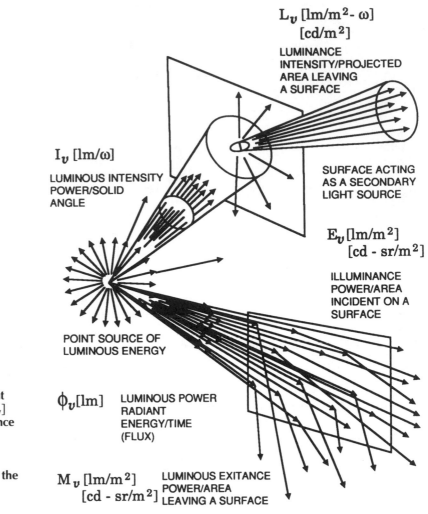

L_v [lm/m^2- ω]
[cd/m^2]

LUMINANCE
INTENSITY/PROJECTED
AREA LEAVING
A SURFACE

I_v [lm/ω]

LUMINOUS INTENSITY
POWER/SOLID
ANGLE

SURFACE ACTING
AS A SECONDARY
LIGHT SOURCE

E_v [lm/m^2]
[cd - sr/m^2]

ILLUMINANCE
POWER/AREA
INCIDENT ON A
SURFACE

POINT SOURCE OF
LUMINOUS ENERGY

ϕ_v[lm]   LUMINOUS POWER
RADIANT
ENERGY/TIME
(FLUX)

M_v [lm/m^2]   LUMINOUS EXITANCE
[cd - sr/m^2]   POWER/AREA
LEAVING A SURFACE

FIGURE 4-8
Illustration of the definitions for photometric terms. The origin is a point source of light with a luminous flux [ϕ_v] that falls on a surface with an illuminance E_v [cd-sr/m^2] or [lm/m^2]. The power leaving the surface is called luminous exitance Mv [lm/m^2] or [cd-sr/m^2]. Luminance is the luminous intensity of the projected area leaving a surface [lm/m^2 − Ω] or [cd/m^2].

comparison against the standard candle may be kept, but such a choice would not allow updating to the newer knowledge base. Alternatively, all old photometric definitions could be eliminated and redefined in terms of physical measurements and a standard method established for evaluating these measurements. The purpose of the following discussion is to demonstrate how the problem has been handled. The radiometric-photometric-visibility or luminosity curve will be brought into a unit concept relating the human eye and its visual response to radiant energy.

The measurement of an incandescent lamp in radiometric terms is an acceptable, precise method of expressing the radiant power or radiant energy of

the lamp, but it says nothing about the visual effectiveness of the light. An example may serve to illustrate the term *visual effectiveness*. If one were to observe a red lamp, a green lamp, and a blue lamp simultaneously, each having the same radiant power of 25 W, the lamps would not appear to possess the same visual intensity. The green lamp would appear brighter or more intense than the blue lamp or the red lamp under photopic conditions. Each lamp possesses the same 25 W in radiant power, why are they not seen as the same visual brightness? The answer lies in the fact that the human eye is a selective spectral receiver, and radiant power measurements in the VIS spectrum denote nothing about the visual effectiveness of that energy. To convert

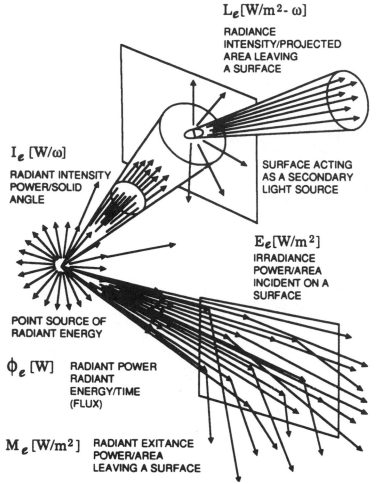

$L_e[W/m^2 \cdot \omega]$

RADIANCE
INTENSITY/PROJECTED
AREA LEAVING
A SURFACE

$I_e [W/\omega]$

RADIANT INTENSITY
POWER/SOLID
ANGLE

SURFACE ACTING
AS A SECONDARY
LIGHT SOURCE

$E_e[W/m^2]$

IRRADIANCE
POWER/AREA
INCIDENT ON A
SURFACE

POINT SOURCE OF
RADIANT ENERGY

$\phi_e [W]$ RADIANT POWER
RADIANT
ENERGY/TIME
(FLUX)

$M_e [W/m^2]$ RADIANT EXITANCE
POWER/AREA
LEAVING A SURFACE

FIGURE 4-9
Radiometric terms defined from a point source. The point source possesses a radiant power ϕ_e in watts and falls on a surface with an irradiance E_e [W/m^2]. The radiant power leaving the surface is radiant exitance [W/m^2]. The source falls on the upper surface where it becomes an extended or secondary source. The radiance leaving the extended source is defined by its intensity per projected area [W/m$^2 - \omega$].

radiometric measurements from an incandescent lamp, i.e., W/unit area, into photometric units and hence into its effectiveness to evoke a visual stimulus, the relative visibility of the visual spectrum must be taken into account. The relative spectral visibility curve relates the visible spectrum to its ability to produce the same physiologic response and has been termed the *luminosity curve* or the *spectral sensitivity curve*.

To establish the spectral sensitivity of the human eye requires a method that produces the same physiologic response to the luminosity of different wavelengths of light. Three different methods of measurement have been used traditionally to measure the luminosity curve. The first method involves a bipartite field with half of the field illuminated with white light and the other half by a monochromatic

wavelength. The two halves are made to appear equal to the observer by adjusting the intensity of the monochromatic field. This method suffers from several experimental errors because it relies on the subjective ability of the observer. When the standard and test sources are of widely different spectral colors, the observer's task of equating the luminous attributes of the bipartite field is very difficult, and large errors exist for the subject and between different subjects.

The second method involves the comparison of bipartite fields in which one field of λ_1 is matched by the second field of λ_2. The wavelengths on the bipartite field are adjacent to each other in the VIS spectrum, and it is easier for subjects to make matches. This method is termed the *step-by-step method*. Thus, the energy necessary for λ_2 to match

		Nit	Stilb	Bougie Hectomètre Carré	Apostilb	Milli-apostilb	Micro-apostilb	Lambert	Milli-lambert	Micro-lambert	Foot-lambert	Candle Per Sq ft	Candle Per Sq Inch
1 Nit = (nt)	$\dfrac{1\ Candela}{m^2}$	1	10^{-4}	10^4	3.14	3.14×10^3	3.14×10^6	3.14×10^{-4}	3.14×10^{-1}	3.14×10^2	2.919×10^{-1}	9.29×10^{-2}	6.452×10^{-4}
1 Stilb = (sb)	$\dfrac{1\ Candela}{cm^2}$	10^4	1	10^8	3.14×10^4	3.14×10^7	3.14×10^{10}	3.14	3.14×10^3	3.14×10^6	2.919×10^3	9.29×10^2	6.452
1 Bougie Hectomètre Carré	$\dfrac{1\ Candela}{(100m)^2}$	10^{-4}	10^{-8}	1	3.14×10^{-4}	3.14×10^{-1}	3.14×10^2	31.4×10^{-8}	3.14×10^{-5}	3.14×10^{-2}	2.919×10^{-5}	9.29×10^{-6}	6.452×10^{-8}
1 Apostilb = (asb)	$\dfrac{1\ Candela}{\pi\times m^2}$	3.183×10^{-1}	3.183×10^{-5}	3.183×10^3	1	10^3	10^6	10^{-4}	10^{-1}	10^2	9.29×10^{-2}	2.957×10^{-2}	2.054×10^{-4}
1 Milli-apostilb = (masb)	$\dfrac{1\ Candela}{\pi\times1000\times m^2}$	3.183×10^{-4}	3.183×10^{-8}	3.183	10^{-3}	1	10^3	10^{-7}	10^{-4}	10^{-1}	9.29×10^{-5}	2.957×10^{-5}	2.054×10^{-7}
1 Micro-apostilb = (μ asb)	$\dfrac{1\ Candela}{\pi\times10^6\times m^2}$	3.183×10^{-7}	3.183×10^{-11}	3.183×10^{-3}	10^{-6}	10^{-3}	1	10^{-10}	10^{-7}	10^{-4}	9.29×10^{-8}	2.957×10^{-8}	2.054×10^{-10}
1 Lambert = (L)	$\dfrac{1\ Candela}{\pi\times cm^2}$	3.183×10^3	3.183×10^{-1}	3.183×10^7	10^4	10^7	10^{10}	1	10^3	10^6	9.29×10^2	2.957×10^2	2.054
1 Milli-lambert = (mL)	$\dfrac{1\ Candela}{\pi\times10^3\times cm^2}$	3.183	3.183×10^{-4}	3.183×10^4	10	10^4	10^7	10^{-3}	1	10^3	9.29×10^{-1}	2.957×10^{-1}	2.054×10^{-3}
1 Micro-lambert = (μL)	$\dfrac{1\ Candela}{\pi\times10^6\times cm^2}$	3.183×10^{-3}	3.183×10^{-7}	3.183×10	10^{-2}	10	10^4	10^{-6}	10^{-3}	1	9.29×10^{-4}	2.957×10^{-4}	2.054×10^{-6}
1 Foot-lambert = (ftL)	$\dfrac{1\ Candela}{\pi\times ft^2}$	3.426	3.426×10^{-4}	3.426×10^4	10.764	1.0764×10^4	1.0764×10^7	1.0764×10^{-3}	1.0764	1.0764×10^3	1	0.3183	2.14×10^{-3}
1 Candle Per Sq ft =	$\dfrac{1\ Candela}{ft^2}$	1.0764×10	1.0764×10^{-3}	1.0764×10^5	3.382×10	3.382×10^4	3.382×10^7	3.382×10^{-3}	3.382	3.382×10^3	3.14	1	6.944×10^{-3}
1 Candle Per Sq Inch =	$\dfrac{1\ Candela}{inch^2}$	1.55×10^3	1.55×10^{-1}	1.55×10^{-5}	4.869×10^3	4.869×10^6	4.869×10^9	4.869×10^{-1}	4.869×10^2	4.869×10^5	4.524×10^2	1.44×10^2	1

NOTE: The value of the unit in the lefthand columns must be multiplied by the conversion factor contained in the table to obtain the value of the unit given at the top of the appropriate column (unit in lefthand column × conversion factor = value of unit in top column). Note that the candela/m² is the SI unit, and it has been named the nit.

TABLE 4-8
Units of Luminance and Conversion Table for Luminance

Equals Unit x	lm/m^{-2} (lux) Factor	Phot	Milliphot	Foot-candle
lm/m^2	1.0	0.0001	0.1	0.0929
Phot	10,000.0	1.0	1,000.00	929.0
Milliphot	10.0	0.001	1.0	0.929
Foot-candle	10.764	0.00108	1.076	1.0

The unit in the left-hand column times the conversion factor equals the value of the unit at the top of the column. The unit of lux or 1lm/m^2 is the SI unit.

TABLE 4-9
Conversion Factors for Units of Illuminance

λ_1 is determined, and λ_1 is replaced by λ_3, and the process repeated until the entire VIS spectrum has been covered. The plot of the l/E$_{e\lambda}$ against the waveband results in a luminosity curve or a relative spectral sensitivity curve.

The final method is a comparison method based on flicker. The flickering field is alternately illuminated with a monochromatic standard and the wavelength λ. Because the flicker due to color difference disappears prior to the flicker due to luminance of the field, the rate of alternation can be adjusted to eliminate flicker. In reality, the observer varies the irradiance of the monochromatic standard, changing its intensity until the flicker disappears, and establishes the E$_\lambda$ for that wavelength λ. The luminosity curve of the observer is determined by plotting l/E$_{e\lambda}$ versus the wavelength λ for the VIS spectrum.

Figure 4-10 illustrates the relative amounts of radiant energy required to stimulate the cones under light-adapted conditions and to stimulate the rods under dark-adapted conditions. These curves are not usually presented in this form but are important in illustrating some very real differences between rod vision and cone vision. First, rod vision requires less radiant energy at all wavelengths than does cone vision; however, rod vision is colorless while normal cone vision possesses the full colors of the spectrum. Second, rod vision requires the least energy at 507 nm and cone vision requires the least energy at 555 nm, a shift known as the Purkinje shift. Finally, rod vision is more sensitive in the blue end of the spectrum and less sensitive than cone vision beyond

about 670 nm. Calculating the reciprocal of E$_{e\lambda}$ and replotting the curves result in the relative sensitivity curve shown in Figure 4-11. The relative sensitivity curve retains all of the features of the original data with the upper rod curve illustrating the greater sensitivity of the scotopic visual receptors. The ordinate of the relative sensitivity curve has been plotted with a maximum value of 1.00.

When the conditions of observation have not been constant, wide variations in the luminosity curves of groups of observers have been found. The spread for normals shows the blue end of the spectrum to have values nearly 10 times higher than for other portions of the VIS spectrum. Comparison of data from different researchers demonstrates a 3:1

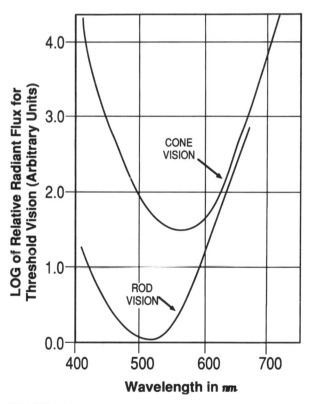

FIGURE 4-10
Relative amounts of radiant flux required for light of different wavelengths to be seen using photopic (cone) and scotopic (rod) vision. Modified from Wulfeck JW, Weiz A, Rahen MW. Vision in Military Aviation. WADC Technical Report 58–399. Wright-Patterson Air Force Base, Wright Air Development Center, 1958.

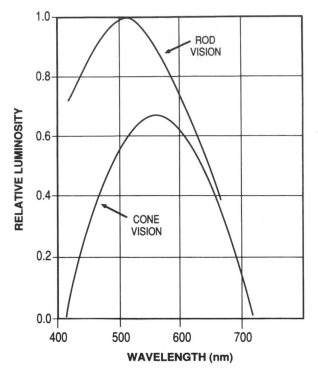

FIGURE 4-11

Relative luminosity or relative spectral sensitivity curve for different wavelengths of light using rod and cone vision. Modified from Wulfeck JW, Weiz A, Rahen MW. Vision in Military Aviation. WADC Technical Report 58–399. Wright-Patterson Air Force Base, Wright Air Development Center, 1958.

variation for normal observers. Observers with defective color vision demonstrate a shift of the peak wavelength of their luminosity curves and wide variations in the overall photopic curve values. These variations make it advisable to standardize on an "average spectral sensitivity curve" for use in calculations relating radiometric data to its ability to cause vision.[71]

In 1924, the Commission Internationale de l'Eclairage (CIE) adopted standard luminosity curves (Fig. 4-12). The curves were established using an average of the data from a large number of individuals reported by many different investigators using the flicker photometry methodology. The photopic luminosity curve relates specifically to foveal vision adapted to photopic conditions but has been assumed to represent the parafoveal and peripheral retinal sensitivities under photopic conditions. The

CIE relative luminosity curve is bell-shaped with the photopic maximum at 555 nm. The symbol V_λ has been adopted to represent the relative luminous efficiency for a defined wavelength over the entire curve under photopic conditions.

The scotopic or V'_λ curve applies to luminance levels from 1.076×10^{-2} cd/m² (10^4 cd/ft²) to the absolute threshold. At the upper scotopic luminance levels, the spectral sensitivity curve becomes less stable and the Purkinje shift occurs. These empiric findings probably indicate that both the rods and cones are operating simultaneously. The V_λ data for the CIE standard photopic luminosity factors adopted by the CIE in 1931 and the V'_λ data for scotopic luminosity factors as adopted by the CIE in 1951 are provided in Table 4-10.

The relative spectral sensitivity curve or luminosity curve expresses the ability of radiant power to produce the same physiologic response for vision. The luminous efficiency or luminous efficacy K is the ratio of the photometric unit (lumens/cm²) to the radiometric unit (W/cm²) at the same wavelength required to produce a physiologic response and can be expressed thusly:

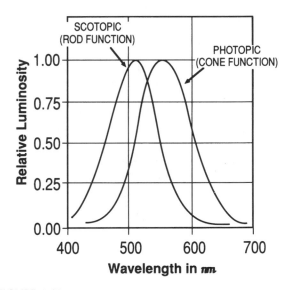

FIGURE 4-12

The standard observer or standard luminosity curves for scotopic and photopic levels of adaptation. Modified from Wulfeck JW, Weiz A, Rahen MW. Vision in Military Aviation. WADC Technical Report 58–399. Wright-Patterson Air Force Base, Wright Air Development Center, 1958.

Wavelength (nm)	$V_\lambda *$	$V_\lambda' *$	Wavelength (nm)	$V_\lambda *$	$V_\lambda' *$
380	0.0000	0.000589	580	0.8700	0.121200
390	0.0001	0.002209	590	0.7570	0.065480
400	0.0004	0.009292	600	0.6310	0.033150
410	0.0012	0.034834	610	0.5030	0.015930
420	0.0040	0.096610	620	0.3810	0.007374
430	0.0116	0.199800	630	0.2650	0.003335
440	0.0230	0.328100	640	0.1750	0.001497
450	0.0380	0.455000	650	0.1070	0.0006772
460	0.0600	0.567200	660	0.0610	0.0003129
470	0.0910	0.675600	670	0.0320	0.0001480
480	0.1390	0.793000	680	0.0170	0.00007155
490	0.2080	0.904300	690	0.0082	0.00003533
500	0.3230	0.981800	700	0.0041	0.00001780
507	—	1.000000	710	0.0021	0.000009143
510	0.5030	0.996600	720	0.00105	0.000004783
520	0.7100	0.935200	730	0.00052	0.0000025462
530	0.8620	0.811000	740	0.00025	0.0000013794
540	0.9540	0.649700	750	0.00012	0.0000007596
550	0.9950	0.480800	760	0.00006	0.0000004249
555	1.0000	—	770	0.00000	0.0000002413
560	0.9950	0.328800	780	0.00000	0.0000001390
570	0.9520	0.207600			

*V_λ is the photopic luminosity function for the standard Observer (CIE, 1931) and V_λ' for the scotopic luminosity function (CIE, 1951).

TABLE 4-10
Relative Luminosity Function Chart

$$K = \frac{\text{Photometric units}}{\text{Radiometric units}} = \frac{1\,\text{lm/cm}^2}{\text{W/cm}^2} = [\text{lm/W}] \quad (4\text{-}13)$$

The fact that the most efficient part of the VIS spectrum producing a visual stimulus is 555 nm allows us to use the luminous efficacy K_{max} for relating radiometric and photometric data. It has been shown empirically that 1 W of radiant power at 555 nm produces 683 lm/cm^2 of luminous power.[72] Therefore, $K_{max} = 683$ lm/W. K_{max}, $E_{e\lambda}$, and V_λ may now be used to relate radiometric and photometric quantities.[72]

The spectral irradiance E_e of a designated wavelength interval $\Delta\lambda$ of the spectrum is expressed by

$$E_{e\lambda} = \sum_{\lambda_1}^{\lambda_2} E_{e\lambda} \cdot \Delta\lambda \quad (4\text{-}14)$$

The irradiance or total power E_e is found by integrating the spectral irradiances $E_{e\lambda}$ over the wavelength range $\Delta\lambda$ of the VIS spectrum:

$$E_e = \sum_{380}^{760} E_{e\lambda} \cdot \Delta\lambda \quad (4\text{-}15)$$

where E_e is the total irradiance [W/cm^2], $E_{e\lambda}$ the irradiance for each waveband [W/cm^2], and $\Delta\lambda$ the wavelength interval [nm].

The standard observer curve is used in photometry to calculate photometric values from radiometric (physical) measurements of the spectral composition of light. To accomplish this conversion requires the inclusion of the luminous efficacy K_{max} and the photopic luminosity factor V_λ into the above formulas. Thus, the radiometric measurement of a source is converted into a visual stimulus by weighting each radiometric spectral component by the luminosity factor Vλ and the relative efficacy K_{max} at 555 nm, then summing the result for the wavelength range of concern. The calculation of the total illuminance within the 380- to 760-nm wavelength range or within a single waveband located in the VIS spectrum is expressed by

$$E_v = K_{max} \sum_{380}^{760} E_{e\lambda} \cdot \Delta\lambda \ [\text{lm/m}^2] \qquad (4\text{-}16)$$

where E_v is the illuminance of the VIS spectrum [lm/m^2], $E_{e\lambda}$ the irradiance of waveband [W/m^2], K_{max} the maximum luminous efficacy of 683 lm/W, V_λ the relative spectral luminosity curve for the human eye, and $\Delta\lambda$ the wavelength interval of the measurements [nm]. Since K_{max} is equal to 683 lm/W, this value may be placed in front of the summation sign in equation (4-16) because the wavelength values for the luminosity factors V_λ reduces K_{max} to the proper value for a specified wavelength. The luminosity factors represent data at 10-nm wavelength intervals, and radiometric measurements of the source should contain the same waveband intervals.

Historically, there has been confusion as to the exact meaning of the relative luminosity curve. The luminosity curve does not give a measure of sensation, a measure of seeing ability due to radiation of different wavelengths, nor does it give an indication of the relative amount of radiant energy at different wavelengths required to give threshold vision.[73] The luminosity curve does not represent the magnitude of the reaction to equal amounts of light but the organism's same physiologic response to various levels of light of different wavelengths. One should also be warned that the luminosity curve applies only to the test conditions actually used in deriving the data, including the experimental methods, changes in field size, and conditions of the surround.

The important concept is that the luminosity factor V_λ and luminous efficacy factor K_{max} are used to calculate the magnitude of a visual stimulus E_v from the radiometric spectral measurement $E_{e\lambda}$ of the source.[74-76] Photometric and radiometric spectral measurements may now be used in the evaluation of a visual stimulus or the effects of radiant exposure on the eye.

4.3 Practical Applications—Visual Performance

Contrast and Glare

THE OCCUPATIONAL VISUAL TASK

Often it is forgotten that the basis for vision is light—without light we cannot see. This is important in the clinical and occupational setting where vision must be assessed or monitored. In fact, the definition of light is based on its ability to stimulate vision. To illustrate the importance of light to vision refer to Figure 4-13 for Konig's data[77] derived in 1897, which gives the level of luminance required for different levels of visual acuity. The intensity of light must reach 0.5 log cd/m^2 before Snellen acuity of 20/20 is achieved.[78] The graph also shows that the acuity for rods, while poor, improves over about a 4.0 log unit increase in luminance. The relation between visual acuity and color or hue is given in Figure 4-14.[79] The background hue for the extremes of the VIS spectrum do not materially affect visual acuity until the low levels of background luminance are achieved.

A basic principle for vision is that there be an object in the visual field that is either darker than or lighter than the background so that contrast can be established. It is contrast that creates the variations in light intensity across the retinal image and allows us to differentiate between the object and the background. An abundance of light without objects or complete darkness with the absence of objects results in the visual system performing abnormally. The eye focuses for about 25 inches or two thirds of a meter, a phenomenon known as *night or space myopia*, which occurs as the result of the lack of contrast in the visual field. The words *perform* or *performance* are key to our problem. As long as the visual system is normal, the lighting is normal, and the contrast is normal, the performance of vision is optimum. Disrupt or degrade any one of the three and visual performance suffers. Glare is an additional parameter that creates visual problems and degrades visual performance. The interactions between light, contrast, and glare constitute the triad for maximizing visual performance.

In this section, the visual task and those attributes of vision that allow us to function optimally will be considered. The quantities will be expressed in object space to make the task easier to describe and evaluate. For example, the quantity of light necessary to accomplish a given task will not be expressed as a quantity of light on the retina but at the physical

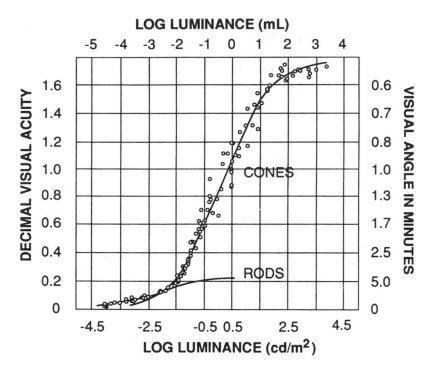

FIGURE 4-13
Relation between visual acuity and luminance determined by using a U-shaped target. The curve at the bottom is for the rods, and the open circles fitted by the sigmoid curve is for cones. The data is from Konig,[77] and the graph is modified from Riggs.[2] The rod and cone curves were fitted to the Konig data by Hecht. From Hecht S. The relation between visual acuity and illumination. J Gen Physiol 11:255–281, 1928; by copyright permission of the Rockefeller University Press.

object. Contrast and glare will be defined and related to visual performance.

Visual tasks or visual displays are usually specified in terms of quantities in object space that can be physically measured:[80] L_o is the luminance of the object, L_b the luminance of the background, λ the spectral distribution of source, C the contrast of the visual task calculated from L_o and L_b, A the size of units in linear measure or visual angle, T the duration in seconds, θ the location relative to the line of sight, f the temporal frequency characteristics, movement in the visual field, and nonuniformities in luminance between the background and the object. Other factors such as attention, expectation, and habituation affect the ability to discriminate a target. All environmental parameters necessary for a visual task to be seen may be perfect but if the observer is day-dreaming, the task may be completely missed or not seen. Thus, both the observer and the visual task must be considered in the evaluation of visual performance.

As a rule objects are seen because they differ in luminance or color (or a combination of both) from the background. When there is a difference in luminance between the background and the object, the condition is called *contrast* or *luminance contrast*. Chro-

matic contrast is the condition described when there is a color difference between the object and its background. Both luminance and chromatic contrast depend somewhat on the spectral distribution of the source.

Another area that is related to contrast but is not the same is *glare*. Glare has become a confusing term because the literature does not clearly differentiate glare from brightness contrast, contrast sensitivity, or differential contrast. Glare is always used with modifiers such as discomfort, disability, veiling, or luminance, but it is most precisely identified as opposite to the term *contrast*. Glare is simply any source or light within the visual field that causes discomfort or disturbing effects to vision or results in lowering visual performance. The limit of the luminance is not determined by the ability of the eye to see but by the disturbing effects of the excessive light. An example is that 1500 cd/m^2 (500 ft L) of light in a bank is considered excessive and disturbs both the employee and the customer but is perfectly acceptable for the surgical lamps in a hospital operating room.

A closer look at contrast and glare will be made in an attempt to understand their relationship to the visual environment and performance.

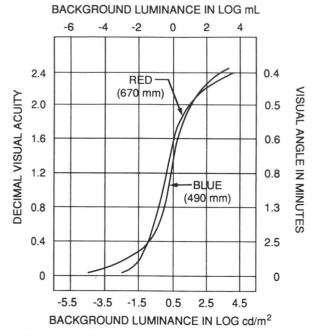

BACKGROUND LUMINANCE IN LOG mL

FIGURE 4-14
Relation between visual acuity and wavelength of background luminance for the extremes of the visible spectrum. Differences are not great except for low background luminances. From Shlaer S, Smith EL, Chase AM: Visual acuity and illumination of different spectral regions. J Gen Physiol 25:553–569 1942; by copyright permission of the Rockefeller University Press.

CONTRAST

LUMINANCE CONTRAST.   For purposes of defining the term contrast, visualize a large-area screen on which a small spot of light whose intensity can be changed is projected. The ability to just see the small spot of light for different levels of screen background intensities is measured. The small spot of light is seen because of its contrast against the background. The following formula may be used to describe or calculate the contrast:[81]

$$C = \frac{L_o - L_b}{L_b} \qquad (4\text{-}17)$$

where C is the contrast in decimal form, L_o represents the intensity of the object or target on the screen, and L_b the intensity of the screen used as the background. From formula 4-17, the following statements can be made: For objects darker than the background (i.e., negative contrast), contrast ranges

from 0 to 1, and for objects brighter than the background (positive contrast), contrast ranges from 0 to infinity. In measuring contrast threshold, the value is the same for objects darker or lighter than the background.[82] The formula for contrast has been used classically to calculate visibility or relative visibility by taking the reciprocal of contrast:

$$\text{Relative visibility} = \tfrac{1}{C} \qquad (4\text{-}18)$$

Finally, there is a formula that applies to periodic patterns or targets such as the sine wave grating, the square wave grating, or gratings that possess maximum and minimum luminances. This formula has existed in optics for many years and is termed *modulation*. The formula for modulation is

$$M = \frac{L_{max} - L_{min}}{L_{max} + L_{min}} \qquad (4\text{-}19)$$

where M is the modulation, L_{max} the maximum luminance, and L_{min} the minimum luminance of the grating pattern. Recently, the term *contrast sensitivity* has been used instead of modulation sensitivity to express the ability of the eye to see certain modulated patterns.

$$\text{Modulation sensitivity} = \tfrac{1}{M} \qquad (4\text{-}20)$$

The contrast threshold varies with target intensity (Fig. 4-15), size of the stimulus (Fig. 4-16), region of the retina (Fig. 4-17), hue (Fig. 4-18), exposure duration, and age (Fig. 4-19). If all other stimulus factors are held constant, the contrast threshold varies as the brightness of the background is changed from dark to extreme light. Research relating brightness contrast with age needs special emphasis.[83]

The acuity and contrast discrimination of 141 subjects from 16 years to 90 years of age was tested with a background brightness range from 34 cd/m² (1.0 ft L) to 0.034 cd/m² (0.01 ft L), with the contrast varying from 95% to 11%, as shown in Figure 4-20. With a luminance of 34 cd/m², the curves overlap, indicating that some of the older subjects performed at the same level as younger subjects, but most young eyes performed better than the older eyes. As the background brightness level was reduced to 0.34 cd/m² and 0.034 cd/m², the performance of younger subjects greatly exceeded that of the older subjects. The older subjects could not perform at the 0.034 cd/m² level of background luminance. As the

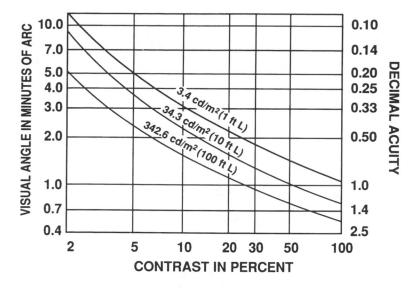

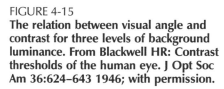

FIGURE 4-15
The relation between visual angle and contrast for three levels of background luminance. From Blackwell HR: Contrast thresholds of the human eye. J Opt Soc Am 36:624–643 1946; with permission.

contrast of the test letters decreased below 30% to 40%, vision decreased rapidly, with the 60-year-old subjects requiring a 25% increase in contrast to see the same target at the same brightness as the 20-year-old subject. These data clearly demonstrate that the old eye does not perform at the same level as the young eye, especially under low levels of light (Fig. 4-19).

The contrast functions using the forced-choice method and 35 subjects in the 20- to 30-year age group were related to the brightness contrast data obtained from 68 subjects in the 40- to 70-year age range using the method of adjustment.[85,86] In spite of the differences between the research methodologies, the data can be related by contrast

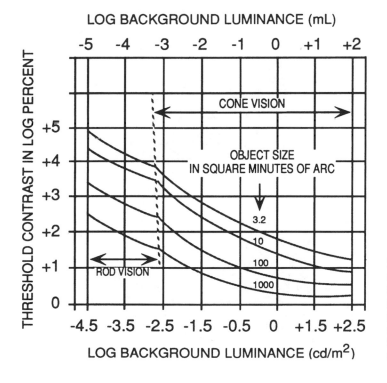

FIGURE 4-16
Contrast threshold as a function of the size of the object. The contrast required to see is drastically reduced as the object increases in size when the background luminance remains the same. From Blackwell HR: Contrast thresholds of the human eye. J Opt Soc Am 36:624–643 1946; with permission.

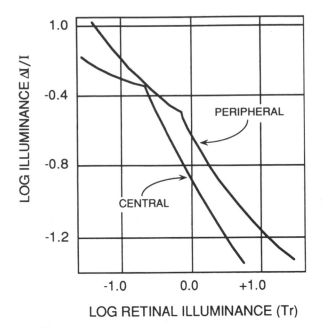

FIGURE 4-17
Contrast as a function of the region of the retina. The curves represent a JND in retinal illuminance for the central and peripheral retina. Contrast discrimination is generally poorer in the periphery compared to the central retina. Modified from Wulfeck JW, Weiz A, Raben MW: Vision in Military Aviation. WADC Technical Report 58–399. Wright-Patterson Air Force Base, Wright Air Development Center, 1958.

CHROMATIC CONTRAST. The objects in the visual field are usually not black and white but are seen in color. The measurement of color (colorimetry) has demonstrated that the percept of color includes three attributes: the luminance or brightness, which describes the intensity of the stimulus; hue or color, which describes the spectral composition or dominant wavelength of the stimulus; and saturation, which describes the amount of the hue or color in the

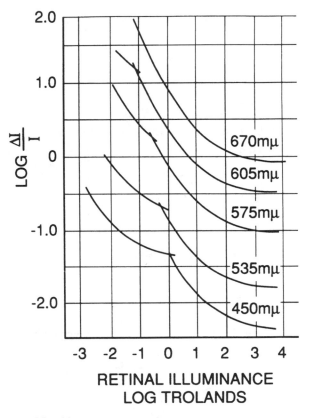

FIGURE 4-18
Contrast threshold as a function of wavelength for different levels of retinal illuminance. The breaks in the curves divide rod and cone functions. The ordinate has been labeled for the yellow 575-nm curve. The 605-nm curve has been elevated 0.5 log unit, the 670-nm curve has been elevated 1.0 log units, whereas the 535 nm and 450 nm curves have been lowered 0.5 and 1.0 log unit, respectively. These alterations allow the data to be compared more easily. From Hecht S, Peskin JC, Patt M: Intensity discrimination in the human eye. II. Relation between $\Delta I/I$ and intensity for different parts of the spectrum. J Gen Physiol 33:7–19 1938; by copyright permission of the Rockefeller University Press.

multiplicative factors (Fig. 4-19). The contrast multiplier indicates the amount that contrast must be increased for the object to just be seen. The data show several factors relating contrast and age that can be gained from studying Figures 4-19 and 4-20. Observer variability increases with age, especially above the age of 40. As the variability increases some observers in each age group overlap with the preceding younger ages. Some of the eyes of the 60- to 70-year age group perform equal to the 55- to 60-year age group and the worst performers in the 40- to 50-year age group, but most younger subjects perform better than 60- to 70-year-old observers. An increase in contrast by a factor of 2.50 for the 60- to 70-year age group, 1.7 for the 50- to 60-year age group, 0.5 for 40- to 50-year age group, and 0.3 for the 30- to 40-year age group is required to allow a visual target stimulus to just be seen.

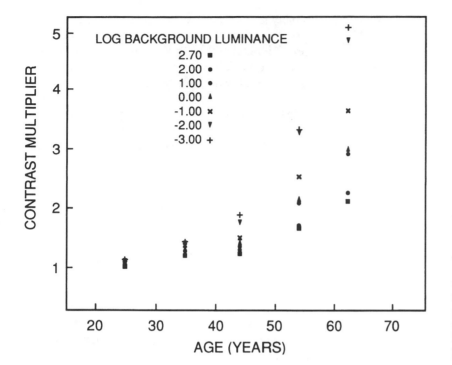

FIGURE 4-19
Contrast thresholds versus age for 156 normal subjects using seven background luminances. The contrast multiplier indicates the required increase in contrast for the target to be seen. From Blackwell OM, Blackwell HR: Visual performance for 156 normal observers of various ages. J Illumin Eng Soc 1:3–13, 1971; with permission.

stimulus relative to the white component. It is difficult to vary any of the three attributes of color vision without affecting the remaining attributes. For example, if luminance or brightness is changed sufficiently, a change can be demonstrated in both saturation and hue. If an object possesses the same luminance as its background but differs in color or hue, the visibility of that object results from the differences in hue and saturation rather than luminance. Chromatic contrast is a term that describes the visibility of objects due to the hue differences with the background.

Chromatic contrast cannot be predicted from luminance contrast because the borders between two colors may be distinct even though the luminances are the same and border phenomena enter into the evaluation.[88] Chromatic contrast produces maximum visibility when its value is 20% of the luminance contrast.[80] Care must be taken when measuring the luminances for chromatic contrast because the measured luminance may not reveal a perceptual brightness equivalent.[89] For example, you may measure $10\,cd/m^2$ of red light, which will not appear as bright as $10\,cd/m^2$ of green light. Chromatic contrast is very difficult to define and study because so many color

phenomena occur simultaneously such as brightness, hue, saturation or purity, afterimages, adaptation level, spatial relationships, and position in the visual field. There is a tendency for the eye or visual system to accentuate differences between chromatic objects that are juxtaposed in visual space. If the phenomenon is spatial in extent it is called *simultaneous contrast*, but if the stimuli are presented in time, the phenomenon is known as *successive contrast*.

The following general statements may be made relative to juxtaposed chromatic objects:

- Juxtaposed objects that produce high or low luminances appear brighter or darker than if viewed at some distance apart or separated in time.
- The same hue possessing high or low saturations appears higher or lower when compared to achromatic objects.
- Sharp contours or borders separating two areas containing colors tend to increase the saturation or brightness of the areas.
- High luminance contrast tends to reduce chromatic contrast, whereas equal luminances tend to maximize hue contrast.

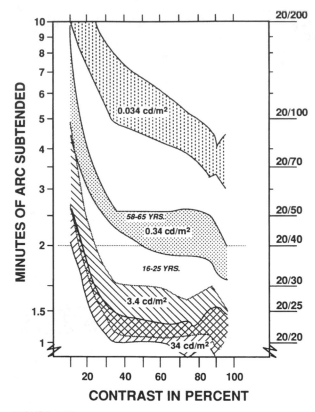

FIGURE 4-20

The visual acuity and contrast sensitivity of 141 subjects from 16 to 90 years of age. At the higher background luminances, the data for the different ages overlap, but the younger subjects performed better at all levels of background luminance than the older subjects. From Richards, OW: Vision levels of night road illumination. XII. Changes in acuity and contrast with age. Am J Optom Physiol Opt 43:313–319. (c) The American Academy of Optometry, 1966, with permission.

GLARE

Glare is the loss in visual performance or visibility, or annoyance or discomfort produced by a luminance in the visual field greater than the luminance to which the eyes are adapted. There are three types of glare: veiling or disability glare, discomfort glare, and reflection glare. *Veiling or disability glare* occurs when the excessive light in the visual field interferes with visual performance and visibility. *Discomfort glare* occurs when the excessive luminance in the visual field results in annoyance or discomfort. Visual performance and visibility may be affected with or without annoyance or discomfort; i.e., veiling or

disability glare may be experienced independent of discomfort glare. Conversely, discomfort glare may be experienced without a decrement in visual performance or visibility but is usually accompanied by losses in visibility and performance.

The third type of glare, *reflection glare*, is often confused with disability glare and discomfort glare. Reflection glare results from excessive luminance reflected from surfaces. Typical examples include reflection from the automobile windshield that prevents the driver from seeing the street, reflections from water that prevent the fisherman from seeing below the water's surface, and reflections from the VDT.

DISABILITY GLARE OR VEILING GLARE.   Veiling glare or disability glare occurs because the eye is not a perfect optical system and does not produce a precise point-to-point image on the retina. Instead, the optical media obeys Rayleigh's law ($1/\lambda^4$) in which the inhomogeneities scatter the light across the retina onto the retinal image of the object. The scattered light across the retinal image reduces retinal luminance contrast and interferes with normal visibility or visual performance. Disability glare affects the visual system because light scattered in the ocular media reduces visual acuity and the differential light threshold is raised.

There are many different sources of disability glare. The classic example is the glare that is created by discrete sources of light such as streetlights or automobile headlights.[90] In fact, it may be argued that every luminous line or point in the visual field may be capable of creating a disability glare because its glare effect is directly proportional to the intensity of the glare source and the angle of the source from the line of sight.[91] Large sources such as windows, doors, and the sky also act as sources for disability glare. It has also been demonstrated that two or more glare sources in the field of vision are additive.

Headlights from an oncoming automobile at night provide an excellent example of disability glare because the retina must re-adapt to resume vision after the car has passed. Sometimes automobile headlights result in discomfort glare. The same automobile with headlights on during daylight hours is usually more easily seen but cannot be classified as a disability or discomfort glare source.

Regional variations or fluctuations of luminance in the visual field are uncomfortable and result in the retina constantly readjusting the level of adaptation. Such a condition is called *transient adaptation*.[92,93] To reduce transient adaptation to a comfortable ratio, the target luminance should not exceed the luminance of the background by more than a factor of 3 or 4. Shadows should be limited to a ± 10% difference from the background in order to not be annoying. These levels are ideal for those using the VDT.

Research on veiling glare has shown that the total scattered light at the fovea is proportional to the number of the scattering particles per unit volume of the ocular media.[94] The glare source results in an actual veil of light over the fovea that changes its adaptation or sensitivity to visual stimuli. The results are confirmed by the fact that the disability glare is more serious for eyes above the age of 40 and especially so for cloudy ocular media.[95,96] The cause appears to be the lens and entopic scatter of the ocular media where scatter from the wavelength range from 420 to 650 nm are independent of wavelength.[97]

The role of the luminance of the source and the angle of the source to the eye in disability glare has taken the following mathematic form:[98–101]

$$L'_v = k\, E_v/\theta^n \qquad (4\text{-}21)$$

where L'_v represents the disability of the glare source, E_v the illuminance at the observer's eye of the glare source, θ the angle of the glare source from the line of sight, and k and n are constants. This formula is known as the Stiles-Holladay formula for disability glare. When the glare source luminance L'_v is in foot lamberts and the illuminance E_v is in lm/ft^2, the value for k is 10π and the value for n is 2. The glare data of Holladay, LeGrand, and Walraven are plotted in Figure 4-21.[102] Fry[103,104] proposed a modified formula to express disability glare, but the Stiles-Holladay formula gives closer agreement with empiric data.[105] The Stiles-Holladay formula constants were re-examined and the constant n was found to have a mean value of 2.3 that did not vary with age.[105] The constant k was related to age and the background luminance with k = (0.2A + 5.8)π, where A is the age of the observer and 5.8 the factor for the background luminance.

DISCOMFORT GLARE.   If the eye is suddenly exposed to a light much higher in luminance than the source to which the eye is adapted, the observer experi-

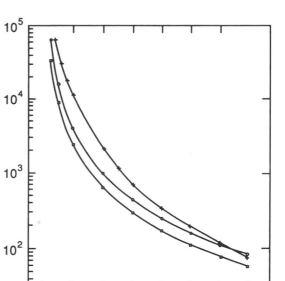

FIGURE 4-21
Veiling or disability glare produced a certain luminance at an angle θ from the line of sight. The data are from Holladay (□), LeGrand (o), and Walraven (+), and although spanning a half century are in remarkable agreement. From Sliney D, Wolbarsht, M: Safety with Lasers and Other Optical Sources. New York, Plenum Press, 1980; with permission.

ences discomfort. The discomfort is usually manifest by pupillary constriction, closure of the palpebral aperture, and aversion by turning the head. This sensation of annoyance, discomfort, or pain caused by high or nonuniform distribution of light in the visual field is known as discomfort glare. The cause is not fully understood but has been related to pupillary activity.[106,107] Discomfort glare varies with six different factors:

1. Size of the glare source[80]
2. Luminance of the background[108]
3. Luminance of the glare source[80]
4. Number of glare sources[90,109]
5. Angle of the glare source to the line of sight[110]
6. Age of the person[95,111,112]

Research on discomfort glare uses the acronym BCD, which indicates the borderline between comfort and discomfort. The BCD is presented as a

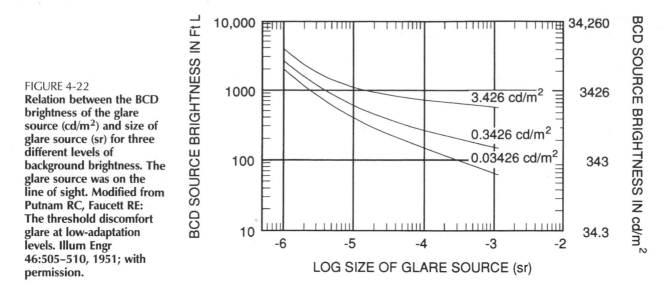

FIGURE 4-22
Relation between the BCD brightness of the glare source (cd/m²) and size of glare source (sr) for three different levels of background brightness. The glare source was on the line of sight. Modified from Putnam RC, Faucett RE: The threshold discomfort glare at low-adaptation levels. Illum Engr 46:505–510, 1951; with permission.

curve but represents the region in which the mean or median values for discomfort are found.

The size of the glare source interacts with its brightness to produce discomfort. Generally, the larger the glare source, the lower will be the brightness of the glare source needed to produce discomfort (Fig. 4-22). The sky is a vast extended source, and the sunlight necessary to cause discomfort approaches 100,000 cd/m², but discrete sources such as a searchlight or a laser can create discomfort with brightnesses as low as 10 cd/m². With the background kept constant, the smaller the angle of the glare source with the line of sight, the lower the brightness of the source required to produce

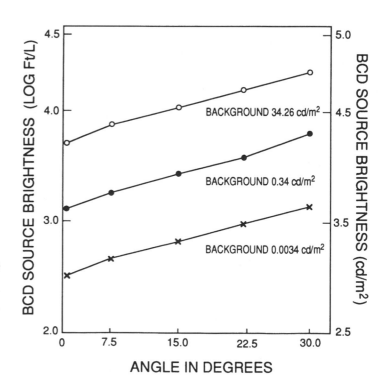

FIGURE 4-23
Relation between BCD source brightness and the angle of the glare source in degrees for three selected levels of adaptation. The data illustrate that as the angle from the line of sight increases, large increases in the glare source intensity are required. Data from Bennett CA: Discomfort glare: Concentrated sources—parametric study of angularly small sources. J ILLUM Eng Soc 6:2–15, 1977; with permission.

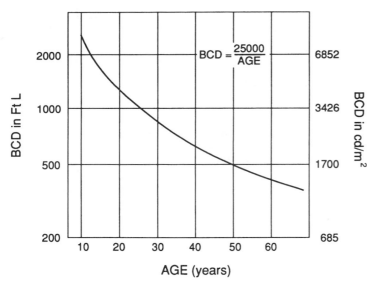
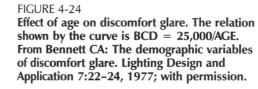

FIGURE 4-24
Effect of age on discomfort glare. The relation shown by the curve is BCD = 25,000/AGE. From Bennett CA: The demographic variables of discomfort glare. Lighting Design and Application 7:22–24, 1977; with permission.

discomfort (Fig. 4-23). At the same time, the number of glare sources in the visual field are additive.[109,113]

Finally, the brightness of the source necessary to produce glare decreases as age increases when the background brightness is kept constant (Fig. 4-24). The aged eye does not ever perform to the same level as the young eye. Wolf[95] found an increase in discomfort glare above the age of 40 and claims the cause is the lens and entopic scatter. Several interesting correlations have been found on the relation of glare and age.[112] The median BCD for ages 20 years to 68 years was 3,940 cd/m^2 (1150 ft L), with those performing outdoor occupations showing a median of 6500 cd/m^2 (1900 ft L) compared to 3400 cd/m^2 (1000 ft L) for those who worked indoors. Brown-eyed subjects showed a median BCD of 4450 cd/m^2 (1300 ft L), whereas blue-eyed subjects had a median BCD of 3770 cd/m^2 (1100 ft L). The BCD at age 10 was about 8500 cd/m^2, which decreases to about 1700 cd/m^2 at 50 years of age. The cause of this loss is probably due to changes in the ocular media and neural retina.[114]

The cause of most glare problems can be reduced to three variables: angle θ the glare source makes to the line of sight, the intensity L_v of the glare source, and the age of the person. If the line of sight and intensity of the source can be controlled, discomfort glare can be reduced to a comfortable level. If a glare source makes an angle of 30° or greater to the line of sight, the source may no longer be considered a glare source.

REFLECTION GLARE.   As has been noted, reflection glare is the result of excessive light being reflected from shiny surfaces. In addition to the typical examples of glare mentioned earlier reflection glare includes reflection from the auto windshield, water, and the VDT screen glare. In each example, the reflections prevent the observer from seeing.... The most obvious correction for reflection glare is polaroid lenses because the reflected light is polarized and the proper polaroid lens prevents the reflected polarized light from reaching the eye while allowing restoration of normal vision.

References

1. Moss CH, Ellis RJ, Parr WH, Murray WE. Biological Effects of Infrared Radiation. DHHS (NIOSH) Publication No. 82-109. Washington, DC, U.S. Dept. Health and Human Services, 1982.
2. Riggs LA. Light as a stimulus for vision. *In* Graham CH (ed): Vision and Visual Perception. New York, John Wiley & Sons, 1966.
3. Stair R, Schneider WE, Jackson JK. New Standard of spectral irradiance. Appl Opt 1963; 2:1151–1154.
4. Deuterium lamp of standard spectral irradiance. Opt Radiat News, No. 11 and No. 32. National Bureau Standards. Washington, Sept. 1975, July 1980.
5. A new diagnostic standard for UV-B region. Opt Radiat News, National Bureau Standards, No. 20. Washington DC, April 1977.

6. Selection Guide for Quality Lighting. Form 9200. Nela Park Research Center, Cleveland, General Electric, 1988.
7. Sylvania Fluorescent Lamps Engineering. Bulletin 0341. Danvers, MA, May 1982.
8. Laue EG, Drummond EG. Solar constant: First direct measurements. Science 1968; 161:888–891.
9. Thekaekara MP. Survey of literature on the solar constant and the spectral distribution of solar radiant flux. NASA SP-74. Greenbelt, MD, Goddard Space Flight Center, 1965.
10. Thekaekara MP. Solar irradiance: Total and spectral irradiance—its possible variations. Appl Opt 1976; 15:915–920.
11. Mercherikunnel AT, Gatlin JA, Richmond JC. Data on total and spectral solar irradiance. Appl Opt 1983; 22:1354–1359.
12. Frohlich C. Data on total and spectral solar irradiance: Comments. Appl Opt 1983; 22:3928.
13. Mercherikunnel AT. Data on total and spectral solar irradiance: Reply to comments. Appl Opt 1985; 24:8.
14. Frohlich C, Brusa RW. Solar radiation and its variation in time. Solar Phys 1981; 74:209–215.
15. Kuhn JR, Libbrecht KE, Dicke RH. The surface temperature of the sun and changes in the solar constant. Science 1988; 242:908–913.
16. Foukal P, Lean J. An empirical model of total solar irradiance variation between 1874 and 1988. Science 1990; 247:556–558.
17. Solar Electromagnetic Radiation. NASA Special Publication 8005. Greenbelt, MD, Goddard Space Flight Center, NASA, 1971.
18. Standard Specification for Solar Constant and Air Mass Zero Solar Spectral Irradiance. ASTM Standard, E490-73a, 1974. Annual Book of ASTM Standards, Part 41. Philadelphia, ASTM, 1974.
19. Johnson FS, Mo T, Green AES. Average latitudinal variation in ultraviolet radiation at the earth's surface. Photochem Photobiol 1976; 23:179–188.
20. Coblentz WW, Grady FR, Stair R. Measurements of ultraviolet solar and sky radiation intensities in high latitudes. J Res Natl Bur Stds 1942; 28:581–591.
21. Diffey BL. Environmental exposure to UV-B radiation. Rev Environ Health 1984; 4:317–337.
22. Condon TP, Toolin RB, Stakutis VJ. Visibility, Chap 14. In Campen CF, Jr, Cole AE, Condron TP, Ripley WS, Sissenwine N, Solomon T (eds): Handbook of Geophysics for Air Force Designers (1st ed). Geophysics Res. Direct., A.F. Cambridge Research Center, Air Research and Development Command, USAF, 1957.
23. Mercherikunnel AT, Richmond AT. Spectral Distribution of Solar Radiation. NASA Technical Memorandum 82021. Greenbelt, MD, Goddard Space Flight Center, 1980.
24. Labs D, Neckel H. Transformation of the absolute solar radiation data into the "International Practical Temperature Scale of 1968." Solar Phys 1970; 15:79–87.
25. Neckel H, Labs D. Improved data of solar spectral irradiance from 0.33 to 1.25 m. Solar Phys 1981; 74:231–249.
26. Henderson ST. Daylight and Its Spectrum. New York, American Elsevier Publishing Company, Inc, 1970.
27. Kondratyev KYA. Radiation in the Atmosphere. New York, Academic Press, 1969.
28. Petitt E. Measurements of ultraviolet solar radiation. Astrophys 1932; 75:185–221.
29. Kostkowski HG, Saunders RD, W, JF, Popenoe CH, Green AES. Measurement of solar terrestrial spectral irradiance in the ozone cut-off region, Chap 1. In Self-Study Manual on Optical Radiation Measurements: Part III, Applications. NBC Technical Note 910-5. Washington, DC, U.S. Govt Printing Office, 1982.
30. Shettle EP, Green AES. Multiple scattering calculation of the middle ultraviolet reaching the ground. Appl Opt 1974; 13:1567–1581.
31. Shettle EP, Nack ML, Green AES. Multiple scattering and the influence of clouds, haze and smog on the middle UV reaching the ground. In Impacts of Climatic Change in the Biosphere, Part 1, Ultraviolet Radiation Effects. Final Report. PB 247 724, DOT-TST-75-55. Washington, DC, Department of Transportation, 1975.
32. Nachtwey DS. Impacts of climatic change on the biosphere. Climatic Impact Assessment Program, Monograph 5, Part 1, Ultraviolet Radiation Effects. Chaps 4–10. PB-247-725, DOT-TST-75-25. Washington, DC, Department of Transportation, 1975.
33. Berger DS, Urbach F. A climatology of sunburning ultraviolet radiation Photochem Photobiol 1982; 35:187–192.
34. Green AES, Swada T, Shettel EP. The middle ultraviolet reaching the ground. Photochem Photobiol 1974; 19:251–259.
35. Willson RC, Gulkis S, Janssen M, Hudson HS, Chapman GA. Observations of solar irradiance variability. Science 1981; 211:700–702.
36. Bener P. Approximate Values of Intensity of Natural Ultraviolet Radiation for Different Amounts of Atmospheric Ozone. Final Tech Report. London, European Research Office, US Army, 1972.
37. Sutherland RA, McPeters RP, Findley GB, Green AES. Sunphotometry and spectral radiometry of wavelengths below 360 nm. J Atmos Sci 1975; 37:427–436.
38. Kollias N, Baquer AH, Isad IQ. Measurements of solar middle ultraviolet radiation in a desert environment. Photochem Photobiol 1988; 47:565–569.
39. Pettit E. Spectral energy-curve of the sun in the ultraviolet, Astrophys J 1940; 91:159–185.
40. Baker KS, Smith RC, Green AES. Middle ultraviolet radiation reaching the ocean surface. Photochem Photobiol 1980; 32:367–374.

41. Blumthaler M, Ambach W, Canaval H. Seasonal variation of solar UV-radiation at a high mountain station. Photochem Photobiol 1985; 42:147–152.
42. Grosbecker AJ (editor-in-chief). Impacts of Climatic Change on the Biosphere. Climatic Impact Assessment Program, Monograph 5, Part 1, Ultraviolet Radiation Effects. Chaps 1–3. PB-247-724, DOT-TST-75-55. Washington, DC, Department of Transportation, 1975.
43. Farman JC, Gardiner BG, Shanklin JD. Large losses of total ozone in Antarctica reveal seasonal CLO_x/NO_x interaction. Nature 1985; 315:207–210.
44. Molina MJ, Rowland FS. Stratospheric sink for chlorofluoromethane: Chlorine atom-catalysed destruction of ozone. Nature 1974; 249:810–812.
45. Halpern P, Dave JV, Braslau N. Sea-level solar radiation in the biologically active spectrum. Science 1974; 186:1204–1207.
46. Brasseur G, Hitchman MH. Stratospheric response to trace gas perturbations: Changes in ozone and temperature distributions. Science 1988; 240:634–637.
47. Cicerone RJ, Stolarski RS, Walters S. Stratospheric ozone destruction by manmade chlorofluoromethanes. Science 1984, 185:1165–1167.
48. Rowland SF. Chloroflurocarbons and the depletion of stratospheric ozone. Amer. Sci 1989; 77:36–45.
49. Alyea FN, Cunnold DM, Prinn RG. Stratospheric ozone destruction by aircraft-induced nitrogen oxides. Science 1975; 188:117–121.
50. Maugh TH, II. Research News: The threat to ozone is real, increasing. Science 1979; 206:1167–1168.
51. Schiff HI. Stratospheric Ozone Depletion by Halocarbons. Washington, DC, Panel on Chemistry and Transport, National Academy of Sciences, Chairman of the Panel, 1979.
52. Gille JC, Smyth CM, Heath DF. Observed ozone response to variations in solar ultraviolet radiation. Science 1984; 225:315–317.
53. Kerr RA. Research News: Stratospheric ozone is decreasing. Science 1988; 239:1489–1491.
54. Kerr RA. Research News: Taking shots at ozone hole theories. Science 1986; 234:817–818.
55. Kerr RA. Research News: Artic ozone is poised for a fall. Science 1989; 1007–1008.
56. Bowman D. Global trends in total ozone. Science 1988; 239:48–50.
57. Kerr RA. Does the ozone hole threaten Arctic life? Science 1989; 244:288–289.
58. Kerr RA. Evidence of Arctic ozone destruction. Science 1988; 240:1144–1145.
59. Reck RA. Stratospheric ozone effects on temperature. Science 1976; 192:557–559.
60. Frederick JE, Lubin D. Possible long-term changes in biologically active ultraviolet radiation reaching the ground. Photochem Photobiol 1988; 47:571–578.
61. Environmental Effects Panel Report Pursuant to Article 6 of the Montreal Protocol on Substances That Deplete the Ozone Layer. Nations Environment Programme (UNEP), November 1989. Available from U.S. Environmental Protection Agency, Washington, DC.
62. Solomon S, Mount GA, Sanders RW et al. Observations of nighttime abundance of OCIO in the winter above Thule, Greenland. Science 1988; 242:550–555.
63. Mount GH, Soloman S, Sanders RW, et al. Observations of stratospheric NO_2 and O_3 at Thule, Greenland. Science 1988; 242:555–562.
64. Crawford M. EPA to cut U.S. CFC production to protect ozone in stratosphere. Science 1989; 238:1505.
65. Urbach F. Geographic pathology of skin cancer. In Urbach F (ed): The Biologic Effects of Ultraviolet Radiation with Emphasis on the Skin, pp 635–650. New York, Pergamon Press, 1969.
66. Taylor HR, West SK, Rosenthal FS, Mudoz B, Newland HS, Abbey H, Emmett EA. Effect of ultraviolet radiation on cataract formation. N Engl J Med 1988; 319:1429–1433.
67. Montreal Protocol on Substances that Deplete the Ozone Layer. United Nations Environment Programme (UNEP), Na 87-6106. Final Act. 1987. Available from U.S. Environmental Protection Agency, Washington, D.C.
68. Dickson D, Marchall E. Europe recognizes the ozone threat. Science 1989; 243:1279.
69. Wyszecki G, Stiles WS. Physical data, Section One. In Color Science: Concepts and Methods, Quantitative Data and Formulas. New York, John Wiley & Sons, Inc, 1967.
70. Wulfeck JW, Weiz A, Raben MW. Vision in Military Aviation. WADC Technical Report 58-399. Wright-Patterson Air Force Base, Wright Air Development Center, 1958.
71. Wright WD. The luminosity curve of the eye, Chap 2, pp 25–42. In Photometry and the Eye. London, Hatton Press Ltd, 1949.
72. International body recommends value for Km. Opt Radiat News, No. 22. Washington, Department of Commerce, National Bureau of Standards, 1977.
73. Moon P. The Scientific Basis of Illuminating Engineering (rev ed). New York, Dover Publications, Inc, 1961.
74. LeGrand Y. Light, Color and Vision. Translated by Hunt RWG, Walsh JWT, Hunt FRN. London, Chapman Hall Ltd., 1957.
75. Pirenne MH. Measurement of the stimulus, Chap 1. In Davson H (ed): The Eye, Vol 2, The Visual Process. New York, Academic Press, 1962.
76. Crawford BH, Jones OC. Physical measurements and calibration of apparatus, Chap 7. In Crawford BH, Gringer GW, Weale RA (eds): Techniques in Photostimulation in Biology. New York, John Wiley & Sons, 1968.

77. Konig A. Die Abhangigkeit der Sehscharfe von der Belauchtungsinstensitat. Sitzber Akad Wiss (Berl) 1897; 35:559–575.

78. Hecht S. The relation between visual acuity and illumination. J Gen Physiol 1928; 11:255–281.

79. Shlaer S, Smith EL, Chase AM. Visual acuity and illumination of different spectral regions. J Gen Physiol 1942; 25:553–569.

80. Lewis AL, Douglas CA. Light and vision. In Kaufman JE, Haynes H (eds): Illuminating Engineering Society Handbook. Reference Volume, Section 3:14, 1981.

81. Fry GA. The optical performance of the human eye. In Wolf E (ed). Progress in Optics, Vol III, pp 70–71. Amsterdam, North Holland Publishing Co, 1970.

82. Blackwell HR. Contrast thresholds of the human eye. J Opt Soc Am 1946; 36:624–643.

83. Hecht S, Peskin JC, Patt M. Intensity discrimination in the human eye. II. Relation between $\Delta I/I$ and intensity for different parts of the spectrum. J Gen Physiol 1938; 33:7–19.

84. Richards OW. Vision at levels of night road illumination. XII. Changes of acuity and contrast with age. Am J Optom Arch Am Acad Optom 1966; 43:313–319.

85. Blackwell OM, Blackwell HR. Visual performance data for 156 normal observers of various ages. J Illumin Eng Soc 1971; 1:3–13.

86. Blackwell HR, Taylor JH. A Consolidated Set of Foveal Contrast Thresholds for Normal Human Binocular Vision. The Ohio State University and University of California, San Diego, Report, Columbus OH, 1970.

87. Guth SK. Effects of age on visibility. Am J Optom Am Acad Optom 1957; 34:463–477.

88. Eastman AA. Color contrast vs luminance contrast. Illumin Eng 1968; 63:613–619.

89. Eastman AA, Allen CJ, Brecher GA. The subjective measurement of color shifts with various light sources. J Illum Eng Soc 1972; 2:23–28.

90. Bennett CA. Discomfort glare: Concentrated sources—parametric study of angularly small sources. J Illum Eng Soc 1977; 6:2–15.

91. Bouma PJ. The problem of glare in highway lighting. Phillips Tech Rev 1936; 1:225–229.

92. Rinalducci EJ. Early dark adaptation as a function of wavelength and pre-adapting level. J Opt Soc Am 1967; 57:1270–1271.

93. Rinalducci EJ, Beare AN. Losses in night time visibility caused by transient adaptation. J Illum Eng Soc 1974; 3:336–345.

94. Wolf E, Gardiner JS. Studies on the scatter of light in the dioptric media as a basis of visual glare. Arch Ophthalmol 1965; 74:338–345.

95. Wolf E. Glare and age. Arch Ophthalmol 1960; 64:502–514.

96. Vos JJ, Bouman MA. Disability glare; theory and practice. Proc CIE [B] 1959; 298–307.

97. Wooten BR, Geri GA. Psychophysical determination of intraocular light scatter as a function of wavelength. Vision Res 1987; 27:1291–1298.

98. Holladay LL. Action of a light-source in the field of view in lowering visibility. J Opt Soc Am 1927; 1–15.

99. Stiles WS. The effect of glare on the brightness difference threshold. Proc Roy Soc [Biol], 1929; B104:322–350.

100. LeGrand Y. Recherches sur la diffusion de la lumiere dans l'oeil humain. Revue d'Optique 1937; 12:201–214, 241–266.

101. Walraven J, Spatial characteristics of chromatic induction; the segregation of lateral effects of straylight artifacts. Vision Res 1973; 13:1739–1753.

102. Sliney D, Wolbarsht M. Safety with Lasers and Other Optical Sources. New York, Plenum Press, 1980.

103. Fry GA. A re-evaluation of the scattering theory of glare. Illum Eng 1954; 49:98–102.

104. Fry GA. Physiological bases of disability glare. Proc CIE 1955; 1:1.4.2 Paper U-F.

105. Fisher AJ, Christie AW. A note on disability glare. Vision Res 1965; 5:565–571.

106. Fry GA, King VM. The pupillary response and discomfort glare. J Illum Eng Soc 1975; 5:307–324.

107. Fugate JM, Fry GA. Relation in changes in pupil size to discomfort. Illum Eng 1956; 56:537–548.

108. Putnam RC, Faucett RE. The threshold discomfort glare at low adaptation levels. Illum Eng, 46:505–510, 1951.

109. Putnam RC, Bower KD. Discomfort glare at low adaptation levels. Part III. Multiple sources. Illum Eng, 53:174–184, 1958.

110. Putnam RC, Gillmore WF, Jr. Discomfort glare at low adaptation levels. Part II. Off axis sources. Illum Eng 52:226–232, 1957.

111. Reading VM. Disability glare and age. Vision Res 1968; 8:207–214.

112. Bennett CA. The demographic variables of discomfort glare. Lighting Design and Application 1977; 7:22–24.

113. Bennett CA. Discomfort glare: Concentrated sources—parametric study of angularly small sources. J Illum Eng Soc 1977; 6:2–15.

114. Guth SK. Effects of age on visibility. Am J Optom Arch Am Acad Optom 1957; 47:463–477.

Appendix 4-1

Units And Symbols

A system of units and symbols is necessary to allow the orderly presentation and interchange of information with the literature. The International System of Units (SI) is used throughout the book for the base units and for units that are derived from the base units.[1] Appendix Table 4-1 presents the base units for the SI system. Note that only the symbol for temperature [K] and for electric current [A] are represented by capital letters. SI symbols do not require punctuation and the symbol for temperature [K] does not require the superscript for degrees. The SI unit should be enclosed between brackets [ ] when used within an equation. Appendix Table 4-2 illustrates the SI prefixes, their symbols, and mathematic factors. The symbols and mathematic prefixes of the SI units may be used in combination to form decimal multiples and submultiples of the SI system.

The symbol used to designate the wavelength of optical radiation is λ and the unit of measure is the nanometer (nm). The nm is equal to 10^{-9} m which is equivalent to 10^{-7} cm, 10^{-6} mm and 10Å. The wavelength of optical radiation has historically been called the angstrom (Å), the millimicron (mμ), and the micrometer (μm). The micrometer (μm) was formerly the micron and is equal to 10^{-6} m, 10^{-4} cm, and 10^{-3} mm.

The new definition of the SI photometric unit, the candela, was approved internationally by the 16th General Conference on Weights and Measures

Factor	Prefix	Symbol	Factor	Prefix	Symbol
10^{18}	exa	E	10^{-1}	deci	d
10^{15}	peta	P	10^{-2}	centi	c
10^{12}	tera	T	10^{-3}	milli	m
10^{9}	giga	G	10^{-6}	micro	μ
10^{6}	mega	M	10^{-9}	nano	n
10^{3}	kilo	k	10^{-12}	pico	p
10^{2}	hecto	h	10^{-15}	femto	f
10^{1}	deka	da	10^{-18}	atto	a

APPENDIX TABLE 4-2
SI Prefixes, Symbols, and Mathematic Factors

(GCPM) meeting in October 1979, at Paris, France, with the following definition:[2]

1. The candela is the luminous intensity, in a given direction, of a source emitting monochromatic radiation of frequency 540×10^{12} hertz and whose radiant intensity in this direction is 1/683 watt per steradian.
2. The candela so defined is the base unit applicable to photopic quantities, scotopic quantities, and quantities to be defined in the mesopic domain.

This action by the GCPM was the final step in the process of approving a definition of photometric units that will allow the same terminology and formulas to be used for both radiometric and photometric measurements.

In radiometry, the watt (W) is the unit of power which is usually used with a unit of area, thusly: W/cm^2 and W/m^2. The joule (J) is the unit of energy and is equal to W · s. Occasionally, the unit used to express the energy of a source is in calories per centimeter squared and minute (cal/cm^2 · min) with the conversion factor to joules being 1.0 J = 0.239 calories.

Throughout the text both radiometric and photometric terms are used with e and v as subscripts. The subscript e (E_e) designates units that are radiometric and the subscript v (E_v) indicates photometric quantities. If a biologic system is exposed to a certain irradiance per unit area (W/m^2) for a selected duration of time in seconds (s), the process is known as a radiant exposure and its symbol is H. The radiant exposure H is expressed mathematically as a

Physical Quantity	Name of Unit	Symbol of Unit
length	meter	m
mass	kilogram	kg
time	second	s
electric current	ampere	A
thermodynamic temperature	kelvin	K
amount of substance	mole	mol
luminous intensity	candela	cd

APPENDIX TABLE 4-1
Base Units for the International System of Units (SI)

W·s/cm^2; however, W·s defines the unit of energy or the joule, using the symbol J; thus, a radiant exposure H is expressed in J/m^2. Subscripts to the symbol for radiant exposure H are used to represent the anatomic portion of the eye that has been exposed. H_c, H_l, and H_r represent exposures to the cornea, the lens and the retina, respectively. The word *dose* is an additional term encountered in the literature for radiant exposure, but since the term *dose* has been traditionally used to designate the amount of a pharmaceutical agent to be taken, the term radiant exposure (H) is used throughout the text.

The SI derived units and conversion tables for both radiometry and photometry are presented in Chapter 4, which also explains their use. This is a matter of convenience because it eliminates searching for a table that is being explained in another portion of the book.

Appendix Table 4-3 presents the physical quantities, unit name, and unit symbol for other units derived from the SI base units that are commonly used. Voltage or electromotive force and magnetomotive force are often found associated with units of area such as V/m^2 or A/m^2. An example occurs when microwaves are measured: both the electric vector and the magnetic vectors are measured and expressed as V/m^2 and A/m^2.

During reading it is often necessary to be able to convert from one physical quantity to another within a reasonable period of time. Appendix Table 4-4 is designed for that purpose and presents selected SI and derived SI conversion factors for quantities used in the text. In solving problems, it is convenient to make a quick comparison of the physical stimulus to its retinal equivalent. Appendix Table 4-5 provides the relationship of the physical angle and the physical solid angle to the distance or area on the retina.[3] Using Appendix Table 4-5, a source of 1.0 sr in physical space occupies an area of 278 mm^2 on the retina. The area of the total retina calculates to be 1145 mm^2 for an eyeball with an inside diameter of 23.5 mm, for a retina that occupies the poster two thirds of the globe, and an optic disc that is 1.5 mm in diameter. This calculation illustrates that the total retina encompasses 4.1 sr (1145 mm^2/278 mm^2).

CIE Standard Light Sources

During the era of intensive colorimetry research, it was discovered that the light source played a significant role in the responses obtained in color matching experiments. In order to eliminate the illuminant as a source of major error, the Committee Internationale d'Eclairage (CIE) has established five standard light sources. Figure 4-4 provides the relative spectral energy of CIE standard sources A, B, C, and E.

Standard Source A is a gas-filled, tungsten filament lamp operating at 2854 [K] on the international temperature scale of 1948 (Judd, 1950), possesses CIE chromaticity coordinates of $x = 0.448$ and $y = 0.4075$, and, in addition, the constant $C_2 = 1.4380$ cm/deg [K] for spectral energy calculations. It may be of interest that the normal 40-W incandescent, tungsten filament lamps may be as low as 2800 [K] while 100-W tungsten filament lamps may be as high as 2900 [K].

Standard Source B utilizes standard source A transmitted through a Davis-Gibson liquid filter to achieve an approximate color temperature of 4870 [K]. Standard Source B has the CIE chromaticity coordinates of $x = 0.349$ and $y = 0.352$. The filter is composed of two 1-cm layer cells with each containing one of two solutions:

Physical Quantity	Name of Unit	Symbol of Unit
area	square meter	m^2
frequency	hertz	Hz (s^{-1})
speed	meter per second	m/s
angular speed	meter per radian	m/rad
force	newton	N(kg·m/s^2)
pressure	pascal	Pa (N/m^2)
plane angle	radian	rad
solid angle	steradian	sr
voltage, electromotive force	volt	V
magnetomotive force	ampere	A

APPENDIX TABLE 4-3
Physical Units, Names and Symbols of Units Derived from the SI System That Are Commonly Used

To convert from	To	Multiply by
angstrom	meter	1×10^{-10}
calorie (thermochemical)	joule	4.184
minute (plane angle)	radian	2.909×10^{-4}
joule	calorie (thermochemical)	0.239
curie	disintegration/s	3.7×10^{10}
day (mean solar)	second (mean solar)	8.64×10^4
degree (plane angle)	radian	1.745×10^{-2}
radian	degrees (plane angle)	57.3
kilocalorie	joule	4.184×10^3
second (plane angle)	radian	4.84×10^{-6}
radian	seconds (plane angle)	206,280
electron volt	joule	1.602×10^{-19}
erg	joule	1.0×10^{-7}
erg/cm^2	watt/m^2	1.0×10^{-3}
gauss	tesla	1.0×10^{-4}
rad (radiation absorbed dose)	Gy (joule/kilogram)	1.0×10^{-2}
roentgen	coulomb/kilogram	2.5798×10^{-4}
W/cm^2	W/m^2	1×10^{-4}
SBU (sunburn unit) at 297 nm	J/m^2	200

APPENDIX TABLE 4-4
Factors for Converting Miscellaneous SI Units and Numbers Including Derived Units and Numbers into Additional Units and Numbers

Solution B1

Copper sulfate (CuSO$_4 \cdot$ 5H$_2$O)	2.452 g
Mannite (C$_6$H$_8$(OH)$_6$)	2.452 g
Pyridine (C$_5$H$_5$N)	30.0 cc
Distilled water to make	1000.0 ml

Solution B2

Cobalt ammonium sulfate (CoSO$_4 \cdot$ (NH$_4$)$_2$SO$_4 \cdot$ 6H$_5$O)	21.71 g
Copper sulfate (CuSO$_4 \cdot$ 5H$_2$O)	16.11 g
Sulphuric acid H$_2$SO$_4$ (1.835 density)	10.00 ml
Distilled water to make	1000.0 ml

Standard Source C also uses Standard Source A in combination with the Davis-Gibson two-solution filters to achieve 6500 [K] on the international temperature scale. Standard source C has the CIE chromaticity coordinates of $x = 0.3135$ and $y = 0.3236$. The two solutions are individually contained in 1-cm layer cells. The solutions are made up as follows:

External Angle	Distance on Retina
1.0 radian	16.383 mm
0.05994 radian	1.0 mm
1.0 degree	0.2912 mm
3.434 degrees	1.0 mm
1.0 minute	4.853 μm
0.2061 minute	1.0 μm

External Solid Angle	Area on the Retina
1.0 steradian	278.3 mm^2
0.003593 steradian	1.0 mm^2
1.0 square degree	0.08478 mm^2
11.80 square degrees	1.0 mm^2
1.0 square minute	23.55 μm^2
0.04246 square minute	1.0 μm^2

(Data from Wyszecki and Stiles, 1967).

APPENDIX TABLE 4-5
Relationship Between the Distance or Area on the Retina with the Visual Angle in Physical Space and the Areas on the Retina with Plain or Solid Angles in Physical Space

Wavelength (nm)	Irradiance ($Wm^{-2}\,nm^{-1}$)			Wavelength (nm)	Irradiance ($Wm^{-2}\,nm^{-1}$)		
	Solar O	Air mass 1	Air mass 2		Solar O	Air mass 1	Air mass 2
200	0.009	0.0	0.0	605	1.647	1.420	1.225
205	0.009	0.0	0.0	610	1.653	1.417	1.227
210	0.009	0.0	0.0	620	1.602	1.401	1.225
215	0.011	0.0	0.0	630	1.570	1.386	1.224
220	0.020	0.0	0.0	640	1.544	1.376	1.226
225	0.040	0.0	0.0	650	1.511	1.359	1.222
230	0.053	0.0	0.0	660	1.486	1.359	1.216
235	0.055	0.0	0.0	670	1.456	1.325	1.206
240	0.057	0.0	0.0	680	1.427	1.306	1.196
245	0.059	0.0	0.0	690	1.402	1.291	1.189
250	0.068	0.0	0.0	700	1.369	1.268	1.087
255	0.091	0.0	0.0	710	1.344	1.248	1.076
260	0.148	0.0	0.0	712.5	1.338	1.241	1.196
265	0.215	0.0	0.0	715	1.329	1.149	1.102
270	0.234	0.0	0.0	717.5	1.322	0.988	0.851
275	0.223	0.0	0.0	720	1.314	0.942	0.787
280	0.265	0.0	0.0	722.5	1.308	1.113	0.998
285	0.380	0.0	0.0	725	1.302	1.004	0.865
				727.5	1.296	1.012	0.877
290	0.482	9.8 E-7	0.0	730	1.290	1.013	0.880
295	0.584	2.2 E-4	0.0	732.5	1.283	1.094	0.984
300	0.514	0.005	0.0	735	1.275	1.149	1.058
305	0.603	0.013	0.0	737.5	1.268	1.143	1.053
310	0.689	0.034	0.002	740	1.260	1.145	1.059
315	0.764	0.088	0.010	742.5	1.254	1.141	1.056
320	0.830	0.222	0.059	745	1.248	1.160	1.083
				747.5	1.241	1.164	1.092
325	0.975	0.296	0.090	760	1.211	1.139	1.072
330	1.059	0.364	0.125				
335	1.081	0.420	0.163	762.1	1.206	0.854	0.695
340	1.074	0.473	0.208	765	1.198	1.129	1.063
345	1.069	0.492	0.227	785	1.147	1.086	1.028
350	1.093	0.527	0.254	790	1.134	1.058	0.996
355	1.083	0.546	0.275	795	1.122	1.044	0.984
360	1.068	0.563	0.297	800	1.109	1.109	0.939
365	1.132	0.615	0.334	805	1.097	1.020	0.961
370	1.181	0.661	0.370	810	1.085	0.986	0.921
375	1.157	0.667	0.385	815	1.073	0.822	0.715
380	1.120	0.666	0.395	820	1.060	0.864	0.772
385	1.098	0.667	0.406	825	1.048	0.841	0.747
390	1.098	0.683	0.425	830	1.036	0.853	0.766
395	1.189	0.756	0.481	835	1.025	0.913	0.848
				840	1.013	0.946	0.895
400	1.429	0.093	0.605	845	1.002	0.945	0.899
405	1.644	1.086	0.717	850	0.990	0.948	0.918
410	1.751	1.174	0.787	890	0.908	0.875	0.843
415	1.774	1.207	0.822	895	0.900	0.875	0.734
420	1.747	1.207	0.834	902	0.899	0.678	0.594
425	1.693	1.187	0.833	907	0.883	0.663	0.577
430	1.639	1.167	0.830	912	0.878	0.642	0.552
435	1.663	1.202	0.868	916	0.873	0.598	0.501
440	1.810	1.327	0.973	920	0.869	0.701	0.628
445	1.922	1.431	1.065	924	0.865	0.685	0.610
450	2.006	1.515	1.145	928	0.860	0.573	0.475
455	2.057	1.566	1.192	935	0.853	0.274	0.168
460	2.066	1.584	1.215	943	0.844	0.400	0.288
465	2.048	1.582	1.222	950	0.837	0.374	0.262
470	2.033	1.582	1.232	954	0.830	0.357	0.247
475	2.044	1.603	1.257	957	0.825	0.457	0.351
480	2.074	1.638	1.294	965	0.811	0.550	0.459
485	1.976	1.573	1.252	975	0.794	0.624	0.554
490	1.950	1.563	1.253	981	0.783	0.678	0.628
495	1.960	1.583	1.279	984	0.778	0.709	0.671
				990	0.767	0.736	0.711
500	1.942	1.580	1.286	995	0.757	0.735	0.714
505	1.920	1.568	1.280	1018	0.719	0.658	0.602
510	1.882	1.542	1.263	1082	0.620	0.544	0.477
515	1.833	1.507	1.239	1094	0.602	0.506	0.464
520	1.833	1.512	1.247	1098	0.596	0.534	0.479
525	1.852	1.533	1.286	1101	0.592	0.535	0.506
530	1.842	1.530	1.270	1128	0.560	0.143	0.083
535	1.818	1.515	1.262	1131	0.577	0.161	0.095
540	1.783	1.491	1.246	1137	0.550	0.152	0.088
545	1.754	1.471	1.234	1144	0.542	0.203	0.135
550	1.725	1.452	1.222	1147	0.539	0.185	0.117
555	1.720	1.450	1.223	1178	0.507	0.432	0.353
560	1.695	1.432	1.210	1189	0.496	0.426	0.366
565	1.705	1.443	1.222	1193	0.492	0.449	0.427
570	1.712	1.452	1.232	1222	0.464	0.415	0.371
575	1.719	1.461	1.242	1236	0.451	0.414	0.380
580	1.725	1.461	1.244	1264	0.427	0.349	0.314
585	1.712	1.461	1.247	1276	0.417	0.363	0.338
590	1.700	1.453	1.243	1288	0.407	0.368	0.332
595	1.682	1.441	1.234	1314	0.386	0.316	0.258
600	1.666	1.430	1.227	1335	0.370	0.202	0.155

APPENDIX TABLE 4-6
NASA/ASTM Standard for Solar Spectral Irradiance

Wavelength (nm)	Irradiance ($Wm^{-2} nm^{-1}$)			Wavelength (nm)	Irradiance ($Wm^{-2} nm^{-1}$)		
	Solar O	Air mass 1	Air mass 2		Solar O	Air mass 1	Air mass 2
1572	0.257	0.235	0.224	2320	0.068	0.060	0.056
1599	0.245	0.228	0.219	2338	0.066	0.057	0.053
1608	0.242	0.220	0.209	2356	0.065	0.054	0.050
1626	0.234	0.218	0.210	2388	0.063	0.038	0.030
1644	0.226	0.208	0.200	2415	0.061	0.034	0.026
1650	0.223	0.206	0.198	2453	0.058	0.031	0.024
1676	0.212	0.191	0.173	2494	0.055	0.021	0.014
1732	0.188	0.170	0.153	2537	0.052	0.005	0.002
1782	0.167	0.144	0.124	2900	0.035	0.003	0.001
1862	0.138	0.004	0.001	2941	0.033	0.006	0.003
1995	0.113	0.045	0.039	2954	0.033	0.006	0.003
2008	0.102	0.073	0.060	2973	0.032	0.009	0.005
2014	0.101	0.078	0.068	3005	0.031	0.008	0.005
2057	0.096	0.073	0.063	1384	0.334	0.006	0.001
2124	0.087	0.073	0.061	1432	0.321	0.047	0.021
2156	0.084	0.069	0.057	1457	0.309	0.090	0.054
2201	0.079	0.069	0.065	1472	0.301	0.082	0.047
2266	0.072	0.064	0.061	1542	0.270	0.252	0.235

Column 1 gives the wavelength in nanometers (nm). The solar spectral irradiance for air mass 0 outside the Earth's atmosphere is presented in column 2. The solar spectral irradiance is at the average sun-Earth distance per unit area normal to the sun's rays. The spectral irradiance values for air mass 1 and air mass 2 are given in columns 3 and 4. Air mass 1 and air mass 2 values were calculated using the standard spectral irradiance data and the U.S. standard atmosphere (20-mm precipitable water vapor, 3.4-mm ozone, and turbidity values corresponding to a clear atmosphere). The wavelength intervals were adjusted to illustrate the absorption bands and the rapid changes in irradiance in the IR region of the spectrum. The UVB, UVA, VIS, and IR spectra are designated by dashed lines. To calculate the total irradiance E_e or the irradiance for a given waveband, the values of the spectral irradiance in W/m^2-nm must be multiplied by the wavelength interval in nm and the results summated. Adapted from Mercherikunnel and Richmond[6]; Green et al.[8]

APPENDIX TABLE 4-6
NASA/ASTM Standard for Solar Spectral Irradiance, continued

Solution Cl

Copper sulfate ($CuSO_4 \cdot 6H_2O$)	3.142 g
Mannite ($C_6H_8(OH)_6$)	3.412 g
Pyridine (C_5H_5N)	30.0 ml
Distilled water to make	1000.0 ml

Solution C2

Cobalt ammonium sulfate ($CuSO_4 \cdot (NH_4)_2 \cdot 6H_2O$)	30.580 mg
Copper sulfate ($CuSO_4 \cdot 5H_2O$)	22.5 mg
Sulphuric acid H_2SO_4 (density 1.835)	10.1 ml
Distilled water to make	1000.0 ml

Source A was intended to be the typical tungsten, gas-filled filament, incandescent lamp commonly in use. Source B was intended as an approximation of noon sunlight. Source C was intended to approximate the overcast sky light. The major difference between source B and source C is that the overcast sky eliminates the longer wavelengths of the spectrum and results in an increase of the color temper-ature from the relative increase in shorter wavelengths of the radiation.

Standard Source E corresponds to the most frequently encountered daylight with a color temperature of 6500 [K] and CIE chromaticity coordinates $x = 0.313$ and $y = 0.329$. Standard source D5500 corresponds to the natural sunlight plus the sky radiation. Source D5500 possesses a color temperature of 5500 [K] and the CIE chromaticity coordinates $x = 0.333$ and $y = 0.347$.

Solar Radiation Tables

Standard NASA/ASTM solar irradiance for air mass 0, air mass 1, and air mass 2 with their spectral radiance values for the sun on earth.[4,5] The data for the 200- to 295-nm waveband in Appendix Table 4-6 was modified from Shettle and Green.[6] The wavelength range for the NASA/ASTM data has arbitrarily been set for 200 to 3005 nm because this waveband contains 99.03% of the sun's energy. To calculate the spectral irradiance

$E_{e\lambda}$ for a given waveband or the total solar irradiance E_e, the spectral irradiance in W/m²-nm must be multiplied by the wavelength interval $\Delta\lambda$ in nanometers and summed over the waveband of concern:

$$E_e = \sum_{\lambda 1}^{\lambda n} E_{e\lambda}\, \Delta\lambda$$

Data on global and direct ultraviolet radiation (UVR) reaching the Earth in the 280- to 340-nm wavelength range for radiation falling on a horizontal surface at different degrees of solar elevations and a variety of conditions that have been published recently[6-9] are presented in Appendix Tables 4-7, 4-8, and 4-9.

Wave-length [nm]	Solar Elevation (90°)		
	Ozone Thickness		
	0.24 atm-cm	0.32 atm-cm	0.40 atm-cm
	Irradiance in Wm⁻² nm⁻¹		
280	1.54×10^{-14}	9.09×10^{-19}	5.44×10^{-23}
285	1.78×10^{-8}	9.50×10^{-11}	5.12×10^{-13}
290	3.58×10^{-5}	2.14×10^{-6}	1.29×10^{-7}
295	2.36×10^{-3}	5.15×10^{-4}	1.13×10^{-4}
300	2.45×10^{-2}	1.07×10^{-2}	4.72×10^{-3}
305	9.25×10^{-2}	5.91×10^{-2}	3.79×10^{-2}
310	2.02×10^{-1}	1.58×10^{-1}	1.24×10^{-1}
315	3.24×10^{-1}	2.48×10^{-1}	2.49×10^{-1}
320	4.39×10^{-1}	4.09×10^{-1}	3.81×10^{-1}
325	5.41×10^{-1}	5.20×10^{-1}	5.01×10^{-1}
330	6.30×10^{-1}	6.17×10^{-1}	6.05×10^{-1}
340	7.87×10^{-1}	7.82×10^{-1}	7.77×10^{-1}
290–320	5.41 Wm²	4.61 Wm²	3.99 Wm²
280–340	15.2 Wm²	14.2 Wm²	13.4 Wm²

*A solar elevation of 90° is equivalent to the sun at zenith or a zenith angle of 0°. Data from Shettle and Green.[7,8]

APPENDIX TABLE 4-7
Global Solar UVR Reaching a Horizontal Surface on the Ground for a Solar Elevation of 90° and Ozone Thickness of 0.24 atm-cm, 0.32 atm-cm, and 0.40 atm-cm*

Wave-length [nm]	Solar Elevation (60°)		
	Ozone Thickness		
	0.24 atm-cm	0.32 atm-cm	0.40 atm-cm
	Irradiance in Wm⁻² nm⁻¹		
280	1.54×10^{-14}	9.09×10^{-19}	5.44×10^{-23}
290	1.29×10^{-9}	3.16×10^{-12}	7.85×10^{-15}
290	7.84×10^{-6}	3.06×10^{-7}	1.21×10^{-8}
295	9.38×10^{-4}	1.63×10^{-4}	2.85×10^{-5}
300	1.34×10^{-2}	5.20×10^{-3}	2.03×10^{-3}
305	6.08×10^{-2}	3.63×10^{-2}	2.18×10^{-2}
310	1.46×10^{-1}	1.10×10^{-1}	8.36×10^{-2}
315	2.48×10^{-1}	2.13×10^{-1}	1.83×10^{-1}
320	3.46×10^{-1}	3.19×10^{-1}	2.94×10^{-1}
325	4.34×10^{-1}	4.15×10^{-1}	3.97×10^{-1}
330	5.11×10^{-1}	4.99×10^{-1}	4.87×10^{-1}
340	6.44×10^{-1}	6.40×10^{-1}	6.35×10^{-1}
290–320	4.08 Wm⁻²	3.42 Wm⁻²	2.92 Wm⁻²
280–340	12.03 Wm⁻²	11.19 Wm⁻²	10.52 Wm⁻²

*A solar elevation of 60° is equivalent to a zenith angle of 30°. The standard atmospheric ozone thickness is taken to be 0.32 atm-cm. Data from Shettle and Green.[7,8]

APPENDIX TABLE 4-8
Global Solar UVR Reaching a Horizontal Surface on the Ground for a Solar Elevation of 60° and Ozone Thickness of 0.24 atm-cm, 0.32 atm-cm, and 0.40 atm-cm*

Appendix References

1. Nicodemus FE, Kostkowski HJ, Hattenburg. Introduction, *In:* NBS Technical Note 910-1, Self-Study Manual on Optical Radiation Measurements, pp 56–61. Washington, DC, U.S. Government Printing Office, Department of Commerce, National Bureau of Standards, 1976.
2. McSparron DA. Redefinition of the photometric units approved. Opt Radiat News 1980; 30:5.
3. Wyszecki G, Stiles WS. The eye. In: Color Science Concepts and Methods, Quantitative Data and Formulas, Section 2, pp 225–227. New York, John Wiley & Sons, 1967.
4. Standard Specification for Solar Constant and Air Mass Zero Solar Spectral Irradiance. ASTM Standard E490-73a-1974, Annual Book of ASTM Standards, Parts 41, Philadelphia, ASTM, 1974.
5. Solar Electromagnetic Radiation. NASA Special Publication 8005. NASA, 1971.

Wave-length [nm]	Solar Elevation (40°)		
	Ozone Thickness		
	0.24 atm-cm	0.32 atm-cm	0.40 atm-cm
	Irradiance in $Wm^{-2} nm^{-1}$		
280	1.35×10^{-18}	2.97×10^{-23}	7.06×10^{-28}
285	9.40×10^{-12}	2.07×10^{-14}	5.90×10^{-17}
290	2.30×10^{-7}	4.16×10^{-9}	9.84×10^{-11}
295	1.05×10^{-4}	1.06×10^{-5}	1.11×10^{-6}
300	3.30×10^{-3}	9.42×10^{-4}	2.72×10^{-4}
305	2.31×10^{-2}	1.17×10^{-2}	5.92×10^{-3}
310	7.07×10^{-2}	4.87×10^{-2}	3.37×10^{-2}
315	1.37×10^{-1}	1.12×10^{-1}	9.16×10^{-2}
320	2.06×10^{-1}	1.85×10^{-1}	1.66×10^{-1}
325	2.70×10^{-1}	2.54×10^{-1}	2.39×10^{-1}
330	3.25×10^{-1}	3.15×10^{-1}	3.05×10^{-1}
340	4.20×10^{-1}	4.16×10^{-1}	4.12×10^{-1}
290–320	2.20 Wm^{-2}	1.79 Wm^{-2}	1.49 Wm^{-2}
280–340	7.28 Wm^{-2}	6.72 Wm^{-2}	6.27 Wm^{-2}

*A solar elevation of 40° is equivalent to a zenith angle of 50°. The standard atmospheric ozone thickness is taken to be 0.32 atm-cm. Data from Shettle and Green.[7,8]

APPENDIX TABLE 4-9
Global Solar UVR Reaching a Horizontal Surface on the Ground for a Solar Elevation of 40° and Ozone Thickness of 0.24 atm-cm, 0.32 atm-cm, and 0.40 atm-cm*

6. Mercherikunnel AT, Richmond AT. Spectral distribution of solar radiation. NASA Technical Memo 82021. Greenbelt, MD, Goddard Space Flight Center, 1980.
7. Shettle EP, Green AES. Multiple scattering calculation of the middle ultraviolet reaching the ground. Appl Opt 1974; 13:1567–1581.
8. Green AES, Sawada T, Shettle EP. The middle ultraviolet reaching the ground. Photochem Photobiol 1974; 19:251–259.
9. Baker KS, Smith RC, Green AES. Middle ultraviolet reaching the ocean surface. Photochem Photobiol 1980; 32:367–374.
10. Kollias N, Baquer AH, Isad IQ. Measurement of solar middle ultraviolet radiation in a desert environment. Photochem Photobiol 1988: 47:565–569.

CHAPTER FIVE

Basic Concepts in Environmental Lighting

Alan L. Lewis, O.D., Ph.D.

Lighting serves several functions in producing an environment where visual performance is optimized. In general, it provides

- an adapting luminance that determines the dynamic range of vision
- task contrast by differential reflection from non–self-luminous objects
- color, by supplying a spectral power distribution suitable for chromatic contrasts
- form and texture by producing shadows and highlights

Since the energy crisis of the early 1970s, lighting has taken on increased importance as a key component of environmental design. In the past poor lighting design could be compensated for by increased lighting levels, but the present day requirement to limit the amount of energy devoted to lighting has created a need to use light wisely and efficiently. Whereas it was once acceptable to use 3 to 4 watts per square foot (35 W/m^2) to light a building interior, current guidelines in some parts of the United States are rapidly heading toward mandatory limits of less than 1 watt per square foot (10 W/m^2). With such constraints, lighting must be designed knowledgeably or the ability to perform visually demanding tasks will be severely impaired. One positive result of better lighting design will be the replacement of many of the bad lighting practices of the past, which often were the work of persons with little or no training in lighting or vision, with installations that are more visually effective, energy efficient, and aesthetically pleasing.

The traditional role of the optometrist and ophthalmologist has been to assess the integrity of the individual's visual system and to take steps to optimize its performance over the long term. Increasingly, especially since the use of visual display terminals (VDT) has become common, the role of the visual environment in which people function has taken on a greater importance. Because so many visually taxing tasks must be performed in interior spaces or while an individual is driving at night, knowledge of the principles of good lighting practice has become necessary for clinicians if they are to assess the cause of patient complaints and to prescribe adequate remedies.

5.1 Elements of Lighting

Lighting design has two major components: (1) quantity, or the amount of light, is usually specified in photometric terms such as intensity, illuminance, exitance, and luminance; the first part of this chapter will discuss these terms in greater detail and (2) quality or the geometry and spectral composition of lighting which determines such factors as the degree of comfort in a space, the color rendering properties of a lighting system, the absence or presence of veiling reflections, and the amount of glare and flicker present in a space. Quality is much more difficult to design and to measure than quantity and is too often not adequately addressed in many lighting installations. The quality of a lighting system can directly affect the requirements for quantity.

Proper lighting design requires that attention be paid to both quantity and quality; one without the other often yields a visual environment that is uncomfortable to its inhabitants, inefficient in its energy utilization, and inadequate in its ability to maximize visual performance.

It is not the role of clinicians to be lighting designers, but they should understand the principles of lighting so that their patients' visual problems that are of environmental origin can be addressed.

5.2 Photometry

Photometry is the measurement of light, that component of the electromagnetic spectrum that most efficiently stimulates vision (see Chapter 4). It generally includes the wavelengths between 380 and 760 nm over which it provides a range of sensitivity of about five orders of magnitude. Photometry makes a number of simplifying assumptions about the way in which the visual system functions, and therefore it only approximates what we really see; however, it serves well as a means to specify and measure light (except at mesopic luminances) and provides the basis for all current light units and measurement techniques.

Photometric Lighting Units

To understand the relationships among the photometric units, it is easiest to start with a point source—a theoretic source of light so small that it has no area—that radiates light equally in all directions into a sphere surrounding the point (Fig. 5-1). The total light output from the point source in a given time (per second) is measured in lumens. Lumens are a measure of *flux* (F), the time rate flow of visually evaluated energy. Because for real sources we are usually concerned with the amount of light being emitted in a particular direction, we specify the directional amount by indicating how many lumens are being emitted into a unit solid angle in that direction. This quantity is called *intensity* (I) and is measured in lumens per steradian, or alternatively, in *candelas* (cd). Because there are 4π steradians contained in a sphere, our uniformly radiating source has an intensity of

$$I = \frac{F}{4\pi} \qquad (5\text{-}1)$$

Before light can be effective, it must interact with matter; that is, it must fall onto a surface such as the cornea, a work table, a roadway, or a book. The amount of light (lumens) that falls *onto* a unit area of surface is called *illuminance* (E) and is measured in lumens per square meter. It is this quantity that is most commonly specified in lighting recommendations. The relationship between intensity and illuminance is given by the inverse square law:

$$E = \frac{I\cos\theta}{r^2} \qquad (5\text{-}2)$$

where θ is the angle between the normal to the surface and a line connecting the source to the point at which the illuminance is measured and where r is the distance from the source to the surface at the point at which the illuminance is measured.

Illuminance of a surface (except perhaps the retina) is not a useful visual concept; it is a measure of how much light falls *onto* a surface. We usually want to know how much light comes *off* the surface. The measure of the total number of lumens that leaves a unit area of surface is *exitance* (M), and like illuminance, is specified in lumens per square meter. For a given surface reflectance, the exitance is given by

$$M = E\rho \qquad (5\text{-}3)$$

where ρ is the reflectance of the surface.

Because exitance measures the light leaving a surface in all directions, it is not a visually useful term. We want to know how much light comes off the surface in a particular direction—usually toward the eye. As in intensity, the directional component is handled by indicating how many lumens are radiated into a unit solid angle in the preferred direction from each elemental area of surface. This measure is called *luminance* (L) and is specified in lumens per steradian per square meter (or candelas per square meter). It is luminance that is most visually meaningful; it is the photometric analog of perceptual *brightness*—what we actually perceive as light. For diffusely reflecting surfaces, the luminance can be approximately calculated from the exitance by

$$L = \frac{M}{\pi} \qquad (5\text{-}4)$$

Of these units, usually only illuminance and luminance are directly measured with physical meters. Illuminance meters are usually far less expensive ($100 and up) than are luminance meters, may be self-powered (photovoltaic cells), and may include a cosine-correcting diffuser that automatically compensates for the cosine law effect. Luminance meters, because they usually include viewing optics to define the area being measured, are usually expensive (over $1000 at publication time) but are more versatile and often more accurate. In recent years, solid state detectors have made photometers more rugged, stable, and accurate. Photodiodes and charge coupled devices (CCD), enhanced by state of the art electronics, now compete with photomultiplier tubes (PMT) in terms of cost, response speed, and sensitivity. However, where very low light levels are to be measured, the PMT remains the detector of choice. Several instruments are available that can function as either luminance or illuminance meters, and, in some cases, as spectroradiometers as well.

Although illuminance meters are adequate to monitor lighting levels in most spaces employing

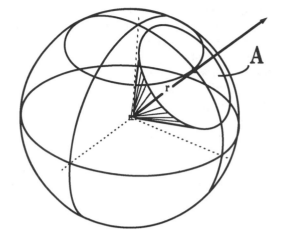

FIGURE 5-1
The steradian or unit solid angle. A theoretic point source of light radiates equally in all directions into a surrounding sphere. The sphere has a radius r equal to unity (r = 1) and an area on the surface of the sphere defined by the radius r. Lines connecting the circumference of the circle with the center of the sphere define a cone of one solid angle or steradian.

general lighting, they cannot be used to survey highly specular surfaces or to determine actual contrasts (which are ratios of luminances); for those measurements a luminance meter must be used. Most recently, CCD cameras, which record and digitize luminance information for an entire scene, have shown promise in providing a much more complete assessment about visual tasks and the luminous environment in which they exist.[1] Such systems greatly simplify the analysis of complex visual scenes and make possible more sophisticated procedures for predicting visual performance in the real world.

5.3 Determining Lighting Levels

The Quality of Light

One of the most controversial questions in lighting for the last century has been, How much light is enough? In the early days of electric lighting, when lamps were expensive and short-lived and when power was scarce, the answer was, All you can get. Lighting recommendations for offices in the 1910s and 1920s were often less than 50 lux.[1] As lamps became more efficient and power was more readily available and cheaper, lighting levels gradually rose. It was during World War II that the role of lighting in productivity was first studied intensively, and it was found that speed of production increased and errors decreased as lighting levels were increased. In Great Britain, one of the first of the human factors' engineers, H. C. Weston, using Landolt C's of varying size and contrast as tasks, performed systematic studies on the effect of illuminance on speed and accuracy and established the basic principles that hold true today:[3]

- When contrasts are low and/or the task is small, increases in illuminance have a large effect on performance;
- When contrasts are high and/or the task is large, increases in illuminance have little effect on performance.

A typical visual performance function is shown in Figure 5-2. A large number of empiric studies to determine the lighting needs of particular visual tasks has been done but the area lacks a unifying theory.

Similar conclusions using reading material was found in the United States (Fig. 5-3).[4] This type of research led to the oversimplified phrase, "More light—better sight."

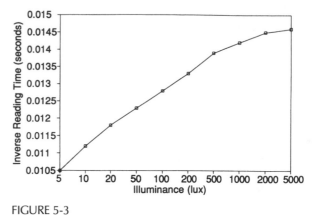

FIGURE 5-3
Visual performance (inverse of the time to read a passage) as a function of illuminance for a reading task. Data from Tinker M.

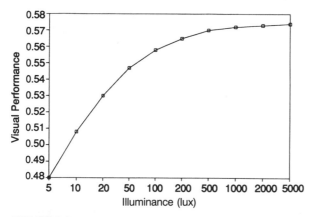

FIGURE 5-2
Visual performance as a function of illuminance for a Landolt C task. Data from Weston HC: The Relation Between Illumination and Visual Efficiency; The Effect of Brightness Contrast. Industrial Health Research Board, Report No. 87. London, HMSO, 1945.

A comprehensive method for assessing the difficulty of a visual task and for determining the level of illuminance necessary to optimize visual performance was developed in 1959.[5] It was reasoned, based on research done in the 1940s,[6] that task contrast and size, combined with the viewer's sensitivity to contrast, were the critical variables in determining visual performance. The notion of visibility level (the ratio of task contrast to its contrast threshold) was developed into a comprehensive system of illuminance specification.[7] Illuminance recommendations were determined by calculating the light levels that would place a visual task at a given visibility level (VL) (e.g., eight times above its own contrast threshold—VL=8). This system was adopted by the Illuminating Engineering Society of North America (IESNA) as the basis for its lighting recommendations and was in use until 1980. With the advent of the energy crisis, a combination of the pressures to reduce the amount of energy used for lighting and technical problems in the computation of the visibility level caused the visibility level procedure to be replaced by a system that is based on consensus rather than experimental data.

Recognizing the need to allow for variables other than the physical characteristics of the task and data documenting the reduction of visual capacity with increased age, a revised system was adopted by the IESNA that allowed greater flexibility in the specification of lighting levels.[8]

The current system involves several steps:

- Determing the task characteristics (size and contrast) to provide a range of target illuminances
- Determining the criticality of the task (the consequences of visual mistakes)
- Determining the age of users

Tables 5-1 to 5-3 demonstrate the use of the current North American illuminance selection procedure. First, the visual task must be identified and classified into one of the categories listed in Table 5-1. For example, if the task is simply walking through a lobby, the task category would most likely be B. If the task is reading #2 pencil handwriting in a classroom, the task category would probably be E. In the first case, the entire space would be lighted to between 50 and 100 lux; in the case of the classroom, only areas where the task of reading was performed would be lighted to between 500 and 1000 lux. This illustrates the difference between general and task lighting.

Once the illuminance range is identified, the specific target illuminance is determined by taking into account the modifying factors stated in Tables 5-2 and 5-3. In the classroom case (Table 5-3), the users are likely to be young; a weighting factor of − 1 is assigned. The need for speed and accuracy is probably not important (that is, the consequences of an error are not serious) and, therefore another weighting factor of − 1 is given. If the writing is done on yellow-lined paper, the background reflectance is about 65%, so a weighting factor of 0 is assigned. All of the weighting factors are then algebraically added,

giving a resultant weighting factor of − 2. Thus, the lowest of the three illuminances within the range becomes the design target: 500 lux.

The actual procedure is discussed more fully in the *IES Lighting Handbook*,[9] including more complete definitions of the descriptive categories and suggestions for using the weighting factors. The system, empirically rather than scientifically based, was intended to be an interim procedure until it could be replaced with one more solidly grounded in research data; it remains to be superseded.

The Quantity of Light

Determining the quantity of light is simply the first step in designing a lighting system. It is important to ensure that a visual task can be performed. Equally as important, however, are the quality aspects of light:

- Spectral power distribution (SPD)
- Disability glare potential
- Discomfort glare potential
- Flicker characteristics
- Noise characteristics
- Aesthetic properties

SPECTRAL POWER DISTRIBUTION
The sources used for lighting today vary significantly in the amount of light emitted at each wavelength. The SPD will affect both the appearance of the lamp/

Type of Activity	Illuminance Category	Illuminance (lux)	Work Plane
Public spaces	A	20-30-50	General
Orientation	B	50-75-100	General
Occasional tasks	C	100-150-200	General
Tasks of high contrast or large size	D	200-300-500	Task lighting
Tasks of medium contrast or small size	E	500-750-1000	Task lighting
Tasks of low contrast or very small size	F	1000-1500-2000	Task lighting
Category F tasks of long duration	G	2000-3000-5000	Supplementary lighting
Very prolonged and exacting tasks	H	5000-7500-10000	Supplementary lighting
Special tasks	I	10000-15000-20000	Supplementary lighting

TABLE 5-1
Illuminance categories and ranges for various visual tasks (interiors). Illuminances for categories G to H should be accomplished by a combination of general (ambient) and task lighting

Room and Occupant Characteristics	Weighting Factors*		
	− 1	0	+ 1
Ages	< 40	40–55	> 55
Room Reflect.	> 70%	30%–70%	< 30%

*An algebraic sum is computed. If the sum is − 2, the low end of the illuminance range is used. If the sum is + 2, the high end of the range is used. Otherwise, use the middle value.

TABLE 5-2
Weighting Factors to Be Used with Categories A to C of Table 5-1

luminaire and of the space illuminated by the lamps. Although not routinely provided by lamp manufacturers, the SPD is one of the most important characteristics of a lamp because many other properties can be derived from it.

COLOR TEMPERATURE
The color temperature of a lamp is the temperature, in kelvin [K], of a blackbody radiator that matches the lamp in appearance. It merely tells you what the lamp looks like; even though it is determined by the SPD, it does not provide any information about the SPD. When virtually all sources were incandescent, with smooth and continuous SPDs, the color temperature was useful to predict how surfaces would appear when illuminated by the source. For example, a lamp with a low color temperature, say

Task and Worker Characteristics	Weighting Factor*		
	− 1	0	+ 1
Ages	< 40	40–55	> 55
Speed/Accuracy	Not important	Important	Critical
Reflectance	> 70%	30%–70%	< 30%

*If the sum is between − 1 and − 3, the low end of the illuminance range is used. If the sum is between + 1 and + 3, the high end is used. Otherwise, the middle of the range is used.

TABLE 5-3
Weighting Factors to Be Used with Categories D–I of Table 5-1

Standard Source A, would enhance reds, whereas a lamp with a high color temperature, say Standard Source C, would enhance blues (see Chapter 4). With the advent of lamps with very discontinuous and restricted spectra, tri-phosphor fluorescent lamps or high pressure sodium discharge arcs, for example, a given lamp color can be produced using any number of narrow phosphor bands or gases that have markedly different effects on the color of a surface although they are identical in appearance to the eye.

The concept of color temperature is useful only for "white" sources because the source must visually match a blackbody. Many "white" lamps, however, such as most fluorescent lamps, never visually match a blackbody and therefore do not strictly meet the conditions required to have a color temperature. Because these lamps come very close to a match, however, they are assigned a color temperature that is close to their actual appearance; this is termed a *correlated color temperature*. Color temperatures are not usually assigned to nonwhite sources.

COLOR RENDERING INDEX
The color rendering property of a source is a measure of the degree to which it changes the appearance of colors in a space from those seen if the space is illuminated with a source with an "ideal" continuous SPD; the index is on a scale of 0 to 100. By definition, standard incandescent lamps, which have continuous SPDs, have a maximum color rendering index (CRI) of 100. The index is assigned by computing the shift in position, in Commission Internationale de L'Eclairage (CIE) chromaticity space, of a selected group of Munsell papers when they are illuminated by a standard source as compared to the source of interest. Because the resultant shift is the average of the component shift of all the papers, the CRI does not tell anything about what any particular color will look like; a low index can result from one color being shifted a great deal or all the colors being shifted a smaller amount. Because of this, and because many of the more energy-efficient lamps with discontinuous spectra do not have high CRIs (an index of at least 80–85 is usually considered desirable for interior lighting where color appearance is important), the CRI has been criticized as inadequate and other indices have been proposed. None has received much industry-wide support at this time, and the CRI remains the most commonly specified standard.

Glare

Glare has been defined as "that condition of vision in which there is discomfort or a reduction in the ability to see significant objects, or both, due to an unsuitable distribution or range of luminances or to extreme contrasts in space or time."[9] Glare is a catch-all term that usually includes three separate effects:

- Disability glare
- Discomfort glare
- Reflected glare (veiling reflections)

These three effects are often linked because each is caused by bright lights in the field of view that create undesirable seeing conditions. Each acts on vision quite differently, however, and should be distinguished from one another when lighting systems are being analyzed and designed.

DISABILITY GLARE

Disability glare causes objects to appear to have lower contrast than they would have if there were no glare. As shown in Figure 5-4, light that should have contributed to the brightness of the retinal image is instead scattered to adjacent parts of the retina; this lowers the brightness of the retinal image and increases the brightness of the background, lowering contrast. The effect is similar to one's turning on the lights in a room while trying to view a slide presentation or a motion picture. In both cases, the addition of light to both the target and its background, a veiling luminance, reduces contrast. For example, assume a simple target with a luminance of 100 cd/m² on a background with a luminance of 25 cd/m². This target would have a contrast of

$$C = \frac{L_{max} - L_{min}}{L_{min} + L_{max}}$$
$$C = \frac{100 - 25}{25 + 100} = 0.60 \qquad (5\text{-}5)$$

If disability glare now adds a veiling luminance of 10 cd/m² to both the target and the background, we get

$$C = \frac{110 - 35}{35 + 110} = 0.52$$

Thus the veiling luminance has reduced the contrast. The same effect occurs when stray light is added to the retinal image of a visual task. Indeed, disability glare is measured in terms of the veiling

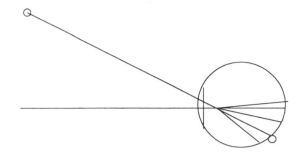

FIGURE 5-4
Diagram of stray light in the eye. Light that should be focused in the image of the object is instead spread over the retina, reducing contrast by decreasing image illuminance and increasing background illuminance.

luminance that would produce an equivalent reduction in contrast as that produced by the glare source.

Several investigators have derived expressions to predict the effect of a glare source on the contrast of an image.[11-14] Although they differ in details, all have the form

$$L_v = k\frac{E_O}{\theta^c} \qquad (5\text{-}6)$$

where E_o = corneal illuminance from the glare source(s), k = dimensional constant, θ = angle between the glare source and the line of sight, and c = 2 (or very close).

In practical terms, this means that bright sources that are close to the line of sight will cause the most visual glare. Figure 5-5, which uses the Stiles-Holliday constants (k = 9.14; c = 2), shows the dropoff in veiling luminance as a source (in this example a 100-W incandescent lamp at 6 m) that produces a corneal illuminance of about 20 lm/m² is moved away from the fixation point; except for very bright sources, the effect becomes negligible beyond about 10°. All the disability glare formulas assume a young, relatively clear eye and therefore significantly underestimate the effect of glare sources on the vision of older persons and others with medial opacities.

Because for small particles (Rayleigh scatter) the amount of scatter is significantly greater for short wavelengths than for longer wavelengths, some suggest that the effects of disability glare might be reduced by restricting the short wavelength output of lamps by filtering or by use of yellow-tinted spectacle

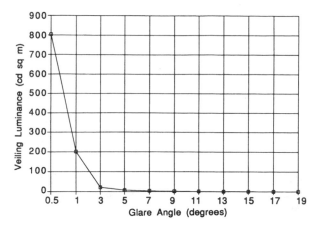

FIGURE 5-5
Equivalent veiling luminance as a function of glare source angle to the line of sight. Based on the Stiles-Holliday formula.

lenses. However, most research indicates that the greatest amount of scatter in the eye is of the large particle type (Mie scattering) and is not wavelength selective.[15-17] This is empirically confirmed by studies that find little or no effect of source spectrum on visual performance.[18]

All areas of space within the central 10° of the visual field contribute to disability glare. Whereas bright lights are the most offensive because they significantly contribute most to corneal illuminance, other sources, such as white walls, desk tops, and windows can also cause loss of contrast and must be considered in control of disability glare.

DISCOMFORT GLARE

Discomfort glare is a sensation of irritation or pain from sources of light in the field of view. Unlike disability glare, the cause of which is mostly understood, the physiologic basis of discomfort glare is unknown. Because so little is known about the origin and measurement of discomfort glare, there is little international agreement on how it should be specified.

The most common measure of discomfort glare is the *border between comfort and discomfort (BCD)*. It is the middle of a range of subjective judgments about how uncomfortable a light source or system is. As an example, a person may be shown a range of lights of varying brightness and asked to evaluate each in terms of its discomfort by placing it on the following type of semantic scale:

- It is unnoticeable
- It is just noticeably uncomfortable
- It is uncomfortable
- It is very uncomfortable
- It is intolerable

The luminance of the light that satisfies the middle of the range is termed the *BCD luminance*. Although not much is known about the physiologic cause of the glare sensation, the parameters that aggravate the response are generally agreed upon:

- Source size
- Source luminance
- Angle of the glare source to the line of sight
- Background luminance

A number of formulas[19] have been proposed to relate the physical parameters of a source to its glare-producing potential; each takes the general form of

$$G = \frac{L_s^a \times W^b}{L_f^c \times f(\theta)} \tag{5-7}$$

where L_s = source luminance toward the eye; W = the solid angle subtended by the source at the eye; θ = the angle of the source from the line of sight; L_t = general field luminance (adaptation level), a, b, and c = weighting constants, and $f(\theta)$ = a function of the displacement angle. North America, the United Kingdom, the Baltic nations, and the former Soviet Union, as well as many other countries, have adopted different versions of the general formula to be used by lighting designers. Very recently, in an attempt to bring some order to the field, CIE has proposed (in draft form)[20] a Uniform Glare Rating method for assessing the glare potential of luminaires but it remains to be seen if it will be used widely.

To evaluate the degree of discomfort in existing spaces, a simple test can be performed: shield the eyes with the hand at the level of the brows, like the visor of a baseball cap. If the space becomes noticeably more comfortable, it was producing discomfort glare. This technique is useful for demonstrating to employers and building managers the degree to which their buildings are potentially fatiguing to their occupants. It can also be used by patients to test whether or not discomfort glare in their working environments might be a cause of visual or asthenopic symptoms.

Preventing discomfort glare is accomplished by avoiding large bright areas within a space, by limiting luminance ratios to less than 10:1, and by shielding luminaires so that lamps are not directly viewed. Indirect lighting systems, where all the light in a space is reflected to the work plane from the ceiling and walls, have been used as a means to produce a discomfort glare–free environment; however, unless carefully designed, such spaces may suffer from a dullness and lack of texture because of the diffuse nature of that arrangement. Lighting systems that incorporate some direct component with a general indirect system can be a good compromise. Where low ceilings make indirect lighting difficult, sharp cutoff luminaires can usually be used effectively.

Fortunately, in most cases, the design techniques that limit discomfort glare also reduce disability glare. Low brightness luminaires with well-controlled cutoff angles, window treatments, and high ceilings all work to reduce both types of glare and make a more pleasant, functional environment.

VEILING REFLECTIONS
Veiling reflections are the specular reflections from working surfaces of bright areas within a visual space, including light sources, that reduce the contrast of the visual task. The classic problem of trying to find a suitable angle to hold a book with a shiny page so that it can be read is a perfect example of the problem of veiling reflections. The VDT, with its specular screen, has also brought the problem of veiling reflections to the forefront of lighting design. Major advances in both design technique and equipment have made the control of veiling reflections easier than ever. If all surfaces were diffusely reflecting or if all lighting was diffusely illuminating, there would be no veiling reflections. However, even if diffuse papers are used, some inks, and certainly pencil writing, have specular properties that must be considered.

The ability of a lighting system to be free of veiling reflections is measured by its *contrast rendering factor (CRF)*. The CRF is essentially the ratio of the contrast of an object under actual viewing conditions to the contrast of the same object under diffuse illumination. The CRF is highly dependent on the lighting geometry of a space: It may be high when viewing in

one direction and very low when viewing in another direction. Commercial computer programs have been written and are available to assess the CRF of a space in as many viewing situations as desired by the user. In addition, CRF meters are now available that measure the actual contrasts and compare them in real spaces. CRFs are not now currently used in the specification of lighting systems, but with the availability of meters that will allow verification of a design, they may be included when lighting quality is important.

5.4 Exterior Lighting

Exterior lighting serves several purposes:

- Roadway/walkway illumination for way-finding and object avoidance
- Safety
- Security and crime prevention

Many of the criteria used for lighting interiors are also applicable to exteriors, but with important differences. Most exterior lighting is designed for a much lower level of adaptation, glare control is more critical, and except for signage, a detection or recognition visibility criterion is more appropriate than is resolution.

Since 1990, the roadway lighting recommendations of IESNA have been based on the visibility of a specified target on the road rather than simply on illuminance.[21] The new system uses procedures that place increased emphasis on the geometry of the lighting system, the reflectance of the pavement, and the contrast of the object to be seen. Rather than simply specifying an illuminance on the horizontal road surface, the new system addresses the visibility of a standard vertical target (Fig. 5-6) seen against a particular pavement. The system recognizes that visibility occurs with either positive or negative contrast and that low visibility occurs when the target and its background have nearly the same luminance. Another impact of the system is that, instead of treating all light equally, it takes into account the direction from which the light comes and the degree to which it reduces contrast because of disability glare.

Objects made visible by lighting at night appear either in positive contrast (light object—dark background) or negative contrast (dark object—light

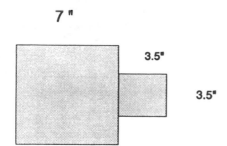

7 "

3.5"

3.5"

FIGURE 5-6
Schematic diagram of the IESNA Roadway Visibility Target. The task is to detect the target on the roadway and to identify its orientation.

background), depending on whether they are illuminated from the front or from behind (Fig. 5-7); either condition is sufficient to make the object detectable or recognizable. An object becomes difficult to see when its brightness approaches the brightness of the background against which it is seen, usually the pavement. This will occur at the point of transition from positive to negative contrast (Fig. 5-7). The challenge to the designer is to minimize the area of roadway or walkway where such zones of low contrast might occur.

If recognition, rather than detection, is the primary visual task, back lighting is insufficient to pro-

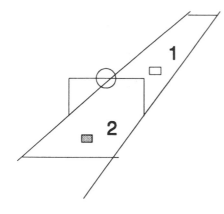

FIGURE 5-7
Schematic diagram of positive (1) and negative (2) contrast of a roadway obstacle illuminated by a single light source. Somewhere between the two positions, the obstacle will have zero contrast and will disappear.

vide the needed information, and more conventional approaches, as used in interiors, are more appropriate.

There are many outdoor applications where color discrimination is a significant requirement and so make the choice of light source important. The ability to locate automobiles by color in parking lots, the correct identification of sign colors for direction and safety, and the need for color in sports facilities are examples that demonstrate the need for broad spectral power distributions. The need for good color rendering is usually less critical in outdoor applications than in interiors, but the ability to recognize colors accurately is always desirable within the constraints of energy and economic realities.

5.5 Light Sources

The array of light sources available today has resulted in the ability of today's designers to produce almost any environment at a reasonable cost and with excellent energy efficiency. The price for this flexibility is that both the designer and the end user need to be knowledgeable about the advantages and disadvantages of each type of source, as well as the types of hardware necessary to optimize their performance in each application. This section will briefly outline some of those characteristics. In general, the choice of source will involve the following elements:

Source size. The closer a source is to a point source, the easier it is to control optically. Large sources require more elaborate and expensive luminaires to limit beam spread and, concurrently, glare. Also, large sources tend to produce a more diffuse lighting environment, reducing highlights and shadows that may be desirable to create visual interest in some installations.

Source efficacy. This is the number of lumens produced for each watt of energy consumed. Although the highest efficacy is desirable, it often occurs at the expense of color rendering, ease of installation and maintenance, or wattage requirements. Table 5-4 lists the efficacy ranges of commonly available sources.

Color properties. The requirements for color rendering and spectral content must be considered.

Source Type	Efficacy Range (lm/W)
Incandescent	4–10
Tungsten-halogen	10–25
Halogen IR reflecting	15–30
Compact fluorescent	15–80
Full-size fluorescent	65–100
Mercury vapor	25–50
Metal halide	45–100
Compact metal halide	45–80
High pressure sodium	45–115
Low pressure sodium	120–185

TABLE 5-4
Efficacy of Various Light Sources

For example, flesh tones appear more attractive when lighted with the redder warm white fluorescent than with the yellower cool white fluorescent. No colors can be discriminated under the monochromatic light from low pressure sodium lamps. These properties are especially critical in merchandising and when recognition of safety colors is involved.

Electrical requirements. Many sources, including fluorescent and high intensity discharge (HID) lamps, require transformers to provide sufficient starting voltages. In addition, some HID sources require several minutes of warm-up time before providing full light output or up to 15 min to relight after being extinguished.

Characteristics of Sources for Lighting

INCANDESCENT.   These lamps are small in size and universally available. Low initial cost; large variety of wattages, voltages, configurations; easy dimming; and excellent color rendering make the incandescent lamp the most popular for noninstitutional use. Their major disadvantages are poor efficacy and short life (about 800 h for a standard 75-W household lamp). Improved quartz-halogen lamps and lamps with infrared (IR) reflectors have made the incandescent source more efficient and longer lived, and despite the higher initial cost, they are less expensive over the life of the lamp.

FLUORESCENT.   Among the most efficient of all sources, fluorescent lamps provide excellent lighting although they have the potential to produce glare, veiling reflections, and flicker. Their large size makes them difficult to control, they require special ballasts to allow dimming, and they are adversely affected by modest changes in voltage and temperature. On the other hand, they are very long lived (up to 20,000 h), are available in a wide variety of colors and color rendering indices, and are moderately priced. Furthermore, the size problem has been partially solved by the introduction of only slightly less efficient and shorter lived compact fluorescent sources, many of which come with integrated optical control and ballasts that allow them to be used in standard incandescent lamp sockets. A 7-W compact fluorescent lamp can replace a 60-W incandescent source and provide similar light output; however, care must be taken to assure that luminaires in which the lamps are used are compatible with both types of sources.

Flicker is sometimes a problem with fluorescent lamps. The lamps normally flicker at twice the line frequency (120 Hz in North America and 100 Hz in Europe and Australia), usually well above the flicker fusion frequency of the human eye. However, when lamps are operated under other than optimal conditions, lower flicker rates occur and can be perceived. It is also possible that neighboring lamps can interact and generate beat frequencies low enough to be seen. Similar interactions have been reported between fluorescent lamps and VDTs.

HIGH INTENSITY DISCHARGE (HID).   Three major categories of HIDs are commonly used:

High Pressure Mercury (HPM). Moderately efficient, reasonably priced, and easily available, HPM lamps lack good color rendering and give objects a greenish appearance. They are best suited for outdoor applications or high bay installations in interiors. Their high brightness demands good glare control wherever they are used.

High Pressure Sodium (HPS). Very efficient and long-lived, HPS lamps have poor color rendering and impart a yellow appearance to objects. Used mostly in roadway applications, they are also used in interiors where color is not critical. Because of their economy of operation, they are often misused and are a significant source of glare and sky glow. With properly designed luminaires that limit their distribution, they can be very effective sources.

A recent development, the white HPS lamp, promises much better color properties at the expense of some efficacy. Available in low wattages (e.g., 50 W), they may have significant impact on interior lighting applications.

Metal Halide. A class of several different sources that use rare earths to achieve a "whiter" distribution than other HID lamps. They are less efficient and shorter lived (10,000 h) than HPS lamps, but are used where color is important, such as in sports arenas, on the sets of television shows, and for merchandise lighting. Metal halide lamps also suffer from significant color changes during their lives and can be operated in limited positions, which restricts their usefulness in general applications. Metal halide lamps emit large amounts of ultraviolet radiation (UVR) and must be used behind UV absorbing glass or polycarbonate shields to protect persons exposed to the lamps. Available in a very large range of wattages, metal halide sources can often replace incandescent lamps if energy efficiency and small size are important.

LOW PRESSURE SODIUM (LPS). These monochromatic (589 nm) sources are among the most efficient lamps ever designed, but the inability to distinguish colors under LPS lamps severely limits their use. The most common applications for LPS are roadway, tunnel, and underpass lighting. Because their monochromatic light is easily filtered out of telescopes, LPS lamps have been mandated in some communities that are located near astronomical observatories which experience serious sky glow from roadway and other exterior lighting. Such measures are usually unnecessary if adequate beam control is included in luminaires with more broad-band lamps.

5.6 Lighting for the Partially Sighted

Lighting for persons with partial sight requires a knowledge of the conditions that caused the disability.[22] In most cases, if the rules of good lighting practice are followed, the principles of lighting for persons with special visual needs are not very different from those used for designing environments for the normally sighted. The main differences are in the areas of the amount of light required (often many times more than normal), the need for very careful attention to sources of disability and discomfort glare, and the problem of lighting the task in the presence of optical aids such as telemicroscopes and stand magnifiers. Patient education is also critically important to assure that the supplemental lighting is used correctly. Poor use of supplemental lighting can often make the situation worse rather than better.

For the purpose of designing lighting, it is useful to divide the partially sighted population into two groups according to the cause of their low vision:

Those whose problem is caused by preretinal anomalies, which reduce the contrast of the retinal image through increased intraocular scatter, such as corneal scarring, cataract, or viteous opacities.

Those whose problem is caused by retinal injury, pathology, or degeneration, which reduce the resolving power or contrast sensitivity of the eye, especially at high spatial frequencies, such as age-related maculopathy, diabetic and hypertensive retinopathy, or other similar conditions.

Persons in the first group are helped most by increasing the physical contrast or, more correctly, the brightness difference of the task while limiting the total flux entering the eye. Because the problem is primarily one of increased disability glare, and because that glare is directly related to the amount of light in the eye available to be scattered, simply increasing illuminance is often counterproductive. Because persons in this group often have normal retinas and contrast sensitivity, the problem is not one of insufficient light but rather one of too much light going to the wrong places. The key to successful lighting design for such persons is careful light control and, if possible, appropriate task selection. Some of the techniques that can be used to improve the visual performance of this group are

• Removal of obvious and unnecessary sources of glare such as unshielded windows, lamps, and luminaires; the use of drapes, sharp cutoff luminaires, indirect lighting, and baffles are helpful.

- Use of high contrast print and chromatic contrast to permit lower illuminances and therefore reduce the light entering the eye.
- Elimination of contrast-reducing veiling reflections by positioning light sources to avoid specular reflections in the direction of the eyes and by using diffusely reflecting materials when possible.
- Reduction of the amount of light reflected from the task by using reverse contrast (light on dark) or apertures in low reflectance backgrounds (such as the Typoscope) or by illuminating only the portion of the task being viewed by controlling the source with optics and/or baffles.

Persons in the second group are usually suffering from retinal disease or injury that has reduced the ability of the visual system to process information either because the receptors are damaged or because the synaptic connections are faulty. The problem is to bring on-line the remaining visual elements and to maximize their information-processing abilities. This may require considerably more light than is necessary for the normally functioning retina. In such conditions, increases in visual performance have been reported for illuminances of more than $10,000 \, cd/m^2$. Levels of this sort require supplementary task lighting, very careful glare control, and often, the use of innovative methods to deliver the light to the task. Because persons with macular problems often use optical magnifying aids, getting the needed light between the device and the task is a special problem.

Persons who have received laser treatment in the macular area occasionally report a disability glare–like sensation at moderate to high retinal illuminances. This may result from a reduction in the normal rod inhibition by cones, which is allowing the rods to saturate. These persons are an exception to the more commonly found acceptance of high light levels in macular dysfunction.

Solutions to the need for high illuminances nearly always include a lamp mated to an optical system, either dioptric or reflective. Without some sort of optical control, the lamp power required and the glare created is simply too great. Lamps of small physical size, such as tungsten-halogen incandescent lamps or some metal halide HID sources, are best suited for these applications. Because they are often used in close proximity to the impaired person's hands or face, low voltage sources (12 V) should also be considered for safety. Small halogen lamps with integral dichroic reflectors, such as the MR-16 or MR-11 lamps, have proven very effective in such cases. They are compact, readily available through commercial lamp distributors, and come in a variety of beam widths and light outputs to suit nearly any working distance. Furthermore, because they require 12 V, they can use rechargeable batteries where portability is important. Head-mounted versions have been successfully used.[23]

In many cases, especially among the elderly, a combination of the above two types of visual impairment is found. The increase in the aged population has caused an attendant rise in the prevalence of age-related maculopathy; except in those in whom cataracts have been removed, elderly persons also invariably suffer from significant intraocular scatter. Their problems remain a challenge to both the clinician and the lighting designer.

Even when conventional lamps can be used to provide the needed illuminance, care must be taken. Incandescent lamps emit about 90% of their energy as heat and can produce burns if they contact the hands or face. To reduce the chances of accidental contact with hot surfaces, the use of metal lamp-shades should be avoided and attention should be given to the placement and ease of use of switches.

5.7 Summary

Lighting remains the weak link in efforts to optimize visual performance. Most lighting is "designed" by persons with little or no formal training in illuminating engineering, vision, or both. Most building codes in North America, if lighting is specified, use outmoded illuminance standard without regard to the qualitative aspects of the lighting environment. There are, however, many very well qualified and experienced lighting designers who have superb records of innovative, energy-efficient, visually pleasing and effective designs that make more enjoyable and functional the spaces in which we work. Both professionals and the general public need to be educated as to what constitutes inadequate lighting and how it can be remedied. The eye care professions have a significant role in that process.

References

1. Rea MS, Jeffrey LG. A new luminance and image analysis system for lighting and vision. I. Equipment and calibration. J Illum Eng Soc 1990; 16:128.
2. Illuminating Engineering Society. Code of Lighting. Trans Illum Eng Soc 1915; 10:605.
3. Weston HC. The Relation Between Illumination and Visual Efficiency; the Effect of Brightness Contrast. Industrial Health Research Board, Report No. 87. London, HMSO, 1945.
4. Tinker MA. Brightness contrast, illumination intensity and visual efficiency. Am J Optom 1959; 36:221–236.
5. Blackwell HR. Specification of interior illumination levels. Illum Eng 1959; 54:317.
6. Blackwell HR. Contrast threshold of the human eye. J Opt Soc Am 1946; 36:624–643.
7. Commission Internationale de L'Eclairage. Unified Framework of Methods for Evaluating Visual Performance Aspects of Lighting. CIE Publication No. 19. Paris, CIE, 1972.
8. Committee on Recommendations for Quality and Quantity of Illumination. RQQ Report No. 6, Selection of illuminances for interior lighting design. J Illum Eng Soc 1980; 9:188.
9. Kaufman JE (ed): IES Lighting Handbook. Reference Volume. New York, Illuminating Engineering Society of North America, 1981.
10. Commission Internationale de L'Eclairage. International Lighting Vocabulary. CIE Publication No. 17. Paris, CIE, 1970.
11. Holliday LL. The fundamentals of glare and visibility. J Opt Soc Am 1926; 12:271–319.
12. Stiles WS. The effect of glare on the brightness difference threshold. Proc R Soc Lond 1929; 104B:322–355.
13. Stiles WS. The scattering theory of the effect of glare on the brightness difference threshold. Proc R Soc Lond 1930; 105B:131–141.
14. Fry GA. A re-evaluation of the scattering theory of glare. Illum Eng 1954; 49:98–102.
15. Boynton RM, Enoch JM, Busch WR. Physical measures of straylight in excised eyes. J Opt Soc Am 1954; 44:879–886.
16. DeMott DW, Boynton RM. Sources of entoptic straylight. J Opt Soc Am 1958; 48:120–125.
17. Boynton RM, Clarke FFJ. Sources of entoptics scatter in the human eye. J Opt Soc Am 1963; 53:869–873.
18. Hopkinson. Visual performance with sources of differing spectral quality.
19. Commission Internationale de L'Eclairage. Discomfort glare in the working environment. CIE Publication No. 55. Paris, CIE, 1983.
20. CIE Technical Committee 3-13. Draft Report. Melbourne, CIE, 1991.
21. Roadway Lighting Committee RP-5. New York: Illuminating Engineering Society of North America, 1990.
22. Lewis AL. Lighting considerations for the low vision patient. Problems in Optometry 1992; 4:20–33.
23. Jampolsky A, Brabyn J, Lewis A, Winderl M. Two experimental low vision illumination aids. J Vis Rehabil 1989; 3:33–37.

CHAPTER SIX

Ocular Effects of Radiant Energy

Donald G. Pitts, O.D., Ph.D.

Ultraviolet radiation (UVR) has become increasingly more common in the manufacturing process in many industries. Table 6-1 lists a series of occupations that expose the worker to UVR and require ocular protection. The electronic industry constitutes one of the major users of UVR because the size of a computer memory chip is dictated by the input and output leads. The narrower, more precise the leads to the chip, the smaller the total size of the chip and, in addition, the greater its memory capacity. As memory sizes increased and the demands for smaller, more precise leads increased, the UV wavelengths used to produce the chip have become shorter. The latest technology uses X-rays in the development of computer memory chips.

Curing Processes	Nondestructive Testing
Dentists	Metal casting inspectors
Food Irradiators	Accelerated weather
Paint curers	testing
Plastics curers	**Outdoor Solar Exposure**
Wood curers	Agricultural workers
Germicidal Exposure	Astronauts
Barbers	Aviators
Hospital workers	Construction workers
Meat cutters	Fishermen/women
Medical profession	Military
Nurses	Oilfield workers
Optometrists	Open-pit miners
Opticians	Pipeline workers
Printing Processes	Railroad workers
Computer chip	Seamen/women
developers	Snow skiing
Electronics workers	Sportsmen/women
Graphic arts	Sunbathers
Lithographers	**Researchers**
Printers	Chemists
Welding Industry	Microbiologists
Foremen/women	Microscopists
Maintenance workers	Photomicrobiologists
Materials handlers	Photoimmunologists
Metal cutters	Phototherapy
Welders	Physicists
Welders' helpers	

TABLE 6-1
Occupations That Expose the Eye to Excess UVR and Require Ocular Protection

6.1 Factors Affecting Ocular Exposure

Transmittance of the Ocular Media

A knowledge of the transmittance properties of the eye for optical radiation is important in explaining some of the observed biologic effects. Radiation must be absorbed by a molecule before a biologic effect may be observed (Grotthus-Draper law), and the absorption spectrum and photochemical properties are specific for a given molecule (see Chapter 4).

Transmittance data for the rabbit,[1-6] the primate,[6-9] and the human[7-14] in the wavelength range from 200 to 2500 nm are similar and are presented in Figure 6-1. The transmittance of radiation incident at the various surfaces of the human ocular media (Fig. 6-2) illustrates that the longest wavelength impinging on the retina is 1400 nm and that most of the IR (infrared) radiation above 1000 nm incident on the eye is absorbed by the cornea and the aqueous humor. The mammalian ocular media transmits 70% to 90% of the visible (VIS) spectrum and IR below 1400 nm to the retina. The cornea transmits more than 90% of the radiation between 400 nm and about 1200 nm but shows IR absorption bands at 1430 nm and 1950 nm. Beyond 3000 nm, the corneal absorption of IR is almost complete.

In the UV portion of the optical spectrum the cornea absorbs almost all radiation below 230 nm (Fig. 6-3).[1,3,15] The epithelium shows a gradual increase in transmittance to 25% at 240 nm, between 30% to 35% to 280 nm, and 90% above 280 nm. The total cornea begins transmitting at 280 nm, increasing transmittance to maximum greater than 90% at 310 nm. The waveband between 230 nm and 290 nm for the total cornea illustrates an increasing penetration of the stroma with UVR reaching the endothelium and crystalline lens at the 295- to 300-nm wavelengths.

The UVR incident on the different surfaces of the ocular media for the 280- to 400-nm wavelengths show that a small but significant UV waveband reaches the retina of the phakic eye beginning at 305 nm, peaking at about 3% at 320 nm and decreasing to less than 1% above 340 nm (see Fig. 6-2). Thus, the retina is provided partial protection against UVR because the crystalline lens absorbs the major portion of the UV as it passes through the ocular media

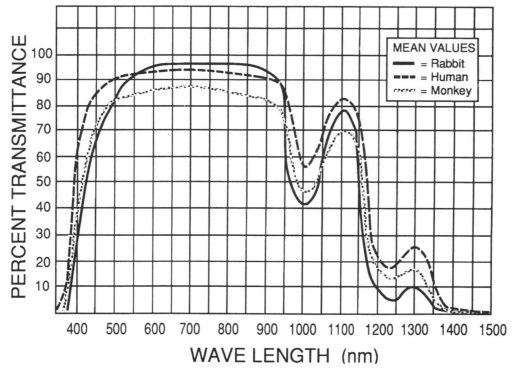

FIGURE 6-1

Spectral transmittance of optical radiation through the ocular media of the rabbit, primate, and human. The data illustrate that transmittance does not differ greatly in the 500 nm to 900 nm wavelength range. However, a 10% difference can affect retinal irradiance significantly. *From* **Geereats WS, Berry ER. Ocular spectral characteristics as related to hazards from laser and other light sources. Am J Ophthalmol 66:15–20, 1968; published with permission from the American Journal of Ophthalmology. Copyright by the Ophthalmic Publishing Company.**

to impinge on the retina. The UV that reaches the retina of the aphakic eye is comparatively substantial and necessitates protective measures.

The transmittance of the VIS spectrum begins at about 380 nm and increases very rapidly to 70% at 450 nm, whereas an 80% to 90% transmittance is maintained throughout the rest of the VIS spectrum (see Figs. 6-1 and 6-2).

The ocular media transmit about 90% of the near infrared (IRA) waveband to the retina (Fig. 6-4).[16] However, the ocular media are essentially opaque to the far infrared (IRB and IRC) wavebands. Corneal absorption bands are found at 1430 nm and 2000 nm, but transmittance remains high between the absorption bands. Beyond 3000 nm, the IR absorption by the cornea appears to be almost complete. When measured alone, the aqueous humor shows absorption bands at 908 nm, 1320 nm, 1453 nm,

and 1950 nm but continues to transmit to about 2400 nm. The crystalline lens has IR absorption bands at 980 nm and 1200 nm, and transmits to about 1400 nm. The IR transmittance of the vitreous humor exceeds 90% to about 900 nm with essentially no transmittance beyond 1400 nm. Nearly all IRA in the 760- to 1400-nm wavelength range impinging on the iris is absorbed by the iris pigment epithelium. The IR that is transmitted to the retina is absorbed primarily by the pigment epithelium.

Occasionally, extremely intense sources are encountered, and this requires knowledge of the transmittance of the eyelid because it serves as a protector for the retina during blinks. Voss and Boogaard[17] used a two projector hetero-brightness match to determine the transmittance of the eyelid. Figure 6-5 presents the spectral transmittance of the eyelid for three subjects.

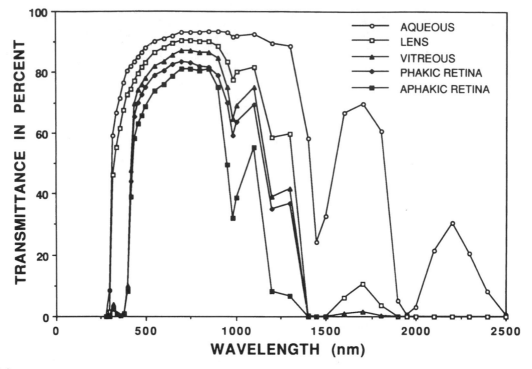

FIGURE 6.2
Spectral transmittance of the optical radiation incident on the cornea that reaches the anterior surfaces of the individual ocular components of the human eye. The transmittance of the phakic and aphakic eye to the retina is included. Note that the longest wavelength reaching the retina is about 1400 nm, while there is a window in the UV centered at 320 nm. *Data from* **Boettner, EA.**[7]

The Pupil

The pupil acts as the limiting aperture of the eye and controls the amount of radiant energy that reaches the lens, vitreous, and retina. In the dark-adapted state, the pupil diameter averages 7 to 8 mm for the younger person, whereas under light-adapted conditions the diameter of the pupil may become as small as 2 mm (Fig. 6-6). The ratio of the diameters of the pupil from light to dark is 1:4; the ratio of the areas of the pupil is 1:16. The size of the pupil is affected by many different variables, including accommodation, intensity of light, and drugs. The theoretic limit of resolution of the eye varies with the wavelength of radiation and the size of the pupil, with maximum performance achieved with a 2.5-mm diameter pupil.[18]

Exposure Duration and Mechanisms of Damage

Exposure duration is an important parameter for determining the effects of radiant energy on the eye. As the exposure duration increases, the radiant power (in watts) incident on the eye decreases until time becomes ineffective and the lesion appears to depend on the irradiance (in watts) reaching the eye. Data for extended duration exposures are rare.

In addition to the duration of exposure, the ocular response to exposure from optical radiation may be related to the level of power of the optical beam and ocular blood flow. The interactions of these three parameters taken individually and simultaneously make the evaluation of retinal research data most difficult. For example, a radiant power of a given level and a small image size may not produce a

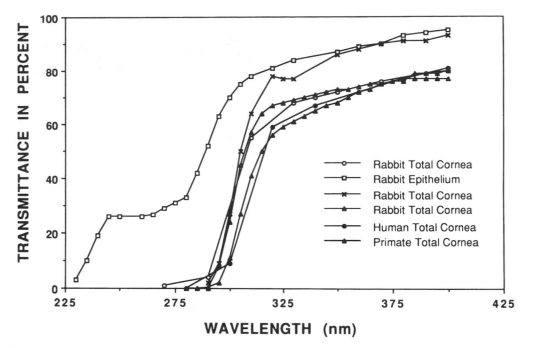

FIGURE 6-3
Spectral transmittance of UV radiation by the cornea. The corneal epithelium absorbs almost all UV below 230 nm and most UV below 280 nm. *Data from* Barker FM, II;[1] Bachem A;[15] and Kinsey ZV.[3] The American Journal of Ophthalmology 41:969–975, 1956, copyright by the Ophthalmic Publishing Company; and Archives of Ophthalmology 39:508–513, 1948, copyright by the American Medical Association.

retinal lesion, but if the power remains constant and the image size increases until the area is larger than the ability of the vascular system to efficiently conduct the heat away, a lesion will result. A radiant exposure that would normally be safe now produces retinal damage.

There are four mechanisms of damage from exposure to optical radiation: (1) optomechanical, (2) thermomechanical, (3) thermal, and (4) photochemical. These mechanisms are related by a number of exposure parameters. The mechanisms of damage and their interactions are summarized in Table 6-2.[20,21]

Optomechanical damage occurs when extremely high power densities are delivered to biologic systems in picosecond to nanosecond time duration (10^{-12} to 10^{-9} s). These exposures occur with the laser and produce nonlinear optical phenomena expressed as a breakdown in normally expected optical behavior.[22] With longer or nanosecond exposure durations and lower power levels, effects from ultrasound may occur. Damage from ultrasound is usu-

ally to the choroid and the pigment epithelium but is not related to a rise in temperature. Damage from direct electric field effect usually results in the Raman effect or Brillouin effect optical modulation phenomena. The photoablation process produced by the excimer laser in refractive sculpturing of the cornea produces nonlinear optical phenomena. The Brillouin effect results when monochromatic radiation is passed through liquids. The resulting scattered radiation produces doublet wavelengths located on each side and at the same distance from the wavelength of the original radiation. The Raman effect occurs when light of a certain wavelength passes through liquids or solids and produces scattered light. The scattered light is analyzed by the Fourier transform and plotted on a curve of frequency versus amplitude. The transformed graph becomes a "fingerprint" of the material being tested.

Self-phase modulation (SPM) occurs when a single primary laser pulse propagating through a medium disturbs the refractive index. The disturbance of the

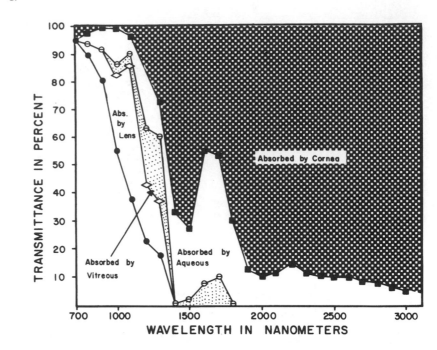

FIGURE 6.4
Transmittance of IR by the components of the rabbit eye. *Data from Kutscher CF.*[16]

index results in changes of the phase and frequency of the original incident laser pulse. *Coupled modulation* (CM) is found when intense and weaker laser pulses of different wavelengths are propagated simultaneously in a nonlinear medium. The intense laser pulse alters the phase and frequency of the weak pulse. *Induced-phase modulation* (IPM) occurs when the delays and pulse walkoff between strong

and weak laser pulses that are generated and controlled outside the interactive medium lead to induced frequency shifts. The frequency shift induces spectral broadening on the weaker laser pulse. *Cross-phase modulation* (XPM) results when the principal wavelength pulse generates a new frequency inside a medium by the Raman process or by harmonic generation. The new frequency interacts with the

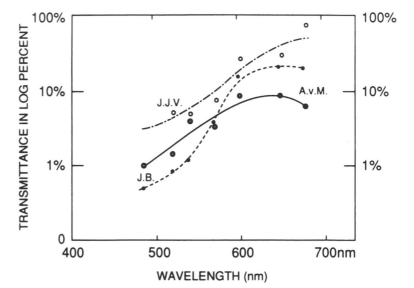

FIGURE 6-5
The spectral transmittance of the eyelid for three subjects. Note the variability of the data for the different subjects. *Redrawn from* **Voss JJ, Boogaard J: A Few Experiments on the Spectral Transmission of the Eyelid. Report No. 12F 1966-15. Soesterferg, the Netherlands, National Defence Research Council TNO, Institute for Perception TND, 1966.**

incoming wavelength pulse to become both frequency- and amplitude-modulated. The spectral width of the exiting beam is broadened by coupling the principal laser wavelength with the internally generated Raman wavelengths.

An example may serve to illustrate that these phenomena are not esoteric. The Nd;YAG laser is used extensively in the eye care professions. This laser has a wavelength of 1064 nm and a pulse duration of 30 ps when used in the mode-locked pulse configuration. The electric field strength incident on the retina when the Nd;YAG laser is operated at threshold is 9×10^{10} V/m^2 at 1064 nm and 1.3×10^{11} V/m^2 at the 532-nm frequency doubled wavelength. Both values are greater than the electric field strength needed to break down biologic membranes.

Thermomechanical damage occurs when the exposure duration lies between 1 ns and 0.1 ms. *Mechanical damage* to retinal structures results from the high power densities delivered in short pulses with the resulting sonic transients. As the power levels decrease and the exposure durations become longer than about 20 ms, the injury becomes thermal in nature. Sonic transients and heat result in a rise in retinal temperature greater than 10 C, primarily in the retinal pigment epithelium (RPE) and choroid, which disrupts the choroid, RPE, receptors, and surrounding tissue. *Thermal damage* mechanisms occur when the power is of medium or moderate intensities delivered between 0.1 ms and 5 s. The absorption of the energy by the RPE and choroid produces temperature rises above 10 C, which results in lesions to all retinal layers. An increase in retinal temperature of 10 C to 20 C above the normal retinal temperature is required to produce an irreversible thermal retinal lesion.[23,24] Pure thermal effects appear to be independent of wavelength; however, the VIS spectrum demonstrates both thermal and photochemical responses. The photochemical portion of the lesion is wavelength-dependent.

Photochemical or actinic damage results from lower power levels and long exposure durations. Damage is found at the molecular level of the cells and involves the DNA, enzymes, and chromophores. True photochemical damage follows the law of reciprocity; i.e., the intensity of the radiation times the duration of the exposure is constant ($I \times t = k$) and is strongly wavelength-dependent. This characteristic is best demonstrated by the action spectra of the

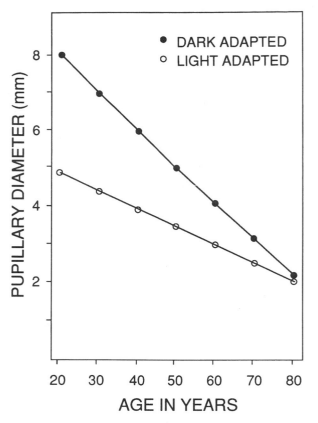

FIGURE 6-6
Diameter of the pupil for dark-adapted and light-adapted conditions as a function of age. The data demonstrate that the pupil diameter above the age of 70 changes very little and may account for the poor visual performance of aged people in the dark. *Data from Kornzweig AL.[18]*

individual anatomic components of the eye. The action spectra demonstrate different thresholds of the various spectral wavebands for the cornea, lens, and retina. For example, photochemical cataractogenesis results from UV exposure in the 295- to 320-nm waveband.

Size of the Retinal Image

The size of the retinal image for extended sources may be calculated from concepts of geometric optics (Fig. 6-7) by using similar triangles and assuming that the chord of a circle and the arc of a circle are

Exposure Parameter	Mechanisms of Optical Radiation Damage to the Retina*			
	Optomechanical	Thermomechanical	Thermal	Photochemical
Duration	ps–ns $(10^{-12}$–10^{-9} s)	1.0 ns–0.1 ms $(10^{-9}$–10^{-3} s)	0.1 ms–5 s $(10^{-3}$–10^{0} s)	10 s–h $(10^{-1}$ s–10^{2} h)
Level of power	Extremely high power levels	High power levels	Medium power levels	Low power levels
Mode	Optical transients Sonic transients Non-linear optical phenomena	Heat Sonic transients	Heat	Molecular level (DNA, enzymes, chromophores)
Temperature rise	Not temperature related	>10 C	>10 C	<10 C
Lesion site	RPE, choroid	RPE, choroid	RPE, choroid OS of receptors	OS-IS receptors Minimal RPE ONL nuclei
Wavelength-dependent	No	No	Partially	Yes

*Boundaries among the mechanisms overlap because there are interactions between the different mechanisms when the exposure parameters are appropriate. An example is that a thermophotochemical interaction occurs between 600 and 1000 nm when high power energy densities delivered in picosecond pulses produces damage to the retina. The damage is related to the electric field strength of the optical radiation.

TABLE 6-2
Mechanisms of Damage from Exposure of the Retina to Optical Radiation

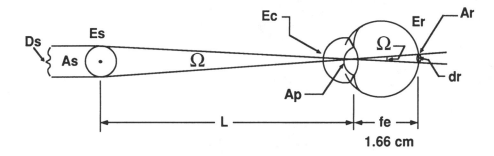

FIGURE 6-7
Schematic for calculating retinal illuminance and determining source–retinal image relationships. A sources of area As and irradiance or illuminance Es is located a distance L from the eye and forms an image Ar on the retina at a distance fe from the posterior nodal point of the eye. The angular subtense of the source Ω is the same for object and image space. The diameters of the source and its retinal image are in ratio of the distances 1 and fe. The source areas As and Ar are in ratio to the square of their respective distances, L^2 and fe^2.

approximately equal for small angles of Ω. The retinal image size is described by:

$$d_r = \frac{D_s f_e}{1_s} \qquad (6\text{-}1)$$

where d_r is the diameter of the retinal image (cm), fe the posterior focal length of the eye or 1.66 cm, 1_s is the distance from the source to the posterior nodal point (cm), and D_s the diameter of the source (cm). Sliney and Wolbarsht[25] have shown that source angles of 60° result in about a 5% error when using formula 6-1.

There are several important concepts to keep in mind about retinal image size (see Fig. 6-7). The first is that the solid angle Ω_s for the source or object in physical space and the solid angle of the image on the retina Ω_r is the same. The second is that because the solid angles are the same the source area A_s is always proportional to the area of the retinal image A_r in the ratio of the square of their distances, or

$$\frac{A_s}{1_s^2} = \frac{A_r}{f_e^2} \qquad (6\text{-}2)$$

This relationship is good for small angles with the error being about 5% for retinal image sizes of 20°.[25]

The third concept is that the retinal irradiance E_r or retinal illuminance E_V and the source radiance L_s or source luminance E_V are also proportional. Irradiance and radiance may be replaced by illuminance and luminance without affecting these concepts. The radiance of the source L_s may be determined from the irradiance E_c measured at the cornea and the solid angle of the source Ω_c at the cornea; thus

$$L_s = \frac{E_c}{\Omega_c} \text{ but } \Omega_c = \frac{A_s}{1_s^2};$$
$$\text{therefore, } E_c = \frac{L_s A_s}{1_s^2} \qquad (6\text{-}3)$$

The area of the pupil A_p limits the irradiance passing through to the retina. Because L_s and E_r are proportional, the retinal irradiance E_r becomes

$$E_r = \frac{L_s A_s}{1_s^2 A_r} \times A_p, \text{ but } A_r = \frac{A_s f_e^2}{1_s^2}$$
$$\text{and } E_r = \frac{L_s A_p}{f_e^2} \qquad (6\text{-}4)$$

To complete the formula, the losses of energy due to transmittance of the ocular media τ and reflectance ρ at the various optical interfaces need to be incorporated:

$$E_r = \tau \cdot \rho \cdot \frac{L_s A_p}{f_e^2} \qquad (6\text{-}5)$$

The posterior focal length f_e^2 is small compared to the distance to the source; therefore, little error is introduced by stating that retinal irradiance may be calculated by

$$E_r = L_s A_p \cdot \tau \cdot \rho \qquad (6\text{-}6)$$

This derivation illustrates the invariant nature of radiation, i.e., retinal irradiance or retinal illuminance is independent of the distance of the source 1_s but varies directly with the area of the pupil A_p. If the pupil remains constant in size and the source is brought closer to the eye, the angle Ω subtended by the pupil at the cornea increases and the area A_r of the retinal image increases. The retinal irradiance or retinal illuminance per unit area on the retina decreases but the total retinal irradiance contained in the beam remains constant. These conditions hold for all viewing conditions until the Fraunhofer diffraction limit of the eye has been achieved.

To determine the retinal irradiance or retinal illuminance without a knowledge of the viewing angle or viewing distance, formula 6-6 becomes

$$\begin{aligned} E_r &= L_s \cdot A_p \cdot \tau \cdot \rho \\ &= \tau \cdot \rho \cdot L_s \cdot \pi \, [d_p^2/4] f_e^2 \qquad (6\text{-}7) \\ &= 0.27 \, d_p^2 \, L_s \tau \rho \end{aligned}$$

where d_p (in centimeters) is the diameter of the pupil, τ the transmittance of the ocular media, and ρ the reflectance of the optical interfaces.

The unit of retinal illuminance, called the *Troland*, is defined as the retinal illuminance produced by a luminance L_v of 1 cd/m^2 passing through a 1-mm^2 pupillary area. Calculations using the retinal irradiance formula would be in Trolands when the radiation is expressed in photometric units of cd/m^2 and the pupillary area is in mm^2. According to Fry,[26] one Troland is equal to 8.46×10^{14} lm/mm^2.

Quality of the Retinal Image

For retinal image sizes below about 10 μm, the use of Formula 6-6 is not appropriate. Figure 6-8 illustrates that as the image size on the retina is decreased, the irradiance across the image decreases until, at about

FIGURE 6-8
Distribution of retinal irradiance for different retinal image sizes. The ordinate represents the retinal irradiance E_r and the abscissa the distance from the center of the retinal image. Note that 60 μm represents 12 min of arc. A retinal image smaller than about 10 μm contains less than 50% of the irradiance incident at the cornea of the eye. An image of about 30 μm contains the maximum retinal irradiance, larger images do not contain higher levels of irradiance but allow the maximum irradiance to be spread over a larger retinal image. *From* **Fry KA: The Blur of the Retinal Image. Columbus, the Ohio State University Press, 1955; with permission.**

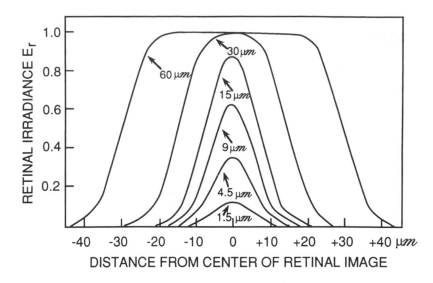

10 μm, the intensity of the retinal irradiance is approximately 50% of the radiance of the source.[29] The decrease in retinal irradiance results from the blur of the retinal image due to the diffraction by the pupil. Scattering by the ocular media, spheric aberration, and chromatic aberration all contribute to the quality of the retinal image, but the major effect is the diffraction determined by the diameter of the pupil. The wavelength of the source, size of the beam, divergence of the beam, and the profile of the beam are all necessary to evaluate the quality of the retinal image and the subsequent effect on the retina.

DISPERSION OR CHANGE IN THE INDEX OF REFRACTION OF THE OCULAR MEDIA WITH THE WAVELENGTH OF RADIATION

One of the basic principles of optical radiation is that the speed of light *c* varies with the index of refraction *n* in the ratio of c/n. The variation of the speed of light with the index of refraction is called *dispersion*. Dispersion is easily demonstrated with a prism when white light is dispersed into the familiar rainbow pattern. In the case of the eye, the classic description of dispersion is that the short wavelength (blue) light has a higher index and is focused in front of the retina, whereas the long wavelength (red) light focuses behind the retina. Only one of the multiple of 10-nm bandwidth images is in exact focus on the retina, whereas the remainder are out of focus.[29] Although the classic blue/red relationship is not or-

dinarily seen by the eye, a monochromatic light will be out of focus if accommodation remains constant or fixed. This phenomenon is known as *axial or longitudinal chromatic aberration.*

Normal dispersion has four important properties:[30] (1) The index of refraction n increases as the wavelength λ decreases; (2) the rate of increase becomes greater for shorter wavelengths with small changes occurring in the VIS spectrum; (3) the higher the index of refraction, the steeper will be the curve for a given wavelength; and, (4) the curve of the index refraction cannot be generalized from one material to another by changing ordinate scales. Because there is no simple relationship between the dispersion curves of different materials, the dispersion of different materials is said to be irrational. Dispersion is important when the effects of retinal exposure are being evaluated because it is one of the parameters that determines the size of the retinal image.

Fry[31] used the chromatic aberration data of Wald and Griffin[32] and Bedford and Wyszecki[33] to calculate the relation between n and λ for the entire eye in the wavelength from 400 to 700 nm, using Cauchy's equation: $n = 1.32546 + 0.002154 \ (10^6/\lambda^2) + 0.000176 \ (10^{12}/\lambda^4)$ when λ is in nanometers. The calculated dispersion curve for the human ocular medium is curvilinear. A dispersion curve will show marked deviations where strong absorption bands exist, indicating anomalous dispersion, but because such absorption bands are not found from the VIS wavelengths and in the UV to 300 nm, the extension of the Cauchy calculation for the eye to 300 nm is acceptable for calculating ocular dispersion.

The calculated index of refraction of the ocular medium varies from 1.329 at 800 nm to 1.371 at 300 nm (0.042 unit) and 1.354 at 555 nm (Fig. 6-9). The rate of change of n shows large increases below 400 nm and small decreases as the wavelength approaches 700 nm in the VIS spectrum. The basic question now concerns the effect of the change of n on the diameter or area of the optical image on the retina. This is important because the size of the retinal image controls the exposure necessary to cause damage and affects the threshold value.

SIZE OF RETINAL IMAGES WITH CHANGES
IN THE INDEX OF REFRACTION

A reduced eye model was used to calculate the change in the size of the geometric retinal blur circle as a function of the index of refraction. Using a corneal radius of 5 mm, axial length of 20 mm, a 7-mm pupil located 1.34 mm behind the apex of the cornea,[26] and the indices of refraction from Figure 6-9, we calculated the diameter of the blur circle for light from an infinitely distant object that fills the pupil to be 0.137 mm for 436 nm and 0.460 mm at 325 nm. These calculations demonstrate that the diameter of a 325-nm retinal image is 3.4 times the diameter of a retinal image at 405 nm.

6.2 Ocular Effects of Ultraviolet Radiation

A review of the information relative to the transmittance of UVR by the eye is provided in Figure 6-10. This figure illustrates that UVR is divided into three segments: UVA from 380 or 400 to 320 nm; UVB from 320 to 290 nm, and UVC from 290 to about 200 nm. UVC is completely absorbed by the ozone in the stratosphere, whereas UVB and UVA are transmitted through the atmosphere to reach the Earth. UVA is transmitted by the cornea and absorbed primarily by the lens, but small amounts are transmitted and are incident on the retina. UVB below 295 nm is absorbed by the cornea, and most of the UV from 295 to 320 nm is absorbed by the lens. Begin-

ning at about 305 nm, a small but significant amount of UVB impinges on the retina.

The previous section on radiant energy discussed the complicated question of mechanisms of ocular damage by using the exposure duration, intensity, and size of the source. Figure 6-11 simplifies these concepts by presenting the waveband, wavelengths, mechanisms, and damage that may occur from a radiant exposure of a threshold or a suprathreshold level in the exposure durations and energy levels ordinarily experienced by humans. The mechanisms of action by UVR are photochemical and thermal. Photochemical mechanisms predominate in the UVC and UVB wavebands, and as UVA is approached, the thermal mechanism becomes involved. Through the VIS spectrum, the photochemical mechanism begins to decline while the thermal

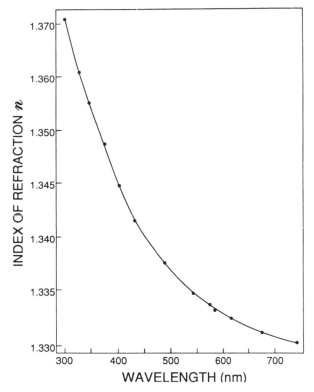

FIGURE 6-9
The dispersion curve of the human eye resulting from a change in the index of refraction of the ocular medium. The curve was calculated by using Cauchy's equation.

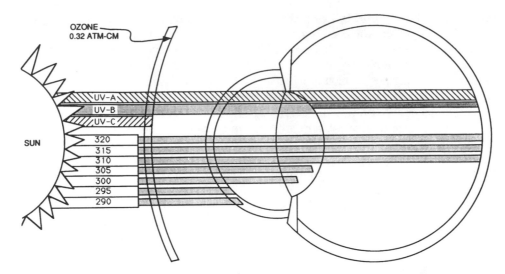

FIGURE 6-10
Diagrammatic representation of UV absorption by the eye. UVR is divided into three segments: UVA, which is absorbed primarily by the lens although small percentages penetrate the ocular media to reach the retina; UVB, which is absorbed by the cornea and lens but also reaches the retina above 305 nm; and UVC, which is absorbed by the ozone in the stratosphere. The wavelength penetration and absorption are illustrated by the shaded lines.

mechanism assumes a more predominant role, until at about 760 nm the process is almost totally thermal.

Action Spectrum for UV Exposure

The threshold effect of radiant exposure of the eye to UVR in the UV wavelength constitutes the action spectrum of the eye to UV radiant exposure (see Fig. 6-12). An action spectrum defines the radiant exposure that produces a defined biologic effect at a specified wavelength of radiation. The criterion biologic effect for the data was minimal damage to the cornea, iris, or lens as determined by the biomicroscope after exposure to different wavebands of UV for a predetermined duration. The action spectrum

FIGURE 6-11
Mechanisms of damage from exposure of the eye to the wavebands of the EMS. Photochemical mechanisms predominate cornea, lens, and retinal damage to about 340 nm. Above 340 nm, the photochemical mechanism becomes increasingly smaller whereas thermal mechanisms increase. Somewhere in the near IR, the response of the eye to exposure is entirely thermal.

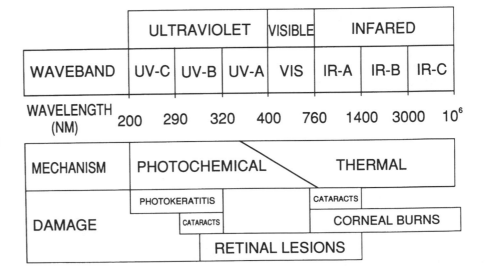

shows the efficiency of the radiation in producing minimal damage and is necessary for establishing protection requirements against exposure. The threshold values for the action spectra were based on a minimal damage criterion rather than a no-damage criterion. In other words, for each threshold value a minimal ocular damage was found from acute exposures that should demonstrate full recovery at some later date. The following paragraphs will describe the effects of exposure of the eye to UVR beginning with the cornea and proceeding to the retina.

Animal studies can be representative of the human exposure to UVR. Blumthaler et al[36] reconstructed human exposures to solar UVR experienced from snow skiing that produced photokeratitis. Their solar UV values were 1200 to 5600 J/m^2 (0.12–0.56 J/cm^2), but they concluded that these lev-

els were too high by a factor of 2 to 4 and estimated the threshold for photokeratitis to be from 300 to 600 J/cm^2 (0.03–0.06 J/cm^2). The UVB data give a threshold value of 0.350 J/cm^2 or 350 J/m^2 and lie within their human values.[37-38] Thus, the carefully reconstructed, real-life situation compares very satisfactorily with laboratory-generated data and can be used for the solution of human problems from exposure to UVR.

Figure 6-12 presents the action spectrum for human, primate, and rabbit eyes, with the ordinate giving the threshold radiant exposure in $J/m^2 \times 10^4$ and the abscissa the wavelength from 200 to 400 nm. The original data of Cogan and Kinsey are shown by the open, upright triangle.[39] The x's provide the threshold for photokeratitis for the human cornea for the wavelength range from 210 to 320 nm.[40-47]

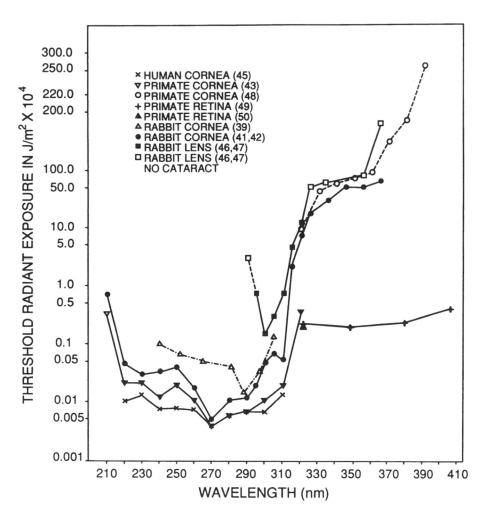

FIGURE 6-12
The action spectrum of the eye to UVR exposure. The ordinate presents the threshold radiant exposure in $J/m^2 \times 10^4$ and is in scaled log units. The abscissa gives the wavelength in nanometers beginning at 200 nm and terminating at 410 nm. The data symbols represent human, primate, and rabbit exposures and include exposures to the cornea, retina, and lens. The sources of the data are listed in the figure.

The open, inverted triangles represent threshold data for the primate.[43] Note the break at 320 nm, which is continued by the open circles to 400 nm. The open circle primate data take the same form and values as the rabbit data and indicate that the data for the three species (human, primate, and rabbit) are essentially the same above 310 nm. If a value 500 times minimum threshold were used as the upper cut-off for the action spectrum, the corneal action spectrum begins at 210 nm and extends to 320 nm. Obviously, corneal damage can be induced with UVR above 320 nm, but the threshold exposure levels are quite high, i.e., much higher than can be found in man-made and natural radiation sources if the laser were excluded.

The solid squares represent the radiant exposure that establishes the UV-induced cataractogenesis in the pigmented rabbit lens. The open squares are exposures in which cataracts could not be induced.[46–47] The wavelength range for UV-induced cataractogenesis begins at 295 nm and extends to 320 nm. No cataracts were noted in either the pigmented rabbit or the primate for the wavelengths above 320 nm, even though exposures as high as 275 J/cm^2 were made.

UVR data for retinal exposures are shown by the plus signs for aphakic primates.[49] The aphakic primate exposures have been recalculated to the plane of the cornea for direct comparison. The retinal threshold of 0.36 J/cm^2 for the phakic primate measured at the plane of the cornea is presented as the solid triangle.[50] The two sets of retinal threshold values will be discussed more fully in the section on UV retinal exposures.

Exposure to the Cornea

EFFECTS ON THE CORNEAL EPITHELIUM
The appearance of the cornea using the biomicroscope demonstrates the response of the cornea to UV exposure. For subthreshold exposures, the initial response is a vast number of small glistening particles called *epithelial debris* that are located within the precorneal tear film. A second prominent observation is termed *granules;* they are the most repeatable and reliable damage criterion found in the cornea. Granules appear as small, discrete, white, round dots located predominantly in the columnar cell layer of the corneal epithelium and secondarily in the wing cell layer.[41] Granules result from the breakdown of the primary lysosome membrane, which releases hydrolytic enzymes that form secondary lysosomes.[51] The function of the lysosome is primarily autophagic and indicates that the immune system has initiated its restorative processes early in the UV exposure history.

Corneal changes from UV exposure follow a rather consistent pattern that is related to wavelength, duration, and level of radiant exposure. Above-threshold UV exposures produce an increase in epithelial debris from 210 nm up to 320 nm, but above 320 nm, debris remains relatively constant regardless of the exposure level. Epithelial damage in the form of haze, stippling, and granules increases in severity as exposure level increases, regardless of the UV wavelength. Epithelial granules increase in number and then coalesce to form a syncytium or network, with the network increasing in density as radiant exposure level increases. Corneal damage shifts from the external epithelial layers to the internal stroma and endothelium as the wavelength increases above 290 nm. The stroma becomes hazy with stromal granules and stromal opacities that continue to become more severe as exposure levels increase. Damage to the endothelium is manifested by an increased thickness of the cornea and the appearance of a flare and cells in the aqueous. Thus, there appears to be both a wavelength and a radiant exposure response to UVR with the depths of the cornea becoming more involved at longer wavelengths and higher exposure levels.

PHOTOKERATITIS
The primary response of the eye to the UV waveband from 210 to 320 nm is the condition called *photo-ophthalmia* or *photokeratitis.*[52–55] This is the "welder's flash" that has been experienced by every arc welder who has struck the arc prior to lowering the protective helmet. It is also the "snowblindness" experienced after unprotected corneal exposure from outside activities in the snow. After exposure to UVR, there is a latency period that depends on the intensity of the exposure but is typically 6 to 12 h. The anterior aspect of the eye, the eyelid, and the adnexa surrounding the eye becomes reddened. There is an ocular sensation of a foreign body or "sand," and the eyes become photophobic, produce excess lacrimation, and undergo blepharospasm to avoid pain. These acute symptoms last usually from 6 to 24 h, but almost all discomfort disappears within

48 h. The radiant exposures necessary to produce photokeratitis are very low because about 4 mJ/cm^2 at 270 nm causes minimal or threshold damage in the human cornea (Table 6-3; see Fig. 6-12). Only radiant exposures that are twice the threshold value (2 × H$_c$) result in permanent damage to the cornea, and such exposures are very rare.

The worker or skier is incapacitated visually during the acute symptom stage; it should be noted that the eye does not develop a tolerance to UV exposure as does the skin but becomes more sensitive with repeated exposures. The visual acuity of human subjects shows a transitory decrement of one or more Snellen acuity lines for most wavelengths within 4 h after exposure, continuing for a period of 24 h (Table 6-4).[45] Subthreshold levels of UV exposure result in an improved visual acuity that corresponds to the biomicroscopic observation of the clearing of epithelial debris from the anterior epithelium. The loss in acuity should not be sufficient to prevent a person from accomplishing most visual tasks unless the exposure is severe enough to result in ocular discomfort, photophobia, and blepharospasm.

Ocular transmittance measurements made after actinic keratitis was induced show that wavelengths below 310 nm are not appreciably reduced.[56] This indicates that UVR is able to penetrate to the anterior chamber, lens, and the retina after photokeratitis is evident. The VIS spectrum shows a 15% to 20% loss in transmittance after photokeratitis occurs, which probably results from the scatter of light by the damaged corneal epithelial cells.[56]

The corneal radiant exposure data from 315 to 400 nm are not considered part of the action spectrum of the cornea because the levels of exposure necessary to produce a corneal threshold are quite high.[37,38] The threshold exposure level at 315 nm is 450 times the corneal threshold at 270 nm. Therefore, UV exposure at 325 nm and for wavelengths up to 400 nm are relatively innocuous to the cornea when compared to the corneal UV action spectrum. These statements should not be taken to indicate that the long wavelength UV exposure cannot damage the cornea because corneal damage is found with extremely high exposure levels.

Wavelength (nm)	Corneal Radiant Exposure (H$_c$[J/cm^2])			Relative Efficiency S$_\lambda$ for Cornea			Conjunctiva (H$_{cj}$[J/cm^2])
	Human	Primate	Rabbit	Human	Primate	Rabbit	Human
210	—	0.33	0.7	—	0.012	0.007	—
220	0.01	0.027	0.046	0.40	0.19	0.11	—
230	0.013	0.022	0.03	0.31	0.18	0.17	—
240	0.008	0.012	0.033	0.53	0.33	0.15	—
250	0.008	0.020	0.041	0.50	0.20	0.12	—
260	0.008	0.011	0.018	0.53	0.36	0.28	—
270	0.004	0.004	0.005	1.00	1.00	1.00	0.0025
280	0.006	0.006	0.011	0.68	0.67	0.45	0.0035
290	0.007	0.007	0.012	0.57	0.57	0.42	0.035
295	—	—	0.02	—	—	0.25	—
300	0.007	0.011	0.05	0.57	0.36	0.10	0.045
305	—	—	0.07	—	—	0.07	—
310	0.014	0.02	0.055	0.29	0.20	0.09	0.0185
315	—	2.25	—	—	—	0.002	—
320	—	7.25	9.6	—	0.0004	0.0007	—

Data from Pitts DG, Kay KR,[42] Pitts DG,[45] and Collen AP, Perera S.[77]

TABLE 6-3
Threshold UV Exposure (H$_c$) to the Cornea and Conjunctiva in Producing Damage from Broadband UV Sources

Wavelength (nm)	Decimal Acuity*
220	0.6
230	0.6
240	0.6
250	0.5
260	1.0
270	0.8
280	0.5
290	0.6
300	0.8
310	0.6

*Acuity is in decimal form where 20/20 is 1.0, 20/25 is 0.8, 20/30 is 0.6, 20/40 is 0.5, and 20/50 is 0.4 decimal acuity.
Data from Pitts DG.[45]

TABLE 6-4
Visual Acuity Following a Threshold Exposure to UVR

OXYGEN DEPENDENCE OF CORNEAL EXPOSURES
The UVB exposure threshold has been shown to be oxygen-dependent (Table 6-5).[57] The threshold for air is 82 J/cm^2, while eyes flushed with oxygen (O_2) give 66 J/cm^2 and eyes flushed with nitrogen (N_2) show an exposure level of 133 J/cm^2. More importantly, there is a major morphologic difference between the O_2-exposed and N_2-exposed corneas. Virtually every cell of the epithelia of the O_2-exposed eyes was damaged, whereas only an occasional swollen epithelial cell was found with N_2-exposed eyes.

The O_2 corneal exposure illustrates an important physiologic response of ocular tissue to exposure to an altered environment simultaneously with UVR. The pure O_2 environment supplies an excess of O_2 to the epithelial tissue and the reduction of O_2 through univalent steps:

$$O_2 + e^- + HO_2 \rightarrow H_2 + O_2 \quad (6\text{-}8)$$

$$HO_2 + e^- + H^+ \rightarrow H_2O_2 \quad (6\text{-}9)$$

This produces the highly reactive species O_2 and H_2O_2. Free radicals have been shown to be responsible for producing irreversible damage to enzyme proteins and membrane lipids. This appears to be the case in these experiments because the oxygen

radicals in the epithelial tissue resulted in a lower threshold value, and in addition nearly every epithelial cell of the O_2-bathed cornea was damaged.

CUMULATIVE EFFECTS OF CORNEAL EXPOSURES
Cullen[51] and Zuclich[59] have studied the cumulative effects of UV exposure at 295 nm to the cornea. Cullen reaffirmed the corneal threshold H_c of 0.02 J/cm^2 at 295 nm and repeated UV exposures of 0.5-H_c + 0.5-H_c, with the second exposure delayed by an interval of 4 to 24 h.[58] A second experiment used a 0.5-H_c exposure level followed by a threshold exposure H_c at varying intervals within 24 h. The 0.5-H_c + 0.5-H_c experiment produced no greater corneal damage than an exposure of H_c only. The 0.5-H_c + 0.5-H_c exposure was as severe as a 2-H_c exposure when the delay between exposures was 4 h or less. When the delay between exposures was 8 h or more, the response of the cornea was as though a single H_c exposure had been made. Cullen's research demonstrates that a reparative mechanism for the cornea is effective in reducing the severity of the corneal damage and that the duration of time between exposures is important.

Zuclich[59] exposed the cornea to subthreshold levels using the UV krypton-ion laser (357.7 nm + 356.4 nm) and varied the interval between the two pulses from 1 h to 10 d. The corneal threshold, as a function of interpulse interval, is plotted in Figure 6-13 along with a single-pulse threshold and two-pulse threshold. The two-pulse data show a geometric increase in threshold as the duration between exposures increases. The threshold curve approaches but does not reach the 2 × H_c value because complete repair could not be achieved during the time interval between exposures. These data

Atmosphere	Threshold Dose (J/cm^2)	95% Confidence Limits (J/cm^2)
Air (control)	82	58–104
O_2	66	56–77
N_2	133	116–155

Data from Zuclich JA, Kurtin WE.[57]

TABLE 6-5
Oxygen Dependence of the Corneal Epithelium

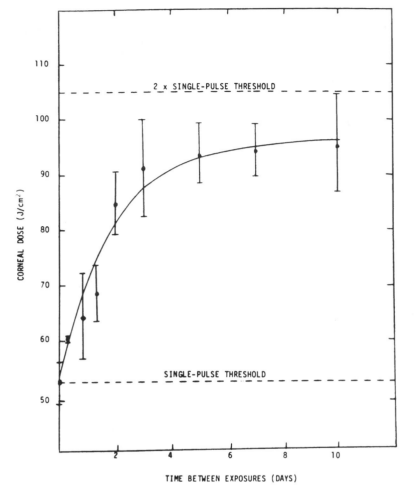

FIGURE 6-13
Repair of corneal epithelial tissue from two identical subthreshold 350 nm UV exposures spaced at intervals varying from 1 h to 10 d. The threshold value never achieves the level of the two-pulse threshold because of the corneal repair mechanism. The curve represents a least-squares fit to the data. *From* Zuclich JA: Cumulative effects of near-UV induced corneal damages. Health Phys 38:833–838, 1980; with permission.

suggest that the cornea follows an exponential repair process. Zuclich derived the following formula for corneal repair using a nonlinear regression calculation:

$$\text{Threshold} = C_1 + C_2(1 - e^{-kt}) \qquad (6\text{-}10)$$

where C_1 is the single-pulse threshold limit of (53.1 J/cm^2), C_2 the limit for the second exposure but less than $2 \times H_c$(43.5 J/cm^2), and k the repair rate constant (0.022/h ± 0.010/h). Evaluation of this formula shows that complete repair requires about 46 h, a value that is the inverse of the rate of recovery factor, k = 0.022. If C_1 equals C_2, complete repair of the cornea would be achieved. The exponential repair rate has been extended to analyze repeated exposures of UVR to the cornea, and the formulas are presented here.[59] If a UV exposure (E_{uv}) is deliv-

ered at time zero (t = 0), at some time later (t_i), the effect of the exposure would be equal to $F_{uv}ie^{-0.022}$. When a series of exposures are given to the cornea, the cumulative effective dose D at any given time t_i can be found by summating the individual exposures:

$$D_{(t)} = \sum_{i=o}^{\infty} E_{uv}e^{-0.022t_i} \qquad (6\text{-}11)$$

where $D_{(t)}$ is the cumulative exposures (W/cm^2), E_{uv} the irradiance of the UVR (W/cm^2), and t_i the duration of time of the individual exposures (in seconds). The cumulative exposures $D_{(t)}$ must remain at or below threshold for the calculation to be valid. Formula 6-11 may be integrated to determine the cumulative effect for a continuous exposure level of UVR:

$$D_{(t)} = \frac{xE_{uv}}{0.022}(1 - e^{-0.022t}) \qquad (6\text{-}12)$$

where x is the continuous exposure to a dose level of x.

Formula 6-12 indicates that as the exposure duration t approaches infinity ∞, $D_{(t)}$ becomes $D(\infty) = 46 \times (1 - e^{-0.022y})$, where y is the duration of the daily exposure in a working environment. Because the single exposure threshold H_c is 52.5 J/cm^2, this equation means that the cumulative effect D remains below threshold if the threshold 52.5 J/cm^2, divided by the 46-h recovery time, is 1.14 J/cm^2-h. A 24-h exposure to UVR should not reach threshold for the cornea if the rate of exposure, 1.14 J/cm^2-h × 24 h = 27.4 J/cm^2, is not exceeded. Zuclich demonstrates that the "worse case" radiant exposure for an 8-h work day must be less than 21.35 J/cm^2 or 2.66 J/cm^2-h or below 0.41 of the single pulse threshold of H_c = 52.5 J/cm^2. This exposure level holds regardless of the variations in the exposure duration or irradiance for each 24-h period of duration. It has been previously reported that if a 1-s exposure were 0.41 H_c or less, the corneal response was as if no UV exposure had been given.[58]

RECIPROCITY OF UV EXPOSURE TO THE CORNEA

Studies on corneal threshold with variations in the pulse width for multiple pulses and single pulses using the argon laser (351.1 nm and 363.8 nm) support complete reciprocity between the irradiance and pulse width (Fig. 6-14).[60] The complete reciprocity relationship provides evidence that the photochemical process is operative over the entire range of parameters. Reciprocity implies an additive effect with no physiologically significant repair up to a 10^4 s-exposure duration (2.8 h). Clinically, this should mean that a UV exposure to the cornea should not result in symptoms until 2.8 h after the cornea has been exposed to a suprathreshold level of UVR.

METABOLIC EFFECTS OF UV EXPOSURE TO THE CORNEA

Exposure of the cornea to UV at different levels of radiation demonstrates a decrease in O_2 uptake, an accumulation of both glucose and glycogen in the epithelium and endothelium, no change in adenosine triphosphate (ATP), and a drastic decrease in phosphocreatine (PCr).[63] The metabolic effects are wavelength-dependent, i.e., the 290-nm waveband gave the largest effect with the 360-nm waveband showing little effect on the phosphates. This suggests that when the O_2 uptake level decreases below 0.3 mm Hg O_2/s, the glycolytic metabolic activity increases in an attempt to sustain the epithelial tissue.

There is an almost immediate response to UV exposure by the corneal epithelium that is manifest by a frank decrease in O_2 uptake. The constant level of the ATP indicates that there is a decrease in the metabolic activity in the epithelium. The abnormal accumulation of epithelial and endothelial glucose

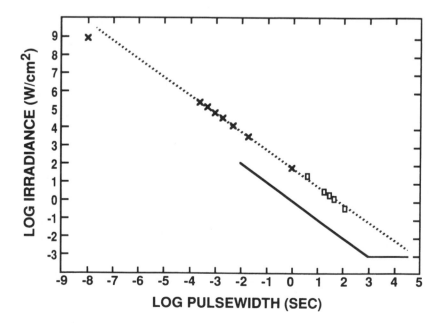

FIGURE 6-14
Reciprocity between irradiance and pulse duration are shown using single pulse thresholds and multiple pulse thresholds. Experimental data are compared to the ANSI standard shown by the solid lines. *From* **Zuclich JA, Connolly JS: Ocular damage induced near-ultraviolet laser radiation. Invest Ophthalmol 15:760–764, 1976; with permission from J.B. Lippincott Co., Philadelphia, PA.**

argues for an active glucose delivery process that accumulates glucose against the concentration gradient. The decreased O_2 uptake rate portends decreased metabolic activity and thus greater corneal damage from subsequent UV exposures.

UV EXPOSURE TO THE CORNEAL STROMA

The corneal stroma appeared to be resistant to UVR because stromal damage was not found with radiant exposures as high as 1 J/cm^2.[41,42,64] The corneal recovery from an exposure of 300 nm UVR after 8 d showed that the epithelium had regained its normal thickness, but the number of cells were decreased and some abnormal cells were still evident.[64] Spaces seen around stromal keratocytes and between some of the lamellae indicate that stromal edema was present. There was a loss in the number of keratocytes demonstrated by spaces containing electron-dense amorphous material instead of a normal or damaged keratocyte. Doughty and Cullen[65,66] describe large, "breadcrumb"-like amorphous opacities in the stroma that persisted throughout the 336 d of their study. It is now certain that UVR of 300 nm and longer wavelengths damages the stroma and that such damage may be permanent.

UV EXPOSURE TO THE CORNEAL ENDOTHELIUM

The effects of UVR on the endothelium are particularly important because of the role of the endothelium in maintaining the passage of metabolically required constituents to the cornea and because of the role of the endothelium and internal limiting lamina in maintaining the proper hydration of the cornea. The waveband responsible for endothelial damage begins at 300 nm and extends to 315 nm. A 0.085 J/cm^2 exposure at 300 nm results in large variations in thickness, loose adherence to the basement membrane, and small vacuoles in the cytoplasm.[66] Higher levels of UV exposure results in a separation of the endothelium from the posterior limiting lamina, numerous large vacuoles, and fewer mitochondria and endoplasmic reticula up to 8 d after exposure. The endothelium was presumed to have resumed its physiologic hydration function because the stroma was free from edema. The epithelial basement membrane, the anterior limiting lamina (Bowman's membrane), and posterior limiting lamina were not damaged.

The physiologic effects of a 300-nm UV exposure on the endothelium measured by the pachometer shows a double time course in the swelling response (Fig. 6-15) and corneal swelling related to the level of radiant exposure (Fig. 6-16).[66] There is an initial swelling of the cornea of less than 20% that peaks at about 22 h postexposure and a maximum thickness increase of over 100% found at 43 h. The initial swelling occurs with radiant exposures of 0.1 J/cm^2 or less, but the maximum thickness is found with radiant exposures above 0.1 J/cm^2. The initial swelling response is the result of damage to the epithelium and anterior stroma, whereas the later response is due to endothelial damage that allows fluid to enter the posterior stroma. The mechanisms of corneal hydration suggest how UVB exposure causes corneal thickness changes. The damage to the corneal epithelium results in an edema of the anterior stroma of less than 20% that usually resolves within 24 h. Higher UV exposure levels result in damage to the endothelium with the subsequent disruption of the endothelial pump mechanism, which in turn results in a severe edema located primarily in the posterior half of the stroma. These findings are supported by both pachometry and electron microscopic studies. The recovery of the cornea to an almost normal state of hydration requires 5 to 6 d,[65] but the endothelial cellular morphology still demonstrates the loss of mitochondria, endoplasmic reticula, and some vacuoles.[64] The threshold for corneal swelling from exposure to UVR at 300 nm was 0.1 J/cm^2, and the corneal swelling increased by a factor of 10 as the radiant exposure increased to 0.5 J/cm^2. The severity of endothelial damage probably results in the permanent loss of endothelial cells.

The most pronounced change in the endothelium from UV exposure is the increase in number and prominence of microvilli protruding into the anterior chamber.[67,68] The microvilli indicate endothelial damage and probably result in the aqueous "leaking" into the cornea to account for increased thickness of the stroma. A marked decrease in ascorbic acid but increases in glutathione and protein concentrations in the aqueous humor at 18 h after exposure to UVR are found. The increase in protein was related to the exposure of the iris because a dilated pupil markedly reduces protein concentration. Endothelial scrapings show no significant changes in ATP and ascorbate, but glutathione increases by a factor of 2, whereas the fraction in the oxidized state (GSSG) increases threefold. The lack of changes in ATP could mean that the endothelium

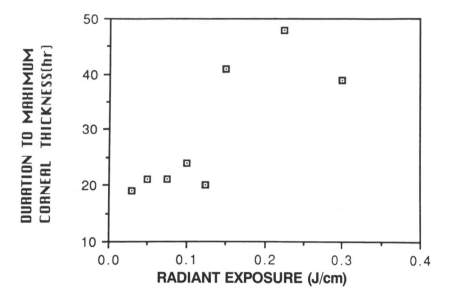

FIGURE 6-15
The relationship between radiant exposure to 300 nm UVR and the time to achieve maximum thickness of the cornea as measured with a pachometer. The initial swelling reaches maximum in about 22 h at radiant exposures of 0.1 J/cm² and lower, whereas higher radiant exposures require about 43 h to achieve maximum thickness. *From* **Cullen AP, Chou BR, Hall MG, Jany SE. Ultraviolet-B damages corneal endothelium. Am J Optom Physiol Opt 61:473–478. ©American Acad of Optometry, 1984, with permission.**

has lost its ability to function and does not use the available ATP. The loss of endothelial function is probably accurate, because corneal swelling indicates a compromise in endothelial function. Ascorbate, an important intracellular antioxidant whose peak absorption is 290 nm, is apparently not required by the UV-exposed endothelium. Glutathione has been shown to be necessary for endothelial cellular function,[69–71] and its increase in both

the aqueous and the endothelium implies that the metabolic system designed to protect the cellular integrity of the cornea is functioning. The increased concentration of GSSG should cause a sharp rise in the supply of NADPH for the production of glutathione reductase through activation of the hexose monophosphate shunt.[69]

UV data on the exposure to the endothelium raise some very important questions concerning

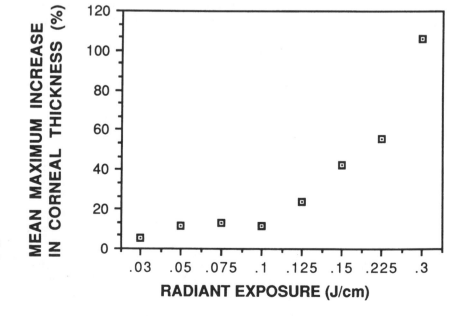

FIGURE 6-16
Percent change in corneal thickness with increase in radiant exposure at 300 nm. The corneal swelling response below 0.1 J/cm² is epithelial, whereas the large increases in thickness from suprathreshold radiant exposures above 0.1 J/cm² result from damage to the endothelial pump mechanism. *From* **Cullen AP, Chou BR, Hall MG, Jany SE. Ultraviolet-B damages corneal endothelium. Am J Optom Physiol Opt 61:473–478. ©Amer Acad of Optometry, 1984, with permission.**

whether these changes actually represent the effects of pleomorphism and cell loss related to the aging process or are related to UV exposure. Endothelial cell density decreases with age, and concomitantly, the number of hexagon-shaped cells decreases while the number of pentagon- and heptagon-shaped cells increase.[72-74] The Japanese endothelium has a higher cell density than the American (Caucasian) endothelium, but cellular polymegathism, pleomorphism, and the loss of hexagonal cells related to the normal aging process do not differ.[75] The welder who is occupationally exposed to greater levels of UVR presents an endothelium in which the size of the cell increases, whereas the number of hexagonal cells decreases as the person ages.[76] Both changes are consistent with normal endothelium aging studies and lead to the conclusion that exposure of the endothelium to UVR at subthreshold, chronic, and cumulative levels plays an important role in the aging of the endothelium.[76] Therefore, it is clinically important that people be provided ocular protection against UVR exposure.

UV Exposure to the Human Conjunctiva

A 5-mm circular area of the lower bulbar conjunctiva approximately 5 mm below the corneoscleral junction exposed to UVR in the wavelength range from 270 to 310 nm in 10-nm wavebands with the threshold response H_{cj} is presented in Table 6-3.[77] The conjunctival response began 4 to 5 h postexposure with a localized injection, chemosis, and rose bengal staining of the irradiated area. Impression cytology demonstrated direct damage to the organelles of the conjunctival cells and the presence of a localized immune response. These findings are consistent with pathologic changes observed in pterygia and pingueculae.

UV Exposure to the Crystalline Lens

The UV waveband from the sun and the daily absorption of small amounts of UV may be responsible for inducing senile cataracts or accelerating the formation of other types of cataracts. The daily level of exposure of the eye to UVR was discussed fully in the section on outdoor risks from solar UV.

The response of the crystalline lens to UV exposure is shown in Figure 6-17, which defines the action spectrum for the production of UV-induced cataracts.[46,47] The threshold radiant exposures cause transient cataracts that disappeared in 7 to 14 d. The wavelength range between 295 nm and 320 nm is efficient in producing UV-induced cataracts, but cataracts could not be induced with radiant exposures below 295 nm or above 320 nm despite very high radiant exposures (Table 6-6). Permanent lenticular changes were induced with radiant exposure levels twice the threshold minimal damage value ($2 \times H_L$).

The first biomicroscopic signs of lens damage are the reduction or loss in the "orange-peel" appearance of the anterior capsule and an increase in the prominence of the anterior suture line. These changes usually regress to a normal appearance

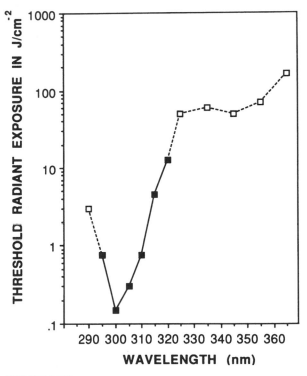

FIGURE 6-17
The action spectrum for UVR-induced cataracts. The solid squares indicate exposures that resulted in a cataract within 24 h after exposure. The open squares represent exposures that did not result in lenticular opacities. (*Data from* Pitts DG, Cullen AP;[46] Pitts DG, Cullen AP, Hacker PD.[47])

Wavelength (nm)	Anterior Uveitis Exposure Threshold (J/cm^2)	Cataract Exposure Threshold (J/cm^2)	Cataract Effectiveness (S_λ)
290	0	> 3.00	< 0.05
295	0.75	0.75	0.20
300	0.50	0.15	1.00
305	0.30	0.30	0.50
310	1.00	0.75	0.20
315	0	4.50	0.03
320	0	12.60	0.01
325	0	> 50.00	—
335	0	> 60.00	—
345	0	> 50.00	—
355	0	> 70.00	—
365	0	> 162.00	—

TABLE 6-6
UV Threshold for Anterior Uveitis and Transient Cataracts in the Lens of the Rabbit Eye

within 24 h after exposure. As the radiant exposure approaches threshold, many small, discrete, white dots appear in the anterior epithelium of the lens, which usually disappear within 24 h. The appearance of anterior subcapsular opacities of the lens is similar to the previously described corneal epithelial granules. The change from the small, discrete, white anterior subcapsular dots into a permanent opacity or cataract develop in an orderly manner. Opacities become larger and less dense, coalesce to form a network, and migrate toward the anterior suture line, where they disappear into the depths of the anterior stroma. At the same time, there is an increase in the stromal haze, and the permanent opacity spreads laterally from the anterior suture line. Occasionally, anterior stromal vacuoles are seen over the anterior subcapsular surface of the lens. Suprathreshold UV exposures result in permanent lenticular opacities.

EPIDEMIOLOGY OF UV-INDUCED CATARACTS. The ophthalmic community has found it difficult to accept the cause-effect relationship of UV exposure in producing cataracts. Conversely, the role of UVR in the induction of skin cancer has received worldwide acceptance by both dermatologists and the public. This is difficult to understand because the crystalline lens is embryonically derived from the surface ectoderm and has been shown to respond similarly to harmful physical stimuli. However, there is ever-increasing evidence in the epidemiologic literature in recent years that implicates UVR as a causative factor in the production of age related cataracts.

When the causes of human cataracts cannot be related to congenital, toxic, traumatic, chemical, or other known factors, they are usually attributed to senility. The prevalence of cataracts has not been definitively determined, but the Framingham study[78-80] has provided cataract prevalences of 4.5% for people aged 52–64 years, 18% for people aged 62–74 years, and 45.9% for people of ages of 75 to 85 years. Cataract prevalence increases with age, is more prevalent in females than in males, and is common above the age of 65. Many metabolic factors such as diabetes, high blood pressure, poor nutrition, increased levels of phospholipids, certain drugs, and a reduced vital capacity have been associated with senile cataracts. Ionizing radiation, IR radiation, UVR, and microwave (MW) radiation are thought to increase the risk of cataracts, but long-term, low dose effects have not yet been established.[81]

The prevalence of cataracts is related to the areas of the world that receive the greatest levels of sunlight.[82] The National Health and Nutritional Examination Survey (HANES) and the Model Reporting Area for Blindness Statistics (MRA) studied the epidemiologic risk factors for senile cataracts, including sunlight. Age related cataracts were positively associated with sunlight and particularly with UVB in sunlight.[83,84] The prevalence of cataracts was significantly higher in those locations with large amounts of sunlight and in the lower latitudes.

The Australian aboriginal is a unique subpopulation that is exposed to a massive amount of sunshine during a lifetime. A study of 350 aboriginals found cataracts associated with the number of hours per day of exposure to sunlight.[84] Those with fewer cataracts were exposed to sunlight less than 8 h per day, and the number of cataracts increased with exposures to greater than 8.5 h of sunlight. The prevalence of cataracts in 64,307 aboriginal and 41,254 nonaboriginal populations residing in five zones of UVB intensity in Australia showed no correlation with sunlight exposure for the nonaboriginal cataract population. However, there was a significant correlation of cataract prevalence in the aboriginal with the climatic UVB and the prevalence of cataracts in the general aboriginal population.[86]

Brilliant et al[87] studied 27,785 Nepalese individuals from the plains, the hills, and the mountains who were rural village residents. The number of hours of daily sunlight were determined for each location. They found that persons exposed to 12 h of sunlight daily were 3.8 times more likely to develop cataracts than those who were exposed to only 7 h of sunlight daily. They also reported a 2.7 times higher prevalence at altitudes of 185 m and below than at 1000 m and above. Chatterjee[88] reported that the Punjab population who lived at higher altitudes were less susceptible to cataract. Brilliant et al[87] were able to account for the apparent discrepancy among previous studies by noting that those who lived higher in the Himalayas were shadowed from sunlight many hours each morning and subsequently received a smaller UVB daily exposure than the Nepalese living below 185 m or on the plains. A study on association of cataracts with the hours of exposure to sunlight in the Nepal population has been repeated recently and has substantiated the association of UVR and cataracts.[89]

The only epidemiologic study designed to investigate the relationship between solar UVR and cataracts used 838 watermen who worked on the Chesapeake Bay.[90] Field measurements of solar radiation allowed the calculation of annual UV exposure, while cataracts were graded by type and severity.[91] Cortical cataracts were associated with exposure to the UVB levels in sunlight. A serially additive UVB exposure model demonstrated that watermen with cortical cataracts received a 21% higher exposure to UVR annually. Watermen in the upper quartile who were exposed to sunlight had a relative risk factor of 3.3 when compared to those in the lowest quartile. There was no association between UVB exposure and nuclear cataracts or between UVA and any type of cataract. The positive correlation between UVB exposure and cortical cataracts illustrates that the ocular lens needs to be protected against UVB exposure. In addition, an increase in pterygia and climatic droplet keratopathy was found in the watermen. The data demonstrate that there is a 1% increase in cortical cataracts for each year of exposure to UVB in sunlight.[90]

In a case control study of 864 patients in the age range from 40 to 69 years, solar radiation exposure showed an increase in the risk of anterior cortical or posterior subcapsular cataracts (PSC) but was not related to nuclear cataracts.[92] In a matched-pair prospective study of 168 patients with posterior subcapsular opacities and 168 controls, it was found that PSC were related to UVB exposure and associated with both diabetes and the use of steroids.[93] Nuclear opacities were not related to UVB exposure. An analysis to characterize UVB exposure at various stages of life suggests that one becomes equally susceptible to UVB damage to the lens at any stage of life, and this finding infers a cumulative effect. There was a positive association between people with blue eyes and PSC but not with UVB radiation. It may be that blue-eyed people are more susceptible to PSC from lower doses of UVB and have a faster progression rate of a PSC because of the selective pigmentation loss in blue-eyed people. The data suggest that UVB exposure may be an important factor in inducing PSC.

In summary, the data demonstrate a correlation between senile cortical cataract and exposure to UVB solar radiation. Despite the variety of methods used to determine the type and severity of cataract, the measurement of solar radiation, the differences in the populations studied, and the disparities in the statistical evaluations of the data, the epidemiologic evidence of the causal relationship between UVB and cataracts is consistent, the evidence is biologically plausible, and it is supported by laboratory data that exhibit a dose-response relationship. The epidemiologic data support the conclusion that senile cataract—cortical senile cataract—is associated with UVB exposures from sunlight and that protection against UVB solar exposure is not only prudent but necessary. Likewise, UVB exposure was not found in nuclear cataracts and UVA was not linked to any type of cataract.

LASER-INDUCED UV CATARACTS. The lens does not appear to be affected by the photochemical processes that result in photokeratitis because minimal lens effects are seen with broadband sources above 320 nm, whereas the corneal photochemical affects appear to extend to 400 nm.[47] The induction of cataracts by a photochemical process appears to occur only with UVR between 295 nm and 320 nm and is concentrated near the anterior surface of the lens.[46] Studies with the 337-nm nitrogen laser found that a 1.1 J/cm² radiant exposure produced immediate lens opacities that resulted from a thermal

Laser	Wavelength (nm)	Pulsewidth (s)	Threshold Irradiance (W/cm^2)
HeCd	325	240	1.1
Nitrogen	337	10^{-8}	1.1×10^8
Argon	351.1, 363.8	1	18.7
Argon	351.1, 363.8	4	19.1
Excimer (XeF)*	351	2.5×10^{-8}	6.2×10^{-8}

*The excimer laser was a multiple-pulse exposure with a pulse repetition rate of 1 Hz.

From Zuclich JA, Connolly JS: Ocular damage induced near-ultraviolet laser radiation. Invest Ophthalmol 15:760–764, 1976; with permission from JP Lippincott, Philadelphia, PA.

TABLE 6-7
Laser Thresholds for Inducing Thermal Cataracts in the Rhesus Monkey

mechanism.[60] Table 6-7 provides a list of lasers, indicating the wavelengths, pulse width, and irradiance that causes UV-induced thermal cataracts.

To ensure that the mechanism is thermal, cataracts induced by exposure to near UV lasers require a minimum level of irradiance that produces an immediate cataract. Exposures at or slightly above the irradiance required to produce thermal cataract result in a nebulous cloudiness of the anterior surface of the lens, whereas exposures at higher irradiances produce bright milk-white opacities that are located in the subcapsular area. The milk-white opacities are permanent and did not change during the 5 y in which they were monitored.[60] The nebulous clouding found after threshold exposure faded over several months to a normal appearance, and subsequent recurrence was not observed. Subthreshold exposures did not result in cataracts even with repeated subthreshold exposures that resulted in a cumulative irradiance as much as 10 times the threshold value.

Anterior Uveitis from UV Exposure

One of the damaging effects to the eye from UVB exposure is secondary anterior uveitis manifested as an inflammation of the posterior limiting layer (De-scemet's membrane) and corneal endothelium.[46,47] The condition is characterized by a localized redness of the eye just lateral to the cornea, aqueous flare, and fibrinous materials deposited on the endothelial side of the cornea. The eye appears seriously affected, but the condition regresses to normal spontaneously within 2 d after exposure. This response is important because it had been postulated previously that the anterior uveitis preceded and was the cause of UV-induced cataracts. The UV waveband that produces anterior uveitis begins at 295 nm and extends to 310 nm (see Table 6-6). The radiant exposure levels are comparable to the levels that produce cataracts. Cataracts are found both simultaneous with and independent of anterior uveitis, but anterior uveitis is not considered the causative agent.

UV Exposure to the Retina

The effect of UVR on the retina has been an area of controversy for many years. Duke-Elder states, "On the whole, it is probably safe to say that the ultraviolet radiations which might harm the retina do not reach it, and those radiations of this spectral region which do reach it have not been shown to do organic or functional harm of any practical importance to this tissue."[81] Duke-Elder appears to have overlooked several important facts. It is known that UVR in the region of 320 nm reaches the retina of the phakic eye, the transmittance of UVB to at least 313 nm reached the retina of the phakic eye,[53] and the aphakic eye can see UV to at least 365 nm.[94-96] Duke-Elder also concluded that UVR above 305 nm was not abiotic, but it is known now that the DNA molecule is affected by UVR to at least 320 nm and possibly longer wavelengths.

The ability of UVR to produce retinal damage in the aphake and pseudophake has been well documented.[97,98] This is not surprising since Goodeve et al[94] have shown the visual limit of UVR in the phakic eye to be 309 nm and in the aphakic eye, 298 nm. If these wavelengths can be seen, they may be transmitted to the retina in sufficient quantities to produce photochemical damage from overexposure.

The UVR reaching the retina does both functional and morphologic damage. The albino rat's absolute visual threshold is 3 to 5 log units higher immediately after exposure to an average 0.381 ×

10^{-3} W/cm^2 of 350-nm UVR.[99] The visual thresholds recover slowly and stabilize at approximately
0.5 log unit above the pre-exposure absolute threshold within 3 to 5 d after exposure. A 15% to 20%
reduction in the outer segments and cell nuclei of
the retinal receptors appears to explain the reduction in sensitivity; however, it has been argued that
photoreceptor damage and behavioral thresholds
are different and separate processes that cannot be
reduced to a causal process.[100]

Beginning near 300 nm, a small amount of UV
that is of the proper energy level to ensure a photochemical lesion reaches the retina (Figure 6-18).[101]
In Figure 6-18, the dashed line represents the direct
and scattered radiation reaching the retina, whereas
the solid line provides the direct transmittance,
which is the irradiance forming the ocular image.
The narrow window of transmitted UVR peaks at
320 nm with about 1% transmittance and decreases
to about 0.2% at 340 nm. The maximum transmittance at 320 nm is essentially the same transmittance
as 400 nm; however, the retina is more sensitive to
damage in the shorter 320-nm window wavelengths
when compared to the 400-nm VIS spectrum wavelengths. The pigment epithelium absorbs UVR very
strongly near the VIS spectrum from 375 to 400
nm,[8] and the lens absorbs it below 295 nm and in a
waveband beginning at 360 nm and ending at 380
nm. The combination of crystalline lens and pigment epithelium absorption ordinarily affords some
protection to the retina.

The HeCd laser (325 nm) threshold for the retina
measured at the plane of the cornea was 0.36 J/cm^2
(Table 6-8), when the criterion was an ophthalmoscopically visible lesion at 24 h.[101] If the criterion
were changed to an ophthalmoscopically visible lesion immediately postexposure, the threshold was
raised to 3.83 J/cm^2, a factor of 10.6. However, the
threshold became 0.15 J/cm^2 or a factor of 2 below
that measured at the cornea when the lesion was
determined by light microscopy. These data illustrate that, indeed, 325 nm does penetrate the cornea, lens, and vitreous to produce retinal lesions and
that the value called "threshold" depends upon the
criterion. Zuclich predicts that 325 nm is close to the
shortest wavelength in which UV retinal lesions may
be produced.[103] This prediction may have valid research support since retinal lesions could not be produced by the XeCl excimer laser at 308 nm; however, 310 to 340 nm is transmitted to the retina.

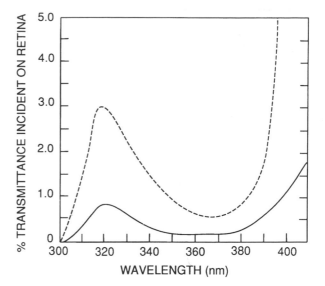

FIGURE 6-18
**Transmittance of UVR to the retina of the monkey eye.
The dashed line represents the total transmittance,
which includes direct and scattered UVR. The solid line
represents the direct transmittance of UVR, which would
form an image on the retina. Note that there is almost
as much UVR reaching the retina at 320 nm as at 400
nm and that the 320-nm peak possesses a bandwidth of
about 40 nm.** *Data from* **Boettner EA, Wolter JR[11]** *and
figure from* Zuclich JA, Taboada J: Ocular hazard from
UV laser exhibiting self-made-lacking. Applied Optics
17:1482–1484, 1978; with permission.

Threshold retinal exposures for the aphakic
rhesus monkey retina using 10-nm wavebands calculated to the plane of the cornea are presented in
Table 6-8.[102] The phakic data differed materially
when the retinal threshold was determined by measuring the radiant exposure at the plane of the
cornea.[102] Calculations make comparisons difficult
because of the difference in transmittance of the
phakic and aphakic eye, the difference in retinal
image sizes due to the change in index of refraction
n with wavelength, and the difference in image size
in the aphakic versus the normal phakic eye. If the
phakic data in Table 6-8 were corrected for the transmittance of the lens, the result is very comparable to
the aphakic data (0.365/cm^2 × 0.42) = 0.21 J/cm^2).

Calculations of the diameter of the retinal image
with the change in the index of refraction illustrate
that the diameter of the retinal image size at 325 nm

Wavelength (nm)	Threshold Radiant Exposure Measured at the Cornea (J)	Calculated Threshold Irradiance on the Retina (W/cm²)
Aphakic Rhesus Monkey Eye		
	—	0.77
405	0.41	0.15
380	0.24	0.081
350	0.20	0.054
325	0.23	0.05
Phakic Rhesus Monkey Eye		
488	0.36	
325	0.21 +	

NOTE: The exposure duration for the aphakic data is 100 s. The data at 325 nm for the phakic eye is from HeCd laser exposures. The 325-nm data have been corrected for ocular transmittance using 3% for the phakic eye and 42% for the aphakic eye.[102]

From Zuclich JA: Ultraviolet-induced photochemical damage in ocular tissue. Health Phys 56:671–682, 1989; with permission.

TABLE 6-8
Threshold Values for Retinal Lesions in the Phakic and Aphakic Rhesus Monkey Eye from Exposures to broadband UVR

is approximately three times the size of a retinal image at 405 nm and is blurred. A photochemical mechanism of damage should not vary in threshold value with changes in the size of the retinal image. Table 6-8 appears to validate the concept because the laser beam provides a retinal image size of approximately 25 μm for 555 nm, but the retinal image at 325 nm would approximate 50 μm when observed fundoscopically.[103] The threshold is essentially the same for the 500-μm broadband data that has been corrected for the index of refraction to be approximately 1000 μm.

The retinal data demonstrate that reciprocity (I × t = k) should hold from 325 to 380 nm because the threshold values are essentially equal. The calculated threshold retinal irradiance may be used to indicate the efficiency with which UVR produces retinal lesions. The wavelengths at 350 nm and shorter are much more efficient than the wavelengths above 350 nm in causing retinal damage. In fact, 325 nm is more efficient by a factor of 3 than 405 nm and more efficient by a factor of 15 than 441 nm.

Thus, the UVB waveband from sunlight proves to be the most hazardous UVR to the cornea, the lens, and the retina of the eye.

Retinal damage to sunbathers' eyes caused by exposure of 2 to 4 h from increased solar radiation due to the reduction of the ozone layer has been reported.[105] Each person suffered the loss of visual acuity varying from 20/40 to 20/80 in the affected eye that returned to between 20/20 and 20/30 within 3 to 9 mo. The eyes still demonstrated a small central scotoma with metamorphopsia, whereas the foveal lesion remained as a permanent reminder of solar retinopathy. The cause of the solar damage to the retina, the ocular transmittance, photochemical mechanisms, and the geophysical conditions present at the time of the exposure were reviewed. The geophysical studies indicate that there was a 15% to 23% decrease in the ozone layer that resulted in an increase in the UVB reaching the Earth. The data of Sundararaman et al,[106] used to calculate the solar flux incident on the Earth's surface at the time of exposure to the subjects, are presented in Table 6-9. Because the loss of ozone results in an increase in UVR below 340 nm and does not affect an increase in the VIS and IR portions of the optical spectrum, the retinal damage must have been initiated by the increase in the UVB portion of the solar spectrum, and consequently, must be photochemical in nature but enhanced by the rise in temperature caused by the VIS and IR radiation reaching the retina.

The threshold radiant exposure for a retinal photochemical lesion was found to be 0.36 J/cm² when measured at the plane of the cornea. The solar irradiance contained in a 5.75-nm waveband centered at 325 mm is 24.55 × 10⁻⁵ W/cm², resulting in an exposure duration of 1466 s or 24.4 min to achieve threshold. The solar irradiance contained in wavebands between 317.6 nm and 329.1 nm is 53.36 × 10⁻⁵ W/cm² and would require only 674.7 s or 11.2 min to achieve a retinal lesion. These calculations indicate that the retinal lesion is within the realm of possibility for the solar UVB available at the plane of the cornea for patients in this study.

The retina is particularly sensitive to damage from exposure to UVR but the crystalline lens absorbs most of the UVB and a considerable amount of the UVA. However, these UV wavebands reach the retina of the aphakic eye in copious amounts. Therefore, spectacle lenses, intraocular lenses, soft contact lenses, PMMA and gas permeable hard contact

Wave-length (nm)	Solar Irradiance Ann Arbor (W/cm² = nm × 10⁻⁶)	Solar Irradiance New York (W/cm² = nm × 10⁻⁶)
297.6	0.071	0.064
300.4	0.070	0.659
305.4	5.36	5.20
308.8	9.5	9.29
311.4	14.6	14.4
317.6	28.1	27.9
325.4	42.7	42.6
329.1	54.2	54.1
332.4	55.9	55.8

NOTE: A total UVB of 0.463 W/cm² and 458.6 W/cm² was available at the cornea of the sunbather's eye for Ann Arbor and New York, respectively. Data are for a latitude of 40° N and a solar zenith angle of 0° at noon.
Data from Yannozi LA, Fisher YL, Krueger A, Slakter J.[105]

TABLE 6-9
Solar Spectral Irradiance on Earth for a 23% Decrease in Ozone Found at Ann Arbor (3/28/86) and a 15% Decrease in Ozone at New York (3/29/86)

lenses that do not absorb the UVB pose a specific hazard to the aphakic eye because they allow an excess of UVB to focus on the retina. It has been argued that retinal damage to human patients has not been documented, but chromatopsia and retinal blanching found clinically in aphakes represents a solar photoretinitis that can be prevented with UV absorptive lenses.

Morphologic damage to the retina in response to UV exposure differs from that caused by the VIS spectrum. Schmidt and Zuclich[101] and Ham et al[49] described UVR damage to the outer segments of the receptors as the initial response to exposure of the primate retina. This contrasts with the pigment endothelium being the affected retinal layer for broadband VIS- and IR-induced thermal burns. The inner segments of the receptors, the RPE, and other parts of the retina may be damaged as UV exposure levels increase. A significant increase in electron-dense bodies are found in the inner segments of the pigmented rabbit eye of the receptors from exposure to UVR at 300 nm. Primate electron microscopic data demonstrate initial damage to the inner segment and outer segments of the receptors along with the cells of Müller, while the remaining cell layers and RPE were the last layers of the retina to be affected.[107]

UV Sensitivity Due to Pharmaceutical Agents

Dramatic increases in the sensitivity of the skin and the eye to UV and other spectral wavebands are induced by a variety of pharmaceutical compounds and the list grows longer each day.[108] The topic is of sufficient magnitude that a book would be required; therefore, the purpose of this introduction is to familiarize the reader with those drugs or medications that are affected by UV with an emphasis on ocular effects. To assist in the understanding of this topic, the important terms need to be defined. *Photosensitive* or *photosensitivity* indicates that a cell or biologic system has an abnormal capacity to react to sunlight. Photosensitivity is defined as a reaction to a compound whose chemical structure endows it with the ability to absorb UV and VIS spectrum light and undergo a photochemical reaction resulting in a generation of highly reactive and relatively long-lived intermediates in the form of triplets, radicals, and ions that cause modifications in other nearby molecules of the biologic system.[109] *Phototoxic* is used when the response time of the biologic system to the physical stimulus of UVR or light is relatively quick following exposure. The term *photoallergic* describes the delayed response of the biologic system resulting from the photosensitized formation of specific compounds that react with proteins to form photoantigenic compounds. The introduction of a photoantigenic compound may result in a photoallergic response from the initial exposure, but in subsequent exposures the response could be a very dangerous anaphylactic response.

A number of commonly prescribed antimicrobial agents or pharmaceutical agents are photosensitizers, phototoxic, or photoallergic in nature. Table 6-10 provides a list of the more common drugs by class, category, generic name, clinical use, and photic effect. A list of 93 specific drugs that are phototoxic, 15 drug categories that are phototoxic and photoallergic, and 61 drugs that are cataractogenic can be found in reference 108. The list is increasing daily as the pharmaceutical agents become more complex.

Class of Drug	Category of Drug	Generic Name	Clinical Use	Photic Effect
Antibiotics	Sulfonamides	Sulfacetamide Sulfanilamide Sulfadiazine Sulfamethizole	Chemotherapy	Phototoxic Photoallergic
		Cholotetracycline Oxytetracycline Doxytetracycline	Bacterial infections	Phototoxic Cataracts
Hyperglycemic	Sulfonylureas	Chloropropamide Tolazamide Tolbutamide	Hypoglycemic Anti-diabetic	Phototoxic
Diuretics	Chlorothiazides	Benzothiadiazide Quinethazone Tricholoromethazide	Diuretic Anti-hypertensive	Phototoxic
Antipsychotics	Phenothiazides	Chlopromazine Promethazine Mepazine	Tranquilizers	Phototoxic Photoallergic
Antianxiety	Chlordiazepoxide	Dalmarc Librium Valium	Tranquilizers	Phototoxic
Photochemotherapy	Furocoumarins	Psoralen 8-Methoxypsoralen Trimethylpsoralen	Vitiligo Psoriasis	Phototoxic Cataracts
	Chlordiazepoxide	8-Methyoxypsoralen	Bacterial infections	Photoallergic
Hormonal	Oral contraceptives	Estrogens Progesterones	Birth control	Phototoxic

Data from Goeckerman WH.[111]

TABLE 6-10
Selected Drugs by Class, Category, Generic Name, Use, and Reactions When Exposed to UVR

It has been known for over 100 years that psoriasis shows improvement during the summer months. UVB or UVA used alone also results in improvement of the condition; however, output limitations of artificial sources and the requirement for increased UVR as the skin tanned became self-defeating for indoor application. Goeckerman[110,111] used crude coal tar to enhance the effects of UVR. It was subsequently shown that the action spectrum for the crude coal tar + UVR was in the UVA waveband. More recently, it has been shown that the psoralens + UVA (PUVA) phototherapy was specific to the treatment of psoriasis and vitiligo.[112] Psoralens are taken orally, 0.6 mg/kg body weight, and after 2 h the person is exposed to UVA in the amount of 1 to 5 J/cm² depending on the spectral distribution of the source, the degree of the patient's tan, and the pa-

tient's sunburn history. Initial experiments indicated that PUVA treatments were safe for the skin and the eyes, but subsequently it has been shown that both skin cancer and cataracts have been induced with PUVA treatment. PUVA has been used to successfully treat mycosis fungoides (MF), an uncommon malignant lymphoma and eczema. PUVA treatments have also been reported to affect the immune system by reducing the number of lymphocytes,[113,114] decreasing the percentage of T lymphocytes circulating in the blood, and depressing the incorporation of thymidine by mononuclear cells.

An increasing number of phototherapy modes are entering into the health care system. It appears that the simultaneous presence of O_2 and other oxygen-derived molecular species are necessary to ensure biologic effectiveness of the treatment in tumor phototherapy.[115] The topical application of indomethacin immediately after irradiation of the skin with UVB reduces the erythemal sensitivity of the skin in patients with actinic prurigo, psoriasis, and atopic dermatitis. Phototoxic reactions associated with nalidixic acid are suspected to be triggered by activated oxygen and may be reduced by melanin.[116] The drugs in the photochemotherapy class are expanding rapidly due to the promising results of cancer treatment by photodynamic cell inactivation. The process includes the oral, intravenous, intramuscular, or topical application of tumor-localizing photosensitizing compounds and their activation by UV or VIS spectrum radiation. This topic deserves separate treatment because of the number of photosensitizing agents and the different mechanisms by which the processes attack cancer cells.

Summary of the Ocular Effects of UV Exposure

A summary of the ocular response to UVR as it varies with the wavelength and the level of radiant exposure is shown in Table 6-11. The exposures up to 290 nm result in damage primarily to the epithelium of the cornea and can be explained by the almost complete absorption of UV below 290 nm by the epithelium. As wavelengths are increased from 290 to 315 nm, corneal damage shifts to the stromal and endothelial layers of the cornea. Exposures above 320 nm require higher levels of radiant exposure to produce damage to the cornea. Thus, the cornea appears to give both a wavelength and radiant exposure response with the depths of the cornea becoming more involved at the UVB wavelengths and at higher exposure levels.

When the minimal-damage action spectra and threshold values are studied, the threshold radiant exposures from broadband optical sources for corneal damage are sufficiently below the radiant exposure levels necessary to produce lens damage and thus the cornea should serve as a protective barrier for the lens. There are two situations in which the concept of the cornea serving as a protective barrier for the lens may fail. The first situation is for long-term, low level repeated exposures that may be in the proper wavelength range but with radiant power levels below the corneal damage level and in which the cumulative effects produce long-term lenticular damage. The second situation occurs when very high radiant exposure levels in the proper wavelength range are delivered in very short durations. These exposures may result in minimal damage to the cornea but extensive damage to the lens in the form of an immediate cataract. Examples of these two exposure situations would be sunlight and the laser. Sunlight would represent the low level, repeated cumulative exposures, and the laser would represent the high radiant exposure source. Sufficient research data are available on the cornea to provide an action spectrum for photokeratits, data on the dependence of the damage on oxygen, decreased visual acuity, repair duration, reciprocity, metabolic disturbances, and the control of corneal hydration. A more focused biochemical research effort on mechanisms of UVR damage levels is needed to complete the picture.

The action spectrum for acute UVB-induced cataracts between 295 and 320 nm clearly demonstrates the fact that UVR can cause cataracts. The epidemiologic literature supports the concept that the UVR in sunlight is one of the many causes of senile cataract in humans. The possibility that UV exposure accelerates other forms of cataracts has not been studied, but recent cataractous animal models allow such studies to be initiated. Biochemically, cataracts appear to occur through three major mechanisms: photo-oxidation of lens crystallins; photo-oxidation of lens membrane lipids; and damage to the lens and bow epithelial DNA, resulting in the production of damaged lens cells and, subsequently, cataracts. Whether any, all, or combinations of the biochemical mechanisms are involved in producing UV cataracts has not been determined experimentally. It is certain that any of the biochemical mechanisms must be proven in vivo for a definitive hypothesis to be developed.

Structure	Waveband	Threshold
Cornea	200–320 nm	0.05 J/cm^2 at 270 nm
Uvea	295–310 nm	0.05 J/cm^2 at 305 nm
Lens	295–320 nm	0.15 J/cm^2 at 300 nm
Retina	310–380 nm	0.36 J/cm^2 at 320 nm

TABLE 6-11
Summary of UV Damage to the Eye

The data on the effects of UVR on the retina should alert the optometrist and other health care professionals to its danger. The threshold irradiance on the aphakic retina required to produce a photochemical lesion using 350-nm radiation requires only 0.054 W/cm^2 for 100 s or 5.4 J/cm^2 (Table 6-8), whereas corneal damage at 350 nm requires nearly 75 J/cm^2 (see Fig. 6-12).[117] These data illustrate that the aphakic retina is about 14 times more sensitive to the ravages of UVA radiation at 350 nm than is the cornea. At 325 nm, the primate cornea requires about 25 J/cm^2 for a threshold response, whereas the aphakic retina requires only 5 J/cm^2, indicating that in UVB radiation, the retina is more easily damaged by a factor of 50 than the cornea. What about the phakic eye? At 325 nm, the 5 J/cm^2 aphakic retinal threshold would become a 12 J/cm^2 phakic retinal threshold (5 J/cm^2/0.42 lens transmittance = 12 J/cm^2), and the phakic retina would be a factor of 2.5 more sensitive to UVR than the cornea. These data clearly illustrate that the retina is more sensitive to UVR than either the lens or the cornea.

Data on multiple exposures, cumulative exposures, and a complete action spectrum are needed to allow the proper retinal protective criteria to be established. Until data are obtained that indicate the contrary, any UV exposure to the retina should be considered dangerous, and steps should be taken to prevent retinal exposure.

Certain commonly used medications are known to be photosensitizers, phototoxic, or photoallergic, and a reasonable number of prescribed medications are cataractogenic. The research in this area has multiplied in recent years, but determining the exposure levels of UVR required to produce the photo-effect and the causal mechanisms involved require slow, laborious laboratory procedures. Nevertheless, the research is necessary in order to establish protective criteria.

Clinical Significance of UV Protection

Research on the effects of exposure of the eye to UVR clearly demands that practitioners possess the knowledge to advise and to provide ocular protection for their patients. The knowledge base must include the life span of the population, changes in human behavioral patterns, changes in the environment, exposure of the eye to sunlight, and the ocular protective devices available to the patient.[118] Each of these topics will be discussed briefly.

The human life span in the United States has increased from 54 years in the 1920s to over 75 years in the 1980s and the same increases are expected throughout the world. In addition, the over 65-year age group is projected to increase by 22.1% through the year 2000 while the total population will increase only 1.7%. These statistics mean that the population will be relatively older as we approach the turn of the century.

Human behavioral patterns have changed dramatically since the World War II era. Today, hats are rarely worn, while short-legged pants and short-sleeved shirts manufactured from lightweight materials have become commonplace in society. The mobility of society and the increase in leisure time have contributed to the increase in UV exposure. Leisure activities have become directed toward tennis, golf, swimming, sunbathing, water sports, winter sports in the snow, and other outdoor activities assuring that a high dose of solar UVR will be received. It appears that society seeks the highest UV-rich climates for their winter and summer playgrounds. The result is that the longer life span combined with more leisure activities ensures higher UV exposure.

Changes in the environment pose the most serious concern for ocular problems from exposure to UV. Ocular damage is caused mainly by UVB,[90,119] which is precisely the region of the solar spectrum affected by losses in atmospheric ozone. The environmental diseases in stratospheric ozone result in dramatic increases in UVA and UVB wavelengths below 340 nm, which emphasizes the requirement for ocular and skin protection. This UVB waveband has been associated with corneal damage,[42-45] pterygium, pinguecula, climatic droplet keratopathy,[119] acute cataractogenesis[46,47,90] and retinal lesions.[100,101,104]

Several attempts have been made to determine the amount of exposure of the eye from solar radiation.[120-127] An intraocular lens within the eye is exposed to an effective irradiance (E_{eff}) of global solar UVR of 0.03 to 0.5 μW/cm^2 at noonday when the sun is at the zenith.[120] The effective UVB in the tropics is 3 to 5 μW/cm^2 at midday, the highest known normal solar UV production. A mathematic model has been developed that predicts UV ocular exposure conditions associated with corneal and skin problems.[124] The model introduces the term

Maryland Sun Year (MSY) which is equal to 2750 SBUs (Sunburn units), while 1 SBU is equal to 20 mJ/cm^2 for a solar elevation of 30° and 36 mJ/cm^2 for a solar evaluation of 69° (the maximum solar elevations for summer and winter in the state of Maryland); therefore, the annual solar radiation varies from 55 to 99 J/cm^2.[123] The outdoor worker spends an average of 8.1 h per day in sunlight while on the job and 4.9 h per day during off-days.[125,127] These data demonstrate that there is sufficient UV in sunlight to cause ocular problems but exact data are difficult because of the many unknown variables.

Based on these arguments, Table 6-12 has been developed to guide the practitioner in providing advice and protection to patients. Protection lies in clinical intervention by prescribing UV-absorbing ophthalmic products and advising the patient to wear the proper clothing. Wearing a brimmed hat reduces ocular exposure to the UV in sunlight by at least 50% and, in certain situations, by a factor of 4. The reduction in UVR from wearing spectacles varies with the properties of the ophthalmic materials. UVA and UVB are reduced by 15.6% by clear glass lenses, to 0.2% with clear UV-absorbing plastic lenses, and to 0.6% with plastic sunglass lenses.[128–130]

Several characteristics of ophthalmic lenses and frames affect their value as protective devices. Ocular exposure increases as the area of the lens increases: a 13 cm^2 lens gives 60% to 65% protection while a 20 cm^2 lens provides a 96% or greater protection. Ocular exposure increases as the vertex distance from the eye increases because radiation can pass between the frame and the eye. The eyebrows, hair, and depth of the cornea from the brow all allow some protection. Thus, the rule of thumb for spectacles is to wear large lenses fitted close to the eyes for maximum protection. In addition to spectacles, soft contact lenses,[130] gas permeable contact lenses,[131] and intraocular lenses[132] afford excellent protection against UVR.

6.3 Ocular Hazards from Exposure to Visible Radiation

Interest in the effects of exposure of the eye to the sun and its retinal damage has spanned the centuries of time.[133] These interests can be divided into three eras of civilization that are not mutually exclu-

Aphakics, pseudophakics, and persons with retinal disorders to prevent retinal damage from exposure to the UV in sunlight and to UV-rich light sources.

People with cataracts to reduce lenticular scatter of the long UV, short blue light found in sunlight.

People with pterygia and pinguecula because these ocular conditions have been related to UVB exposure.

People who are prescribed photosensitizing medications: chlorothiazides, antibiotics, and oral contraceptives.

Workers in vocations that are rich in UV: welding, electronics, graphic arts, watermen, and researchers.

People who spend excessive hours in sunlight because UVB exposures above 8 hours result in a 3.8 times increase in the prevalence of anterior subcapsular cataracts.

People who participate in avocations and vocations that are rich in UV: snow skiing, sunbathing, and mountain climbing.

People who use sunlamps or frequent solariums because the outputs from these sources are rich in both UVA and UVB that are associated with skin cancer.

Children who play outside or exposed to excessive UV in sunlight to delay the photochemical responses in the cornea, lens, and retina.

Examples given are limited but a fuller discussion is given throughout the chapter.

TABLE 6-12
Recommendations for Different Populations Who Require Ocular Protection Against Damage from Exposure to UV

sive, because once discovered, the interest continued. The ancient era included exposure to solar eclipses that resulted in retinal damage and the term *eclipse blindness*. The second era revolved around the high energy of the nuclear age that saw retinal lesions result from exposures at extreme distances. The latest high energy source is the laser with a mega-energy, coherent optical beam capable of causing thermal damage, photochemical damage, mechanical damage, and nonlinear optical phenonenona simultaneously or independently, depending on the characteristics of the exposure. The era of the low level light damage to the retina began in the 1960s and continues as an interesting and fruitful area of research.

The research experimental variables in the production of retinal lesions by optical radiation include the pupil size, spectral transmittance of the ocular media, optical quality of the retinal image, exposure duration, size of the retinal image, size of the source, and the location of the exposure on the retina. Pupil size, ocular media transmittance, and optical quality of the retinal image have been presented earlier in the section on the factors affecting ocular exposure. The literature on ocular exposure is sufficiently enormous that books may be written on the subject. The literature cited in this section has been carefully selected, but those with greater interests are encouraged to read further.[133–135]

During World War II both the Australian[136] and American[137] antiaircraft observers, plane spotters, and gunners in the Pacific Theater of Operations suffered foveomacular retinitis and retinal burns. In an attempt to determine the cause, Eccles and Flynn[138] produced chorioretinal burns in the rabbit using the sun as a source and binoculars to direct the solar beam to the retina. The appearance of the rabbit lesions resembled that of the humans', and the cause was believed to be solar radiation.[139–141] It was thought that the rise in retinal temperature was responsible for the retinal lesion, and considerable research was expended in determining the increases in retinal temperature, from different exposure durations, wavelength distributions, and retinal image sizes.[142–147] The calculated increase in the temperature of the retina from observation of the sun demonstrates that temperature rise alone is not sufficient

to produce a retinal lesion.[148–150] Calculations demonstrated that as the wavelength of the VIS spectrum increased from 400 to 1200 nm, a greater increase in irradiance was required to maintain a constant retinal temperature.[147] Research efforts were directed toward other ocular parameters.

The pupil establishes the area of the entrance beam into the eye. Figure 6-19 provides data on the effect of the pupil on retinal irradiance,[151,152] illustrating that as the pupil diameter increases from 3 to 7 mm, the retinal irradiance required to produce a threshold response must be increased 5.5 times. The ratio of the retinal irradiance required for threshold to the corneal irradiance necessary for threshold defines the optical gain of the eye.[153] In these experiments, the optical gain of the rabbit eye for all pupil sizes was 3.7×10^3. The optical gain allows an estimate of retinal irradiance when the irradiance at the cornea is known. If the irradiance at the plane of the cornea was 20 mW/cm^2, the irradiance on the retina would be 20×10^3 W/cm$^2 \times 3.7 \times 10^3 = 74$ W/cm^2, ignoring the transmittance of the ocular media.

The effect of the size of the retinal image on the threshold retinal irradiance is shown in Figure 6-20. As the retinal image diameter approaches 1000 μm (1 mm) and larger, the irradiance necessary to produce a threshold lesion is essentially a constant value. For retinal areas smaller than 0.16 cm^2 (a diameter of 500 μm), the threshold radiant exposure rises

FIGURE 6-19
The effect of the pupil diameter on the irradiance of light falling on the retina. The data indicate that the retinal irradiance increases from 20 to 140 W/cm^2 as the pupillary diameter increases from 3 to 8 mm. *From Ham WT Jr, Mueller HA, Williams RC, Geeraets WJ: Ocular hazards from viewing the sun unprotected and through various windows and filters. Applied Optics 12:2122–2129, 1973; with permission.*

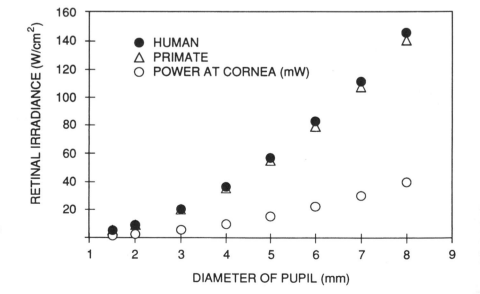

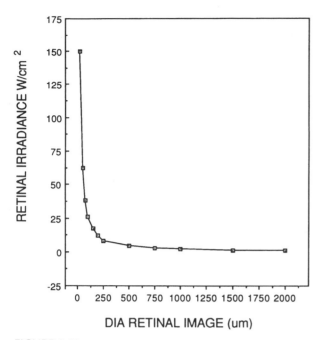

FIGURE 6-20

Maximum permissible exposure for circular retinal images using broadband, extended sources. The data are for rabbit retinal burn thresholds and provide a safety factor of 2.5 because the human thresholds for both the fovea and peripheral retina are higher than the rabbit. *From* **Sliney DH, Freasier BC. Evaluation of optical radiation hazards. Applied Optics 12:1–24, 1973; with permission.**

exponentially until at about 0.0005 cm^2 (100-μm diameter), the slope of the curve increases rapidly.

The effect of exposure duration on the threshold retinal irradiance is shown in Figure 6-21. As exposure duration reaches and exceeds 100 s, the retinal irradiance for a threshold response becomes essentially a constant value and, at that point, the lesion depends on the power of the optical beam.

Figure 6-22 presents the retinal irradiance for threshold using different laser-produced wavelengths and exposure durations of 1 s, 16 s, and 100 s and 1000 s.[154-157] The retinal thresholds show a geometric increase as the wavelength increases from 400 to 700 nm at exposure durations shorter than 100 s; however, the wavelength response becomes linear when the exposure duration exceeds 100 s. All curves for the longer wavelengths become almost parallel to the baseline above 650 to 700 nm, indicating that different mechanisms may be responsible

for the damage. To complete the wavelength picture, Figure 6-23 presents the retinal radiant exposure (J/cm^2) as the y-axis and the exposure duration [s] as the x-axis with the UV retinal thresholds.[158] The data appear to represent three sets of curves: a lower cluster from 325 to 350 nm, a middle cluster from 380 to 514.5 nm, and an upper cluster from 580 to 1064 nm. Note that the slopes of all curves are parallel until the 16-s exposure duration, where the upper cluster continues as a straight line to the 1000-s data point. Except for 441.6 nm, the middle wavelength curves break at the 16-s exposure duration and remain essentially parallel to the 1000-s exposure duration. The UV cluster of curves all remain parallel to each other and essentially parallel to the baseline of the graph.

Figures 6-22 and 6-23 may be used to deduct the mechanisms that caused the retinal damage. Three different types of damage have been proposed for the retina: thermomechanical, thermal, and photochemical.[20,159] Thermomechanical retinal damage is found only after very rapid, intense laser exposures and is not represented in these figures, but Figure 6-23 could be interpreted to illustrate the ratios of thermal/photochemical damage in the 325-nm and 1064-nm wavebands. The upper cluster of curves represents a purely thermal response at 1064 nm with perhaps a small photochemical element. The middle wavelengths are approximately equally thermal and photochemical responses, with the 441-nm curve indicating primarily a photochemical response with a moderate thermal element. The 350- to 325-nm curves illustrate an essential photochemical response with little or no thermal component.

The previous discussion has been based on retinal data derived from laser radiation exposures at specific wavelengths. Can laser data be representative of broadband exposures? Figure 6-24 presents the retinal irradiance (W/cm^2) versus the exposure duration [s] for a threshold retinal response using three wavebands of the VIS spectrum. The exposures clearly demonstrate that the IR portion of the optical spectrum plays a minor role in the production of retinal damage. The radiant exposure required to produce a thermal retinal lesion in the 700- to 1400-nm waveband was 69,100 J/cm^2 (69.1 W/cm^2 for 1000 s).[154] The slope of the 700- to 1400-nm line at long exposure durations is the same slope as the short exposure durations for the 300- to 1400-nm

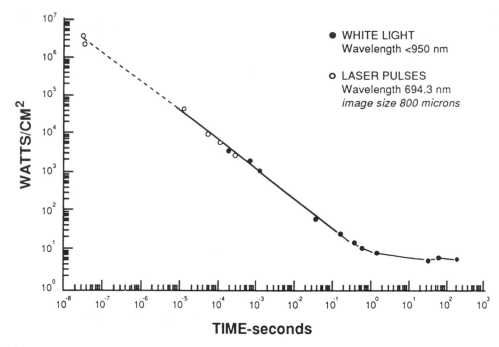

FIGURE 6-21

Retinal irradiance versus the exposure duration for threshold retinal lesions. As exposure duration reaches 100 s, threshold becomes a constant value. *From* **Ham WT et al: Retinal sensitivity to damage from short wavelength light. Reprinted by permission from Nature 260:153–155. © 1976 Macmillan Magazines Ltd.**

and 400- to 800-nm curves and is interpreted as being from a thermal mechanism. The change in slope of the 300- to 1400-nm and 400- to 800-nm curves at 10 s indicate a photochemical mechanism has come into play. The optical spectrum exhibits both photochemical and thermal mechanisms, depending on the exposure duration and the waveband of the exposure. Long exposure durations from short wavelengths favor a photochemical lesion, whereas long wavelength and short exposures result in thermal lesions. Thus, the laser and broad band exposures lead to the same conclusions for the cause of the ocular damage.

Experiments have been done using rats exposed to ambient light levels below that expected to cause thermal damage to the retina.[160] The mechanisms of damage were proposed to be a metabolic poisoning following the production of retinal toxic waste products or photo-oxidation. The radiation from the indirect ophthalmoscope was used to expose a retinal area of 3 mm² with a corneal power density of 4

W/cm² and an exposure duration of 15 min and produced an irreversible retinal lesion.[161] Subsequent low level retinal damage was induced in the monkey,[162] the rabbit,[163,164] and the pigmy pig.[165] The damage from the low light level exposures is proposed to be from photo-oxidation that produces singlet oxygen and free radicals, leading to the oxidation of fatty acids and the subsequent destruction of retinal membranes.[166] Thus, the low-level, long-term retinal damage has been categorized as photochemical damage and can be very damaging to the retina.

Several studies bear on the question of the threshold from exposure to broad spectrum white light. The data appear confusing because of the different methodologies used in arriving at the threshold. The threshold retinal exposure for primates varied from 8.4 to 15.6 J/cm² (mean of 12 J/cm²) for the cones and from 15.6 to 26.6 J/cm² for the rods (mean 21.2 J/cm²) when ocular transmittance was ignored.[167] The integrated transmittance of the monkey was

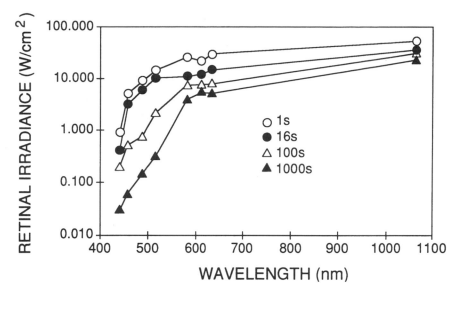

FIGURE 6-22
Threshold retinal irradiance for the indicated wavelengths of the VIS spectrum using 1-s (○), 16-s (●), 100-s (△), and 1000-s (▲) exposure durations. The Nd-YAG, HeNe, Ar-pumped dye, Ar, and HeCd lasers were used. The total diameter of the optical beam entered the 8-mm dilated pupil of the monkey eye. Integrated transmittances of 0.74 for 1064 nm, 0.93 for 632.8 nm, 0.92 for 610 nm, 0.91 for 580 nm, 0.83 for 488 nm, 0.69 for 457.8 nm, and 0.45 for 441.6 nm were used in the retinal irradiance calculations. (*From* Ham WT et al: Sensitivity of the retina to radiation damage as a function of wavelength. Photochem Photobiol 29:735–743, 1979; with permission.

established at 0.794 for the 400- to 800-nm VIS spectrum,[8,9] and correction of the mean data would result in a cone threshold of 9.6 J/cm^2 and a rod threshold of 16.83 J/cm^2. The retinal threshold for the primate using the VIS spectrum with a 500-s exposure duration was found to be 365 J/cm^2. More recently, reflection densitometry from the primate eye established a 230 J/cm^2 threshold radiant exposure for the VIS spectrum (350–800 nm).[168] The value 0.99 was used for the transmittance of the ocular media, but 0.794 has become the standard for the VIS spectrum.[8,9] When correcting for the transmittance differences, the threshold becomes 182.6 J/cm^2. The rabbit retinal threshold varied from 3.2 to 5.2 J/cm^2 when the eye was exposed to cool-white fluorescent light.[169] The mean of these data (4.2 J/cm^2) compare well with the 4.1 J/cm^2 values for the rabbit exposure in Table 6-13.

Table 6-13 presents the retinal burn thresholds for man, the monkey, and the rabbit, using identical exposure parameters.[170] The human retinal threshold varies from 7.9 to 13.8 J/cm^2 with a mean of 10.9 J/cm^2. The primate retinal threshold is 5.9 J/cm^2, and the rabbit is 4.1 J/cm^2. These data give a human: primate:rabbit ratio of 1:2:3; therefore, the interspe-

cies comparison of retinal threshold values is valid if the exposure parameters are constant.

The site of the retinal lesion from exposure to the VIS spectrum appears to be the outer segments and inner segments of the receptor layer of the retina,[169–173] and, as the exposure level increases, the pigment epithelium becomes involved. Within 24 h of exposure, the inner and outer segments of the photoreceptors have lost their irregularity, with the outer segment lamellae broken down into vesicles and tubules.[172] The pigment epithelium shows blanching and derangement of the cells. The lesion progresses until the central area is depigmented and the edges of the lesion take on irregular pigmentation.

Recovery of the retina from exposure to radiant energy appears possible because those who have experienced retinal damage from observing an eclipse follow a characteristic recovery pattern.[105,174–177] Ocular histories of eclipse-damaged retinas showed acuities of 20/40 or better and recovered to 20/20 within 3 mo; acuities of 20/60 to 20/80 required 4 mo but recovered only to 20/25 to 20/30.[105] The recovery process depends on the length and intensity of the exposure. The preservation of the pigment

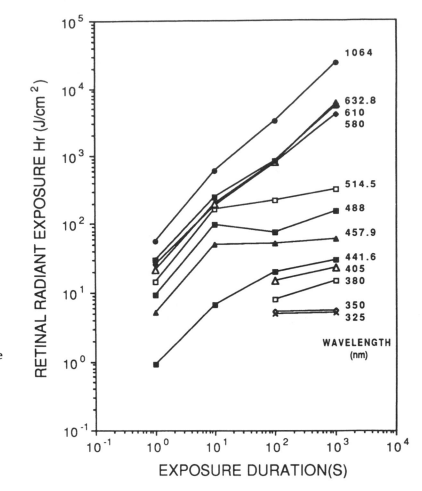

FIGURE 6-23
Threshold radiant exposure in J/cm² required to produce a minimal lesion for the various exposure durations. The top cluster of curves represent a predominate thermal response, the middle cluster of curves both thermal and photochemical, and the lower cluster illustrates the predominate photochemical response. *Modified from* **Ham WT et al: Sensitivity of the retina to radiation damage as a function of wavelength. Photochem Photobiol 29:735–743, 1979; with permission.**

epithelium and the photoreceptor cell body are necessary for recovery to take place.[165] If the outer segments of the receptors are disconnected from the inner segments, recovery does not occur, and a permanent loss of the visual receptors occurs. A slow recovery can be seen by both the electroretinogram (ERG) and histologically if the exposure is not sufficient to disconnect the inner and outer segments of the receptor.[165] Retinal exposures to primates at 441.65 nm show an immediate loss in visual acuity that recovers in 5 d if the exposure is 60 J/cm² or less, while exposure to 90 J/cm² produces permanent loss in acuity to 20/30 or less. These data assist in understanding the recovery of visual acuity by people who have experienced eclipse blindness or solar retinitis. Most eclipse blindness victims recover 20/20 acuity within 6 mo after exposure.[174]

Unfortunately, government standards on exposure of the retina to the VIS spectrum do not exist.[178] The research data indicate that the lowest retinal threshold for the VIS spectrum in the 400- to 800-nm wavelength has a value of 10.9 J/cm², which is equivalent to 7655 lux.[166]

6.4 Ocular Hazards from Exposure to Infrared Radiation

Although there has been interest over the past 80 years or more in investigating and preventing ocular damage from IR, efforts have failed to provide concrete mechanisms of action. Previous evaluators have said, "There is a need for accurate and reliable

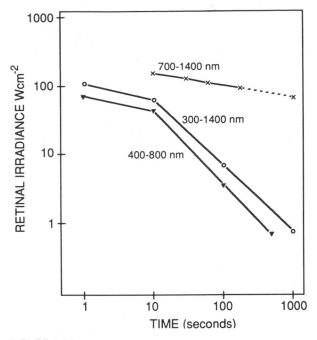

FIGURE 6-24
Retinal thresholds for broadband optical radiation. The curves for all wavebands are parallel until the 10-s exposure duration. The 300- to 1400-nm and 400- to 800-nm wavebands change slope but remain essentially parallel from 10 to 1000 s. The short exposure durations express the thermal nature of the exposure, whereas the longer exposures represent the photochemical component of the radiation. The 400- to 800-nm curve illustrates that the VIS spectrum is most efficient in producing retinal burns. *From* **Ham WT et al: Sensitivity of the retina to radiation change as a function of wavelength. Photochem Photobiol 29:735–749, 1979; with permission.**

Ocular Structure	Expected Damage
Iris	Miosis, hyperemia, swelling, necrosis
Lens	Anterior opacities, prominence of sutures
Vitreous humor	Haze or fire
Retina	Depigmentation, edema, burn

Detailed investigations of very low, prolonged exposures have not been initiated, but industrial epidemiologic studies attempt to describe ocular changes in the context of low dose, prolonged exposures in the workplace. Assessment can be made easily in certain areas, but other areas may not have sufficient data to provide valid conclusions.

A review of IR transmittance (see Fig. 6-4) data reveals three important facts about IR and the eye. First, the wavelength limit of IR reaching the retina is about 1400 nm. Second, because the energy of a

scientific research (occupational and experimental) in the areas of threshold, energy levels, and time of exposure."[179] That need still exists. This review of existing literature is an attempt to establish safe exposure levels.[180-187] A summary chart of expected ocular tissue damage resulting from acute IR exposure follows:

Ocular Structure	Expected Damage
Cornea	Opacification, debris, haze, exfoliation
Aqueous humor	Flare, cells, pigment

	Retinal Area Exposed*		
Species	Paramacula (J/cm²)	Fovea (J/cm²)	Comments
Man	9.0–12.2	13.8	Temporary afterimage
Man	9.5–9.9	9.7	Absolute central scotoma
Man	9.7	—	Foveal detachment
Man (white)	9.3 ± 1.56	—	18 patients
Man (black)	7.9 ± 1.86	—	10 patients
Monkey	5.9 ± 1.5	5.7 ± 0.35	22 rhesus eyes
Rabbit	4.1 ± 0.4	—	100 rabbits

*The optical source was an xenon 2500-W lamp filtered to produce a 400- to 800-nm spectrum. The retinal image diameter was 1 mm and the exposure duration was 135 ms.
From Ham WT, Jr, Muella HA: The photopathology and nature of blue light and near-UV retinal lesions produced by laser and other optical sources. *In* Wolbarsht ML (ed): Laser Applications in Medicine and Biology, pp 227–228. New York, Plenum Publishing Corp, 1989.

TABLE 6-13
Retinal Burn Thresholds for Human, Primate, and Rabbit Eyes

photon of IR is quite low when compared to the VIS and UV spectra and because the lens absorbs a relatively small amount of IR, an exposure necessary to cause lenticular damage would be quite high. Finally, the massive absorption of IR by the cornea and aqueous humor should result in a higher temperature in the anterior segment when compared to that in the posterior segment of the eye. The fall in temperature of the anterior ocular segment on removal of the IR source would be much more rapid than in the posterior segment. A 9 C increase in the aqueous humor from exposure to IR would be near the coagulation threshold of 47 C to 50 C.[52,80]

When the total ocular transmittance data are examined, one finds that a large proportion of incident IR in the 725- to 1400-nm waveband is transmitted through the eye and is incident on the retina (Table 6-14). Acute ocular damage in this waveband requires an extremely high radiant exposure, whereas the levels of energy for this review should more appropriately be concerned with long-term, chronic exposure effects, an area clouded by a lack of quantified data and requiring a cautious approach.

IR Exposure to the Cornea

Transmittance studies have shown minimal absorbance of 715- to 400-nm IR incident on the cornea for both the rabbit and humans (Table 6-15). Threshold values for corneal damage will be relatively high as a result of the low absorbance of IR by the cornea in the 715- to 1400-nm waveband and because of the low energy per quanta in these wave-

Mean % Transmittance	Model	Study
97.4	Human	Hartridge and Hill (1917)[183]
97	Rabbit	Kutscher (1946)[16]
96	Human	Boettner and Wolter (1962)[11]
98	Rabbit	Campbell (1968)[179]
80	Cat	Dawson (1963)[188]

TABLE 6-15
Transmittance of the Cornea for the 750- to 900-nm Waveband

lengths. Potential hazards to the cornea involve loss of corneal transparency, the result of denaturation from the heat. In the course of both coherent and noncoherent IR exposure, the cornea responds with a "burn" and secondary necrotic ulceration similar to that of an ordinary cutaneous burn.[188–192]

The posterior regions of the cornea may show more damage than the anterior regions. It has been suggested that the anterior corneal surface may be sufficiently cooled by the overlying tear film to minimize anterior IR effects.[52] Relatively recent studies monitored corneal epithelial and endothelial temperatures during IR laser exposures.[192,193] The CO_2 laser, with a wavelength of 10,600 nm, produced an initial direct corneal epithelial heating that spread secondarily to the endothelium. The erbium laser, with an output at 1540 nm (still outside the waveband of our concern but within the classification of IRA), was capable of significantly increasing the temperature in both the epithelial and endothelial tissues, but the difference was not statistically significant. It could be assumed that shorter wavelength IR, within the 750- to 900-nm waveband, would heat the endothelium to a greater degree than the epithelium because of the greater ability of this waveband to penetrate the cornea. Because the endothelium is a nonregenerative tissue, attention must be paid to these threshold values.

CO_2 laser radiation to rabbit corneas has been shown to increase the aqueous humor temperature as well, but more important was a concomitant increase in intraocular pressure.[193] Therefore, IR-induced changes in the cornea or anterior segment of the eye cannot be treated as an isolated condition

Total Ocular Transmittance		
Mean % Transmittance	Model	Reference
92.5	Rabbit	Weisinger et al (1956)[5]
91.5	Rabbit	Geeraets et al (1960)[8]
96	Human	Geeraets et al (1960)[8]
91	Human	Boettner and Wolter (1962)[11]
71.6	Human	Ludvig and McCarthy (1938)[10]

TABLE 6-14
Ocular Transmittance Data for IR from 725- to 1400-nm that Is Incident on the Retina

because the secondarily induced changes in intra-ocular pressure may have a detrimental effect on the viability of the retina. The exposure data for cataractogenesis are provided in Table 6-16 and in Figures 6-25 and 6-26.[181,182] The cornea does not serve as a protector to the lens for irradiances below about 3.8 W/cm^2 but protects against exposures above 4 W/cm^2 (Fig. 6-25). The process of damage by IR exposure is a single process and is known to be heat-dependent (Fig. 6-26). When the full spectrum of the source is used, the irradiances of the UV and VIS spectra are added to the IR spectrum to produce a lower threshold than when IR is used alone.[182]

IR Exposure to the Aqueous and the Vitreous

The aqueous and vitreous humors have not been reported to be affected or are minimally affected by IR because their transmittance curves are very much like water. Changes in the quality of the aqueous and

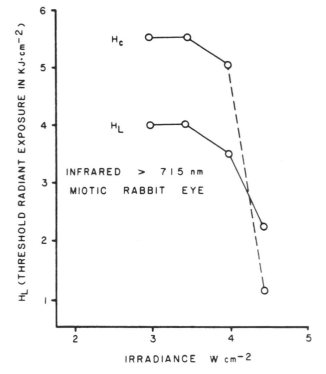

FIGURE 6-25
The threshold radiant exposure versus irradiance for the cornea and lens for the rabbit eye. These data show that the threshold varies with the rate of delivery of IR when the irradiance exceeds about 4 Wcm^2. Each of the curves could be represented by a horizontal line connecting the first points and a diagonal line connecting the last two points. The intersection of these lines is 3.8 and 4 kJ/cm^2 respectively. H_c represents the threshold for the cornea and H_L the threshold for the lens. *Data from* Pitts DG, Cullen AP, Dayhaw-Barker P[180]; Pitts DG, Cullen AP.[181]

vitreous have been attributed to by-products from the iris, lens, or retina.

IR Exposure to the Iris

The human iris absorbs from 53% to 98% of incident IR in the 750- to 900-nm waveband, but iris absorption depends on its pigmentation.[194] The data suggest that the iris is very sensitive to IR; however, melanin absorption decreases markedly above 700 nm and absorbs very little more IR than other ocular tissues at 1060 nm.[185,187] The threshold for physical injury to the iris is about the same as the cornea

Irradiance (W/cm^2)	Cornea (J/cm^2)	Iris (J/cm^2)	Lens (J/cm^2)
Rabbit IR Spectrum, Focused Beam, Miotic Pupil			
2.3–2.9	5500	4000	4000
3.4–3.6	4750	3760	4000
3.8–4.1	5000	3500	3500
4.4–4.7	1250	1250	2250
Rabbit Full Spectrum, Focused Beam, Miotic Pupil			
3.8	750	1000	2000
Primate IR Spectrum, Focused Beam, Miotic Pupil			
4.2–4.9	8000	8000	10,000

NOTE: Measurements were made at the plane of the cornea. The focused beam was 0.8 cm × 1.5 cm at the corneal plane and the dilated pupil allowed simultaneous exposure of both the lens and the iris. The xenon source was filtered by a Schott RG-715 filter that limited the IR spectrum reaching the lens and retina to a wavelength range of 715 to 1400 nm. Full spectrum was the complete optical radiation of the source. (Primate n = 10, rabbit n = 100).
Data from Pitts, Cullen, and Dayhaw Barker[180] and Pitts and Cullen.[181]

TABLE 6-16
Summary of IR Threshold Radiant Exposure (J/cm^2) Data for the Cornea, Iris, and Lens

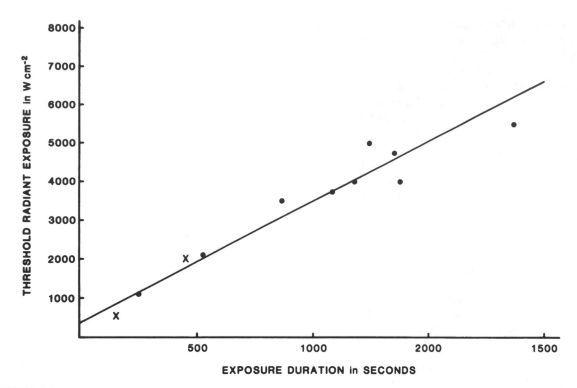

FIGURE 6-26
Radiant exposure required to produce a minimal lesion in the rabbit eye for different exposure durations. H_L in J·cm^{-2} is plotted on the ordinate and exposure duration in second(s) along the abscissa. The symbol (•) represents data for the IR spectrum focused beam and miotic pupil, whereas the (x) is the data for full spectrum focused beam and miotic pupil. The full spectrum data indicate that the process is additive, whereas the line indicates that the damage is from a single process of straight heat. *Data from* **Pitts DG, Cullen AP, Dayhaw-Barker P[180]; Pitts DG, Cullen, AP.[181]**

(Table 6-16), and when sufficient IR is absorbed by the iris, the result is a pupillary miosis, "aqueous flare," and posterior synechiae. An early study found 900 nm IR to be most effective at inducing an aqueous flare.[195] The inflammatory response of the iris to IR results from a secondary breakdown of the blood-aqueous barrier, which allows leakage of protein into the anterior chamber and produces an aqueous flare.[196–200] This IR-induced inflammatory process is inhibited by indomethacin, imidazole, and theophylline and suggests that the aqueous flare is mediated through prostaglandin channels.[197] Indeed, elevated prostaglandin levels are found in the aqueous humor of rabbits immediately after exposure to IR.[200] Quantitative data may be used to set allowable exposure durations;[195] however, some of the studies were concerned with the nature of the inflammatory process and did not quantify IR exposure values.[182,186]

IR Exposure to the Crystalline Lens

The first mention of the epidemiologic effects of IR radiation on the crystalline lens was in 1739, but since that date many authors have pointed out the relationship between certain types of cataracts and occupations requiring prolonged exposure to heat.[183] Meyenhofer[201] was the first to study glassworkers and to provide data on the number of workers who developed cataracts. He described the posterior cortical opacity that has become accepted as representing the early stages of the IR-induced cataract.

The mechanism of the formation of IR cataracts centers on three hypotheses. Vogt[202,203] interpreted his data to indicate that the cataracts obtained experimentally were the result of the direct absorption of the IR by the crystalline lens. Experimental evidence includes ocular transmittance absorption bands of IR in the 800- to 1200-nm bandwidth. Vogt's description of the source was a carbon arc (Bogen lamp) whose light was filtered through water and iodine sulfate ("deren Licht durch Wasser und Jod schwefelkohlenstoff filtriart wurde"). Water absorbs IR in bands much like the aqueous and the vitreous humors and reduces the IR available for absorption by the anterior segment of the eye. The water-iodine combination readily transmits UVR, whereas the carbon arc lamp is rich in UV. Thus, it is suspected that the direct absorption by Vogt's animals was UVR rather than IR and serves to negate Vogt's hypothesis.

Verhoeff and Bell[52] suggested that the outer surface of the cornea was air-cooled and that the anterior capsule of the lens was cooled by circulation of the aqueous humor. Thus, the cataract formed on the posterior surface of the lens because of its elevated temperature. They further postulate that the heat interferes with the function of the ciliary body, which subsequently interferes with the metabolism of the crystalline lens. Nearly all researchers, including Verhoeff and Bell, have reported anterior lenticular opacities and involvement of the cornea. Therefore, the lower temperatures from the air and aqueous are not sufficient to prevent anterior lens and corneal involvement. If the ciliary body were damaged, some evidence should be seen in the aqueous, but very little or no aqueous involvement has been observed. Thus, the model of Verhoeff and Bell is not supported by the experimental evidence.

Goldmann[204-211] stated that IR cataract was due to IR being absorbed by the iris with indirect transmittance of the heat to the lens. Goldmann felt that the effects of the direct absorption of IR were minimal, and the experimental evidence accumulated has been substantially in favor of his hypothesis.[212] Hager et al[213] and Ruth et al[214] suggest that both direct absorption by the lens and indirect heating of the lens through the absorption of the iris account for IR-induced cataracts. Later research supports the hypothesis of Goldmann because lenticular opacities could not be produced by directly exposing the lens but only when the iris was exposed.[180,181] The opacity was located beneath the area of the exposed iris and demonstrated that the contribution of direct absorption of IR by the lens was minimal.

The preponderance of the experimental evidence supports the theory of Goldmann despite speculations that may question this view. For example, the excessive number of "solar cataracts" found in India is most probably due to UVB in sunlight

and/or nutrition and not all workers in the metal industries develop cataracts. The studies attempting to negate Goldmann's theory used sources containing UV that was not filtered out. In addition, researchers attributing posterior lenticular cataracts to IR describe the initial response to IR exposure as anterior subcapsular opacities.

The IR experimental evidence indicates that acute IR-induced lenticular opacities are not the classically described posterior subcapsular opacity but are IR-induced opacities that lie in the anterior subcapsular region of the lens that first appear as discrete "whitish dots" or granules.[180,181,212,215] If sufficient exposure has been given, the granules or whitish dots form into a diffuse, network-like whitish opacity. Exposed eyes have been followed for up to 45 d, and migration of the anterior opacities, either equatorily or toward the posterior subcapsular region into the posterior cortex, was not observed. Instead, the anterior opacities faded and disappeared within 6 w after exposure.[181,216] None of the lenticular opacities induced by using the full spectrum or the IR spectrum exposure were posterior subcapsular opacities; however, the posterior opacity has a latency of 60 to 90 d.[212] For these reasons, it was concluded that acute IR-induced cataract is an anterior subcapsular opacity, whereas the posterior subcapsular opacity is a delayed process of the anterior damage migrating posteriorly during the normal aging process and is probably accelerated by subsequent exposure to IR or other environmental factors.

The anterior subcapsular opacity is common to almost all types of radiation-induced cataracts. Cogan et al[186] describe the characteristics of cataracts induced by X-ray, atomic bomb, and cyclotron exposure as an initial spottiness or attenuation of the anterior subcapsular epithelium. There is a piling up of the equatorial cells, with failure of these cells to "drop off" into the cortex. The advanced stages in humans is a doughnut-shaped, sharply demarcated anterior cataract configuration seen with the ophthalmoscope that progresses in a manner similar to what has been described.[211] The most interesting type of cataract may be caused by ionizing radiation, including X-rays, gamma rays, beta rays, and neutrons.[81] Histologically, the anterior subcapsular epithelium is involved primarily, along with secondary involvement of the cells of the equatorial area of the lens. In contrast, the UV-induced lenticular opacity consists of small, circumscribed white spots located in the anterior epithelium just posterior to the anterior capsule. At near threshold irradiance levels, the experimentally induced IR opacity appears similar to the UV-induced opacity and is located near the anterior lens epithelium.

The early epidemiologic literature appears to leave little doubt that the number of workers in the iron, steel, glass, and rail furnace industries who experienced IR- or heat-induced cataracts exceeded workers in other industries. This is particularly true of the epidemiologic literature of the late 1890s and early 1900s.[201,217,218] However, beginning in the 1950s epidemiologic studies[219,220] indicate that workers in the "heat industries" showed equal or fewer cataracts than control populations. What is the cause of this phenomenon? First, statistical procedures in handling epidemiologic data have improved. An example is the study on the prevalence of cataracts and sunlight.[83,84] Additionally, if sunlight were the causative agent, UVR would necessarily be implicated because the atmosphere transmits radiation to 288 nm, and the 295- to 320-nm wavelength range comprises the UV action spectrum for lenticular damage. Finally, the decrease in incidence of IR cataracts in industry may be due to an improved environment, including protective devices for the eyes and body, automation of the manufacturing processes, improved ventilation, and better dietary habits of the worker including replacement of electrolytes.

A correlation between IR-induced cataract development and an increase in lenticular temperature does not prove causation.[210] To date, studies have not been done using alternative methods of lenticular heat induction to confirm Goldmann's original theory. The crucial question is whether stellate posterior cortical opacities of the lens are characteristic of long-term IR exposure or if such opacities in individuals exposed to IR on a long-term basis are accelerated age-related processes. Logic suggests the latter to be the case, especially because generalized aging and age-related changes have been associated with oxidative processes,[221–222] which appear to have some connection with thermal changes. Heating of tissue above its normal temperature has been linked to an increase in the metabolism of the affected tissue.[179] A metabolic acceleration could lead to premature aging as a result of an abnormal accumulation of metabolic by-products. Indeed, some investigators have suggested an osmotic involvement in the development of senile cataracts,[222] in-

voking an accumulation of water-soluble substances as the means of loss of lenticular transparency. The question of how the temperature elevation may occur, whether by iris absorption or by direct lenticular absorption, is a secondary consideration.

Many industrial sources that are rich in IR also produce small amounts of UVR down to at least 350 nm.[182] Kurtin and Zuclich[48] have shown that cataracts can be produced with lasers in the 350- to 365-nm wavelength range that are due to a thermal mechanism. It may be that the solar and industrial sources of radiation produce radiation in this waveband that contributes to the heat cataract by an undetermined process.

A prospective epidemiologic study of iron workers, steel workers, and glassworkers was done to clarify the role that long-term, chronic exposure to IR plays in producing cataracts.[223–235] For the iron and steel industries, 208 age-matched subjects and controls were used. The spectral irradiances of the industrial source were measured and related to the history of exposure of each worker. The sample size for the glassworker study was 398 workers and 298 controls, weighted with respect to the age distribution of the glassworker. The age, lifetime dose, peak irradiance, spectral irradiance, and length of exposure for iron- and steelworkers are given in Table 6-17. The data for the Swedish glassworkers, including age, maximum and minimum peak irradiances, and radiant exposure levels are given in Table 6-18.

These data will be used in an attempt to establish valid criteria for long-term or chronic exposure analysis. The lowest irradiance was 3.4 mW/cm^2, and the highest irradiance was 130 mW/cm^2 for the glassworkers, but the low peak median irradiance was 350 mW/cm^2, and the high peak irradiance was 870 mW/cm^2 for the steelworkers. These irradiances provide a median lifetime radiant exposure in the 760- to 1400-nm waveband of 1.4×10^5 J/cm^2 and 8.6×10^5 J/cm^2, respectively.

The iron- and steelworkers showed a statistically significant increase in the prevalence of wedge-shaped cataracts for workers at and above the age of 60 and for workers exposed to the high radiant exposures (doses) of IR. The glassworkers showed a statistically significant increase in the prevalence of cataracts for workers age 60 and above. A glassworker 70 years of age who had experienced 20 years of IR exposure demonstrated an increase in risk factor of 12 for cataracts when compared to

Exposure History	Age Range			Dose		Irradiance			
	<50	50–59	60+	Large Dose	Large Dose 60+	High Irradiance	High Irradiance 60+	Long Exposure	Long Exposure 60+
Age (yr) mean	37.6	55.6	65.4	58.7	66.2	54.4	65.7	63.8	66.0
Exposure time (yr)									
Mean	14.4	25.2	35.2	32.6	37.3	27.7	35.9	40.0	40.8
Max	31	43	51	50	50	51	51	51	51
Min	5	5	14	5	16	5	15	31	31
Lifetime dose 300–400 nm ($J \times cm^{-2}$)									
Median	0.066	0.12	0.15	0.30	0.30	0.21	0.23	0.23	0.20
Q1	0.00	0.00	0.020	0.21	0.15	0.029	0.089	0.024	0.024
Q3	0.16	0.48	0.49	0.74	0.68	0.73	0.73	0.51	0.51
Lifetime dose 400–760 nm ($J \times cm^{-2} \times 10^3$)									
Median	1.4	2.1	5.3	7.8	7.8	5.1	5.0	5.6	6.0
Q1	0.063	0.11	0.44	6.0	6.1	1.2	0.27	0.68	0.49
Q3	3.3	6.7	8.9	15	15	9.7	11	9.8	12
Lifetime dose 760–1400 nm ($J \times cm^{-2} \times 10^5$)									
Median	1.4	1.9	5.2	7.9	8.6	5.0	5.0	5.4	6.2
Q1	0.026	0.027	0.58	6.6	7.1	1.1	0.35	0.88	0.63
Q3	3.1	5.5	8.6	11	16	8.2	9.0	9.9	13
Lifetime dose 1400–2600 nm ($J \times cm^{-2} \times 10^6$)									
Median	0.74	0.75	3.3	4.9	5.4	2.1	2.1	3.3	3.9
Q1	0.028	0.084	0.45	3.8	4.7	0.74	0.29	0.51	0.47
Q3	1.7	2.9	5.4	7.5	10	4.8	5.8	6.6	8.4
Lifetime dose 300–2600 nm ($J \times cm^{-2} \times 10^6$)									
Median	0.93	0.94	3.8	5.7	5.9	2.4	5.4	4.0	4.6
Q1	0.031	0.087	0.52	4.6	5.3	0.88	2.4	0.65	0.55
Q3	2.0	3.4	6.2	8.7	12	5.5	10.2	7.5	9.8
Peak irradiance ($mW \times cm^{-2}$)									
Median	350	470	530	530	540	870	710	530	540
Q1	140	240	350	430	430	550	550	260	390
Q3	450	830	630	550	550	1200	1200	550	630

From Lydahl RE: Infrared radiation and cataract. Acute Ophthalmol (Copenh) (Supp) 166; 1–63, 1984 with permission of Scriptor Publisher, ApS, Copenhagen, Denmark.

TABLE 6-17
Exposure Data for Iron- and Steelworkers

Exposure History*	Age Range			Dose*			
	50–59	60–69	70	Large Dose	Large Dose 70+	Long Exposure	Long Exposure 70+
Age (yr)							
Mean	54.8	64.1	75.6	71.3	75.8	74.6	76.3
Time of exposure (yr)							
Mean	34.0	42.7	49.4	48.0	50.8	53.4	53.8
Max	44	53	64	62	62	64	64
Min	20	20	22	28	40	51	51
Lifetime dose 300–400 nm ($J \times cm^{-2}$)							
Median	0.20	0.30	0.28	0.39	0.34	0.28	0.29
Q1	0.17	0.20	0.19	0.20	0.17	0.20	0.20
Q3	0.28	0.53	0.48	0.60	0.56	0.50	0.51
Lifetime dose 400–760 nm ($J \times cm^{-2} \times 10^3$)							
Median	6.4	8.7	9.8	12	11	9.8	9.8
Q1	4.8	7.1	7.4	9.8	9.8	7.4	7.4
Q3	7.4	12	12	15	14	11	12
Lifetime dose 760–1400 nm ($J \times cm^{-2} \times 10^5$)							
Median	6.0	8.1	9.5	12	12	9.5	9.5
Q1	4.8	6.7	7.0	11	11	7.0	7.0
Q3	7.1	10	11	13	13	11	11
Lifetime dose 1400–2600 nm ($J \times cm^{-2} \times 10^6$)							
Median	3.7	4.8	5.7	7.8	7.6	5.6	5.7
Q1	2.9	3.9	4.2	6.8	6.7	4.3	4.3
Q3	4.3	7.0	6.8	9.0	9.0	7.3	7.0
Lifetime dose 300–2600 nm ($J \times cm^{-2} \times 10^6$)							
Median	4.3	5.7	6.8	9.0	8.8	6.5	6.8
Q1	3.4	4.5	5.0	7.9	7.8	5.1	5.0
Q3	5.1	8.1	8.1	11	10	8.4	8.1

*The exposure history provides the age of the worker, duration of the exposure, and the lifetime dose for four wavebands.
From Lydahl RE: Infrared radiation and cataract. Acta Ophthalmol (Copenh) [Supp] 166; 1–63, 1984; with permission of Scriptor Publisher, ApS, Copenhagen, Denmark.

TABLE 6-18
Exposure Data for Groups of Glassworkers

non–IR-exposed controls of the same age. There was a statistically significant difference between the prevalence of cataracts in the right eye and left eye, with the left eye being more affected, but even the right eye was more affected in IR-exposed persons than in the controls.

The differences in the prevalence of cataracts in the glass industry versus that of the steel industry can be explained by the exposure experienced by each group. A glassworker usually begins as an apprentice and progresses through each work category to become a highly skilled worker. The iron- and steelworker study included many workers who experienced a low exposure and a smaller number who were exposed to high levels of IR. The daily dose in the glass industry was more evenly distributed among different jobs than in the iron and steel industry, with 99% of the glassworkers and only 42% of the iron- and steelworkers being exposed to a lifetime dose of 2×10^6 J/cm^2.[226]

IR Exposure to the Retina

Retinal studies have been concerned about an indirect thermal injury to the neural elements of the retina secondary to IR absorption by the RPE.[228-232] RPE thermal injury occurs as a result of laser IR exposure durations ranging from microseconds to several seconds. It has been argued that if the retinal irradiance is high enough to produce an appreciable elevation of temperature within the retina of 10 C, and if the retinal irradiance is kept constant, there is a reciprocity between temperature and duration of exposure (temperature × time = k),[230] but the same principles should hold for non-coherent sources of IR.[231]

The mechanism for retinal injury by sun-gazing was originally thought to be a thermal process.[233] At present, it is recognized that there are two separate processes, a photochemical process that is due to short wavelength radiation and a thermal process that is due to long wavelength radiation.[234-237] The key difference between the two mechanisms is that thermal damage is strongly dependent on retinal image size,[233,234] whereas photochemical damage should be independent of image size but strongly wavelength-dependent.[104,105] Other studies have examined the physics of thermal damage to the retina and quantified tissue temperature elevation as a result of IR exposure.[233] Ham et al[234] used the xenon photocoagulator to produce a retinal image diameter of 159 μm on the retina and interference filters to limit the source spectral irradiance to a waveband from 700 to 1200 nm. The corneal power and retinal irradiances required to produce retinal lesions in the primate eye are presented in Table 6-19.

Exposure Duration (s)	Power at Cornea (mW)	Retinal Irradiance (W/cm^2)	Retinal Exposure (J/cm^2)
10	43.3 ± 5.8	150 ± 20.9	1500
20	37.0 ± 7.0	133 ± 25.2	2660
60	32.0 ± 7.7	115 ± 27.8	6900
180	27.0 ± 4.2	97.4 ± 15.1	17,532

The diameter of the retina image was 159 μm. The spectral distribution of the source on the retina was 700 to 1200 nm. (n = 7 primate eyes.)

From Ham WT, Jr, Mueller HA, Williams RC, Geeraets WJ: Ocular hazards from viewing the sun unprotected and through various windows and filters. Applied Optics 12:2122–2129, 1973; with permission.

TABLE 6-19
Corneal Power and Retinal Irradiance Required to Produce Primate Retinal Burns for IR Exposure Durations from 10 to 180 s

Permissible IR Exposure Levels

The American Conference of Government Industrial Hygienists (ACGIH) in 1984 adopted threshold limit values for IR exposure that are more fully discussed in Section III, Ocular Protection Against Optical Radiation Hazards. However, it must be recognized that IR exposure limits are tentative because of the lack of sufficient quantified data. Notwithstanding, reasonable exposure limits can be established using present experimental data and conservative guidelines. IR exposure levels should use an envelope concept that sets the exposure limit to that portion of the eye most sensitive to IR. The cornea, iris, and lens are almost equally sensitive to IR, but the retina is more resistant (see Table 6-16); therefore, exposure limits for the cornea should protect the retina. The concept of the cornea protecting the retina fails when the irradiance level is below acute threshold, and cumulative effects enter the picture. In addition, when the IR irradiance is high and the exposure duration extremely short, severe damage may occur to the lens and cornea with minimal damage to the retina.

The corneal irradiance from sunlight is about 1×10^3 W/cm^2,[153] and a corneal irradiance of 0.1 W/cm^2 is below the level for acute ocular damage; thus, the

IR in sunlight is not sufficient to cause acute ocular damage. The level of irradiance of the Swedish glassworker is 2.9×10^6 W/cm² [225] and results in cataracts in 49.4 y. A safe chronic exposure of 10 mW/cm² for IRA, 0.1 W/cm² for continuous wave (CW) lasers, and 0.1 J/cm² for pulsed wave (PW) lasers has been suggested.[153] The ACGIH allowable acute ocular IRA exposure calculates to be 1.38 W/cm². It is reasonable to predict that an exposure of 20 mW/cm² will not produce acute or chronic ocular damage from IRA exposure.

6.5 Microwave/Radiofrequency, Ionizing, and Other Radiation

MW/RF Radiation

Microwaves (MWs) are the portion of the electromagnetic spectrum (EMS) with a wavelength range from 1 m to 1 mm, a frequency of 3×10^8 to 3×10^{11} Hz, and a photon energy range from 1.2 meV to 1.2 μeV (See Table 4-2). MWs are divided into three frequency bands: ultra-high frequency (UHF) with a frequency of 300 to 3000 MHz and a wavelength varying from 1 cm to 10 m; super-high frequency (SHF) with a frequency of 3000 to 30,000 MHz and a wavelength varying from 10 cm to 1 cm, and extremely high frequency (EHF) with a frequency of 30,000 to 300,000 MHz and a wavelength from 1 mm to 1 cm.[238]

The rotating antennas at airports, on ocean liners, and the large stationary cup-shaped antennas used for receiving satellite signals are familiar, but our knowledge about MWs is limited. MW radiation may be emitted by CW or by PW. An example of a CW exposure would be the MW oven common to the home. An example of the pulsed MW would be the radar system used as a tracking system by aircraft controllers. An MW pulse is transmitted for a period of time in a predetermined direction, then strikes an object that reflects the beam back to the antenna. The reflected beam is detected and analyzed during the silent period of the pulse. Microwave beams may be spread out over wide areas or concentrated into narrow beams depending on the antenna configuration under use.

The most common military and civilian uses of MW radiation are shown in Table 6-20.[238] Table

Application	Frequency in MHz
Military Uses	
Communications	30–300
Early Warning	300–3000
Ground Control Interception	3000/10,000
Height Finding	3000
Missile Control & Detection	100–10,000
Navigational	3000/10,000
Surveillance	1000–5000
Tracking & Search	300–70,000
Civilian	
Communications, Radio, TV	30–1000
Diathermy and Medical	30–300
Ground Control Approach	3000/10,000/35,000
Industrial Heating/Processing	30/1000–10,000
Navigational Search	3000/10,000
Ovens	30/1000–24,000 3000/10,000
Satellite Relay Stations	3000–24,000

The dash (–) is used to indicate the range of frequencies for a particular use. The slash (/) is used to indicate distinct frequency bands.
Data from Assenheim HM, Hill DA, Preston E, Cairne AB.[238]

TABLE 6-20
Uses of MW Energy Categorized for Military and Civilian Applications

6-21 lists eight categories in manufacturing and about 100 different tasks or processes in which MWs are used in the manufacture of consumer products.[239] The manufacture of plastic products and wood products constitute the majority of the tasks. In most manufacturing processes there is little concern of ocular hazard unless the individual works in a radar systems factory on the development, repair, and calibration of radar systems.[240]

Communications constitutes the greatest use of MWs. The AM radio frequencies (RF) lie between 535 and 1650 kHz but possess effective radiated power (ERP) up to 50 kW in the United States. FM lies between 88 and 108 MHz with an ERP up to 200 kW. Television transmits in the very high frequency (VHF) band and the UHF band. The VHF band for channels 2 to 6 has an ERP up to 100 kW in the 54- to 84-MHz frequency, whereas channels 7 to 13 occupy the 174- to 216-MHz frequency with an ERP of

Automotive Workers
   Drying of trim base panels
   Embossing of heel pads to carpets
   Heat sealing body interior trim panels
   Heat sealing convertible tops and vinyl roofs
   Heat sealing upholstery covers for seats and backs

Furniture and Wood Workers
   Decking assembly
   Door lamination
   Fabrication of posts and rafters
   Fiberboard fabrication
   Laminated beams
   Lumber edge gluing
   Plywood panel patching
   Plywood or particleboard scarf gluing
   Ski lamination
   Veneer panel gluing

Glass Fiber Workers
   Drying and curing sizing on machine packages
   Drying coatings on continuous moving strands
   Drying glass fibers on forming tubes
   Drying roving packages

Paper Product Workers
   Correcting moisture profile on continuously moving webs
   Drying resin coatings
   Drying twisted twine packages
   Gluing paper
   Heating coating on continuous webs

Rubber Products Workers
   Drying latex foams
   Gelling latex foams
   Preheating prior to curing latex foams
   Preheating prior to molding

Textile Workers
   Drying continuous webs
   Drying impregnated or coated yarns
   Drying rayon cake packages
   Drying slasher coatings
   Drying wound packages

Plastic Heat-Sealing Workers for Manufacture/ Fabrication of

Acetate box covers	Machine covers
Advertising novelties	Mattress covers
Appliance covers	Mild cartons
Aprons	Oxygen tents
Baby pants	Packages
Beach balls	Pharmaceuticals
Belts and suspenders	Pillowcases
Blister packages	Pillow packages
Book covers	Plastic gloves
Capes	Pool liners
Charge cards	Protective clothing
Checkbook covers	Racket bags
Convertible tops	Rain apparel
Cushions	Refrigerator bags
Diaper bags	Shoe bags
Display boxes	Shoes
Electric blankets	Shower curtains
Food packages	Slipcovers
Fountain pens	Splatter mats
Garment bags	Sponge backings
Gas masks	Sport equipment
Goggles (industrial)	Tobacco pouches
Handbags	Toys
Hat covers	Travel cases
Index cards	Umbrellas
Lampshades	Wallets
Liquid containers	Waterproof containers
Luggage	Wire terminal covers

RF/Microwave Application Workers
   Advertising. RF-excited gas display signs
   Ceramics. Drying of ceramic objects
   Chemical. Activation of chemical reactions
   Electronics. Tube aging and testing
   Laser. RF-excited gas lasers
   Medical. Diathermy and (experimental) cancer therapy
   Scientific equipment. Low temperature ashing of samples
   Welding. RF-stabilized welding

Data from Radiofrequency (RF) Sealers and Heaters: Potential Health Hazards and Their Prevention.[239]

TABLE 6-21
Manufacturing Categories and Specific Tasks that Use RF Heating and Sealing in the Manufacturing Process

about 316 kW. The UHF television stations from channel 14 to 83 use the 470- to 890-MHz waveband with an ERP of 5 megawatts. Amateur radio and citizen's band radio transmitters use the 3- to 30-MHz frequency and are limited to 1-kW and 5-W input into the antenna, respectively.

MW ovens usually operate at 2450 MHz with power output from 400 to 2300 W. Some MW ovens use an additional frequency at 9800 MHz for browning the surface of meat. The MW oven used in the home operates in the power range of 400 to 700 W.

Certain wavebands of MW have been reserved for Industrial, Scientific and Medical (ISM) use, including 13.56 MHz, 27.12 MHz, 40.68 MHz, 915 MHz, 2450 MHz, 5.80 GHz, and 22.125 GHz. The medical uses include diathermy (27.12 MHz), whole body hyperthermia (122 MHz) for elevation of the body temperature after open heart surgery, and in dermatology where 9800-MHz penetration is limited to about the same thickness as the skin.

The generation of MWs had its origin in the early 1940s, and fears concerning possible harmful effects from exposure to MWs were expressed during World War II. There was little research on the effects of MW exposure after the war until 1948, when MW exposure was reported to result in cataracts in the dog.[241,242] It was not until the middle of the 1950s that the need for MW standards was recognized. In the meantime, reports on a number of conferences and surveys, and reviews on MW exposure and the possible hazards from MWs have been published.[243-253] Generally, the surveys reported that the prevalence of cataracts between the exposed and nonexposed was not statistically different, which inferred that MWs did not cause cataracts or other ocular damage in humans. The results of these conferences and the reviews should be studied by the serious student of MW hazards.

Dosimetry

Dosimetry has been a critical issue in the experiments on the biologic effects of MW radiation. Power output varied with the type of generator, conditions of exposure, and methods of measurement. Investigators used their own systems for measuring exposures, including core temperature increases, temperature increases in the organ of exposure, and models to estimate power. Exposures have been made in the near field, with the results based on average power density (W/m^2) measurements made with far field instruments.[238,250] Exposure procedures varied from the use of waveguides to free field. One of the more serious concerns is that the specific absorbed rates (SARs) of animals and organs vary with the size of the body and organ. For example, comparisons between ocular exposures for the rabbit eye and rat eye would be impossible due to their vast difference in size, which in turn affects the SAR. Thus, it is difficult to extrapolate data from one species to another. The variables in dosimetry have resulted in confusion in interpreting the data and in comparing research from different laboratories,[251] but the difficulties are being resolved with the use of new density power meters.

The exposure units of the MW incident on biologic systems are usually expressed as the power density of the beam in W/m^2 or $\mu W/cm^2$ (1 $mW/cm^2 = 10 \ W/m^2$) with the exposure duration in minutes. Thus, the radiant exposure is in J/cm^2 and because most MW exposure durations are measured in minutes, care must be taken to convert to seconds in calculating the radiant exposure. MW radiation is also measured in units that represent the electric field strength ($\overline{E}$) and the magnetic field strength ($\overline{H}$) of the radiation. The electric field strength $\overline{E}$ is measured in volts per meter or V/m and the magnetic field strength $\overline{H}$ is measured as ampere per meter or A/m.

When a biologic system is exposed, it is inferred that the radiation has been absorbed. MW research uses two terms to define the energy absorbed: the Joule (J) defines the total energy absorbed and the SAR, the specific absorption rate, defines the energy absorption rate.[238]

Ocular Damage from MW Radiation

CORNEAL DAMAGE

Studies on the damage to the cornea from MW exposure are difficult to understand because there is an interaction between frequency and the temperature of the eyeball. For example, corneal damage does not ordinarily result from exposure to 3.10 to 2.45 GHz frequencies because MWs at these frequencies do not penetrate the depths of the cornea. However, if the ocular temperature is raised to 44 C, anterior segment damage to the iris, and ciliary epithelium and cortical cataracts are produced. It is generally accepted that frequencies at or above 10 GHz are required to produce ocular damage.[254]

Exposing the cornea to 2450 MHz CW and 2860 MHz PW with an average power density of 225 $\mu W/cm^2$ did not damage the cornea nor affect the healing process of the wounded cornea.[255,256] A granular corneal opacity was seen 24 h after exposure using 10 GHz at 225 $\mu W/cm^2$, but the lesion disappeared within 4 d.[257] Permanent corneal, iritic, and eyelid damage was produced from exposure to 10 GHz at 350 $\mu W/cm^2$, but only transient damage occurred using 35 GHz, 70 GHz, and 170 GHz.[258,259] Corneal exposures indicate that the threshold for damage lies between 225 and 350 $\mu W/cm^2$.

MW CATARACTOGENESIS

The formation of cataracts from exposure to MW radiation has received the greatest research effort. Not all experimenters agree on the description of the MW-induced cataract, but a compilation of a number of papers leads to the following description. The anterior epithelium of the lens shows changes described as granular opacifications. The initial changes at the posterior cortex may be seen faintly at this time, but the classic posterior subcapsular cortical opacity does not appear until 24 to 48 h after exposure. Posterior lens changes vary considerably according to the power and frequency of the radiation, from small granules along the posterior suture line to globules, patches, or the dispersion of granules across the entire posterior capsule.[252,260,261]

A 100% frequency of cataract formation in the rabbit eye has been found with 2.45-GHz MWs at 180 mW/cm^2.[262–266] However, the data demonstrate that the MW exposure that produces cataracts is a power density and exposure duration phenomenon. Figure 6-27 presents the power density necessary to produce threshold cataract response in the rabbit eye for different exposure durations.[262] As the power density decreases, there is an increase in the exposure duration necessary to produce a cataract. Extrapolation of the curve indicates that 110 mW/cm^2 would require at least a 60-min exposure to achieve cataract threshold. Thus, a threshold value must include the frequency, power density, and exposure duration to be valid. Chronic exposures of the rabbit eye from 0.5 to 5 mW/cm^2 of 2450-MHz continuous MW radiation results in no difference between the controls and exposed eyes.[267,268] The lenticular damage for the rabbit eye has been modeled by McRee.[269]

Cataract formation induced by MW exposure differs with species. Primates exposed to 500 mW of 2450 MHz up to 60 min and observed for 1 yr failed to develop cataracts.[270] Investigators using operant conditioning techniques exposed primate eyes to 9.31 GHz with an average power density of 150 mW/cm^2 and an exposure duration that varied from 15 to 22 min, no cataracts were induced. Thus, it would appear that the primate eye is immune to MW cataracts at the level and rate of exposure that has caused cataracts in the rabbit eye.[271–274]

The dog was the first animal used to establish that MWs were capable of causing cataracts.[241] Since the initial study, mixed results have been reported with

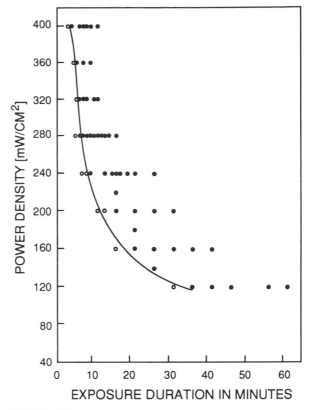

FIGURE 6-27

Exposure durations and power densities necessary to produce cataracts in the rabbit eye from a single exposure of 2450-MHz MW radiation. The open circles indicate no ocular damage, and the solid circles the exposures that produced cataracts. Extrapolation of the curve indicates that 110 mW/cm^2 would require a 60-min exposure duration to produce a cataract. *From Carpenter RL, Biddle DK, Van Ummersen CA: Opacities in the lens of the eye experimentally induced by exposure to microwave radiation. IRE Transactions on Medical Electronics ME7:152–157, 1960. © 1960 IRE (now IEEE).*

experimental exposure of dogs. Acute or chronic whole-body exposure of the dog does not produce lenticular changes at MW frequencies of 200 MHz, 400 MHz, 2800 MHz, and 24,000 MHz;[225–228] when the eyes of dogs were exposed to 2450 MHz at 300 mW/cm^2 for 30 min no cataracts were found, but when the power density was increased above 460 W/cm^2 for 30 min, an ophthalmoscopically visible anterior cortical cataract developed.[241] Table 6-22 compares the exposure parameters and effects for

Species	Power Density (mW/cm²)	Exposure Duration (min)	Frequency (MHz)	Effect*
Rabbit	180	240	2450	Cataract
	180	140	2450	Cataract
	120–180	60 min × 20 d	2450	Cataract
	150	100	2450	Cataract
	~40	60	35,000	Keratitis
	~40	60	10,700	No cataract
	100	15	3000	No ocular effects
	200	30		
	300	15	3000	
	400	15	3000	No lens changes
	500	15	3000	Miosis, hyperemia of lids and conjunctiva, iris vessel enlargement, anterior chamber flare
Monkey	300	22	2450	No cataract
	400	30,60	2450	No cataract
	500	60	2450	No cataract
Dog	350–470	20 min × 7 d	2450	No cataract or damage
	300	30	2450	
	460	30 min × 8 d	2450	Anterior cortical cataract
	165	180 / 360 min × 21 d	2800	No damage

*Note that exposure intensity, duration, and frequency interact to produce a given effect. A frequency of 2450 MHz, an intensity of 150 mW/cm², for an exposure duration of 100 min is the threshold for cataracts.

TABLE 6-22
Summary of Ocular Exposure to MW Radiation

the rabbit, dog, and primate and illustrates that cataract production in the monkey and the dog is difficult to achieve, but the rabbit cataract threshold is about 150 mW/cm² for a 100-min exposure.

There is a suggestion that MW exposure is cumulative for the rabbit eye.[255,257,263,275] Cumulative damage must be demonstrated through repeated subthreshold exposures until threshold cataract damage is achieved. A careful evaluation of the cumulative data illustrate that a power density value greater than 100 mW/cm² with durations of greater than 1 hr are found. These values are close to normal threshold values (Fig. 6-27) and do not represent a true subthreshold exposure; thus, the cumulative effects of repeated exposures are still open to question.

In vitro studies of the rat lens indicate that pulsed MW exposures were more damaging than continuous wave MW exposures when the total exposure was kept constant.[276-278] The depth of damage 918 MHz increased with increasing exposure duration and dose rate for pulsed MWs; i.e., the total dose is an important damage parameter. The lens damage included a fragmented stretching of the lens capsule, holes, foam, and globules. Modern directional antennas deliver power densities in excess of their experimental exposures and could be a hazard.[230] The size of the rat lens and human lens differ considerably, and the rat data must be extrapolated to the human for such conclusions to be applicable.

Biochemical studies on the effects of MW exposure to the eye have only recently been initiated.

These studies have looked at the uptake of ^{3}H thymidine changes in ascorbic acid in the lens epithelium and used pore gradient electrophoretic techniques to study the lens proteins. A marked suppression in the uptake of ^{3}H thymidine was found as early as 6 h after exposure, but uptake returned to normal within 48 h. Ascorbic acid decreased within 18 h after acute exposure in both the rabbit and monkey eye.[279] Electrophoresis demonstrated a shift to the higher molecular proteins in the lens cortex after irradiation to 300 W/cm^2 for 20 min on 2 consecutive days.[280] These studies indicate that there is an early induced change in lens physiology, followed by a reduction in ascorbic acid and shifts toward higher molecular weight proteins, which supports the argument that MW exposure is capable of inducing lenticular cataracts.

RETINAL DAMAGE

The retina has received very little attention in spite of the enormous amount of research related to cataractogenesis. The rabbit retina was exposed to 3100 MHz pulsed MWs at 0.055 W/cm^2 for 60 min, providing a radiant exposure of 198 J/cm^2. Fundus photographs revealed no retinal changes, but ultrastructural examination showed extensive changes in the retinal synaptic terminals, neuronal cell bodies, and neuronal processes. Thus, there is little doubt that MW radiation at 3100 MHz is able to penetrate and damage the retina.

Human Exposure to MW Radiation

Information on human exposure to MW radiation is derived from the occasional case report that appears in the literature, surveys conducted on a selected population of occupationally "exposed" workers, and from retrospective epidemiologic studies. Russia and the Eastern European nations have been the most active in reporting human problems from MW exposure.

The first indication that MWs were capable of inducing human cataracts was in 1952. The MW-induced cataract has been described as a bilateral, posterior subcapsular cataract (PSC);[282,283] however, haziness of the posterior suture line[284] and anterior subcapsular cataracts[285] have also been reported. A few case histories serve to demonstrate the difficulty in establishing a cause-effect relationship:

A 38-year-old electronics technician suffered bilateral PSCs after being exposed to 200- to 300-MHz MW radiation with powers ranging from 40 to 380 μW/cm^2.[282] In addition, he had nuclear cataracts and a recurrent chorioretinitis. The question arises whether the cataracts were secondary to chronic infection or the result of MW exposure. A technician, aged 51, had worked in electronics for 7 yr, and 8 yr after quitting his job, he developed PSCs. Was MW radiation or advancing age the cause? Finally, a 22-year-old microwave technician was exposed to 2500- to 3000-MHz MW radiation for 2 mo at unknown powers and durations. The technician developed bilateral anterior cataracts and PSCs.[285]

A number of surveys on radar workers have been conducted that emphasized lenticular and retinal examinations, but none have found damage from MW exposure.[286-295] Workers in a factory where radar and other MW equipment was tested and calibrated were surveyed, but it was impossible to separate MW and non-MW cataracts because of the lack of controls.[296] However, retinal lesions resembling the chorioretinal scars that remain after a chorioretinal inflammation were found in the posterior central portion of the fundus and were reported to be due to MW exposure. The problem of human exposure to MW radiation was reviewed, and it was concluded that inadequate scientific methodology and confounding multiple factors have made human reports unreliable.[297,298] The available literature does not support cataract formation or retinal damage in the human from low-level, long-term MW exposure.[261]

MW Standards

The subject of MW standards is interesting because the standards process usually recognizes the problem, research is accomplished to establish the experimental hazard parameters, and safety or tolerance levels based on the research are established. Table 6-22 illustrates the dilemma relative to MW radiation, however, because there is an interaction between frequency, exposure duration and power density that has not been fully determined safety or tolerances are difficult to defend.

The United States MW radiation standard is based on the ability of the human body to dissipate heat under normal physiologic conditions and on certain assumptions about the way MWs interact with living tissue. The human body is estimated to dissipate 100 W of heat, or a body of 20,000 cm^2 loses 0.005 W/cm^2 of heat.[298,299] A UHF radar system with a power density of 0.1 W/cm^2 provides 20 times more energy to the body than the body dissipates. Thus, an exposure of 0.01 W/cm^2 or 10 mW/cm^2 provides a safety factor of 10. The 10 mW/cm^2 figure has stood since the original conference in 1953. The present U.S. exposure limits for MW radiation in the frequency range from 300 kHz to 100 GHz from ANSI C95.1-1982[300] and adopted by OSHA[239] are as follows:

1. CW exposure. Total exposure is 10 mW/cm^2 for an 8-h workday or the equivalent free-space electric field strength of 200 V/m root mean square (RMS) and 0.5 A/m RMS, respectively.
2. PW exposure. The power density and RMS of the field intensities are averaged over 0.1-hr period (6 min) of time. In any 6-min period, the exposure levels should not exceed a power density of 10 mW/cm^2 or 1 mW/cm^2 energy density and an electric field strength of 40,000 V^2/m^2.

The present U.S. standard of 10 mW/cm^2 CW is approximately one tenth the threshold level for the cataract from a single acute exposure of 100 to 150 mW/cm^2 of 2450 MHz for 100 min. U.S. standard levels are used by Canada and Britain but have not been accepted by all countries. Russia limits MW exposure to 0.1 μW/cm^2 for a full day but allows up to 0.1 μW/cm^2 for a 2-h period and 1 μW/cm^2 for up to 20 min. Sweden, Germany, and the U.S. electronics industries use 1 mW/cm^2 as the safe exposure limit for all MW frequencies. Russia and Eastern European countries base their standards on a different philosophy from Western countries, who base standards on the presence of an effect from a biologic exposure (MPE), whereas the Eastern European figure is the level toward which the industry should strive rather than a level that must not be exceeded.[244]

6.6 Ionizing Radiation

Interest in the effects of exposure of biologic tissue to ionizing radiation heightened tremendously after the two atomic bombs were dropped on Hiroshima and Nagasaki to end World War II. It was realized that the scientific community knew very little about the biologic effects of exposure to ionizing radiation. The Cold War era elevated the interest further because nuclear weapons became the major deterrent to hostilities. The literature is vast in both the number and the content of the publications, so this section on ionizing radiation will concentrate on ocular damage, after a short introduction on the definition of ionizing radiation units. Damage threshold values for the anatomic portions of the eye from exposure to the different types of ionizing radiation will be provided. The weight, mass, and charge of particulate and electromagnetic radiation[301] are shown in Table 6-23.

Ionization occurs when the electrical balance of atoms is disrupted by the transfer of energy from the ionizing particle to the orbital electrons of the atom. The quantity of energy transferred depends on the velocity, mass, and charge of the particle. In the energy-transfer process of the neutral atom, the free electron becomes negatively charged and the atom becomes positively charged. The negative ion (free electron) and positive ion (positively charged atom) produced in the ionizing process are termed an *ion pair*. The initial or primary negative ion will impart energies to other orbital electrons and produce secondary electrons with lower energies but capable of producing further ionization. Some of the energy transferred from the ionizing particle will not cause ionization but is sufficient for the orbital electron to exist in an excited state. The orbital electron may accumulate absorbed energy and become ionized. The energy is normally dissipated by the direct transfer of the excitation to other nearby atoms by a process called nonradiative de-excitation or by the production of electromagnetic radiation.

The gamma radiation and X-radiation of the EMS may produce ionization through secondary means. The atom absorbs the electromagnetic radiation and emits a charged particle that is ordinarily an electron having sufficient velocity to produce ion pairs. Electromagnetic radiation transfers or dissipates its energy by the photoelectric effect, the Compton effect, or by pair production. The photoelectric effect occurs when low energy electromagnetic radiation is absorbed by matter with high atomic weight (large number of orbital electrons) and becomes excited or ejects an electron that produces ionization by impact. In the Compton effect,

Radiation	Weight (g)	Atomic Mass Unit	Charge*
Particulate			
Alpha	6.642×10^{-24}	4.000279	2 pos
Deutron	3.343×10^{-24}	2.01417	1 pos
Neutron	1.6744×10^{-24}	1.00894	No
Proton	1.6722×10^{-24}	1.00758	1 pos
Meson	18.0×10^{-26}	0.11	Pos or neg
Electron (beta)	9.19×10^{-28}	0.0005486	1 neg
Positron	9.19×10^{-28}	0.0005486	1 pos
Neutrino	A few hundredths of the mass of the electron	Less than a few thousand eV	No
Electromagnetic			
Gamma and x-radiation (photon)	1.762×10^{-27}	0.00107 1.0 MeV	No

*One charge equals 4.8201×10^{-10} electrostatic units. Pos = positive, neg = negative.
Data from Nuclear Radiation Guide. Report No. MRL-TDR-62-61. Aerospace Medical Division, Aerospace Medical Research Laboratories, Wright-Patterson Air Force Base, Ohio, 1962.

TABLE 6-23
Weight, Mass, and Charge of the Particulate and Electromagnetic Ionizing Radiation

the incident photon of moderate energy produces a free electron in almost any element and continues to produce secondary ions of decreased energy. The secondary ions recoil and deflect through the atoms of the material until the photon undergoes photoelectric absorption. Pair production results when electromagnetic radiation of high energy interacts with matter of high atomic weight. The energy penetrates almost to the nucleus so that the nucleus recoils; this results in the formation of a positron-electron pair with high acceleration. The ionization results from the particles of the positron-electron pair.

The absorption of radiation by soft biologic tissue results in the cellular H_2O being transformed into hydrogen dioxide (HO_2), hydrogen peroxide (H_2O_2), and the OH^- radical. Each of these constituents is capable of further destructive interaction with biologic systems. The cellular enzymes are rendered ineffective, and cell division is slowed. Cells may grow to abnormal size and die or by mutation divide into two daughter cells that are genetically different from the parent cell. Some general rules relating cellular response to the absorption of ionizing radiation have been formulated. The higher the metabolic rate of a cell, the lower its resistance to radiation. Young cells or newly divided cells are more sensitive to radiation than are older cells. Normal healthy cells are more resistant to ionizing radiation than undernourished cells.

Units of Measurement

Ionizing radiation cannot be measured directly but is measured by the ionization produced as the radiation passes through a medium. The measurement may be expressed as energy, a charge, or by the biologic effect that an exposure produces.[301]

The roentgen is the basic unit and is the quantity of X-ray or gamma radiation necessary to produce ions carrying 1 electrostatic unit of electricity of any kind. Table 6-24 defines the roentgen and provides units equivalent to the roentgen.

In recent years, the radiobiologic units used to define the roentgen in terms of its biologic effect have changed from the curie RAD, and REM to the Becquerel (Bq), the Gray (Gy), and Sievert (Sv) (Table 6-25). The radiobiologic effectiveness (RBE) is an integer that expresses the effectiveness of ionizing radiation in producing biologic damage. The RBE of gamma rays and X-rays is 1; that of beta particles

Roentgen Equals

93 ergs of energy absorbed per gram of soft tissue
5.23×10^{13} eV of energy absorbed per gram of air
6.77×10^{10} eV of energy absorbed per cubic
centimeter (0.00129 gm) of air

Roentgen is equivalent to

2.083×10^9 ion pairs (1 esu) created per cubic
centimeter (0.00129 g) of air by X-rays or gamma rays
1.61×10^{12} ion pairs created per gram of air
87 ergs of energy absorbed per gram of air

TABLE 6-24
Definition of the Roentgen and Its Equivalent Measures

(electrons) and positrons is close to 1 but not greater than 2; for neutrons it is 2 to 5; protons 8 to 10; and α particles 10 to 20. An additional term is the roentgen equivalent physical (REP), which is equal to the absorption of 93 ergs/g of soft tissue and is used in biologic research. A capital N represents the exposure of biologic tissue to neutrons and is equivalent to 1 roentgen induced by X-rays in the ionization chamber.

Effects of Ocular Exposure

Table 6-26 provides the threshold values for different portions of the eye exposed to ionizing radiation. These data are from a review of the literature and illustrate that a single number cannot represent a

Old Units	New Units
Curie (Ci) = 3.7×10^{10} disintegrations per second	Becquerel (Bq) = 1 disintegration per second
RAD (roentgen absorbed dose) = 0.01 J absorbed energy per kg of any medium	Gray (Gy) = 1 J absorbed energy per kg of any medium (100 RAD = 1 Gy)
REM (roentgen equivalent man) = RAD × RBE	Sievert (Sv) = Gy × RBE

TABLE 6-25
Radiobiologic Units Used to Define the Roentgen

threshold. The data provide a range of values representing all of the many variables of the source and the research methodology required.[302]

At or near threshold and after a 3- to 9-d latent period, the corneal apex loses its normal bright, shiny luster and the conjunctival vessels become engourged with blood.[303–307] Higher levels of exposure result in exfoliation of epithelial cells, corneal ulcers, and keratitis with increased fibroblasts in the stroma and a loss of the superficial nerve fibers.[305] The corneal signs are accompanied by a flare in the anterior chamber and loss of pigment by the iris. In addition, the lacrimal gland may cease to function, which results in drying of the cornea and conjunctiva. All of these signs are reversible for the pigmented rabbit eye. Aqueous humor damage results in an inflammatory exudation in the anterior chamber and a partial reduction in the production of aqueous.

Cataract formation follows a logical sequence in development over a 3- to 5-mo latent period after exposure.[307–309] The anterior and bow epithelial cells are damaged, and the entire anterior lens surface just below the capsule takes on a granular appearance. The damaged cells at the lens bow fail to form normal fibers, and the aberrant fibers migrate toward the anterior and posterior poles of the lens. The lens opacities continue to become more dense as the time progresses. Clinical observation with the biomicroscope on the rabbit demonstrates vacuoles in the equatorial region of the lens that spread anteriorly and posteriorly from the equator. The vacuoles are thought to represent the early stage of the epithelial and lens fiber damage. Most changes found in the radiation type of cataract can also be found in other types of cataracts. Specific to the human radiation cataract is the migration of cells beneath the posterior capsule and the thickening of the posterior capsule, which are responses that occur prior to changes in the lens cortex.[310–316]

Recent research has been directed toward establishing the basic mechanisms of cataractogenesis using biochemistry. It is contended that cataractogenesis mediated by ionizing radiation is through cell membrane damage.[317] Alternatives include altered proteins, damage to lens DNA, damage to the sulfur-sulfur bond, and the prevention of the production of protective enzymes. This appears to be the same criteria for cataractogenesis that results from any type of radiation insult to the lens.

Type of Radiation	Species	Cornea	Aqueous	Lens	Vitreous	Retina	Reference
X-ray	Human	—	100–1300 r	600 r	1800 r	2000 r	306–309
	Rabbit	1000–1500 r 40 Gy	100–1300 r —	1500–2000 r —	1800 r —	<2000 r —	303–307 305
Gamma	Rabbit	1000 r	—	1350 r	—	2000 r	318, 319
	Primate					2000 r	320
Deutrons	Rabbit	—		125–250 rep			321
Electron (Beta)	Rabbit	35,000 rep 30–50 Gy	— 75–100 Gy	— —	— —	— —	322 304–306
Alpha	Rabbit	—	—	125–250 rep	—	—	322–324
Neutron	Man	—		8.4×10^9 W/cm^2 200–1200 rep 1.4 N*			325–328
	Rabbit	400 rep		60–120 rep (1.5×10^{11} N/cm^2)			329, 330

*N is the amount of ionization induced by neutrons equal to that induced by 1 r of X-rays in the ionization chamber.
Units: r = roentgen, rad = radiation absorbed dose, rep = radiation equivalent physical, and Gy = Gray (100 rad = 1 Gy).

TABLE 6-26
Comparison of Threshold Ionizing Radiation Levels for Different Species, Types of Radiation, and Units

Exposure of the posterior segment of the human eye to ionizing radiation, particularly X-ray, results in a visual sensation resembling a luminous glow called a *phosphene*. The intensity of the stimulus varies from 1.6 to 8.7 mr/s for the normal human eye.[331] As the level of X-radiation increases to 2000 r and above, morphologic changes are found in the retina of the rabbit indicating radiation damage. There is a pyknosis in the outer nuclear layer of the retina accompanied by fragmentation of the outer segments of the visual receptors within 4 h after exposure.[332] Higher levels of exposure result in increasing damage to the retina. Cibis et al[308] contemplated the sequence of events from exposure to a single X-ray from 2000 r or more. The first symptom would be nightblindness followed quickly by congestion, exudation, and hemorrhages of the uveal and retinal vessels. The rods and cones would degenerate leaving the macular area and "tunnel" visual fields. Extremely high doses would result in immediate blindness.

The question of whether a threshold exists for exposure to neutrons and gamma rays has been discussed. Human culture cells were exposed to gamma rays with the data evaluated using the linear hypothesis, and it was concluded that the results appeared to show no threshold for a lethal cellular response.[333–335]

Current OSHA standards for permissible exposure of the body and parts of the body to ionizing radiation are presented in Table 6-27.[336] It should be noted that persons below 18 years of age are limited to 10% of the adult values. The level of permissible exposure depends on the history of the exposure experienced by the worker. The intent of the standard is to ensure that the worker is not exposed to ionizing radiation in levels that would affect personal health and welfare.

6.7 Ultrasound

Ultrasound is not electromagnetic radiation but mechanical energy that operates in the 4- to 18-MHz frequency range. Ultrasound has proven to be useful in differential diagnosis and in the evaluation of ocular constants, detachments of the retina, choroid, and vitreous,[337] location and size of intraocular tumors,[338] location and size of intraocular foreign

Part of Body	Rem per calendar quarter*
Whole Body: head, trunk, blood forming organs, crystalline lens, gonads†	1.25
Skin—whole body	7.5
Hands, forearms, feet, and ankles	18.75

Persons below 18 yr of age are limited to 10% of the above.
*U.S. background is 120 mrem/yr. REM = roentgen equivalents man.
†Where adequate past and current exposure records are available, a whole-body dose of up to 3 REM per quarter is allowed if accumulated dose is less than 5 (N − 18) REM, when N is the person's age in years.

TABLE 6-27
Current OSHA Permissible Exposure Limits for Ionizing Radiation

bodies,[337] study of orbital tumors,[339] study of optical dimensions of the eye,[340,341] axial length irregularities,[340–342] and phacoemulsification of cataracts.[343–345] The accuracy of localization depends on the density of the media relative to the object to be located, the frequency of the ultrasound, and a knowledge of the velocity of ultrasound as it passes through the tissue. The purpose of this discussion is to provide values for the safe levels of exposure of the eye to ultrasound and descriptions of damage so that these data can be used in assuring safe exposure levels.

An exposure of 0.25 W/cm^2 of ultrasound for 5 min creates minimal ocular damage that is reversible and considered a safe exposure.[346] This value was accepted as safe until the early 1970s, when cataract removal by phacoemulsification became the method of choice, and endothelial damage from the procedure resulted in severe corneal edema. Reversible increases in corneal permeability were reported at 0.2 W/cm^2;[347] however, no damage was reported for ocular exposures at intensities of 0.0337 W/cm^2 for 4 h, which is considered a safe clinical level.[348] The effects of ultrasound in the phacoemulsification procedure are related to the irrigating solution, bubbles arising from the tip of the blades, and ultrasound. When correct procedures are used, the extent of endothelial damage is consistent with other surgical methods.[349]

Ultrasound of 0.25 W/cm^2 for 5 min is safe for external application to the eye. The diagnostic ultrasound intensity of 0.0337 W/cm^2 is safe for external application to the eye for longer periods of time. Ultrasound intensities within the globe should be kept to a minimum, and 0.0034 W/cm^2 is safe, but care must be taken to keep the exposure duration as short as possible to maintain the integrity of the corneal endothelium.

6.8 Electromagnetic Fields

When an electric current moves through a wire or any other conducting object, an electromagnetic field (EMF) is produced that surrounds the object. The strength of the EMF varies with the voltage and the frequency of the electricity. If the frequency varies from 3000 to 30,000 Hz, it is called very low frequency (VLF), whereas if the frequency lies between 30 and 3000 Hz, it is termed extremely low frequency (ELF).

EMFs have been measured in gauss (G), which is one line of magnetic force per square centimeter, but recently that has been changed to the tesla (T) or one line of magnetic force per square meter; therefore a tesla (T) is equal to 10^{-4} G. The SI units for EMFs are given in Table 6-28. Most EMF data in the United States is still reported in milligauss (mG), and this unit will be used in this section with the conversions to T in parenthesis.

People are constantly surrounded by EMFs in their homes and at the workplace, because most environments are wired with electricity that produces ELF-EMF as it travels through wires. A vast array of

Physical Quantity	Name of Unit	Symbol of Unit
Magnetomotive force	ampere	A
Magnetic flux	weber	Wb (V·s)
Magnetic flux density	tesla	T(Wb/m^2)
Magnetic field strength	ampere perimeter	A/m

TABLE 6-28
SI Physical Quantities, Names of Units, and Symbols of Units for Electromagnetism

common household appliances produce EMFs: can openers, toasters, food blenders and processors, irons, garbage disposals, dishwashers, clothes dryers, refrigerators, freezers, ovens, MW ovens, vacuum cleaners, hair dryers, electric blankets, sewing machines, radios, computers, and televisions constitute a partial list of the common appliances that produce rather high outputs of EMF. Table 6-29 gives the measured EMFs for many of these appliances. The Earth's magnetic field is 0.5 G (5×10^{-5} T).

Human-Generated EMFs

The electric activity of the human heart produces from 10 to 100 mA/m^2 of EMF, which exceeds the magnetic fields found in measurements from high voltage power lines by a factor of 100 to 1000.[350] The human visual system produces magnetic fields[351,352] from the transretinal potential (recorded by ERG),[353] eye movements (recorded by the electro-oculogram, or EOG),[351] eye blinks, and the visual

Human Visual Electrical Activity	EMF (T $\times 10^{-13}$)
Electroretinogram (ERG)	0.5–1
Visually evoked response (VER)	3
Blinking	3
Electro-oculogram (EOG)	10–12

From Armstrong RA, Janday B: A brief review of magnetic fields from the human visual system. Ophthalmic Physiol Opt 9:298–301, 1989; with permission by Butterworth–Heinemann Ltd, Oxford, England.

TABLE 6-30
Electromagnetic Fields for Different Activities of the Human Visual System

cortex (recorded by the visual evoked response, or VER).[351-356] The EMFs generated by the eye are shown in Table 6-30.[356]

Whole Body Exposure to EMFs

Beischer[357] reviewed the literature on the human tolerance to magnetic fields and reported that Faraday discovered that the human muscle was diamagnetic, whereas Kohlrausch found the human hand to be diamagnetic. A diamagnetic object is repelled by both poles of a magnet and aligns itself perpendicular to the lines of force of the magnet. Edison's laboratory exposed a boy to 2000 cgs lines/cm^2 with no apparent effect.[358] Anecdotal quotations from personnel working in the Lawrence Radiation Laboratory, Brookhaven National Laboratory, Argonne National Laboratory, and other laboratories that create very high magnetic fields have led Beischer to the observation that magnetic fields up to 20,000 G can be tolerated by man without sensation and that exposures up to 5000 G for 3 d per man per year appears to have no cumulative effect. These observations are not based on well-defined research and should not be used to establish human exposure tolerances.

Animal experiments are difficult to interpret and to extrapolate to the human. Barnothy[359] exposed mice to uniform magnetic fields of 5000 G and reported death to young animals, retarded growth, elevation in body temperature, changes in food consumption, problems in fertility, and an elevated white blood count. Higher levels of exposure to

Item	*EMF (mG)	Item	*EMF (mG)
Can opener	30–225	Ovens	1–8
Toaster	0.6–7	Microwave ovens	3–40
Food blenders and processors	5–100	Vacuum cleaners	1–20
Irons	1–3	Hair dryers	1–75
Garbage disposals	1–5	Electric blanket	3–50
Dishwashers	1–15	Sewing machine	1–23
Clothes dryers	1–24	Lamps	6–20
Refrigerators	1–8	Computer monitors	0.93–2.04
Freezers	1–3	Television	<1.5

*EMF decreases rapidly with distance. An example is a measurement of 18.1 mG at 15 cm (6 in) from the EMF source becomes 1.4 mG at 76 cm (30 in) from the source.

TABLE 6-29
Electromagnetic Fields of Different Household Appliances

Swiss white mice (8000–14,000 G) failed to demonstrate significant biologic changes.[360] Other studies have shown an enhanced DNA synthesis in human fibroblasts with an exposure level of 0.5 to 2.5×10^{-5} T/s,[361] a reduction in the b-wave of the isolated retina of the turtle using magnetic fields of 10 to 100 G,[362] and the induction of cellular transcription from repetitive 15-Hz pulse trains producing a magnetic field of 0.1 G.[363]

More recent studies on the effects of magnetic fields on the human body[364] have reported a reduction of melatonin produced by the pineal gland[350,365] by 30% to 50%; an increase in cellular uptake of calcium;[350] an increase in breast cancer in male electricians, power plant workers and utility linemen; and an increase in cancer of the brain,[368] leukemia, and lymphomas.[367,368] Neurologic effects from exposure to EMFs have also been reported.[364] The perception threshold for EMFs is about 12 kV/m. The most disturbing fact is that these effects have been attributed to magnetic fields of 2 mG.[349]

Ocular Exposure to EMFs

When an alternating current is passed between two electrodes applied externally, flickering phosphores are seen. The same visual phenomena are observed when the head is placed in a pulsating EMF.[370,371] The fusion frequencies for EMF stimulation of the eye lie between 50 and 70 Hz, depending on the strength of the magnetic field and the level of adaptation of the retina.[372–374]

The influence on vision from exposure to ELF-EMF with a frequency range of 0 to 51 KHz produced by an electric arc welding power supply and electric steel furnaces demonstrated magnetophosphenes.[375] The phosphenes varied with the frequency of the magnetic field and reached threshold at 20 to 25 Hz. With increasing time in the dark, the visual threshold values to produce phosphenes increased instead of decreased, as is found when a normal dark adaptation curve is obtained. This "reverse adaptation effect" is probably due to the elevation of the retinal threshold by the phosphenes, which results in an increased threshold for subsequent magnetic field effects.

Corneal exposure from 0.019 V/m (0.1 G) to 0.19 V/m (1 G) showed no effect on the cellular structure of the cornea using histologic, DNA and protein biochemical synthesis, cellular viability, and mitosis as end-points.[376] Tissue cultures demonstrated that in some wound-healing experiments magnetic fields assisted corneal recovery from the damage. The power and frequency levels of the improvement in wound healing were not given.

The press has created concern in recent times about the effects of exposure of the human to EMF. This area suffers from many of the problems associated with other forms of EMF research: measurement, exposure procedures, end-point for damage, data analysis, and public concern. It is a complex problem that will be solved by ingenious scientists and adequate funding by the government. In the meantime, we must be content to carefully follow the valid data that are forthcoming.

References

1. Barker FM, II. The transmittance of the EMS from 200 nm to 2500 nm through the optical tissues of the eye of the pigmented rabbit. MS Thesis. University of Houston, Houston, Texas, 1979.
2. Burge WE. The effect of radiant energy on the lens and humors of the eye. Am J Physiol 1914; 36:21–36.
3. Kinsey EV. Spectral transmission of the eye to ultraviolet radiations. Arch Ophthalmol 1948; 39:508–13.
4. Prince JH. Spectral absorption of the retina and choroid from 340 to 1700 millimicrons, Final Report on Project 1069, Contract AF41 (657)-306. Aerospace Medical Division, USAF School of Aerospace Medicine, Brooks Air Force Base, Texas, 1972.
5. Weisinger H, Schmidt FH, Williams RC, Tiller CO, Ruffin RS, Guerry D III, Ham WT. The transmission of light through the ocular media of the rabbit eye. Am J Ophthalmol 1956; 42:907–910.
6. Geeraets WJ, Berry ER. Ocular spectral characteristics as related to hazards from lasers and other light sources. Am J Ophthalmol 1968; 66:15–20.
7. Boettner EA. Spectral transmission of the eye. Final Report, Contract AF41 (609)-2966. USAF School of Aerospace Medicine, Brooks Air Force Base, Texas, 1967.
8. Geeraets WJ, Williams RC, Chan G, Ham WT Jr, Guerry D III, Schmidt FH. The loss of light energy in the retina and choroid. Arch Ophthalmol 1960; 64:606–15.
9. Maher EF. Transmission and absorption coefficients for ocular media of the Rhesus monkey. SAM-TR-78-32. Aerospace Medical Division, USAF School of Aerospace Medicine, Brooks Air Force Base, Texas, 1978.

10. Ludvig E, McCarthy EF. Absorption of visible light by the refractive media of the human eye. Arch Ophthalmol 1938; 20:37–51.

11. Boettner EA, Wolter JR. Transmissivity of the ocular media. Invest Ophthalmol 1962; 1:776–783.

12. Said FS, Weale RA. The variation with age of the spectral transmissivity of the living human crystalline lens. Gerontologia 1959; 3:213–231.

13. Keates RH, Gentsler DE, Tarabichi S. Ultraviolet light transmission of the lens capsule. Ophthalmic Surgery 1982; 13:374–376.

14. Werner JS. Development of scotopic sensitivity and the absorption spectrum of the human ocular media. J Opt Soc Am [A], 1982; 72:247–258.

15. Bachem A. Ophthalmic ultraviolet action spectra. Am J Ophthalmol 1956; 41:969–975.

16. Kutscher CF. Ocular effects of radiant energy. Ind Med 1946; 15:311–316 and Trans Am Acad Ophthalmol Otolaryngol 1946; 50:230–241.

17. Voss JJ, Boogaard J. A Few Experiments on the Spectral Transmission of the Eyelid. Report No. IZF 1966-15. Soesterberg, The Netherlands, National Defence Research Council TNO, Institute for Perception TNO, 1966.

18. Kornzweig AL. Physiological effects of use on the visual process. Sight Saving Review 1954; 24:138.

19. Ham WT Jr, Mueller HA, William RC, Geeraets WJ. Ocular hazard from viewing the sun unprotected and through various windows and filters. Appl Opt 1973; 12:2122–2129.

20. Sliney DH. Interaction mechanisms of laser radiation with ocular tissues. In Court LA, Duchene A, Courant D (eds); Lasers et Normes de Protection. First International Symposium on Laser Biological Effects and Exposure Limits, Vol 5, pp 65–82. Fontenay-aux-Roses, France, Commissariat l'Energie Atomique, Dept de Protection Sanitaire, Service de Documentation, 1986.

21. Ham WT, Jr, Mueller HA, Ruffolo JJ, Miller JE, Cleary SF, Guerry RK, Guerry D III. Basci mechanisms underlying the production of photochemical lesions in the mammalian retina. Curr Eye Res 1984; 3:165–174.

22. Alfano RR, Ho PP. Self- and couple-phased modulations of ultrashort laser pulses. Opt News 1989; 15:13–18.

23. White TH, Mainster MA, Wilson PW, Tips JH. Chorioretinal temperature increases from solar observation. Bull Math Biophys 1971; 33:1–10.

24. Mainster MA, White TJ, Tips JH, Wilson PW. Retinal–temperature increases produced by intense light sources. J Opt Soc Am [A] 1970; 60:262–270.

25. Sliney D, Wolbarsht M. Safety with Lasers and Other Optical Sources. New York, Plenum Press, 1980.

26. Fry GA. The optical performance of the human eye. In Wolf E (ed): Progress in Optics, Vol II, pp 118–123. Amsterdam, North Holland Publishing Co, 1970.

27. Le Grand Y, Hunt RNG, Walsh JWT, Hunt FRW, trans. Light, Colour and Vision. New York, Dover Publications Inc, 1957.

28. Crawford BH, Jones OC. Physical measurements and calibration of apparatus. In Crawford BH, Granger GW, Weale RA (eds): Techniques of Photostimulation Biology, Vol 7 pp 201–233. Amsterdam, North Holland Publishing Co, 1968.

29. Fry GA. The Blur of the Retinal Image. Columbus, The Ohio State University Press, 1955.

30. Jenkins FA, White HE. Fundamentals of Optics (4th ed). St. Louis, McGraw-Hill Book Company, 1965.

31. Fry GA. Visual measurements. In Bartelson CJ, Crum F (eds): Optical Radiation Measurements, Vol 5, pp 78–84. New York, Academic Press Inc, 1984.

32. Wald G, Griffin DR. Change in the refractive power of the human eye in dim and bright light. J Opt Soc Am [A] 1947; 37:321–336.

33. Bedford RE, Wyszecki G. Axial chromatic aberration of the human eye. J Opt Soc Am [A] 1957; 47:564–565.

34. Obstfeld H. Optics in Vision. London, Butterworths, 1978.

35. Rockwell RJ, Sliney DH, Smith JF. Laser safety, Part 1. Introduction to hazard calculations. Electro-Optical Systems Design 1978; 10:32–39.

36. Blumthaler M, Ambach W, Daxecker F. On the threshold radiant exposure for keratitis solaris. Invest Ophthalmol Vis Sci 1987; 28:1713–1716.

37. Pitts DG, Cullen AP, Hacker PD. Ocular effects of near ultraviolet radiation: Literature review. Am J Optom Physiol Opt 1977; 54:542–549.

38. Pitts DG. The ocular effect of ultraviolet radiation: Glenn A. Fry Award lecture. Am J Optom Physiol Opt 1978; 55:19–35.

39. Cogan DG, Kinsey VE. Ophthalmic ultraviolet action spectra. Am J Ophthalmol 1956; 41:969–975.

40. Duke-Elder WS, Duke-Elder PM. A histological study on the action of short-waved light on the eye with a note on the 'inclusion bodies.' Br J Ophthalmol 1929; 13:1–37.

41. Pitts DG, Prince JE, Butcher WI, Kay KR, Bowman RW, Richey DG, Mori LH, Strong JE, Tredici TJ. The effects of ultraviolet radiation on the eye. SAM-TR69-10. USAF School of Aerospace Medicine, Brooks Air Force Base, Texas, 1969.

42. Pitts DG, Kay KR. The photo-ophthalmic threshold for the rabbit. Am J Optom Physiol Opt 1969; 46:561–572.

43. Pitts DG. A comparative study of the effects of ultraviolet radiation on the eye. Am J Optom Physiol Opt 1970; 47:235–246.

44. Pitts DG. The ultraviolet action spectrum and protection criteria. Health Phys 1973; 25:559–566.

45. Pitts DG. The human ultraviolet action spectrum. Am J Optom Physiol Opt 1974; 51:946–960.

46. Pitts DG, Cullen AP. Ocular effects from 295 nm to 400 nm in the rabbit eye. DHEW (NIOSH) Publication No. 77-175, 1977. Washington, DC, Department of Health, Education and Welfare, 1977.
47. Pitts DG, Cullen AP, Hacker PD. Ocular effects of ultraviolet radiation from 295 nm to 400 nm. Invest Ophthalmol Vis Sci 1977; 16:932–939.
48. Kurtin WE, Zuclich JA. Action spectrum for oxygen-dependent near-ultraviolet induced corneal damage. Photochem Photobiol 1978; 27:329–333.
49. Ham WT, Jr, Mueller WA, Ruffolo JJ, Jr, Guerry III D, Guerry RK. Action spectrum for retinal injury from near ultraviolet radiation in the aphakic monkey. Am J Ophthalmol 1982; 93:299–306.
50. Schmidt RE, Zuclich JA. Retinal lesions due to ultraviolet laser exposure. Invest Ophthalmol Vis Sci 1980; 19:1166–1175.
51. Cullen AP. Ultraviolet induced lysosome activity in the corneal epithelium. Graefes Arch Clin Exp Ophthalmol 1980; 214:107–118.
52. Verhoeff FH, Bell L: The pathological effects of radiant energy on the eye: An experimental investigation with a systematic review of the literature. Proc Am Acad Arts Sci 1916; 51:630–811.
53. Widmark EJ: Uber der Einfluss des Lichtes aud die Vorderen Medien des Auge. Scand Arch Physiol 1889; 1:264–280.
54. Widmark EJ: Uber die Durchdringlichkeit der Augenmedien for Ultraviolette Strahlen. Scand Arch Physiol 1892; 3:14–46.
55. Widmark EJ: Uber Blendurg der Netzhaut. Scand Arch Physiol 1893; 4:281–294.
56. Schive K, Kavli G, Volden G. Light penetration of normal photokeratitis induced rabbit cornea. Acta Ophthalmol (Copenh) 1984; 62:309–314.
57. Zuclich JA, Kurtin WE. Oxygen dependent on near-ultraviolet induced corneal damage. Photochem Photobiol 1977; 25:133–135.
58. Cullen AP. Additive effects of ultraviolet radiation. Am J Optom Physiol Opt 1980; 57:808–814.
59. Zuclich JA. Cumulative effects of near-UV induced corneal damage. Health Phys 1980; 38:833–838.
60. Zuclich JA, Connolly JS. Ocular damage induced near-ultraviolet laser radiation. Invest Ophthalmol 1976; 15:760–764.
61. Lattimore MR, Jr. Glucose concentration profiles of normal and ultraviolet radiation exposed rabbit corneas. Exp Eye Res 1988; 47:699–704.
62. Lattimore MR, Jr. The effect of ultraviolet radiation on metabolism of the corneal epithelium of the rabbit. PhD Dissertation. College of Optometry, University of Houston, August, 1987.
63. Lattimore MR, Jr. Effect of ultraviolet radiation on the energy metabolism of the corneal epithelium of the rabbit. Photochem Photobiol 1989; 49:175–180.
64. Pitts DG, Bergmanson JPG, Chu LW-F, Waxler M, Hitchins VM. Ultrastructural analysis of corneal exposure to UV radiation. Acta Ophthalmol (Copenh) 1987; 65:263–273.
65. Doughty MJ, Cullen AP. Three month evaluation of rabbit corneal physiology following a single exposure to low dose UV-B. ARVO Abstracts. Invest Ophthalmol Vis Sci [Suppl] 1987; 28:161.
66. Cullen AP, Chou BR, Hall MG, Jany SE. Ultraviolet-B damages corneal endothelium. Am J Optom Physiol Opt 1984; 61:473–478.
67. Ringvold A, Davanger M, Olsen EG. Changes of corneal endothelium after ultraviolet radiation. Acta Ophthalmol (Copenh) 1982; 60:41–63.
68. Riley MV, Giblin FJ. Toxic effects of hydrogen peroxide on corneal endothelium. Curr Eye Res 1983; 2:451–458.
69. Edelhauser HF, van Horn DL, Miller P, Pederson HJ. Effect of thiol-oxidation of glutathione with diamide on corneal endothelial function, junction complexes and microfilaments. J Cell Biol 1976; 68:567–578.
70. Ng MC, Riley MV. Relation of intracellular levels and redox state of glutathione to endothelial function in the rabbit cornea. Exp Eye Res 1980; 30:511–517.
71. Laing RA, Sandstrom MM, Berrospi AR. Changes in corneal endothelium as a function of age. Exp Eye Res 1976; 22:587–594.
72. Laule A, Cable MK, Hoftman CE, Hanna C. Endothelial cell population changes in the human cornea during life. Arch Ophthalmol 1978; 96:2031–2035.
73. Suda T. Mosaic pattern changes in human corneal endothelium with age. Jpn J Ophthalmol 1984; 28:331–338.
74. Matsuda M, Yee RW, Edelhauser HF. Comparison of the corneal endothelium in an American and a Japanese population. Arch Ophthalmol 1985; 103:68–70.
75. Karai I, Matsumura S, Takise S, Horiguchi S, Matsuda M. Morphological change in the corneal endothelium due to ultraviolet radiation in welders. Brit J Ophthalmol 1981; 68:544–548.
76. Good GW, Schoessler JP. Chronic solar radiation exposure and endothelial polymegathism. Curr Eye Res 1988; 7:157–162.
77. Cullen AP, Perera S. Human conjunctival response to ultraviolet irradiation. Suppl to Optom Vis Sci 1990; 67:150.
78. Kahn HA, Leibowitz HM, Ganley JP, Kini MM, Colton TL, Nickerson RS, Dawber TR. The Framingham Eye Study, I. Outline and major prevalence findings. Am J Epidemiol 1977; 106:17–32.
79. Kahn HA, Leibowitz HM, Ganley JP, Kini MM, Colton TL, Nickerson RS, Dawber TR. The Framingham Eye

Study, II. Association of ophthalmic pathology with single variables previously measured in the Framingham heart study. Am J Epidemiol 1977; 106:33–41.

80. Leibowitz HM, Krueger DE, Maunder LR, Milton RC, Kini MM, Kahn HA, Nickerson RJ, Pool J, Colton TL, Ganley JP, Lowenstein JI, Dawber TR. The Framingham Eye Study Monograph. Survey Ophthalmol [Suppl] 1980; 24:350–365.

81. Duke-Elder WS, McFaul PA. System of Ophthalmology, Vol. XIV, Injuries. Part 2, Non-Mechanical Injuries, pp 867–884, 929. London, Henry Kimpton, 1972.

82. Weale RA. The age variation of "senile" cataract in various parts of the world. Br J Ophthalmol 1982; 66:31–34.

83. Hiller R, Giacometti L, Yuen K. Sunlight and cataract: An epidemiological investigation. Am J Epidemiol 1977; 105:450–459.

84. Hiller R, Sperduto RD, Ederer F. Epidemiologic associations with cataract: The 1971–1972 National Health and Nutrition Survey. Am J Epidemiol 1983; 118:239–249.

85. Taylor HR. The environment and the lens. Br J Ophthalmol 1980; 64:303–310.

86. Hollows F, Moran D. Cataract—the ultraviolet risk factor. Lancet 1981; 2:1249–1250.

87. Brilliant LB, Grassett NC, Pokhrel RP, Kolstad A, Lepkowski JM, Brilliant GE, Hawks WN, Pararajasegaram B. Associations among cataract prevalence, sunlight hours and altitude in the Himalayas. Am J Epidemiol 1983; 118:250–264.

88. Chatterjee A. Cataract in Punjab. *In* Symposium on the Human Lens in Relation to Cataract, pp 265–279. CIBA Foundation Symposium 19. Amsterdam, Associated Scientific Publishers, 1973.

89. Mitchell BD, Lepowski JM. The epidemiology of cataract in Nepal. Hum Biol 1986; 58:975–990.

90. Taylor HR, West SK, Rosenthal FS, Munoz B, Newland HS, Abbey H, Emmett EA. Effect of ultraviolet radiation on cataract formation. N Engl J Med 1988; 319:1429–1433.

91. West SK, Taylor HR. The detection and grading of cataract: An epidemiologic perspective. Survey Ophthalmol 1986; 31:175–184.

92. Collman GW, Shore DL, Shy CM, Checkoway H, Luria AS. Sunlight and other risk factors for cataracts: An epidemiologic study. Am J Public Health 1988; 78:1459–1462.

93. Bochow TW, West SK, Azar A, Munoz B, Sommer A, Taylor HR. Ultraviolet light and risk of posterior subcapsular cataracts. Arch Ophthalmol 1989; 107:369–372.

94. Goodeve CF. Vision on the ultraviolet. Nature 1934; 134:416–417.

95. Wald G. The spectral sensitivity of the human eye. J Opt Soc Am [A] 1945; 35:189–196.

96. Wald G. Human vision and the spectrum. Science 1945; 101:653.

97. Kamel ID, Parker JA. Protection from ultraviolet exposure in aphakic erythopsia. Can J Ophthalmol 1973; 9:563–565.

98. Saurux H, Manuet LP, LaRoche L. Erythopsie chez un porteur d'implant. Etude physiologique et electrophysiologique. J Fr Ophtalmol 1984; 7:557–562.

99. Henton WW, Sykes SM. Changes in absolute threshold with light-induced retinal damage. Physiol Behav 1983; 31:179–185.

100. Henton WW, Sykes SM. Recovery of absolute threshold with UVA-induced retinal damage. Physiol Behav 1984; 32:949–954.

101. Schmidt RE, Zuclich JA. Retinal lesions due to ultraviolet laser exposure. Invest Ophthalmol Vis Sci 1980; 19:1166–1175.

102. Zuclich JA. Ultraviolet-induced photochemical damage in ocular tissues. Health Phys 1989; 56:671–682.

103. Zuclich JA, Blankenstein MF. Ocular effects of the Xenon Chloride excimer laser. In Effects of Laser Radiation on the Eye, Vol II, pp 7–29. Technical Report SAM-TR-84-10. USAF School of Aerospace Medicine, Brooks Air Force Base, Texas, 1984.

104. Ham WT, Jr, Mueller WA, Ruffolo JJ, Jr, Guerry III D, Guerry RK. Action spectrum for retinal injury from near ultraviolet radiation in the aphakic monkey. Am J Ophthalmol 1982; 93:299–306.

105. Yannuzi LA, Fisher YL, Krueger A, Slakter J. Solar retinopathy: A photobiological and geophysical analysis. Tr Am J Ophthalmol Soc 1987; LXXXV:120–158.

106. Sundararaman N, St. John DE, Venkateswaran SV. Solar ultraviolet radiation received on the earth's surface under clear and cloudless conditions. DOT-TST-75-101. Washington, DC, Department of Transportation, 1975.

107. Pitts DG, Bergmanson JPE, Chu LW-F. Primate Retinal Responses to 300 nm Ultraviolet Exposure. Presented at the Annual Meeting of American Academy of Optometry, Houston, Texas, Dec. 13–16, 1986.

108. Fraunfelder FT. Drug Induced Ocular Side Effects and Drug Interactions. Philadelphia, Lea & Febiger, 1976.

109. Lerman S. Lens proteins and fluoresence. Isr J Med Sci 1972; 8:1583–1589.

110. Goeckerman WH. The treatment of psoriasis. Northwest Med 1925; 24:229–231.

111. Goeckerman WH. Treatment of psoriasis: Continued observations on the use of crude coal tar and ultraviolet light. Arch Dermatol Syphiol 1931; 24:446–450.

112. Parrish JA, Anderson RR, Urbach F, Pitts DG. UV-A Biological Effects of Ultraviolet Radiation with Emphasis on Human Responses to Longwave Ultraviolet. New York, Plenum Press, 1978.

113. Scherer R. The human peripheral lymphocyte: A model system for studying the combined effect of

psoralen plus black light. Klin Wochenschr 1977; 55:137–140.

114. Scherer R, Kern B, Braun-Falco O. UVA-induced inhibition of proliferation of PHA-stimulated lymphocytes from humans treated with 8-methoxypsoralen. Br J Dermatol 1977; 97:519–527.

115. Henderson BW, Fingar VH. Oxygen limitation of direct tumor cell kill during photodynamic treatment of a murine tumor model. Photochem Photobiol 1989; 49:299–304.

116. Dayhaw-Barker P, Truscott TG. Direct detection of singlet oxygen sensitized by nalidixic acid: The effect of pH and melanin. Photochem Photobiol 1988; 47:765–767.

117. Zuclich JA, Taboada J. Ocular hazard from UV laser exhibiting self-mode-locking. Appl Opt 1978; 17:1482–1484.

118. Pitts DG, Bergmanson JPG. The UV problem: Have the rules changed? J Am Optom Assoc 1989; 60:420–424.

119. Taylor HR. The biologic effects of UV-B on the eye. Photochem Photobiol 1989; 50:489–492.

120. Sliney DH. Estimating the solar ultraviolet radiation exposure to an intraocular lens implant. J Cataract Refract Surg 1987; 13:296–301.

121. Sliney DH. Physical factors in cataractogenesis: Ambient ultraviolet radiation and temperature. Invest Ophthalmol Vis Sci 1986; 27:781–790.

122. Diffey BL. Environmental exposure to UV-B radiation. In Reviews on Environmental Health, Vol IV, pp 317–337. Tel Aviv, Israel, Freund Publishing House, 1984.

123. De Luisi JJ, Harris JM, Tate TK. A determination of the absolute radiant energy of a Robertson-Berger meter sunburn unit. Atmosph Env 1983; 17:751–758.

124. Rosenthal FS, West SK, Munoz B, Emmett EA, Strickland PT, Taylor HR. Ocular and facial skin exposure to ultraviolet radiation in sunlight: A personal exposure model with application to a worker population. Health Phys 1991; 61:77–86.

125. Rosenthal FS, Safran M, Taylor HR. The ocular dose of ultraviolet radiation from sunlight exposure. Photochem Photobiol 1985; 42:163–171.

126. Rosenthal FS, Phoon C, Bakalian AE, Taylor HR. The ocular dose of ultraviolet radiation to outdoor workers. Invest Ophthalmol Vis Sci 1988; 29:649–656.

127. Hoover HL. Sunglasses, pupil dilation, and solar ultraviolet irradiation of the human lens and retina. Appl Opt 1987; 26:689–695.

128. Rosenthal FS, Bakalian AE, Lou C, Taylor HR. The effect of sunglasses on ocular exposure to ultraviolet radiation. Am J Public Health 1988; 78:72–74.

129. Rosenthal FA, Bakalian AE, Taylor HR. The effect of prescription eyewear on ocular exposure to ultraviolet radiation. Am J Public Health 1986; 76:1216–1220.

130. Pitts DG, Lattimore MR. Protection against UVR using the Vistakon UV-Bloc soft contact lens. ICLC 1987; 14:22–29.

131. Dumbleton KA, Cullen AP, Doughty MJ. Protection from acute exposure to ultraviolet radiation by ultraviolet-absorbing RGP contact lenses. Ophthalmol Physiol Opt 1991; 232–238.

132. Werner JS, Spillman. UV-absorbing intraocular lenses: Safety, efficacy, and consequences for the cataract patient. Graefes Arch Clin Exp Ophthalmol 1989; 227:248–256.

133. Lanum J. The damaging effects of light on the retina: Empirical findings, theoretical and practical implications. Surv Ophthalmol 1978; 22:221–249.

134. Ham WT, Jr. The photopathology and nature of the blue light and near UV retinal lesions produced by lasers and other optical sources. In Wolbarsht ML (ed). Laser Applications in Medicine and Biology, Vol. 4, pp 191–246. New York, Plenum Press, 1989.

135. Waxler M, Hitchins VM. Optical Radiation and Visual Health. Orlando, FL, CRC Press, 1987.

136. Flynn J. Photoretinitis in anti-aircraft lookouts. Med J Aust 1942; 2:400–401.

137. Smith HE. Actinic macular retinal pigment degeneration. US Navy Med Bull 1944; 42:675–680.

138. Eccles JC, Flynn AJ. Experimental photoretinitis. Med J Aust 1944; 1:339–342.

139. Cordes FC. Eclipse retinitis. Am J Ophthalmol 1948; 31:101–107.

140. McCulloch C. Changes at the macula due to solar radiation. Am J Ophthalmol 1945; 28:1115–1122.

141. Tso MOM, La Piana FG. The human fovea after sun-gazing. Trans Am Acad Ophthalmol Otolaryngol 1975; 79:788–795.

142. Voss JJ. A theory of retinal burn. Bull Math Biophy 1962; 24:115–128.

143. Voss JJ. Digital Computations of Temperature in Retinal Burn Problems. Report 1ZF, 19650-16. Institute for Perception, RVO-TNO. Soesterberg, The Netherlands, 1963.

144. Hayes JR, Wolbarsht M. Thermal model for retinal damage induced by pulsed lasers. Aerospace Med 1968; 39:474–480.

145. Clarke AM, Geeraets WJ, Ham WT, Jr. An equilibrium thermal model for retinal injury from optical sources. Appl Opt 1969; 8:1051–1054.

146. Mainster MA, White TJ, Allen RG. Spectra dependence of retinal damage produced by intense light sources. J Opt Soc Am [A] 1970; 50:848–855.

147. Mainster MA, White TJ, Tips JH, Wilson PW. Retinal temperature increases produced by intense light sources. J Opt Soc Am [A] 1970; 50:848–855.

148. Allen RG, Richey EO. Eclipse burns in humans and laboratory measurements in rabbits. SAM-TR-66-45.

USAF School of Aerospace Medicine, Brooks Air Force Base, Texas, 1966.

149. White TJ, Mainster MA, Wilson PW, Tips JH. Chorioretinal temperature increases from solar observation. Bull Math Biophys 1971; 33:1–10.

150. Allen RG. Retinal thermal injury. In Wolbarsht M, Sliney DH (eds): Ocular Effects on Non-ionizing Radiation. Proc Soc Photo-Opt Inst Eng 1980; 229:80–86.

151. Ham WT, Jr, Mueller HA, Williams RC, Geeraets WJ. Ocular hazards from viewing the sun unprotected and through various windows and filters. Appl Opt 1973; 12:2122–2129.

152. Ham WT, Jr, Mueller HA, Ruffolo JJ, Jr, Guerry D, III. Solar retinopathy as a function of wavelength: Its significance for protective eyewear. In Williams TP, Baker BN (eds): The Effects of Constant Light on Visual Processes. New York, Plenum Press, 1980.

153. Sliney DH, Freasier BC. Evaluation of optical radiation hazards. Appl Opt 1973; 12:1–24.

154. Ham WT, Jr, Mueller HA, Sliney DA. Retinal sensitivity to damage from short wavelength light. Nature 1976; 260:153–155.

155. Ham WT, Jr, Mueller HA, Ruffolo JJ, Clarke AM. Sensitivity of the retina to radiation damage as a function of wavelength. Photochem Photobiol 1979; 29:735–743.

156. Ham WT, Jr, Mueller HA, Ruffolo JJ, Jr. Retinal effects of blue light exposure. Proc Soc Photo-Opt Inst Eng 1980; 229:46–50.

157. Ham WT, Jr. Ocular hazards of light sources: Review of current knowledge. J Occup Med 1983; 25:101–103.

158. Ham WT, Jr, Mueller HA, Ruffolo JJ, Jr, Guerry D, III, Guerry RK. Action spectrum for retinal injury from near ultraviolet radiation in the aphakic monkey. Am J Ophthalmol 1982; 93:229–306.

159. Ham WT, Jr, Ruffolo JJ, Jr, Mueller HA, Guerry D, III. The quantitative dimensions of intense light damage as obtained from animal studies. The nature of retinal radiation damage: Dependence on wavelength, power level and exposure time. Vision Res 1980; 20:1105–1111.

160. Noel WK, Walker VS, Kang BS, Berman S. Retinal damage by light in rats. Invest Ophthalmol 1966; 5:450–473.

161. Friedman E, Kuabara T. The retinal pigment epithelium, IV. The damaging effects of radiant energy. Arch Ophthalmol 1968; 80:265–279.

162. Tso MOM, Fine BS, Zimmerman LE. Photic maculopathy produced by the indirect microscope, 1. Clinical and histopathological study. Am J Ophthalmol 1972; 73:686–699.

163. Lawwill T. Effects of prolonged exposure of rabbit retina to low intensity light. Invest Ophthalmol 1973; 12:45–51.

164. Lawwill T, Crockett S, Currier G. Retinal damage secondary to chronic light exposure, thresholds and mechanisms. Doc Ophthalmol 1977; 44:379–402.

165. Kuwabara T, Gorn RW. Retinal damage by visible light: An electron microscopic study. Arch Ophthalmol 1968; 79:69–78.

166. Kramers J. Photochemical damage of the retina. PhD dissertation. University of Maastricht, Maastricht, The Netherlands, December 1989.

167. Sykes SM, Robinson WG, Waxler M, Kuwabara T. Damage to the monkey retina by broad-spectrum fluorescent light. Invest Ophthalmol Vis Sci 1981; 20:425–434.

168. Kremers JJM, van Norren D. Retinal damage in macaque after white light exposures lasting ten minutes to twelve hours. Invest Ophthalmol Vis Sci 1989; 30:1032–1040.

169. Pitts DG, Bergmanson JPG, Chu LW-F. Rabbit eye exposure to broad-spectrum fluorescent light. Acta Ophthalmol Suppl (Copenh) 159, 1983.

170. Ham WT, Jr, Mueller HA. The photopathology and nature of blue light and near-UV retinal lesions produced by laser and other optical sources. In Wolbarsht ML (ed): Laser Applications in Medicine and Biology, pp 227–228. New York, Plenum Press, 1989.

171. O'Steen WK, Shear CR, Anderson KV. Retinal damage after prolonged exposure to visible light. A light and electron microscopic study. Am J Anat 1972; 134:5–22.

172. Tso MOM. Photic maculopathy in rhesus monkey: A light and electron microscopic study. Invest Ophthalmol 1973; 12:17–34.

173. Ham WT, Jr, Ruffolo JJ, Jr, Mueller HA, Clarke AM, Moon ME. Histologic analysis of photochemical lesions produced in rhesus retina by short-wave-light. Invest Ophthalmol 1978; 17:1029–1035.

174. Penner R, McNair JN. Eclipse blindness. Am J Ophthalmol 1966; 61:1452–1457.

175. Kuwabara T. Retinal recovery from exposure to light. Am J Ophthalmol 1970; 70:187–198.

176. Farrer DN, Graham ES, Ham WT, Jr, Geeraets WJ, Williams RC, Mueller HA, Cleary SF, Clarke AM. The effect of threshold macular lesions and subthreshold macular exposures on visual acuity in the rhesus monkey. Am Ind Hyg Assoc J 1970; 31:198–205.

177. Moon ME, Clarke AM, Ruffolo JJ, Jr, Mueller HA, Ham WT, Jr. Visual performance in the rhesus monkey after exposure to blue light. Vision Res 1978; 1573–1577.

178. Sliney DH, Conover DL. Nonionizing radiation. In: Industrial Environmental Health. The Worker and the Community (2nd ed), pp 157–177. New York, Academic Press, 1975.

179. Ellis RJ, Moss CE, Parr WH. A Review of the Biological Effects of Infrared Radiation. Publication No. 82-109. Washington, DC, DHHS (NIOSH), 1982.

180. Pitts DG, Cullen AP, Dayhaw-Barker P. Determination of Ocular Threshold Levels for Infrared Radiation Cataractogenesis. Publication No. 80-121. Washington, DC, DHHS (NIOSH), 1980.

181. Pitts DG, Cullen AP. Determination of infrared radiation levels for acute ocular cataractogenesis. Graefes Arch Clin Exp Ophthalmol 1981; 217:285–297.

182. Pitts DG, Cameron LL, Jose JG, Lerman S, Moss E, Varma SD, Zigler S, Zigman S, Zuclich J. Optical radiation and cataracts. In Waxler M, Hitchins VM (eds): Optical Radiation and Visual Health, pp 6–36. Orlando, CRC Press, 1987.

183. Turner HS. The Interaction of Infrared Radiation with the Eye: A Review of the Literature. NSR Contract Report. Columbus, OH, The Aviation Research Laboratory, Ohio State University, 1970.

184. Lydahl E. Infrared radiation and cataract. Acta Ophthalmol Suppl 1984; 166:1–63.

185. Sliney DH. Biohazards of ultraviolet, visible, and infrared radiation. J Occup Med 1983; 25:203–210.

186. Cogan DG, Donaldson DD, Reese AB. Clinical and pathological characteristics of radiation cataract. Arch Ophthalmol 1952; 47:55–70.

187. Sliney DH, Freasier BC. Evaluation of optical radiation hazards. App Opt 1973; 12:1–24.

188. Dawson WW. Experimental ocular pathology related to corneal transmittance and infrared psychophysics. J Appl Physiol 1963; 18:1013–1016.

189. Fine BS, Fine S, Peacock GR, Geeraets WJ, Klein E. Preliminary observations on ocular effects of high-power continuous CO_2 laser irradiation. Am J Ophthalmol 1967; 64:209–222.

190. Fine BS, Fine S, Feigen L, MacKeen D. Corneal injury threshold to carbon dioxide laser irradiation. Am J Ophthalmol 1963; 66:1–14.

191. Mainster MA. Ophthalmic applications of infrared lasers—thermal considerations. Invest Ophthalmol Vis Sci 1979; 18:414–420.

192. Bargeron CB, McCalley RL, Farrell RA. Calculated and measured endothelial temperature histories of excised rabbit corneas exposed to infrared radiation. Exp Eye Res 1981; 32:241–250.

193. MacKeen D, Fine G, Feigen L, Fine BS. Anterior chamber measurements on CO_2 laser corneal irradiation. Invest Ophthalmol Vis Sci 1970; 9:366–371.

194. Prince JH. Spectral Absorption of the Retina and Choroid from 340 to 1700 nm. Publ. 14. Columbus, OH, Institute for Research in Vision, Ohio State University, 1982.

195. Fischer FP, Vermuelen D, Eymers JG. On the minimum quantity of ultraviolet and infrared light required for injury of the eye. Arch für Augen Helk 1935; 109:462–467.

196. Unger WG, Perkins ES, Bass MS. The response of the rabbit eye to laser irradiation of the iris. Exp Eye Res 1974; 19:367–377.

197. Bengtsson E. The inhibiting effect of indomethacin on the disruption of the blood-aqueous barrier in the rabbit eye. Invest Ophthalmol Vis Sci 1975; 14:306–313.

198. Bengtsson E. The effect of imidazole on the disruption of the blood-aqueous barrier in the rabbit eye. Invest Ophthalmol Vis Sci 1976; 15:315–320.

199. Bengtsson E. The effect of theophylline on the breakdown of the blood-aqueous barrier in the rabbit eye. Invest Ophthalmol Vis Sci 1977; 16:636–640.

200. Bengtsson E, Ehinger B. The effect of experimental uveitis on the uptake of prostaglandin. Acta Ophthalmol 1977; 55:688–695.

201. Meyenhofer W. Zur Aetiolgie des graven staars: Jugendliche kataraken bei glasmachern. Klin Monatsbl Augenheilk 1886; 24:49–67.

202. Vogt A. Einige Messungen der Diathermansie des menschlinchen Augapfels und seiner Medien, sowre des menschlichen Oberlides, nebst Bermerkugen zur biologischen Wirkung des Ultrarot. Arch für Ophthalmol 1912; 83:99–1131.

203. Vogt A. Fundamental investigations of the biology of infrared. Klin Monatsbl Augenheilk 1932; 89:256–258.

204. Goldmann H. Kritische und Experimentelle Untersuchungen uber den Sogenannen Ultrarotstar der Kaninchen und der Feverstar. Arch für Ophthalmol 1930; 125:313–402.

205. Goldmann H. Experimentelle Untersuchungen uber due Genese des Feverstarres: uber Arbeitshyperthermie bei Feverarbeiern. Arch für Ophthalmol 1932; 128:648–653.

206. Goldmann H. Genesis of heat cataract. Arch Ophthalmol 1933; 9:314.

207. Goldmann H. Experimentelle Untersuchungen uber due Genese des Feverstarres, I Teil. Arch für Ophthalmol 1933; 130:93–130.

208. Goldmann H. Experimentelle Untersuchungen uber due Genese des Feverstarres: die Physik des Feverstars, II Teil. Arch für Ophthalmol 1933; 130:93–130.

209. Goldmann H. Experimentelle Untersuchungen uber due Genese des Feverstarres: die Physik des Feverstars, III Teil. Arch für Ophthalmol 1933; 130:140–179.

210. Goldmann H. The origin of glassblowers cataract. Ann d'Ocul 1935; 172:13–41, Am J Ophthalmol 1935; 18:590–618.

211. Goldmann H, Konig H, Mader F. Die Durchlassigkeit der Auginlinse fur Infrarot. Ophthalmologica 1950; 120:198–205.

212. Langley RK, Mortimer CB, McCulloch C. The experimental production of cataracts by exposure to heat and light. Arch Ophthalmol 1960; 63:473–488.

213. Hager G, Pagel S, Broschmann D. Fire cataracts among locomotive firemen. Verk Med 1971; 18:443–449.

214. Ruth W, Levin M, Knave B. Occupational Hygiene Evaluation of Infrared Emitters for Drying Automobile Enamel. Study Report AMMP 104/76. Stockholm, 1976.

215. Edbrooke CM, Edwards C. Industrial radiation cataract: The hazards and the protective measures. Ann Occup Hyg 1967; 10:293–304.

216. Jacobson JH, Cooper B, Najac HW. Effects of thermal energy on retinal function. Technical Document Report No. AMRL-TDR-62-96. Life Support System Laboratory, Wright-Patterson Air Force Base, Ohio, 1962.

217. Legge TM. Home Office Report on Cataract in Glassworkers. Report of Medical Inspectors in Factories and Workshops. Annual Report for 1907, pp 250–254. London, HMSO, 1907.

218. Robinson W. Glassworkers' cataract. The Ophthalmolmoscope 1915; 13:538–554.

219. Dunn KL. Cataract from infrared rays (Glassworkers cataracts) AMA Arch Ind Hyg Occup Med 1950; 1:160–180.

220. Wallace J, Sweetnam PM, Warner CG, et al. An epidemiological study of lens opacities among steelworkers. Br J Ind Med 1971; 28:265–271.

221. Kurzel RB, Wolbarsh ML, Yamanashi BS. Spectral studies on normal and cataractous intact human lenses. Exp Eye Res 1973; 17:65–71.

222. Marcatonio JM, Duncan G, Davies PD, Bushell AR. Classification of human senile cataracts by nuclear colour and sodium content. Exp Eye Res 1980; 31:227–237.

223. Lydahl E, Philipson B. Infrared radiation and Ophthalmol, I. Epidemiological investigation of iron- and steelworkers. Acta Ophthalmol 1984; 62:961–975.

224. Lydahl E, Glansholm A, Levin M. Ocular exposure to infrared radiation in the Swedish iron and steel industry. Health Phys 1984; 46:529–536.

225. Lydahl E, Glansholm A. Infrared radiation and cataract, III. Differences between the two eyes of glassworkers. Acta Ophthalmol 1985; 63:39–44.

226. Geeraets WJ, Ridgeway D. Retinal damage from high intensity light. Acta Ophthalmol Suppl 1963; 76:109–112.

227. Johnstone IL. Familial cataract with extensive pedigree chart. Br J Ophthalmol 1947; 31:385–395.

228. Francois J. Genetics of cataract. Ophthalmology 1982; 184:61–71.

229. Chou BR. Retinal protection from solar photic injury. Am J Optom Physiol Opt 1981; 58:270–280.

230. Goldman AL, Ham WT, Jr, Mueller AH. Ocular damage thresholds and mechanisms for ultrashort pulses of both visible and infrared laser radiation in the Rhesus monkey. Exp Eye Res 1977; 24:45–56.

231. Roulier A. Calculation of temperature increase in the eye produced by intense light. Bull Math Biophys 1970; 32:403–427.

232. Ham WT, Mueller HA, Williams RC, Geeraets WJ. Ocular hazard from viewing the sun unprotected and through various windows and filters. Appl Opt 1973; 12:2122–2129.

233. White TJ, Mainster MA, Tips JH, Wilson PW. Chorioretinal thermal behavior. Bull Math Biophys 1970; 32:315–322.

234. Ham WT, Jr, Mueller HA, Ruffolo JJ, Jr, Clarke AM. Sensitivity of the retina to radiation damage as a function of wavelength. Photochem Photobiol 1979; 29:735–743.

235. Wheeler CB. Calculation of retinal temperature distributions resulting from laser irradiation of the eye: Continuous Lasers. Phys Med Bio 1976; 21:616–630.

236. Bredemeyer HG, Wiegmann OA, Bredemeyer A, Blackwell HR. Radiation thresholds for chorioretinal burns. Technical Documentary Report No. AMRL-TDR-63-71. 6570th Aerospace Medical Research Laboratories, Wright-Patterson Air Force Base, Ohio, 1963.

237. Geeraets WJ, Berry ER. Ocular spectral characteristics as related to hazards from lasers and other light sources. Am J Ophthalmol 1968; 66:15–20.

238. Assenheim HM, Hill DA, Preston E, Cairne AB. The Biological Effects of Radio-frequency and Microwave Radiation. NRCC No. 16448. Ottawa, Canada, National Research Council Canada, 1979.

239. Radiofrequency (RF) Sealers and Heaters: Potential Health Hazards and Their Prevention. NIOSH/OSHA Current Intelligence Bulletin 33. Washington, DC, U.S. Department of Health, Education and Welfare, National Institute for Occupational Safety and Health Administration, December 1979.

240. Aurell E, Tengroth B. Lenticular and retinal changes secondary to microwave exposure. Acta Ophthalmol 1973; 51:764–771.

241. Dailey LE, Wakim KG, Herrick JF, Parkhill EM. The effects of microwave diathermy on eye. An experimental study. Am J Ophthalmol 1950; 33:1241–1254.

242. Richardson AW, Duane TD, Hines HM. Experimental cataract produced by 3 centimeter pulsed microwave irradiations. Arch Ophthalmol 1951; 45:382–386.

243. Microwave Hazards Bibliography. U.S. Army Environmental Hygiene Agency, Edgewood Arsenal, Maryland, 1967.

244. Michaelson SM. Effects of exposure to microwaves: Problems and perspectives. Environ Health Perspect 1974; 8:133–156.

245. Czerski P, Ostrowski K, Shore ML, Silverman V, Suess MJ, Waldeskog B, Shalwon E (eds): International Symposium on Biologic Effects and Health Hazards of

Microwave Radiation. The World Health Organization, U.S. Department of Health, Education and Welfare, Scientific Council to the Minister of Health and Social Welfare of Poland. Warsaw, Polish Medical Publishers, 1974.

246. Michaelson SM, Miller MW, Magin R, Carstensen EL (eds): Fundamental and Applied Aspects of Nonionizing Radiation. New York, Plenum Press, 1975.

247. Hazzard DG (ed): Symposium on Biological Effects and Measurement of Radio Frequency/Microwaves. HEW Publication (FDA) 77-8026. Rockville, MD, U.S. Department of Health, Education and Welfare, 1977.

248. Chou CK, Guy AW. Quantitation of microwave biological effects. In Hazzard DG (ed): Symposium on Biological Effects and Measurement of Radio Frequency/Microwave. HEW Publication (FDA) 77-8026. U.S. Department of Health, Education and Welfare, 1977.

249. Wilkening GM. Biomedical effects of microwave radiation. Bull NY Acad Med 1979; 55:1126–1132.

250. Hazards of Microwave Radiation and Radiation Levels Derived Therefrom. Report 66E. Leischendam, The Netherlands. The Health Council of the Netherlands, Ministry of Health and Environmental Protection, 1979.

251. Milroy WC, Michaelson SM. Biologic effects of microwave radiation. Health Phy 1971; 20:567–575.

252. Carpenter RL. Ocular effects of microwave radiation. Bull NY Acad Med 1979; 55:1048–1057.

253. Castren J, Lauteala L, Antere E, Aho J, Torvi K. On microwave exposure. Acta Ophthalmol (Copenh) 1982; 60:647–654.

254. Bollemeijer JC, Lagendijk JJW, van Best JA, de Leeuw AAC, van Delft JL, de Wolff-Rouendaal D, Oosterhuis JA, Schipper JJW. Effects of microwave-induced hyperthermia on the anterior segment of healthy rabbit eyes. Graefe's Arch Clin Exp Ophthalmol 1989; 227:271–276.

255. Williams RJ, Finch ED. Examination of the cornea following exposure to microwave radiation. Aerospace Med 1974; 45:393–396.

256. Hagan GJ, Carpenter RL. Relative cataractogenic potencies of two microwave frequencies 2.45 and 10 GHz. In Johnson CC, Shore ML (eds): Biological Effects of Electromagnetic Waves. HEW Publication (FDA) 77-8010, pp 143–155. Boulder, CO, U.S. Department of Health, Education and Welfare, 1976.

257. Carpenter RL, Van Ummersen CA. The action of microwave power on the eye. J Microw Power 1968; 3:3–19.

258. Birenbaum L, Kaplan IT, Metlay W, et al. Effect of microwaves on the rabbit eye. J Microw Power 1969; 4:232–243.

259. Rosenthal SW, Birenbaum L, Kaplan IT, Metlay W, Snyder WZ, Zaret MM. Effects of 35 and 107 GHz CW microwaves on the rabbit eye. In Johnson CC, Shore ML (eds): Biological Effects of Electromagnetic Waves. HEW Publication (FDA) 77-8010, pp 110–128. Boulder, U.S. Department of Health, Education and Welfare, 1976.

260. Appelton B, Hirsch SE, Brown PVK. Investigation of single-exposure microwave ocular effects at 3000 MHz. Ann NY Acad Sci 1975; 247:125–134.

261. Cohen R. Radiofrequency and microwave radiation in the microelectronics industry. Occup Med 1986; 1:145–154.

262. Carpenter RL, Biddle DK, Van Ummersen CA. Opacities in the lens of the eye experimentally induced by exposure to microwave radiation. IRE Trans Med Electr 1960; ME-7:152–157.

263. Carpenter RL, Biddle DK, Van Ummersen CA. Biological Effects of Microwave Radiation, with Particular Reference to the Eye. Third International Conference on Medical Electronics. OP-401-408. London, HMSO, 1960.

264. Carpenter RL, Hagan GJ, Ferri ES. Use of a dielectric lens for experimental microwave irradiation of the eye. Ann NY Acad Sci 1975; 247:142–154.

265. Van Ummersen CA, Cogan FC. Effects of microwave radiation on the lens epithelium in the rabbit eye. Arch Ophthalmol 1976; 94:828–834.

266. Foster MR, Ferri ES, Hagan GJ. Dosimetric study of microwave cataractogenesis. Bioelectromagnetics 1986; 7:129–140.

267. Chon CK, Guy AW, Borneman LE, Kunz LL, Kramar P. Chronic exposure of rabbits to 0.5 and 5 mW/cm^2 2450-MHz CW microwave. Bioelectromagnetics 1983; 4:63–77.

268. Guy AW, Harris C, Kramer PO, Emery AF. Study of effects of chronic low level microwave radiation on rabbits. 1976 IMPI Symposium Summaries. J Microw Power Electromagn Energy 1976; 11:134–135.

269. McRee DI. Thresholds for lenticular damage in the rabbit eye due to single exposure to CW microwave radiation: An analysis of the experimental information at a frequency of 2.45 GHz. Health Phys 1971; 21:763–769.

270. Kramar P, Harris C, Emery AF, Guy AW. Acute microwave irradiation and cataract formation in rabbits and monkeys. J Microw Power 1978; 13:239–249.

271. Lubin M. Effects of ultrahigh frequency radiation on animals. Arch Ind Health 1960; 21:555.

272. Addington C. Review of work conducted at the University of Buffalo. Studies on the biological effects of 200 mc. In Proceedings of Second Annual Tri-Service Conference on Biological Effects of Microwave Energy. RADC-TR-54, Rome, NY, Rome Air Development Command, 1958.

273. Michaelson SM, Thomson RAE, Howland JW. Physiological aspects of microwave irradiation of mammals. Am J Physiol 1961; 201:351.

274. Michaelson SM, Howland JW, Deichmann WB. Response of the dog to 24,000 and 1285 MHz microwave exposure. ASTIA Doc No. AD 824-242. Rome Air Development Center, Griffis Air Force Base, Rome, New York, 1967.

275. Williams DB, Monaham JP, Nicholson WJ, Aldrich JJ. Biologic effects studies on microwave radiation. Arch Ophthalmol 1955; 54:863.

276. Creighton MO, Larsen LE, Stewart-Dettaan PJ, Jacobi JH, Samual M, Baskerville JC, Bassen HE, Brown DO, Trevithick JR. In vitro studies of microwave-induced cataract, II. Comparison of damage observed for continuous wave and pulsed microwaves. Exp Eye Res 1987; 45:357–373.

277. Stewart-de Haan PJ, Creighton MO, Larsen LE, Jacobi JH, Ross WH, Sanwal M, Guo TC, Guo WW, Trevithick JR. In vitro studies of microwave-induced cataracts: Separation of field and heating effects. Exp Eye Res 1983; 36:75–90.

278. Stewart-de Haan PJ, Creighton MO, Larsen LE, Jacobi JH, Sanwal M, Baskerville JC, Trevithick JR. In vitro studies of microwave-induced cataract: Reciprocity between exposure duration and dose rate for pulsed microwaves. Exp Eye Res 1985; 40:1–13.

279. Merola LO, Kinoshita JH. Changes in the ascorbic acid content in lenses of rabbit eyes exposed to microwave radiation. Proceedings of Fourth Annual Tri-Service Conference on Biological Effects of Microwave Radiation, pp 285–291. New York, Plenum Press, 1961.

280. Oosta GM, Mathewson NS. Effects of high-power density microwave on the soluble proteins of the rabbit lens. Invest Ophthalmol Vis Sci 1979; 18:391–400.

281. Paulsson LE, Hamnerius Y, Hansson HA, Sjostrand J. Retinal damage experimentally induced by microwave radiation at 55 mW/cm^2. Acta Ophthalmol (Copenh) 1979; 57:183–197.

282. Hirsch GF, Parker JT. Bilateral lenticular opacities occurring in a technician operating a microwave generator. Arch Ind Hyg 1952; 6:512–517.

283. Kurz GH, Einaugler RB. Cataract secondary to microwave radiation. Am J Ophthalmol 1968; 66:866–869.

284. Minecki L. The health of persons exposed to the effect of high frequency electromagnetic fields. Medycyna Pracy (Poland) 1961; 12:337–344.

285. Shimkovich IS, Shilyayev VG. Cataract of both eyes which developed as a result of repeated short exposures to an electromagnetic field of high density. Vestn Oftamol 1959; 72:12–19.

286. Barron CI, Baraff AA. Medical considerations of exposure to microwaves (radar). JAMA 1958; 168:1194–1199.

287. Clark LA, Jr. Eye study survey. In Proceedings of Third Annual Tri-Service Conference on Biological Effects of Microwave Radiating Equipment, University of California, Berkeley. RADC-TR-59-140, Rome Air Development Center, Griffis Air Force Base, Rome, New York, 1959.

288. Majewska K. Investigations on the effect of microwaves on the eye. Polish Med J 1968; VII:989–994.

289. La Roche LP, Zaret MJ, Braun AF. An operational safety program for ophthalmic hazards for microwave. Arch Environ Health 1970; 20:350–355.

290. Appleton B, McCrossan CG. Microwave lens effects in humans. Arch Ophthalmol 1972; 88:259–262.

291. Odland LT. Observations on microwave hazards to USAF personnel. J Occup Med 1972; 544–547.

292. Appleton B, Hirsch S, Kinion RO, Soles EM, McCrossan GC, Neidlinger RM. Microwave lens effects in humans: Results of a five-year survey. Arch Ophthalmol 1975; 93:257–258.

293. Shackett DE, Tredici TJ, Epstein DL. Evaluation of possible microwave-induced lens changes in the United States Air Force. Aviat Space Environ Med 1975; 1403–1406.

294. Hathaway JA, Stern N, Soles EM, Leighton E. Ocular medical surveillance on microwave and laser workers. J Occup Med 1977; 19:683–688.

295. Cogan DG, Fricker SJ, Lubin M, et al. Cataracts and ultra-high-frequency radiation. AMA Arch Ind Health 1958; 18:299–302.

296. Tengroth B, Aurell B. Retinal changes in microwave workers. In Czerski P, Silvermen C, Ostrowski K, Shore ML, Suess ML, Shalmon E (eds): Biologic Effects and Health Hazards of Microwave Radiation. Proceedings of an International Conference, pp 302–305. Warsaw, Polish Medical Publishers, 1974.

297. Roberts NJ, Jr, Michaelson SM. Epidemiologic studies of human exposures to radiofrequency radiation. Int Arch Occup Environ Health 1985; 56:169–178.

298. Milroy WC, Michaelson SM. Microwave cataractogenesis: A critical review of the literature. Aerospace Med 1972; 43:67–75.

299. Schwan HP, Li K. Hazards due to total body irradiation by radar. Proc IRE 1956; 44:1572.

300. American National Standards. Safety Levels with Respect to Human Exposure. ANSI C95.1-1982. New York, American National Standards Institute, Inc, 1982.

301. Nuclear Radiation Guide. Report No. MRL-TDR-62-61. Aerospace Medical Division, Aerospace Medical Research Laboratories, Wright-Patterson Air Force Base, Ohio, 1962.

302. Buchanan AR, Heim HC, Krauschaar JJ. Biomedical Effects of Exposure to Electromagnetic Radiation, Part II. Biomedical Effects on the Eye from Exposure to Microwaves and Ionizing Radiation. ASD Technical Report 61-195. Aerospace Medical Laboratory, Air

Force Systems Command, Wright-Patterson Air Force Base, Ohio, 1961.

303. Biegel AC. Experimental ocular effects of high-voltage radiation from the betatron. AMA Arch Ophthalmol 1955; 54:392–406.

304. Simkova M, Prouza Z. Study of the innervation of the cornea after different physical noxious effects, I. Analysis of the problems and methods. Acta Univ Carol [Med] (Praha) 1982; 28:3–24.

305. Simkova M. Study of the innervation of the cornea after different physical noxious effects, II. Effects of ionizing radiation. Acta Univ Carol [Med] (Praha) 1982; 28:25–57.

306. Simkova M. Study of the innervation of the cornea after different physical noxious effects, III. Comparison of effects of ionizing radiation with thermal and mechanical factors. Acta Univ Carol [Med] (Praha) 1982; 28:59–86.

307. Cogan DG, Donaldson DD. Experimental radiation cataracts, 1. Cataracts in the rabbit following single x-ray exposure. AMA Arch Ophthalmol 1951; 45:508–522.

308. Cibis PA, Noell WK, Eichel B. Ocular effects produced by high intensity x-radiation. AMA Arch Ophthalmol 1955; 53:651–663.

309. Hayes BP, Fisher RF. Influence of a prolonged period of low-dosage x-rays on the optic and ultrastructal appearances of cataract of the human lens. Br J Ophthalmol 1979; 63:457–464.

310. Cogan DG, Dreisler KK. Minimal amount of x-ray exposure causing lens opacities in the human eye. AMA Arch Ophthalmol 1953; 30–34.

311. Cogan DG, Donaldson DD, Reese AB. Clinical and pathologic characteristics of radiation cataract. AMA Arch Ophthalmol 1952; 47:55–70.

312. von Sallman L. Early lenticular lesions resulting from ionizing radiation. Trans Am Acad Ophthalmol 1959; 63:439–448.

313. Pirie A, Flanders PH. Effect of x-rays on partially shielded lens of rabbit. AMA Arch Ophthalmol 1957; 57:849–854.

314. Becker B, Constant MA, Cibis PA, Tergossian M. The effect of moderate doses on X-ray radiation on ocular tissue. Am J Ophthalmol 1956; 42:51–57.

315. von Sallman L. Experimental studies on early lens changes after roentgen irradiation, III. Effects of x-radiation on mitotic activity and nuclear fragmentation of lens epithelium in normal and cystein-treated rabbits. Arch Ophthalmol 1952; 47:305–320.

316. Leinfelder PJ, Kerr HD. Roentgen-ray cataract. An experimental clinical and microscopic study. Am J Ophthalmol 1936; 19:739–756.

317. Lipman RM, Tripathi BJ, Tripathi RC. Cataracts induced by microwave and ionizing radiation. Surv Ophthalmol 1988; 33:200–210.

318. Cogan DG. Lesions of the eye from radiant energy. JAMA 1950; 142:145–151.

319. Hunt HB. Cancer of the eyelid treated by radiation with consideration of irradiation cataract. Am J Roentgenol 1947; 57:160–180.

320. Brown DVL, Cibis PL, Pickering JE. Radiation studies on the monkey eye, 1. Effects of gamma radiation on the retina. Arch Ophthalmol 1955; 54:249–256.

321. von Sallman L, Tobias CA, Anger HO, Welch C, Kimura SF, Munoz CM, Drungis A. Effects of high-energy particles, x-rays, and aging on lens epithelium. Arch Ophthalmol 1955; 54:489–514.

322. von Sallman LC, Munoz CM, Drungis A. The effects of beta radiation on the rabbits eye. Arch Ophthalmol 1953; 50:727–736.

323. Shaffer RN. Alpha irradiation. Effect of astatine on the anterior segment and on epithelial cysts. Trans Am Ophthalmol Soc 1952; 50:607–627.

324. Shaffer RN. Alpha irradiation. Effect of astatine on the anterior segment and on an epithelial cyst. Am J Ophthalmol 1954; 37:183–196.

325. Cogan DG, Coff JL, Graves E. Experimental radiation cataract, II. Cataract in the rabbit following single exposure to fast neutrons. AMA Arch Ophthalmol 1952; 47:584–592.

326. Upton AC, Christenberry KW, Melville GS, Furth J, Hurst GS. The relative biological effectiveness of neutrons; X-rays and gamma rays for the production of lens opacities on mice, rats, guinea pigs, and rabbits. Radiology 1956; 67:686–696.

327. Evans TC. Effects of small daily doses of fast neutrons on mice. Radiology 1948; 50:811–834.

328. Cogan DG, Donaldson DD, Goff JJ, Graves E. Experimental radiation cataract, III. Further experimental studies on x-ray and neutron irradiation of the lens. Arch Ophthalmol 1953; 50:597–602.

329. Riley EF, Leinfelder PJ, Evans TC, Rhody RD. Relative cataractogenic effectiveness of fast neutron radiation from different sources. Radiat Res 1955; 3:342.

330. Cogan DG, Goff JL, Graves E. Experimental radiation cataract, II. Cataract in the rabbit following single exposure fast neutrons. Arch Ophthalmol 1952; 47:584–592.

331. Lipetz LE. The x-ray and radium phosphores. Br J Ophthalmol 1955; 39:577–597.

332. Kent SP, Swanson AA. Effects of high intensity x-irradiation on the retina. A histological, histochemical and chemical study in the rabbit. Publication No. 56-85. Air University School of Aviation Medicine, Randolph Air Force Base, Texas, 1956.

333. Furcinitti PS, Todd P. Gamma rays: Further evidence for lack of a threshold dose for lethality to human cells. Science 1979; 206:475–476.

334. Rydin RA. Gamma rays and the concept of a threshold dose. Science 1980; 210:806.

335. Le Page JJ. Gamma rays and the concept of a threshold dose. Science 1980; 210:806.

336. Cheever CL. Ionizing radiation—its safety aspects. National Safety News September 1980, pp 55–60.

337. Baum G, Greenwood I. Ultrasound in Ophthalmology. Am J Ophthalmol 1960; 49:249–261.

338. Baum G, Greenwood I. Orbital lesion localization by three dimensional ultrasonography. NY State J Med 1961; 61:4149–4157.

339. Baum G, Greenwood I. Ultrasonography—an aid in orbital tumor diagnosis. Arch Ophthalmol 1960; 180–194.

340. Lowe RF. Linear A-scan ultrasonography in the measurement of intra-ocular distances: A stand-off technique. Trans Ophthalmol Soc Aust 1967; XXVI:72–77.

341. Young FA, Leary GA. Ultrasound and phakometry measurements of the primate eye. Am J Optom Arch Am Acad Optom 1966; 43:370–386.

342. Jansson F. Measurements of intraocular distances by ultrasound. Acta Ophthalmol Suppl (Copenh) 1963; 74:1–51.

343. Kelman CD. Phacoemulsification and aspiration: A new technique of cataract removal: A preliminary report. Am J Ophthalmol 1967; 64:23–35.

344. Kelman CD. Phacoemulsification and aspiration of senile cataracts: A comparative study with intracapsular extraction. Can J Ophthalmol 1973; 8:24–32.

345. Kelman CD. Phacoemulsification: Summary of personal experience. Trans Am Acad Ophthalmol Otolaryngol 1974; 78:35–38.

346. Baum G. The effect of ultrasonic radiation upon the eye and ocular adnexa. Am J Ophthalmol 1956; 42:696–706.

347. Aristarkhova AA, Nuritoinov VA. The effect of ultrasound on corneal permeability. Vestn Oftalmol 1974; 90:46–48.

348. Ziskin MC, Romayananda N, Harri K. Ophthalmic effect of ultrasound at diagnostic intensities. J Clin Ultrasound 1974; 2:119–122.

349. Olson LE, Marshall J, Rice NSC, Andrews R. Effects of ultrasound on the corneal endothelium, I. The acute lesion. Brit J Ophthalmol 1978; 62:134–144.

350. Pool R. Electromagnetic fields: The biological evidence. Science 249; 199:1378–1381.

351. Armstrong RA, Janday B. A brief overview of magnetic fields from the human visual system. Ophthalmol Physiol Opt 1989; 9:298–301.

352. Katila T, Maniewski R, Poutanen T, et al. Magnetic fields produced by the human eye. J Appl Physiol 1981; 52:2565–2571.

353. Ikeda H. Retinal mechanisms and the clinical electroretinogram. In Halliday AM, Butler SR, Paul R (eds): A Textbook of Clinical Neurophysiology, p 569. Chichester, UK, John Wiley and Sons, 1987.

354. Brenner D, Williamson SJ, Kaufman L. Visually evoked magnetic fields in the human brain. Science 1975; 190:480.

355. Janday BS, Swithenby SJ, Thomas IM. Investigation of pattern reversal response by combined MEG and EEG measurement (Abstr). Electroencephalogr Clin Neurophysiol 1988; 70:132P.

356. Okada Y. Visual evoked fields. In Biomagnetism. An Interdisciplinary Approach, pp 443–459. NATO-ASI Series, 1982.

357. Beischer DE. Human tolerance to magnetic fields. Astronautics 1962; 24–25, 46–48.

358. Peterson F, Kennelly AE. Physiological experiments with magnets at the Edison Laboratory. NY Med J 1892; 56:729–732.

359. Barnothy TM. Biological effects of magnetic fields. In Glasser O (ed): Medical Physics, Vol III. Chicago, Year Book Publishers, Inc, 1960.

360. Eiselen TE, Bowtell HM, Biggs NW. Biological effects of magnetic fields—negative results. Aerospace Med 1961; 32:383–386.

361. Liboff AR, Williams T, Jr, Strong DM, Wistar R, Jr. Time-varying magnetic fields: Effect on DNA synthesis. Science 1984; 223:818–820.

362. Raybourn MS. The effects of direct-current magnetic fields on turtle retinas in vitro. Science 1983; 715–717.

363. Goodman R, Bassett CAL, Henderson AS. Pulsing electromagnetic fields induce cellular transcription. Science 1983; 220:1283–1285.

364. Sheppard AR, Eisenbud M. Biologic Effects of Electric and Low Magnetic Fields of Extremely Low Frequency. New York, New York University Press, 1977.

365. Wilson BW, Chess EK, Anderson LE. 60-Hz electric-field effects on pineal melatonin rhythms: Time course for onset and recovery. Bioelectromagnetics 1986; 7:239–242.

366. Modan B. Exposure to electromagnetic fields and brain malignancy: A newly discovered menace? Am J Ind Med 1988; 13:625–627.

367. Coleman NP, Bell CM, Taylor HL, Primic-Zakelj M. Leukemia and residence near electricity transmission equipment: A case-control study. Br J Cancer 1989; 60:793–798.

368. Cartwright RA. Low frequency alternating electromagnetic fields and leukemia: The saga so far. Br J Cancer 1989; 60:649–651.

369. Bordeur P. The magnetic-field menace. MACWORLD July 1990; 136–145.

370. Hermann L. Hat das magnetische Feld direkte physiologische Wirkungen? Pflugers Arch 1888; 43:217–237.

371. Rohracher H. Uber subjektive Lichterschienungen bei Reizung mit Wechselstromen. Z Sinnesphysiol 1935; 66:164–181.

372. Frankenhauser F. Uber einen neuen Versuch zur Einfuhrung des Magneten in die Therapie. Diat Physik Ther 1902; 6:52–55.

373. Magnusson CE, Stevens HC. Visual sensations caused by magnetic fields. Phil Mag 1914; 28:188–207.

374. Flieschman L. Gesundheitsschadlichkeit der Magnet-Wechselfelder. Naturwissenchaften 1922; 10:434.

375. Lovsund P, Oberg PÅ, Nilsson SEG. Influence on vision of extremely low frequency electromagnetic fields. Acta Ophthalmol (Copenh) 1979; 57:812–821.

376. Basu PK. Effect of electric and magnetic fields on cornea. Indian J Ophthalmol 1987; 35:119–121.

377. Seegal RF, Wolpan JR, Dowman R. Chronic exposure of primates to 60 Hz electric and magnetic fields, II.

Neurochemical effects. Bioelectromagnetics 1989; 10:289–301.

378. Dowman R, Wolpan JR, Seegal RF, Savta-Murti S. Chronic exposure of primates to 60 Hz electric and magnetic fields: Neurophysiologic effects. Bioelectromagnetics 1989; 10:303–317.

379. Olcese J, Reuss S, Stehle J, Steinlechner S, Vollrath L. Responses of the mammalian retina to experimental alteration of the ambient magnetic field. Brain Res 1988; 448:325–330.

CHAPTER SEVEN

Lasers in Industry and the Clinic

Donald G. Pitts, O.D., Ph.D.

The term *laser* is an acronym for the words *l*ight *a*mplification from *s*timulated *e*mitted *r*adiation. When Theodore H. Maiman achieved success in pulsing the ruby rod, a laboratory curiosity was born that possessed the theoretical potential to revolutionize industry. The initial laser was a ruby crystal with a wavelength of 694.3 nm, but advances in applied physics have shown that lasting materials extend to dyes, gases, and semiconductors. The wavelength range of the laser has been extended in bandwidth by gas and dye lasers and covers almost the entire optical spectrum.

This chapter will cover the technical aspects and clinical uses of lasers with emphasis on the vision care field. It is not intended to be a definitive work but instead will provide sufficient technical information to allow an understanding of the basic scientific concepts governing lasers and their clinical usage in the vision health care fields.

Table 7-1 lists 16 uses of the laser in industry and health care. Most of us are familiar with the user of the laser and fiber optics in modern telephone systems. It has been stated that more information can be encoded into a laser beam than is contained in the entire Bell Telephone system of today! Photochromics and lasers are being applied to the computer, and assures computation times shorter than present-day computers. Printing plates, typesetting, graphic arts, and facsimile machines have all used the laser to increase production and to improve the quality of the product. Circuit welding and circuit board production use the ultraviolet (UV) lasers to produce precision parts for the electronic industry. UV lasers produce smaller chips and more precise circuitry for the computer. Research is now underway that will replace the UV laser with X-rays. Little needs to be said about optics, ranging, and guidance because of the recent demonstrations of the accuracy with

Communications	Surveying
Computers	Welding/Drilling
Electronics	Health care
Graphic arts	Dermatology
Guidance	Oncology
Optics	Ophthalmology
Ranging	Optometry
Research	Surgery

TABLE 7-1
Some Present-Day Uses of the Laser

which these technologies delivered "smart weapons" during the recent United States–Iraq conflict.

The use of lasers in health care began in the 1960s but has progressed steadily. As a more thorough understanding of the absorption characteristics of biologic systems and their responses to laser exposure is gained, the laser will assume an ever-increasing position of importance. It is not beyond technology to produce a laser "surgical knife" that opens the abdomen for an appendectomy and "welds" the abdomen together on completion of the surgical procedure—without the loss of blood.

7.1 Laser Theory

Light is produced by electron transitions from a higher energy state to a lower energy state, by heat that creates vibrations and rotational molecular modes, by energy absorption as in the luminescent

paint on a watch dial from photons, and by chemical reactions such as the flame from a log. These changes or transitions occur randomly and produce photons that are noncoherent, i.e., the light that we are accustomed to from the incandescent filament and sunlight. The electron transitions of the laser are stimulated by the precisely correct energy, and the stimulated emissions are of the same wavelength, the same phase, propagated in the same direction, and highly collimated. These characteristics of the laser beam produce what is termed *coherence*.

The laser consists of three major components: (1) the lasing material, which may be a solid, liquid, or gas; (2) a pumping system, which may be optical, electric, or chemical and provides the energy required to lase the material; and (3) the optical cavity that contains the lasing material and is bounded by mirrors placed at each end of the cavity. The mirror at one end is a full reflector and the mirror at the other end is partially reflecting, with the laser beam being emitted through the partially reflecting mirror.[1,2]

7.2 Laser Operation

The pumping system supplies energy to the laser material (Fig. 7-1). The energy is absorbed by the laser material, resulting in the orbital electrons achieving an excited energy level that spontaneously decays without producing radioactivity to a metastable energy level. The storage of electrons in the higher energy state at the metastable level[1-4] sets up a condition known as *population inversion,* in which

FIGURE 7-1
Diagram of the energy changes in the outer-shell orbital electrons for a three-level energy laser system. Energy levels allow the metastable energy state to produce a population inversion and results in the subsequent lasing. *From* Weber MJ (ed). CRC Handbook of Laser Science and Technology, Boca Raton, FL, CRC Press, 1991.

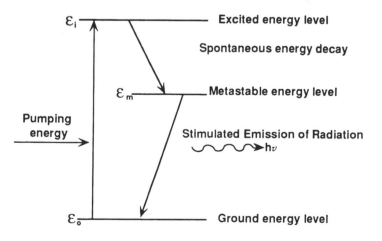

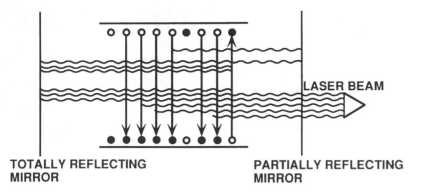

FIGURE 7-2
Photons oscillate between the laser cavity mirrors recruiting photons. The number of photons increases until they are emitted through the partially reflecting mirror as a laser beam. *From* Weber MJ (ed). CRC Handbook of Laser Science and Technology. Boca Raton, FL, CRC Press, 1991.

more electrons are excited to a higher energy level than remain at ground energy level. When a population inversion is achieved, the spontaneous decay of electrons from the metastable energy level to a lower energy level initiates a chain reaction. Photons are emitted that spontaneously stimulate other electrons to complete the transition from the metastable energy level to lower energy levels. The photons are reflected back and forth through the laser material where the chain reaction continues to increase the number of photons. Some of the photons arriving at the partially reflecting mirror are reflected, but many escape to constitute the laser beam (Fig. 7-2), a beam that is the same phase, same wavelength, in phase, highly collimated, and in the same direction, and said to be coherent.

7.3 Laser Beam Characteristics

Spatial Modes

The mode structure of a laser refers to the direction of energy accumulation within the laser cavity. The transverse mode describes the distribution of energy in the laser beam in a direction perpendicular to the long dimension of the laser cavity. Transverse mode laser beams are limited in coherence and in the diameter of the beam when focused. Longitudinal modes result from multiple harmonic oscillations along the length of the laser cavity that produce a wavelength and frequency that differ from the main wavelength.

Laser beams produce wave patterns that are transverse to their direction of propagation. The transverse electromagnetic wave patterns are identi-fied by the acronym TEM and mode numbers such as TEM_{00}. Figure 7-3 illustrates only four TEM modes but will serve to establish the significance of different TEM patterns. TEM_{00} mode results in a single spot that possesses the total power of the laser beam and is used to establish the divergence and diameter of the beam. TEM_{01} and TEM_{10} show two laser beams that are identical except for a 90° rotation. They can be considered as two lasers operating side-by-side with each beam possessing one half the power of the total laser beam. Each of the four beams in TEM_{11} possesses one fourth the power of the total beam of TEM_{00}.

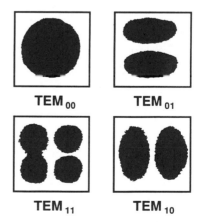

TEM$_{00}$ TEM$_{01}$

TEM$_{11}$ TEM$_{10}$

FIGURE 7-3
Diagram illustrating the transverse electromagnetic spatial modes (TEM) of the laser beam for four different beam cross sections. The TEM subscript numbers can be as high as 33. *From* Weber MJ (ed). CRC Handbook of Laser Science and Technology. Boca Raton, FL, CRC Press, 1991.

The longitudinal mode influences the frequency and degree of coherency of the laser beam. Both the frequency and the degree of coherency depend on the length of the laser cavity such that the wavelength interval is equal to the wavelength squared, divided by twice the distance between the laser cavity mirrors ($\lambda^2/2$ L).

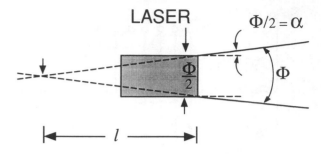

FIGURE 7-4
Divergence of the laser beam. The apparent origin of the laser beam is at a distance 1 from the front mirror of the laser. The angle ϕ represents the full angle of divergence and α the half-angle of divergence.[19]

Diameter of the Laser Beam

The diameter of the laser beam is measured at the exit aperture of the laser cavity with the laser operating in the TEM_{00} mode. The edge of the laser beam is defined as the circle where the power density of the laser beam is ½, $1/e$, or $1/e^2$ of the maximum power density that is assumed to occur at the center of the beam. The diameter of the laser beam has also been defined as a circle that contains 90% of the power or energy of the beam. The diameter must be clearly defined and provided for safe calculation evaluations to be valid.

Divergence of the Laser Beam

Lasers cannot produce a perfectly collimated beam; however, the beam divergence is much less than any known source of radiant energy. The beam diameter is determined by operating the laser in the TEM_{00} mode and defining the edge of the beam. Beam divergence increases with the distance from exit aperture of the laser cavity. The full beam divergence is expressed as ϕ or as the half-angle α (Figure 7-4).

Temporal Modes

The laser beam operates in several time modes. Continuous wave (CW) lasers have a constant output over time and require external timing systems to control "on" and "off." The atoms of the CW laser constantly repeat the energy levels of the laser and continuously emit radiation. Examples of CW lasers are the argon, krypton, CO_2, and Nd:YAG lasers.

The pulsed or long-pulsed operation (PW or P) results when the lasing material is pumped by xenon flash lamps. The duration of the pulse is determined by the duration of the xenon lamp and the laser

materials but is usually in the millisecond range. Examples of the pulsed laser are the ruby crystal and the Nd:glass lasers.

The Q-switched laser contains an electro-optical shutter of acusto-optical crystals that has a plane of polarization perpendicular to the plane of polarization of the laser beam within the laser medium (Fig. 7-5).[17] A short-duration electric voltage pulse is provided to the crystal that rotates its polarization 90°. This shift in polarization of the Q-switched shutter allows the laser beam to pass through the shutter to oscillate within the optical cavity producing the laser beam. A Q-switched laser beam usually lasts from 10 to 30 ns. The "Q" refers to the resonant quality of the laser optical cavity. A Q-switched laser delivers less total energy than a normal laser but the energy is delivered in a short period of time, which results in very high peak powers in the mega- and gigawatt ranges.

The phase or mode-locking shutter is a photovoltaic cell that contains a thin layer of photosensitive dyes (Fig. 7-6). The mode-locking shutter may be placed near the totally reflecting or partially reflecting mirror within the laser cavity. As stimulated emissions recruit more and more photons, the dye is bleached allowing a single pulse of the laser beam to be released. The mode-locking shutter recovers in 4 to 5 ps and repeats the process. The result is a train of laser beam pulses that are 30 to 100 ps in duration separated by 4 to 5 ps for shutter recovery. Mode-locking lasers are usually 1 m or longer to permit cancellation and reinforcement of the harmonic modes in the cavity called *harmonic oscillations.*

The mode-locked operation and the longitudinal modes of the laser cavity are coupled to give specific phase relationships by making the laser cavity longer to synchronize the cavity with the duration of time required for the oscillation to travel one round trip. The longitudinal modes are brought into phase for certain periods of time, which results in constructive addition to give a train of very short pulsed, high powered laser beams. The period T of the mode-locked laser is the duration of time the resonant beam requires to travel twice the length of the laser cavity (2 L). About 20 longitudinal modes can be produced for the argon laser with pulses of 1 ns resulting, but the Nd:YAG laser can produce mode-locked pulses of picoseconds in duration.[1]

7.4 Types of Lasers

Table 7-2 illustrates the wavelength and operation mode of a selected number of lasers listed according to the type of lasting medium: gas, dye, or solid-state. Table 7-3 provides a listing of representative diode lasers. A discussion of the characteristics of each type of laser follows.

Solid-State Lasers

In 1960, Maiman was the first to demonstrate that the ruby laser would lase.[5] Since then, the number of solid-state lasers has grown extensively; the ruby laser and the YAG laser are representative of this group of lasers (see Table 7-2).

The ruby laser (C_r:Al_2O_3) is an optically pumped crystalline sapphire that produces a laser beam wavelength at 694.3 nm.[1] In the normal pulsed mode the beam consists of a train of random pulses that are 30 ns to about 1 ms in duration. The ruby laser can also be operated in the Q-switched mode (~ 20 ns) and in the mode-locked mode (~ 1 ns). Although the ruby laser was the first used, the radiation produced is in the visible (VIS) spectrum, and operates in three of the four laser time modes.

The Nd:YAG laser (Nd:$Y_3 Al_5O_2$) is the most common laser in use. It is optically pumped by a xenon flash lamp for pulsed beams or a continuous xenon arc lamp to produce CW beams. The radiation emitted by the Nd:YAG laser is at 1064 nm in the

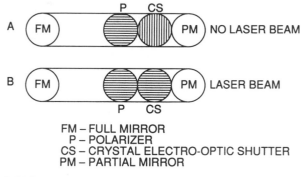

FM – FULL MIRROR
P – POLARIZER
CS – CRYSTAL ELECTRO-OPTIC SHUTTER
PM – PARTIAL MIRROR

FIGURE 7-5
Diagram of the active Q-switching of the laser. *A.* The loss of resonance of the electrons within the laser cavity results from the cross-polarization of the crystal electro-optical shutter. *B.* When the proper electric pulse is applied to the electro-optical shutter, parallel planes of polarization allow the laser beam to be emitted. *Adapted from* Sigleman J. Retinal Diseases: Pathogenesis, Laser Therapy and Surgery. Boston/Toronto, Little, Brown and Company, 1984.

near infrared (near-IR). The use of frequency doubling techniques produces a wavelength in the green VIS spectrum at 532 nm.

Figure 7-1 illustrates the three-level energy system that is employed by the ruby laser. The Nd:YAG possesses a four-level energy system in which the highest excited energy levels quickly decay to the

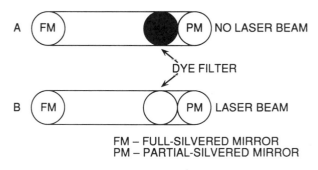

FM – FULL-SILVERED MIRROR
PM – PARTIAL-SILVERED MIRROR

FIGURE 7-6
Diagram of the passive mode-locking of the laser. *A.* An organic dye filter prevents oscillation within the laser cavity from reaching the partial reflecting mirror (PM). *B.* As the stimulated emissions recruit more photons, the dye filter is bleached allowing a single pulse of the laser. The dye filter recovers in 4 to 5 ps and repeats the process. *Adapted from* Sigleman J. Retinal Diseases: Pathogenesis, Laser Therapy and Surgery. Boston/Toronto, Little, Brown and Company, 1984.

Lasing Medium	Wavelength (nm)	Operation Mode
Gas		
F₂	157	P
ArF	193	P
KrCl	222	P
KrF	249	P
XeCl	308	P
HeCd	325 + 442	CW
N₂	337	P
XeF	351	P
Ar	351 + 363.8	CW
Kr	458, 568, 647	CW
HeNe	632.8	CW
CO	5,000–7,000	CW, P, Q
CO₂	9,000–12,000	CW, P, Q
	10,600	CW, P, Q
Dye*		
N2	205–950	Depends on pump source
Rhodamin 6G/	570–640	CW, P
	570–660	
Sodium fluorescein	535–580	CW, P
Solid-state		
Ruby	694.3	P, Q, M
Nd:YAG (Glass)	1064	CW, P, Q

CW = continuous wave, P = pulsed, Q = Q-switched, M = mode-locked.

*There are a number of dye lasers and only three were selected for illustration.

The information for this table was assembled from numerous sources.

TABLE 7-2
A Selected Number of Different Types of Presently Available Lasers

lower levels and make the material less difficult to lase.[4] The energy level necessary to achieve lasing is lower for the four-level and higher-level energy systems.

Gas Lasers

The term *excimer* is derived from "excited dimer" and is used to indicate diatomic molecules whose atoms

are bound in the excited state but are not bound in the zero or ground state.[6] When two atoms of a diatomic molecule are electrically excited, they are attracted to each other and form a stable molecule; however, the same atoms mutually repel each other when at ground state. Thus, when the excited molecule of an excimer laser returns to ground state the molecule self-destructs and ceases to exist. This means that the ground state does not actually exist and that a population inversion is achieved as soon as the molecule is formed because the molecule exists only in the excited state.

The gas halides do not occur in nature but constitute the gases of choice for the excimer laser. The halide gases used in lasers include xenon fluoride (XeF, 351 nm), xenon chloride (XeCl, 308 nm), krypton fluoride (KrF, 249 nm), krypton chloride (KrCl, 322 nm), and argon fluoride (ArF, 193 nm) and are readily produced commercially by electric gas discharge. Helium or neon usually serves as the filler or buffer gas and acts as a catalyst in transferring the energy to the lasing gas but does not participate in the lasing process.

The excimer laser consists of a tube filled with the gas through which an electric discharge is passed transversely. Because the gas halides are consumed in the lasing process, the laser cavity must be refilled from a gas reservoir for continuous laser action. The duration of the excimer laser pulses varies from 1 to 10 ns. Excimer lasers have created considerable excitement in industry and the clinical and basic sciences

Excimer Laser	Wavelength (nm)	Threshold $(H - J/cm^2)$
XeF	352	H_c 0.06[1]
		H_L 15.4
XeCl	308	H_c 0.021
		H_L 0.08
KrF	248	Not available
ArF	193	H_c 15.4
F₂	157	Not available

Data from Zuclich JA and Blankenstein MF[12,13] and Zuclich.[15]

TABLE 7-3
Radiant Exposure Thresholds for the Cornea

Cutting	Microprocessing, noble metals
Drilling	Plastics and noble metals
Surface treatment	Hardening alloys, glazing metals, aluminum planarization Semiconductors, semiconductor annealing
Marking	Metals, plastics, electronics, components
Trimming	IC and hydrid circuits
Scribing	Ceramics and glass
Ablation	Wire skinning, PCBs mask repair
Deposition	IC production, metals on insulators
Doping	Silicon with boron
Lithography	PC direct writing or pattern function IC mask production

From Helzer P. Excimer lens tackle processing. Photonics Spectra 1989; 23:112–113.

TABLE 7-4
Present and Future Uses of the Excimer Laser in Manufacturing

because the wavelengths are in the UVR range.[7,8] A number of present and future uses of the excimer laser in industry are presented in Table 7-4.[9]

The ArF excimer laser at 193 nm appears to be the ideal choice for photoablative procedures on the cornea. The ArF laser induces an optical breakdown of tissue by the formation of a plasma and associated gas waves, a process that has been called *ablative photodecomposition*. The 193-nm excimer laser relies on strong absorption of the UVC radiation by biologic tissues. The advantages of the ArF laser are that it cuts very precise depths with smooth edges when compared to surgical instruments. It can be used to etch or ablate the cornea into the desired shape to eliminate refractive errors and with the precision necessary to eliminate corneal astigmatism.[10] The 193-nm laser does not penetrate the cornea to cause damage to the aqueous humor, crystalline lens, vitreous humor, or the retina. The major disadvantage is that the eye must be completely stabilized to eliminate eye movements greater than 20 μm. The ablated tissue is forced from the area of ablation as a gas that sometimes reaches the temperature of 1000 C. Neighboring tissue is most probably thermally

loaded, which depends on the repetition rate of the laser and the energy of the laser output.[11-13]

A concern exists in the use of the excimer laser because UVR is both mutagenic and carcinogenic. The ArF 193-nm laser at 8.5-mJ energy pulse has been reported to cause a significant DNA repair in yeast.[11] The radiant exposure thresholds using different excimer lasers for the primate cornea and lens are given in Table 7-5.[12] Energies of 84 J/cm^2 were required to penetrate the primate corneal epithelium, and 1 J/cm^2 produces a 1.0-μm thickness of corneal ablation.[8,12,13] The corneal epithelium appears to heal completely within 48 h, but a nebulous corneal opacity remains.[14] A full discussion of the clinical application of the excimer laser will be covered in the next chapter on the clinical application of lasers. The UV laser thresholds for the cornea and lens are presented in Table 7-5.[15]

Dye Lasers

The organic dye laser ordinarily uses a high-power argon laser as the laser pump. The laser cavity is maintained at 40 to 50 psi. The argon laser beam is focused in the laser cavity and a thin stream of organic dye is directed across the laser beam. The dye absorbs the laser radiation, which induces a population inversion and the subsequent laser emission (see Table 7-2).

Lasing Medium	Wavelength (nm)	Operation Modes*
Ga Al As	790–850	P, T
Ga As	820–860	P, T
Al Ga As	850	P, T
In Ga As	1000–1550	P, T
In Ga As P	1000–15,000	P, T
In GaP/In Ga AlP	634	P, T
In Ga As/Al Ga As	1010	P, T

*P = pulsed, T = trains of pulses. Their mode of operation is pulsed or trains of pulses that can be controlled using an external shutter system.
Data from Weber MJ (ed). CRC Handbook of Laser Science and Technology. Boca Raton, FL, CRC Press, 1991.

TABLE 7-5
Representative Laser Diodes

Figure 7-7 illustrates a number of different dyes and their spectral emissions.[4] Dye lasers have successfully produced wavelengths in the entire spectrum from about 195 to 4000 nm. Wavelengths may be selected using a birefringent mirror located within the laser cavity or by using a monochromator or interference filters exterior to the cavity. When diode lasers are used to pump Nd:YAG and Nd:YLF lasers, visible wavelengths of 420 to 542 nm have been produced with the dye laser output achieving about 25% to 30% of the power of the pumping laser.

Laser Diodes

Laser diodes are semiconductor p-n junction solid-state devices that emit coherent radiation when an electrical current is passed through them. The early laser diodes used various combinations of indium, gallium, arsenide, aluminum, and phosphorous vacuum deposited on a substrate. More recently, alternate layers of the diode mixtures have been employed. Laser diodes vary in wavelength according to the materials used in their construction (see Table 7-3) and are tunable by temperature, which causes a 5- to 10-nm shift in the peak wavelength. The diameter of the beam varies from 4 to 200 μm, and the beam divergence is usually 0.1 to 6 mrad. Beam divergence is found by dividing the beam diameter by the distance with the measurement being made from the output facet.

Laser diodes are small in physical dimension, being 0.1 μm $\times$ 5.0 μm in size. They produce a high radiant energy that varies with the applied amperage and the construction of the diode, i.e., whether the diode is a single layer (single stripe) or multiple layer (multistripe) of the diode material deposited on the substrate. Laser diodes consume from 15 to 200 mA of electric current and provide output efficiencies as high as 55%. This is astounding when compared to the Nd:YAG with 1% or other lasers with 2% efficiency, which is more common.

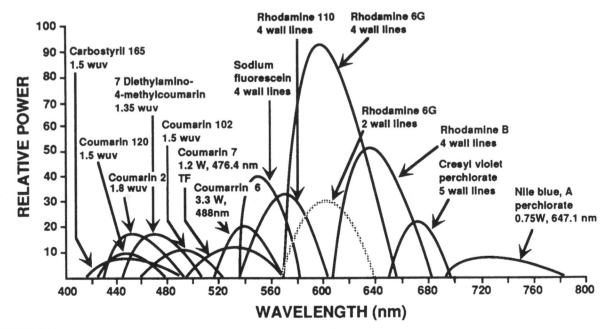

FIGURE 7-7
The different dyes used in dye lasers and their spectral waveband outputs. Wavelengths can be obtained using a birefringent mirror, a monochromator, or by filters. Dye lasers produce broad wavebands across the UV, VIS, and near IR portions of the optical spectrum. *From* L'Esperance FA, Jr. Ophthalmic Lasers (3rd ed). St. Louis, The CV Mosby Company, 1989; reprinted with permission.

7.5 Selecting a Laser for Ophthalmic Therapy

Assuming that the laser possesses adequate power, there are other major concerns in selecting a laser for ocular therapy: the absorption characteristics of the ocular media, the wavelength of the laser, heat caused by the laser, and DNA damage to the tissue. Figure 7-8 illustrates the absorption characteristics of the ocular media, retinal pigment epithelium (RPE), and choroid for selected lasers with wavelengths from 500 to 1064 nm.[4] Table 7-6 presents a list of lasers that may be used for the different ocular therapies. The copper and gold metal vapor lasers are listed because their wavelengths may offer excellent alternative choices. The laser diodes are listed because current research indicates that laser diodes will produce wavelengths from the UVC through the far IR with energy levels sufficient to offer an excellent choice. The physical size, the power output, and the efficiency of laser diodes make them a laser to watch for the future.

Table 7-7 provides the UV laser–induced damage thresholds for the cornea, lens, and retina.[15] This table includes damage thresholds for the corneal epithelium and endothelium, the anterior epithelium, and nucleus of the lens, as well as for different parts

Type of Laser*	Wavelength (nm)
Excimer UV lasers	157–352
Dye lasers	From UV to IR
Argon laser	351, 364, 458, 514.5
Nd:YAG (frequently doubled)	532
Copper metal vapor laser	511, 578
Krypton laser	531, 568, 647
Gold metal vapor laser	628
Ruby laser	694.3
Nd:YAG	1064
Erbium	1228
Ho:AG	1900–2200
CO_2 laser	10,600
Laser diodes	634–15,000

*Listed in descending order of wavelength.
Information for this table was derived from many references on lasers.

TABLE 7-6
Lasers That May Be Used in Ocular Therapy

	Argon	Frequency-doubled Nd:YAG	Dye	Dye	Dye	Krypton	Nd:YAG
Wavelength	500.0 nm	532.0 nm	577.0 nm	590.0 nm	610.0 nm	647.1 nm	1064.0 nm
Ocular media	5%	5%	5%	5%	5%	5%	35%
Retina	--	--	--	--	--	--	--
Pigment epithelium	58%	57%	53%	51%	48%	45%	15%
Choroid	36%	48%	55%	55%	55%	55%	22%
Sclera							

FIGURE 7-8
Absorption of the ocular media, the retina, RPE, and choroid for a selected group of lasers. *From* L'Esperance FA, Jr. **Ophthalmic Lasers (3d ed). St. Louis, The CV Mosby Company, 1989; reprinted with permission.**

Part of Eye	Wavelength (nm)	Laser Pulse Width (s)	Threshold Measured at Cornea (J/cm^2)	Comments
Cornea				
Epithelium	215–315 (UVC + UVB)	10^{-9}–10^5	0.1–1	Usually repairs in 48 h
Epithelium and endothelium	315–400 (UVA)	10^{-9}–10^5	10–100	Usually repairs in 48 h
All layers	193–308 (UVC + UVB)	10^{-8}	1	Photoablation; 1 J/cm^2 ablates 1 mm of corneal tissue
Lens				
Anterior epithelium	295–320 (UVB)	>1	0.1–10	Transient opacity at H_L but 2 × H_L produces permanent cataract
Anterior epithelium	335–380 (UVA)	10^{-9}–1	1–10	Acute thermal cataract
Lens nucleus	300–400 (UVB + UVA)	>>1	??	Chronic cataract accumulates over a lifetime
Retina				
Photoreceptors	315–400 (UVA)	1	0.1–1	No or slow repair
Retina—RPE and photoreceptors (aphakic eye)	>315	>>1	0.1	Photochemical and thermal

Modified from Zuclich JA: Ultraviolet-induced photochemical damage in ocular tissues. Health Phys 1989; 56:671–682; with permission.

TABLE 7-7
UV Laser–Induced Damage Thresholds for the Cornea, Lens, and Retina, Including Layers of These Structures

of the retina. Heat generation and DNA repair data must be established empirically prior to adopting a laser system for biologic exposure.

7.6 Laser Hazard Evaluation and Protection

As we have noted the laser produces an optical beam that possesses the same wavelength, the same phase, is highly collimated, and is said to be coherent. Coherent radiation presents a special problem because very high energy levels transmitted by the ocular media can be concentrated into extremely small areas on the retina. The size of the coherent beam and the area of the pupil are of particular interest in calculating the levels of energy reaching the retina. Rockwell et al[18,19] have presented an excellent pa-

per on laser calculation formulas, and their concepts will be followed. Care must be taken when using the following formulas because they are derived by using the VIS spectrum for which the index of refraction for the eye is reasonably constant. When the exposure is in the UV waveband, however, the index of refraction changes rapidly and affects the size of the retina image.

Laser Hazard Evaluation

Because the laser beam is not totally collimated, the origin of the laser beam is a virtual point located outside or within the laser cavity but posterior to the front mirror of the laser. Let α represent the diameter of the exit beam from the laser, ϕ the full angle beam divergence of the laser (Fig. 7-9), and for small beam

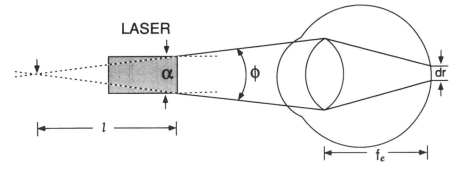

FIGURE 7-9
Diagram of the interaction of the laser and its beam with the eye. The symbol α represents the exit aperture, ϕ the full divergence of the beam, 1 the distance of the origin of the beam from the anterior partially coated mirror, fe the posterior focal length of the eye (1.67 cm) and dr the diameter of the beam on the retina.

divergences it can be assumed that $\tan \phi/2 = (\phi/2)$ or radian measure can be used. The distance l of the origin of the virtual laser beam from the front mirror of the laser is expressed as

$$1 = \frac{\alpha}{\phi} \qquad (7\text{-}1)$$

If the collimated beam is smaller than the pupil, i.e., the pupil allows the total beam to be focused on the retina (intrabeam viewing), the calculation of the diameter of the beam on the retina is found by

$$d_r = \phi f_e \qquad (7\text{-}2)$$

where d_r is the diameter of the laser beam on the retina, ϕ the beam divergence, and f_e the posterior focal length of the human eye (1.67 cm). The diameter of the beam is directly proportional to the posterior focal length of the human eye and the divergence of the laser beam. The divergence of the laser beam is usually expressed in milliradians, and variations in beam divergence can alter the retinal irradiance drastically. The calculation of the area of the beam on the retina becomes

$$A_r = \pi r^2 \text{ or } \pi(d^2/4) \qquad (7\text{-}3)$$

The calculation of the collimated beam on the retina can be solved easily by the relation

$$E_r = \frac{\phi\tau}{A_r} \qquad (7\text{-}4)$$

where E_r is the irradiance on the retina [W/cm^2], ϕ the power of laser beam [W], A_r the area of the beam on the retina [cm^2] and τ the spectral transmittance of the ocular media in decimal form. These formulas

will help the observer to recognize the potential hazards of the laser. The collimated laser beam creates a microscopic lesion on the retina that is diffraction-limited. The larger the area of the laser beam on the retina, the lower will be the retinal irradiance for threshold, and the area or size of the beam on the retina will vary with the index of refraction which, in turn, varies with the wavelength. Therefore, care must be taken when retinal exposures outside the VIS spectrum are evaluated because the retinal irradiance varies indirectly with the area of the retina exposed.

A final laser concept is that of optical gain (OG), which is defined as the ratio of the retinal irradiance E_r to the corneal irradiance E_c. As the laser beam passes through the ocular media, it is spectrally absorbed, and the retinal irradiance E_r must be modified by the ocular transmittance τ to be directly compared with the corneal irradiance E_c. In addition, OG can be related to the diameters of the areas of the beam and the pupil:

$$OG = \frac{\tau E_r}{E_c} = \frac{\tau d_r^2}{d_p} \qquad (7\text{-}5)$$

where τ is the transmittance of the eye, E_r the retinal irradiance (W/cm^2), E_c the corneal irradiance [W/cm^2], d_r the diameter of focused beam on the retina (cm), and d_p the diameter of the pupil. The OG of the human eye is in the 10^5 figure range and alerts one to the fact that low power level lasers incident on the cornea can become greatly increased in power when incident on the retina. A few milliwatts at the cornea becomes hundreds of watts at the retina and approaches the level necessary to produce a permanent retinal lesion. Warning: NEVER LOOK directly into a laser beam because lasers in both direct (or intrabeam) and reflected viewing are potentially hazardous.

When the laser beam is larger than the pupil, the area of the pupil A_p and area on the retina A_r are in direct ratio to the square of the distances l_s^2 and f_e^2, and the evaluation given in the previous discussion for extended sources applies but with a caution that the beam is coherent. Often a source is reflected diffusely from a surface or becomes an extended source, and the rationale for handling this situation becomes more difficult. The extended source relationship between the radiance L_e of the source and irradiance E_e reflected from the diffuse surface follows:

$$L_e = \rho \frac{E_e}{\pi} \qquad (7\text{-}6)$$

where L_e is the radiance of the source [W/cm^2-sr], E_e the irradiance incident on the surface [W/cm^2], and ρ the reflectance factor of the surface. The relationships between L_c, the source radiance, and E_e, the irradiance falling on the surface, depends on the reflectance of the source, whereas π accounts for the angular size of the source (scatter caused by reflection; see Chapter 4). These relationships hold for coherent and noncoherent sources as long as the surface is diffuse and the resulting source is extended.

Classification of Lasers (ANSI Z136.1-1986)

The classification of lasers requires a knowledge of the wavelength or wavelength range average power output and the exposure duration for CW and PW lasers. For PW lasers, the total energy per pulse, pulse width, or duration and emergent beam are additional requirements. Most lasers are point sources, but diode laser arrays and laser output diffuser optics have created extended laser sources. For the extended laser source the angular subtense and radiance of the source must be known.

The ANSI Z136.1-1986 standard[20] requires that both the irradiance of the laser output and the area of the limiting aperture (AEL) be considered when the laser's hazard potential or maximum permissible exposure (MPE) is determined. To decide if hazard must be evaluated, the laser must be classified according to its efficiency in producing damage. The maximum emission level (MEL) is a product of the intrabeam MPE and the area of the limiting aper-

ture for the MPE (MEL = MPE × (area of limiting aperture). The diameter of the limiting aperture is 0.1 cm for UV from 200 to 400 nm; 0.7 cm for VIS radiation and IRA from 400 to 1400 nm; 0.1 cm for IRB and IRC radiation; and 1.1 cm for 0.1- to 1-mm wavelengths. ANSI Z136.1-1986 presents the following classification system for optical radiations:

1. Class 1—Laser or laser system that is limited to the following radiation levels and emission duration:
   a. UV (0.2–0.4 μm) $\leq 0.8 \times 10^{-9}$ W to $\leq 0.8 \times 10^{-6}$ W for 3×10^4 s
   b. VIS (0.4 × 0.7 μm) $\leq 0.4\, C_B \times 10^{-6}$ W for 3×10^4 s, where $C_B = 10^{15(\lambda - 0.550)}$ for $\lambda = 0.550$ to 0.700 μm
   c. Near-IR (0.7–1.06 μm) $\leq 0.4 \times 10^{-6}$ W to $\leq 200 \times 10^{-6}$ for a duration of 3×10^4 s (1.06–1.4 μm) $\leq 200 \times 10^{-6}$ W for durations of 3×10^4 s

The Class 1 laser is exempt from all control measures and surveillance except when used in research and development without a protective housing.

2. Class 2
   a. VIS (0.4–0.7 μm)
      Class 2 lasers have a power output greater than Class 1 but limited to $\leq 1 \times 10^{-3}$ W for both CW and PW lasers. The laser may be designated as Class 2a if its output does not exceed Class 1 lasers and the exposure duration is not greater than 1×10^3 s in any 24-h period.

3. Class 3
   a. UV (0.2–0.4 μm)—emit power greater than Class 1 but limited to 0.5 W for ≥ 0.25 s or a radiant exposure of 10 J/cm^2 for < 0.25 s
   b. VIS (0.4–0.7 μm)—power in excess of class 1 for 0.25 s exposure duration but not greater than 0.5 W, including CW and PW lasers
   c. VIS and near-IR (0.4–1.4 μm)—single PW lasers that emit in excess of Class 1 but do not exceed 10 J/cm^2 or produce a hazardous diffuse reflection
   d. Near-IR (0.7–1.4 μm)—capable of emitting radiant power for the τ_{max} in excess of Class 1 but not greater than 0.5 W for durations of 0.25 s, including CW and PW lasers

All class 3 lasers that do not meet the above requirements are classified as class 3b.

4. Class 4
   a. UV (0.2–0.4 μm)—all lasers that have a radiant power ≥ 0.5 W for 0.25 s or a radiant exposure of 10 J/cm^2 for exposure durations of less than 0.25 s
   b. VIS (0.4–0.7 μm)—lasers emitting an average power ≥ 0.5 W for periods of time ≥ 0.25 s or a radiant exposure of 10 J/cm^2 by intrabeam or diffuse reflection
   c. Near-IR (0.7–1.4 μm)—lasers emitting an average power of ≥ 0.5 W for periods of 0.25 s or a radiant exposure of 10 J/cm^2 by intrabeam or diffuse specular viewing
   d. Far-IR (1.4–1 mm)—same requirements as UVR

Laser Protection Methods

Each laser facility should have a person designated as the laser safety officer who is responsible for and has the authority to establish laser hazards standard operating procedures and to enforce the control of laser hazards. The safety officer should be capable of evaluating laser hazards, training personnel in the safe operation of lasers, and be knowledgeable concerning engineering controls, special controls, administrative and procedural controls, and personnel protective equipment.

To determine the ocular protection required, the laser must first be classified according to Z136.1-1986.[20] The exposure level should then be calculated and, if the values exceed the MPE, additional protection should be required. In a 7-mm diameter pupil, MPE calculates to 2.40 J/cm^2,[20] and the exposure duration (in seconds) for the laser would be

$$\text{Exposure duration} = \frac{\text{MPE (J/cm}^2)}{E_{e\lambda}[\text{W/cm}^2]} \quad (7\text{-}7)$$

The 2.40 J/cm^2 is two magnitudes below the LD 50 threshold for producing a visible retinal lesion in the primate retina. The optical density (OD) required for laser protective eyewear for a specific wavelength is given by

$$D_\lambda = \log_{10}\frac{Ho}{MPE} \quad (7\text{-}8)$$

where Ho is the anticipated worst case exposure in W/cm^2 for CW laser sources and J/cm^2 for PW laser sources and MPE is the maximum permissible exposure determined by ANSI 136.1-1986.[20] To make an initial calculation for the CW laser,

$$MPE = C_B \times 10^{-6} \text{ W/cm}^2 \quad (7\text{-}9)$$

where C_B is 1 for wavelengths less than 400 μm but not greater than 550 μm and is $10^{15(\lambda - 0.550\mu m)}$ for wavelengths between 0.550 and 0.700 μm. For PW lasers,

$$MPE = 320\, C_A \cdot 10^{-6} \text{ W/cm}^2 \quad (7\text{-}10)$$

where C_A varies in the wavelength range of 0.700 to 1.4 μm, from 1 at 0.700 μm, 1.5 at 0.800 μm, 2 at 0.900 μm, and 5 above 1.1 μm. The OD formula may be simplified:

$$OD = \log_{10} I_i/I_t \quad (7\text{-}11)$$

where I_i is the intensity of the radiation incident on the protective filter in any unit and I_t is the intensity of the laser radiation transmitted through the filter.

LASER PROTECTIVE EYEWEAR
Any filter placed before the eye increases the hazards where electric, chemical, and other laboratory equipment are in use. Dark filters and opaque side-shields increase the danger of the laboratory technician making a serious error. The laser protective filter that provides maximum transmittance of the wavelengths in the VIS spectrum and maximum absorbance of the laser wavelength is the protective lens of choice.[22]

Laser protective eyewear should be worn when other control methods do not attenuate the laser beam to or below the MPE and the laser beam has the potential to injure the eye. A Class 4 laser system usually requires protective eyewear in addition to other protective equipment. The most important features of laser protective eyewear is that the device be comfortable, the luminous transmittance be adequate to allow excellent vision, and that the laser beam is absorbed. A minimum attenuation of OD 5 is necessary for a filter to be classified as a laser protective filter.

Laser protective goggles are available in different configurations. Laser protective lenses are designed

| Wavelength (nm) | Manufacturer / Source | American Optical | | | | | | | Fish-Schurmar | |
	Model	581	584	585	588*	598*	599	598	AL-515-7	AL-633-5
< 320	(Actinic)	>2	>2	>2		>2				
325	HeCd	>2	>2	>2		>2				
332	Neon	>2	>2	>2		>2				
337.1	Nitrogen	>2	>2	>2		>2				
347.1	Ruby (2d Harmonic)	>2	>2	>2		>2				
441.6	HeCd	<1	<1	<1	<1	17	10.5		>10	
457.9	Argon	<1	<1	<1	<1	17	10.5	11	>10	
488	Argon	<1	<1	<1	<1	13.5	8.6	10	10	
514.5	Argon	<1	<1	<1	<1	9	5.5	8	7	
530	Neodymium (2d Harmonic)	<1	<1	<1	<1	7	6	4.5		
611.8	HeNe	3	<1	1	1	<1	<1	<1		
632.3	HeNe	4	1	3	2	<1	<1	<1		5
647.1	Krypton	4	1	3	3	<1	<1	<1		
694.3	Ruby	6	4.5	7	6	<1	<1	<4		
840	GaAs	5	11	17	15	<1	<1	<10		>10
905	GaAs	4	11	17	15			11		
1060	Neodynium	2	9.5	14	12.5			7.4		>30
1084	HeNe	2	9	13	12			8		
1152	HeNe	1	8	10	11			6		
% Luminous Transmittance		**10**	**46**	**35**	**33**	**24**	**25**	**5**	**70**	**64**
Cost Range‡		**B**	**C**	**C**	**A**	**A**	**B**	**C**	**A**	**A**

TABLE 7-8
Optical Densities at Various UV, VIS, and Near-IR Wavelengths for Standard Laser Eye Protection from Manufacturer's Specifications

to provide maximum attenuation of the laser wavelength but allow maximum luminous transmittance for good vision. The frames must fit tightly around the nose, forehead, temples, and cheeks to prevent direct or reflected laser beams from entering the eye. Each laser protective goggle has the stock code of the manufacturer identified on the frame, the optical density of the lens, and its wavelength. An example is that a goggle with a greenish-blue color lens possesses an OD of 5 at 633 nm and an OD of 10 at 694 nm. Sliney et al.[23]

have presented an excellent summary of the available laser ocular protection goggles that has been modified as Table 7-8.

OCULAR EVALUATION OF LASER WORKERS
An ocular evaluation of workers using lasers is necessary prior to hiring and should be repeated annually during employment and at the termination of employment.[21] The ocular evaluation for visual hazards in laser areas should include the following:

| Fish-Schurmar | | Fred Reed Optical Co. | | Glendale* Optical Co. | | | | |
| AL-1060-9 | AL-2800-45 | RF6-PL-GG9-GBS† | FR6-PL-KG3-GBS† | LGS, LGU, 7400 or VL Series* (one piece) | | | | |
		(3 mm GG-9)	(3 mm KG-3)	NN	HN	A	R	NDGA
>1	>1	>5	<1	<15	<10	20	10	>25
		>5	<1	15	>10	20	8	25
		>5	<1	15	>10	21	9	25
		>5	<1	16	>10	19	9	24
		>5	<1	16	>10	18	9	23
		2	<1	<1	1	14	<1	7
		<1	<1	<1	1	14	<1	7
			<1	<1	<1	15	<1	1
		<1	<1	<1	11	<1	1	<1
	<1		<1	<1	<1	5	<1	<1
	<1		<1	<1	3	<1	1	<1
			<1	<1	6	<1	3	1
			<1	<1	5	<1	4	1
			<1	<1	2	<1	6	3
2			<2	<1	<1	<1	<1	14
5		3	<1	<1	<1	<1	16	30
9	4		4.5	<1	<1	<1	<1	16
9	4		4.5	<1	<1	<1	<1	10
9	4		4.5	<1	<1	<1	<1	1
64	70	85	70	20	45	20	45	20
A	A	C	C	A	A	A	A	A

*Spectacle type (otherwise goggle)
†Prescription spectacle
‡A is 560–590, B is 590–S120, C is S120–S150
§OD 6 at 1800 nm; OD 5 at 3400 nm

TABLE 7-8 continued
Optical Densities at Various UV, VIS, and Near-IR Wavelengths for Standard Laser Eye Protection from Manufacturer's Specifications, continued

1. Ocular history
2. Acuity 35 cm
3. Patient's Rx, if any
4. External ocular examination
5. Amsler grid
6. Fields
7. Cycloplegic refraction
8. Examination of the fundus
9. Photograph of posterior fundus
10. Slit lamp examination
11. Examination of retina with slit lamp and gonioscope lens

The subject of ocular damage from and protection against laser exposure is a complicated subject that cannot be fully covered in a short treatise. ANSI Z136.1-1986, American National Standard for the safe use of lasers;[20] ANSI Z136.2-1988, American

Wavelength (nm)	Model / Source	Phase-R Corporation				Spectra-Optics	
		LG-A or A* Series — NDGA R NM	LG-B or B* Series — HDGA DOUB. ND A NN	AGR	AGB	Spectro-guard	Custom Made
<320	(Actinic)	25	25		>3	16	
325	HeCd	25	25		2.5	16	
332	Neon	25	25		2	16	
337.1	Nitrogen	25	25		1	15	
347.1	Ruby (2d Harmonic)	25	25		<1	15	
441.6	HeCd	<1	14	4.5	<1	11	
457.9	Argon	<1	14	4.5	<1	11	
488	Argon	<1	11	4	<1	5	
514.5	Argon	7	4	1	5		
530	Neodymium (2d Harmonic)	<1	4	3.5	1.5	5	6
611.8	HeNe	<1	<1	1.5	5	5	<1
632.8	HeNe	<1	<1	<1	<5	5	<1
647.1	Krypton	1	<1	<1	<5	6	<1
694.3	Ruby	6	<1	<1	3.5	9	>1
840	GaAs	30	4		3	12	<1
905	GaAs	5		<3	12	<1	
1060	Neodymium	30	4			13	6
1084	HeNe	10	2			9	
1152	HeNe	1	<1			9	
% Luminous Transmittance		**45**	**15**	**15**	**0.4**	**0.65**	
Cost Range[‡]		**C**	**C**	**B**	**C**	**C**	**A**

*Spectacle type (otherwise goggle)
[†]Prescription spectacle
[‡]A is 560–590, B is 590–S120, C is S120–S150
§OD 6 at 1800 nm; OD 5 at 3400 nm
NOTE: Another characteristic of these goggles, which should be considered in the selection of laser protective eyewear, is one before damage or filter plate.
SOURCES: American Optical Corporation, Optical Products Division, PO Box 1, Southbridge, MA 01550 (617-765-9711)
    Fish-Schurman Corporation, 75 Portman Road, New Rochelle, NY 10802 (914-636-1300)
    Fred Reed Optical Co., Inc., PO Box 1336, Albuquerque, NM 87103 (505-265-3531)
    Glendale Optical Co., Inc., 130 Crossways Park Drive, Woodbury, LI, NY 11797 (516-921-5800)
    Phase-R Corporation, PO Box G-2, New Durham, NH 03855 (603-859-3800)
    Spectra-Optics, 12317 Gladstone Avenue, Sylman, CA 91342 (213-361-0949)
Data from Sliney DH, Griffis DW, and Lyon TL.[23]

TABLE 7-8 continued
Optical Densities at Various UV, VIS, and Near-IR Wavelengths for Standard Laser Eye Protection from Manufacturer's Specifications, continued

National Standard 136.2-1988 for the safe use of optical fiber communication systems utilizing laser diode and LED sources;[24] and ANSI Z136.3-1988, American National Standard for the safe use of lasers in health care facilities should be consulted for additional information.[25]

References

1. Weber MJ (ed). CRC Handbook of Laser Science and Technology. Boca Raton, FL, CRC Press, 1991.
2. Laser Health Hazards Control. AF Manual 161-8. Dept of the Air Force, Hq US Air Force, April 1969.
3. Rhodes CK. Topics in Applied Physics. Vol 30, Excimer Lasers. New York, Springer-Verlag, 1979.
4. L'Esperance FA, Jr. Ophthalmic Lasers, Volume I (3rd ed). St. Louis, CV Mosby Company, 1989.
5. Maiman TH. Stimulated optical radiation in ruby. Nature 1960; 187:493.
6. Brau CA. Rare gas halogen excimers, Chap 4. In Brau CA (ed): Topics in Applied Physics, Vol 30. New York, Springer-Verlag, 1979.
7. Srinivasan R. Kinetics of ablative photodecomposition of organic polymers in the far-ultraviolet. J Vacuum Sci Tech 1983; B-1:923.
8. Trokel SI, Srinivasan R, Braren B. Excimer laser surgery of the cornea. Am J Ophthalmol 1983; 96:710–715.
9. Helzer P. Excimer lasers tackle processing. Photonics Spectra 1989; 23:112–113.
10. Seiler T, Bende T, Wollensak J, Trokel S. Excimer laser keratectomy for correction of astigmatism. Am J Ophthalmol 1988; 105:117–124.
11. Seiler T, Bende T, Winckler K, Wollensak J. Side effects in excimer corneal surgery DNA damage as a result of 193 nm excimer laser radiation. Graefes Arch Clin Exp Ophthalmol 1988; 226:273–276.
12. Zuclich JA, Blankenstein MF. Part I. Ocular effects of ultraviolet and infrared laser radiation. A. Ocular effects of the xenon chloride (XeCl) excimer laser. In Effects of Laser Radiation on the Eye, Vol II, pp 7–33. USAF-SAM-TR-84-10. USAF School of Aerospace Medicine, Brooks Air Force Base, Texas, April 1984.
13. Zuclich JA, Blankenstein MF. Part I. Ocular effects of pulsed ultraviolet and infrared radiation. In Effects of Laser Radiation on the Eye, Vol IV, pp 1–15. USAF-SAM-TR-85-13. USAF School of Aerospace Medicine, Brooks Air Force Base, Texas, 1985.
14. Bende T, Seiler T, Wollensak J. Side effects in excimer corneal surgery. Graefes Arch Clin Exp Ophthalmol 1988; 226:277–280.
15. Zuclich JA. Ultraviolet-induced photochemical damage in ocular tissues. Health Phys 1989; 56:671–682.
16. Taboada J, Mikesell GW, Reed RD. Response of corneal epithelium to KrF excimer laser pulses. Health Phys 1981; 40:677–683.
17. Sigleman J. Retinal Diseases: Pathogenesis, Laser Therapy and Surgery. Boston/Toronto, Little, Brown and Company, 1984.
18. Sliney D, Wolbarsht M. Safety with Lasers and Other Optical Sources. New York, Plenum Press, 1980.
19. Rockwell RJ, Sliney DH, Smith JF. Laser safety, Part 1. Introduction to hazard calculations. Electro-Optical Systems Design 1978; 10:32–39.
20. American National Standard for the Safe Use of Lasers. ANSI Z136.1-1986. New York, American National Standards Institute Inc, 1986.
21. Zweng HC, Rose H. Eye examination standards and treatment. In Sperling HG (ed): Laser Eye Effects, pp 87–89. Washington DC, Armed Forces-National Research Council Committee on Vision, 1968.
22. Swope CH. The eye—protection. Arch Environ Health 1969; 18:428–433.
23. Sliney DH, Griffis DW, Lyon TL. Laser Protective Eyewear. TG-081. Aberdeen Proving Ground, MD, US Army Environmental Hygiene Agency, 1982.
24. American National Standard for the Safe Use of Optical Fiber Communication Systems Utilizing Laser Diode and LED Sources. New York, American National Standards Institute Inc, 1986.
25. American National Standards for Safe Use of Lasers in Health Care Facilities. New York, American National Standards Institute Inc, 1986.

CHAPTER EIGHT

Clinical Applications of Lasers

Jimmy Jackson, M.S., O.D.

The latest changes in ophthalmic treatment have occurred with the application of laser technology to the eye (Table 8-1). Before lasers were developed, treatment of most conditions required intraocular manipulations. Complications of anesthesia and surgically entering an eye are numerous and potentially sight-threatening. Although laser techniques are not without their own unique and potentially serious side effects, most laser procedures have rendered the corresponding surgical procedures obsolete. "The present applications and future investigational developments of ophthalmic lasers are two of the most important topics in ophthalmology"[1] and optometry. Therefore, laser education and training is a vital component in all optometry and ophthalmology programs.

This chapter will be limited to the clinical aspects of anterior segment laser procedures. Patient selection, preoperative and postoperative management, technique(s), and complications will be discussed. Even with this limited focus, this chapter will not be all-inclusive because the field of ophthalmic lasers is

1963	Zweng, Campbell	Clinical ruby laser
1968	L'Esperance	Clinical argon laser
1971	L'Esperance	Clinical frequency-doubled Nd:YAG laser
1972	L'Esperance	Clinical krypton laser
1972	L'Esperance	Clinical CO_2 laser
1972	Beckman	Ruby laser transscleral cyclo-coagulation
1973	Beckman	Clinical CW Nd:YAG laser
1973	Krasnov	Ruby laser goniopuncture
1973	Beckman	Ruby laser iridotomy
1974	Krasnov	Argon laser gonioplasty
1975	L'Esperance	Argon laser photomydriasis
1975	Abraham	Argon laser iridotomy
1977	Bernard	Argon laser transpupillary cyclocoagulation
1977	Simmons	Argon laser goniophoto-coagulation
1979	Wise	Argon laser trabeculoplasty
1980	Fankhauser Aron-Rosa	Clinical pulsed Nd:YAG laser
1981	L'Esperance	Clinical dye laser
1985	Seller, Wollensak	Clinical excimer laser

From Esperance FA (ed.). Ophthalmic Lasers. St. Louis: CV Mosby, 1989:26.

TABLE 8-1
Ophthalmic Lasers: Procedure Landmarks

growing rapidly. This chapter is designed to demonstrate some of the clinical applications of the basic laser information presented in Chapter 7. It is not designed to be a how-to text for practitioners who have not received hands-on experience in laser procedures. Like all clinical procedures, the best way to learn them is by supervised training with an experienced practitioner or in clinical workshop sessions.

At the present time a large number of lasers are either undergoing investigation, being tested in clinical trials, or have been introduced. Some of these include the excimer, diode, tunable dye, erbium:YAG, and holmium lasers. It is beyond the scope of this chapter to discuss these laser systems. A list of additional readings is provided for more detailed information.

8.1 General Techniques in Using Anterior Segment Lasers

Contact Lenses

The use of a contact lens with anterior segment laser procedures varies with the individual practitioner as well as with the particular procedure. In general, benefits of these lenses include prevention of lid closure, stabilization of the eye, absorption of heat energy away from the cornea (in conjunction with gonio solution), and minimization of energy loss by reflection. Due to their high plus buttons (in most lenses), they also magnify the view and increase the laser energy at the target site while decreasing the energy delivered to surrounding tissue. The main drawbacks of contact lens use include complication of the process and fear and discomfort in the patient.

The use of a contact lens is an obvious requirement for the completion of an argon laser trabeculoplasty (ALT) because visualization of the angle is a prerequisite for completion of the procedure. A Goldmann three-mirror is most commonly used. A Goldmann one-mirror or Ritch lens is useful for patients with small palpebral fissures.

Although a laser peripheral iridotomy (LPI) can be performed without a contact lens, most clinicians feel its use is mandatory.[2-6] The two most commonly used lenses are the Abraham iridectomy lens (Fig. 8-1) and the Wise iridotomy lens (Fig. 8-2).

The use of a contact lens in performing a Nd:YAG anterior vitreolysis is strongly recommended. Vitreous is relatively difficult to visualize in the anterior chamber, and the use of an iridotomy lens will aid in the procedure by increasing magnification. The increased cone angle will also decrease collateral damage to surrounding tissue.

The use of a contact lens for capsulotomies is less universal than for iridotomies. The use of a contact lens is preferred in patients with a silicon intraocular lens (IOL) (more likely to sustain laser damage) and in uncooperative patients. There are several laser capsulotomy lenses available. The Abraham Nd:YAG lens has a 66 diopter central button (see Fig. 8-3). The Peyman lens has a front curve that approximates the corneal curvature.

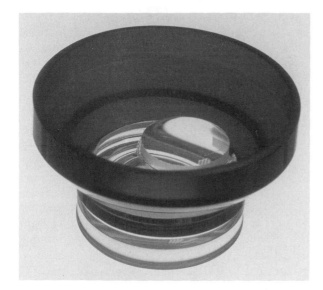

FIGURE 8-1
Abraham Iridotomy Laser Lens. Photo courtesy of Ocular Instruments, Inc., Bellevue, WA

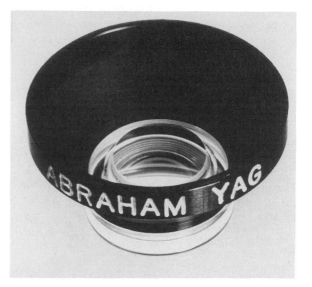

FIGURE 8-3
Abraham Nd:YAG Capsulotomy Laser Lens. Photo courtesy of Ocular Instruments, Inc., Bellevue, WA

Contraindications

A clear visual pathway through which to apply the laser energy is a prerequisite for all anterior segment laser procedures. It is imperative to be able to

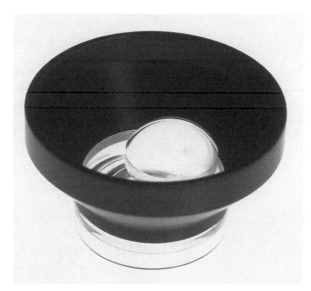

FIGURE 8-2
Wise Iridotomy Laser Lens. Photo courtesy of Ocular Instruments, Inc., Bellevue, WA

clearly visualize the target tissue and precisely focus the laser. Corneal edema is, therefore, a general contraindication to all laser procedures. Likewise, corneal scars, arcus, or other opacities should be avoided. A flat (or extremely shallow) anterior chamber is also a contraindication, because adequate separation between target tissue and adjacent tissue is necessary to prevent coincident destruction of tissue.

Anterior uveitis and cystoid macular edema (CME) are known complications of anterior segment laser procedures; therefore, it is advisable to defer laser treatment until those conditions have resolved. Likewise, patients who are at risk for retinal detachment (RD) should have laser procedures (especially capsulotomy) deferred as long as practical.

Patients who are unable or unwilling to hold their eyes still during the procedure increase the likelihood of an errant shot(s) causing corneal, iris, lenticular, or intraocular lens (IOL) damage and should be approached with caution.

Patient Preparation

The preparation of the patient is minimal. An explanation of the laser procedure with possible complications is mandatory. An informed consent form signed by the patient is recommended. The patient should be told to expect to see flashes of light and colored afterimages. When utilizing the Nd:YAG laser, the patient should be told to expect to hear a snap when the laser is fired. Patients should be reassured that the procedure is relatively painless and to report any sensation of pain.

Topical anesthetic is almost always sufficient for all anterior segment laser procedures. Retrobulbar anesthesia is reserved for the rare uncooperative patient or for patients with severe nystagmus.

Prophylactic use of therapeutic agents to prevent or blunt any postlaser intraocular pressure (IOP) rise is becoming routine. Of all the agents used, only apraclonidine is used preoperatively. It is generally administered one hour before the laser procedure.

Miosis aids in the completion of a LPI. It serves to thin the iris and make penetration easier. Pilocarpine (generally 4%) is given one hour pre-iridotomy.

Most practitioners prefer to dilate a patient's pupil to perform a capsulotomy because this facilitates the procedure and allows visualization of the full extent of the opacification. However, the patient's pupil centration should be noted carefully before dilation to prevent the creation of a capsulotomy that is not coincident with the pupil in the nondilated state. Other practitioners feel that the desire to create the smallest opening that is coincident with the pupil requires performing the capsulotomy nondilated. A capsulotomy that is slightly larger than the pupil may be made easily by having the patient look in different directions.

Postoperative Treatment

If apraclonidine was administered preoperatively, another drop is instilled immediately after completion of the laser procedure. Other recommended therapeutic agents used in lieu of apraclonidine include beta blockers, pilocarpine, and oral carbonic anhydrase inhibitors. All of these agents have been shown to be somewhat effective in blunting the postoperative IOP pressure rise,[7–15] but a majority of clinicians feel that apraclonidine is the most effective agent available. Topical steroids may be used routinely or reserved for cases of observed anterior chamber response.

IOP should be measured 1 to 3 h following the laser procedure. If the postoperative IOP increases more than 6 mm Hg from the preoperative IOP level, steps should be undertaken to reduce it. If no significant elevation is noted at the 1- to 3-h evaluation, the patient is generally released and seen at 1 d to 1 w, depending on practitioner preference and type of procedure performed.

Complications

General complications of anterior segment laser procedures are quite common but not usually sight-threatening. Postoperative IOP rise has been studied by a host of investigators.[4,7–11,16–32] A 10-mm or greater rise in IOP has been reported in up to 43% of eyes that received no prelaser or postlaser medication to prevent such a rise. Risks from the IOP rise can be minimized by prophylaxis[7–11] and careful monitoring. A study by Robin[7] found 96% of all eyes that demonstrated a postiridotomy IOP spike did so within two hours. The final 4% occurred within three hours following the iridotomy, and no eyes without an IOP elevation during the first three hours developed a late (days to weeks) IOP elevation. A recent study reported that a small percentage of patients developed a late-onset (1–3 y) IOP elevation following Nd:YAG laser capsulotomy.[24] No factors to predict which eyes are at risk for this late-onset elevation were identified. The implications of this interesting study remains to be seen.

A mild transient iritis sometimes occurs following laser procedures. Rates of iritis will vary depending on type of laser procedure, postoperative medications, and follow-up schedule.[8,33–34] The iritis usually responds promptly to topical steroids. Occasionally, patients with diabetes will develop a much more intense iritis and require more frequent usage of topical steroids and mydriatics.[35]

Blurred vision is reported to occur after LPI, ALT, and capsulotomy.[35–37] This slight blur is generally associated with released pigment or hemorrhage (LPI and ALT) or capsular debris (capsulotomy). Rapid, spontaneous resolution is almost always noted.

Corneal and lenticular opacities have been reported following LPI.[16,18,33] Use of iridotomy lenses and careful focusing prevents most such opacities. Corneal opacities that do occur usually resolve completely within 24 to 48 h, although in eyes with marginally decompensated corneas, there have been cases of further decomposition.[38] Transient corneal opacities have also been reported with capsulotomy, anterior vitreolysis, and ALT.[26,32,39–42] Lenticular opacities that occur have been found either to be stable and nonprogressive[2] or to resolve altogether.[43]

Iris hemorrhaging can occur with laser procedures. It most commonly occurs when the Nd:YAG laser is used to perform iridotomies. Although the incidence is high (up to 60% in some studies), it can usually be controlled by applying slight digital pressure to the globe. No serious complications related to the hemorrhaging has been reported.[16,18–21,33]

Retinal damage is a rare but potentially severe complication of some anterior segment laser procedures. Using a contact lens, careful focusing, and directing the beam away from the fovea minimize the risk.

8.2 Laser Peripheral Iridotomy

Indications

The primary indication for LPI is angle-closure glaucoma in which primary or secondary pupillary block is presumed to be the causative factor.[2–4,16,17,44] Primary block is seen in acute angle closure, whereas secondary block can occur in iris capture of an IOL or in development of posterior synechiae, which leads to a secluded pupil. Prophylactic LPIs are indicated in all fellow eyes following an acute angle glaucoma attack in the opposite eye.[2–17,44] Intermittent and chronic pupillary block are considered to be relative indications for LPI.[3,4,17] Patients with chronic angle closure not due to pupillary block, e.g., closure due to neovascularization or inflammatory synechiae, are not candidates for LPI.[3] An optical iridotomy, or coreoplasty, is indicated when the visual axis is blocked by the presence of iris tissue or inflammatory membrane. Because the laser treatment is, by definition, in the visual axis, particular care must be taken to avoid creating lenticular or IOL opacities. If a coreoplasty is performed on a phakic eye, minimal power should be utilized (see Figs. 8-4 and 8-5).

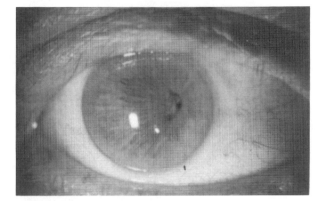

FIGURE 8-4
Ectopic pupil with membrane secondary to postoperative inflammation. V.A. was finger counting.

Both argon and Nd:YAG lasers are used for LPI, and there is no agreement about which is the preferred laser. Practitioner experience, patient parameters, and availability all play a role, along with "expert" opinion. Table 8-2 shows a comparison of argon and Nd:YAG features.

Contraindications

Corneal edema may preclude LPI in the patient with an acute angle closure attack. It is generally preferred to manage this patient medically until the cornea clears and then proceed with the LPI. In cases in which it is judged to be unsafe to wait, one

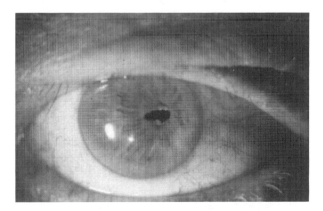

FIGURE 8-5
Same patient as in Figure 8-9 following Nd:YAG coreoplasty. V.A. improved to 20/100.

	Argon	Nd:YAG
Iris color	Factor[2,3,45]	Not a factor[2,3,45]
Number of shots	More	Less
Total energy	More[3,45]	Less[3,45]
Hemorrhaging	Rare[2,46]	20%–60%[16,18–21]
Closure	16%–40%[20–23,45]	Rare[20,23,45]
Margins	Smooth[2,3]	Jagged[2,3]
Lens injury	Possible	More likely ±[2,47]
Corneal injury	Possible	Possible
Pupil distortion	Common[45,48]	Rare[45]
P/O IOP rise	Yes[7,18]	Yes[16,18,20]

TABLE 8-2
**Comparison of Characteristics of Argon and
Nd:YAG LPIs**

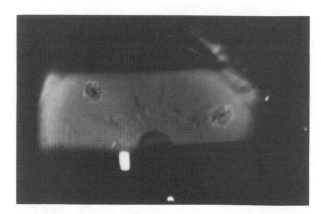

FIGURE 8-7
Patient with two patent LPIs created with argon laser.

can either use topical glycerin in an attempt to clear the cornea or convert to a surgical iridectomy. Another laser option for the attack that is not responding medically is to perform an argon peripheral gonioplasty, which is discussed in more detail later in this chapter. A flat (or extremely narrow) anterior chamber is also a relative contraindication for an LPI because it is very difficult to avoid corneal burns in these patients.

Technique

The placement of the iridotomy should be under the superior lid, in the 11 or 1 o'clock position, to avoid secondary retinal images and poor cosmetic appearances (Fig. 8-6). The 12 o'clock position should be avoided because bubbles caused by the procedure can accumulate and interfere. Superionasal is the preferred site because it minimizes

accidental macular exposure, although it is advantageous to perform two iridotomies to protect against closure (Fig. 8-7).

Placement should be far enough peripherally to avoid the lens (Fig. 8-8), usually two thirds the distance from the pupillary margin to the limbus. Nd:YAG lasers do not require pigmentation and are preferable in patients with lightly pigmented irises. It is advantageous to choose an iris crypt for the iridotomy site because this represents an area of relatively thinner iris.[2,3] When the argon laser is used with a lightly pigmented iris, it is helpful to find an iris freckle because the increased pigmentation will absorb laser energy and aid in penetration.[2,3]

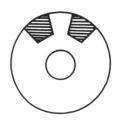

FIGURE 8-6
**Shaded areas represent suitable
areas for placement of LPIs.**

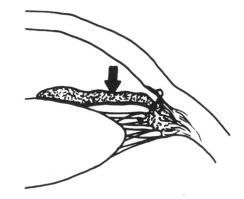

FIGURE 8-8
**Arrow represents correct peripheral placement of LPI to
minimize lenticular damage.**

Because penetration of the iris is not always easy to ascertain, the practitioner must know how to evaluate a "successful" iridotomy. For example, penetration is often signaled by a "plume of pigment" or a "mushroom cloud" (Fig. 8-9) caused by the sudden release of trapped aqueous and dispersed pigment. Transillumination is a good evaluation technique (Fig. 8-10) in medium and dark irises, but not with

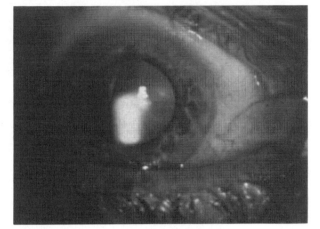

FIGURE 8-10
Retroillumination demonstrating transillumination of LPIs at 11 o'clock and 2 o'clock.

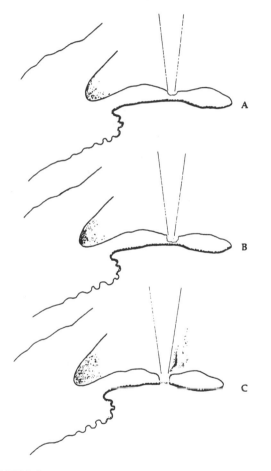

FIGURE 8-9
Typical chipping-away laser iridotomy procedure creating vaporization and destruction of small portions of iris stroma (A and B) until the pigment epithelium is reached and perforated (C). When the pigment epithelium is reached, pigment granules are liberated in a fine plume that is exaggerated at the time of penetration by the flow of aqueous from the posterior chamber into the anterior chamber. This liberation of pigment usually signifies partial or complete penetration of the pigment epithelium. From Ritch and Solomol.[2] Reprinted with permission.

light irises. Direct observation of the anterior lens capsule is clear evidence but often difficult to obtain. Deepening of the anterior chamber is another sign and should be verified by gonioscopy.

Nd:YAG Laser Peripheral Iridotomy—Basic Approach

The Nd:YAG laser is a photodisruptor that creates a shock wave that mechanically cuts tissue. This effect is not pigment-dependent. An advantage of the Nd:YAG laser is its ability to create an iridotomy regardless of iris color. The primary disadvantage of the Nd:YAG laser is the occurrence of bleeding at the iridotomy site. This is primarily self-limiting and can usually be controlled with minimal digital pressure. The hemorrhaging rarely can cause the completion of the iridotomy to be delayed for a day or two. Nd:YAG LPIs should be approached cautiously, however, in patients with neovascularization or in those taking anticoagulants. Alternatively, these patients could be "pretreated" with the argon laser to photocoagulate or seal the iris vessels. The iridotomy could then be completed with the Nd:YAG laser.

Another concern with the Nd:YAG laser that has been voiced by some investigators is its potential to cause more lens damage (with resultant progressive cataract formation) than the argon laser.[47] This has not been appreciated clinically.[2] Because the shock wave created by the Nd:YAG laser travels toward the operator from the point of focus,[48] careful focusing largely avoids this potential complication. The recommended point of focus for the Nd:YAG when an LPI is being performed is generally recognized as just posterior to the anterior iris surface.[3,4]

Because Nd:YAG laser energy is invisible (1064 nm), helium-neon aiming beams are used to focus the laser beam. With most Nd:YAG lasers, two or more aiming beams are brought to a single point to determine visibly the focus point for the laser beam. The basic Nd:YAG LPI technique is given in Table 8-3.

Argon Laser Peripheral Iridotomy

There are many argon LPI techniques suggested by various authors and clinicians.[2,49-51] The direct approach (Table 8-4) is recommended initially in all cases of argon LPI. Adjustments of power and duration are made based upon tissue response. If this approach is not successful, then the contraction burn technique is used (Table 8-5). Contraction burns are achieved with large spot size, long duration, and lower energy. This maximizes the contraction or contour changes caused by the coagulation effect and prepares the site for penetration by the direct technique.

The argon laser is a photocoagulator. The absorption of argon laser energy varies tremendously with different amounts of iris pigmentation. Light-colored irises are the most difficult irises to penetrate with the argon laser. Most clinicians recommend the use of the Nd:YAG laser in these cases. If argon is the only laser available, the direct technique should be used with lower power settings (700–800 mW) and longer durations (0.2 s or longer). If the power setting is too high, it is possible for the laser energy to pass through the iris stroma and destroy the pigment epithelium—leaving the stroma intact and creating a transillumination defect without a patent iridotomy. Longer duration burns can often create heat levels that destroy stroma tissue as well as pigment epithelium. A drawback to the longer duration burns is that they are often uncomfortable for the patient. Light brown irises are the easiest to penetrate and respond well to the direct approach. Dark brown irises can often be quite difficult to penetrate because they may char, which gives an appearance of black, shiny material at the base of the iridotomy site. This is caused by excessive heat generated by long duration burns in the presence of high amounts of pigment. To avoid charring, short exposure times of 0.02 to 0.05 s should be used with a spot size of 50 μm and energy of 400 to 1000 mW.[4] When extensive charring occurs, penetration at that site is almost impossible.

Spot size	25 microns (fixed)
Energy level	1–6 mJ
Burst	1

Note: Select an area of thin iris. Energy level should begin low and be slowly increased. The use of an iridotomy lens with a magnifying button often results in less energy being required. Some practitioners recommend multiple bursts; the author believes this affords less control and should be avoided.

Pre-op: 1 gtt Pilo 4% one hour before iridotomy
1 gtt apraclonidine one hour before iridotomy
Post-op: 1 gtt apraclonidine immediately after iridotomy
1 gtt topical steroid BID–QID × 7 d (optional)

TABLE 8-3
Nd:YAG LPI Technique

Spot size	50 microns
Duration	0.05–0.2 seconds
Energy level	700–1000 mW

Note: The proper tissue response is slight contraction (formation of a pit) with no pain experienced by the patient. Often a small bubble will be created. In general when increasing the power, decrease the duration.

Pre-op and post-op as with YAG LPI.

TABLE 8-4
Argon LPI—Direct Technique

Spot size	100–500 microns
Duration	0.2–0.5 seconds
Energy level	200–500 mW

Note: Significant contour changes should be seen immediately on laser application.

TABLE 8-5
Argon LPI—Contraction Burn Technique

Complications

Monocular diplopia or blurring can occur if the iridotomy site is not well covered by the lid.[36] Therefore, avoid the palpebral aperture when selecting an iridotomy site. Pupil irregularities can occur with the argon laser due to contraction associated with the photocoagulative nature of the laser. These are usually of no consequence.

Closure of the iridotomy site is the most common "serious" complication. Rates of closure of 16% to 40% have been reported following argon LPIs.[20,22,23,45] Closure is most likely to occur in the first 1 to 2 months and almost never after 6 months. Closure with the argon laser can be minimized by performing larger PIs and controlling inflammation. After penetration has been established, enlargement of the opening should be attempted (Fig. 8-11) utilizing the clean-up technique described in Table 8-6. Closure is very rare with the Nd:YAG laser[20,23,45] and is a leading reason why many practitioners choose the Nd:YAG over the argon for LPIs.

8.3 Nd:YAG Capsulotomy

Nd:YAG laser capsulotomy has rapidly replaced riskier, intraocular capsule discission by needle or needle-knife unless it is during cataract surgery.[35]

The primary indication for a capsulotomy is opacification of the posterior capsule causing visual impairment. Capsulotomies are performed routinely as early as four weeks after cataract extraction by some practitioners, whereas others recommend waiting three to

Spot size	50 microns
Duration	0.01–0.05 seconds
Initial energy	200–500 mW

Note: Do not aim the beam directly into the opening created. This can cause lens damage and potential posterior pole damage. Aim the beam so that ⅔ is on the pigment epithelium and ⅓ is in the opening.[4]

TABLE 8-6
Argon LPI—Cleanup Technique

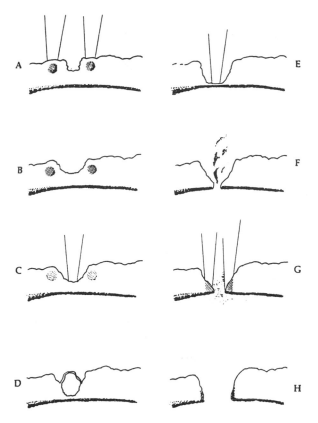

FIGURE 8-11
Multiple diagrammatic representations indicating (A) contraction burns on either side of an iris crypt to (B) draw the edges of the crypt apart, exposing the depths of the crypt to (C) the impact of the laser beam as it "chips away" small portions of the iris stroma with each impact. As the laser beam approaches the depth of the iris stroma, it is not uncommon to produce a vapor bubble (D); when this has disappeared, the chipping-away process continues (E). Eventually the pigment epithelium is perforated, liberating a plume of pigment granules into the anterior chamber (F). The edges of the patent iridectomy are then enlarged in some cases by coagulation to the borders of the iridectomy site (G), with the resultant moderately sized opening in the iris structure (H). From Ritch and Solomol.[2] Reprinted with permission.

six months.[35,52] Patient history, visual acuity, glare testing, and slit-lamp examination are the main indicators used in determining the need for capsulotomy.

The incidence of posterior capsule opacification depends greatly on its definition and method of determination. Rates range from 7% to near 60%, with most studies suggesting the latter.[35,53–55] Children in whom cataract extraction has been performed have an opacification rate of essentially 100%.[56]

Technique

It is preferable to direct the first laser shot away from the visual axis. This allows the practitioner to determine the "marking" or "pitting" characteristics of the IOL without creating a central defect. When it is difficult to open a fibrous capsule, it is advisable to use a contact lens, use minimal laser energy, search for areas of greater separation between the lens and capsule, and work away from the center of the lens.

Several designs or types of capsulotomies have been recommended by various authors (Fig. 8-12), with the cross pattern or variations thereof being the most common. Targeting tension or stress lines in the posterior capsule creates a large opening without unnecessary additional energy being pumped into the eye. Thicker, more densely fibrosed capsules may require a fragmentation process (Fig. 8-13).

Most practitioners now feel that capsulotomies should be made as small as possible.[35,52] The opening should be slightly larger than the pupil in ambient light because capsular remnants remaining within the pupil may cause visual symptoms. Generally, a capsulotomy opening of 3.5 to 4.5 mm is sufficient (Fig. 8-14).

The minimum laser energy that creates an opening in the capsule should be used; this is generally 1 to 3 mJ of power (Table 8-7). Often, capsulotomies

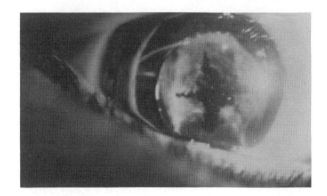

FIGURE 8-13
YAG laser capsulotomy performed on patient with extremely opacified capsule requiring fragmentation process.

can be created with as few as 5 to 10 pulses. A good rule-of-thumb average would be 20 to 30 pulses at 1 to 2 mJ of power. This would represent a total power discharge in the eye of 20 to 60 mJ (number of pulses time power per pulse). Whereas particularly thick capsules can sometimes require over 100 pulses at power settings of 3 mJ or higher, it is an unusual capsulotomy that cannot be completed in one session.

Complications

IOL marks following Nd:YAG laser capsulotomy were found to occur 12% of the time in one study.[57]

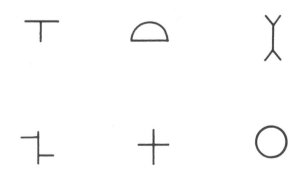

FIGURE 8-12
Several representative laser capsulotomy patterns that have been used by practitioners.

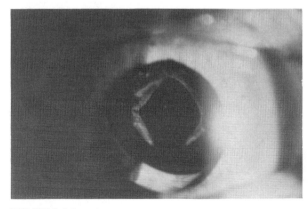

FIGURE 8-14
YAG laser capsulotomy.

Spot size	25 microns (fixed)
Energy level	1–4 mJ
Burst	1

Note: Topical anesthesia is not a requirement, but it is usually helpful. A contact lens is not usually necessary. Steady patient fixation and adequate corneal hydration is vital. Begin by focusing the two HeNe beams on the posterior capsule, and then push the joystick slightly forward so that the focus is just beyond the posterior capsule and into the vitreous. This will help decrease pitting or marking the IOL. Begin at an off-axis point and create a vertical opening of approximately 3 mm. Next create horizontal openings of similar size on either side of the vertical.

Pre-op: 1 gtt apraclonidine one hour before (optional)
Post-op: 1 gtt apraclonidine immediately after
      1 gtt topical steroid BID–QID × 7 d
            or
      1 gtt beta blocker BID × 7 d
      1 gtt topical steroid BID–QID × 7 d

TABLE 8-7
Nd:YAG Posterior Capsulotomy Technique

However, there was no subjective visual loss. Other studies have reported that up to 30% of patients with posterior chamber IOLs sustain damage to the IOL during a Nd:YAG capsulotomy[58–60] but that these markings do not appear to affect visual acuity. Silicone IOLs are most susceptible to marking with the YAG laser. The use of a contact lens during the capsulotomy will help decrease the marking of the IOL.

The incidence of cystoid macular edema (CME) following YAG capsulotomy has been reported by various authors to be slightly higher than the incidence of CME following cataract extraction.[38,59,61,62] However, it appears that the YAG capsulotomy may just allow a clearer view of pre-existing CME secondary to the cataract surgery. An interesting study by Lewis et al[63] examined this question by following 76 patients with no CME before capsulotomy (proven by angiography) for 6 months after capsulotomy. None of the 76 developed CME during this period.

Retinal detachment is the most serious potential complication reported to occur secondary to capsulotomy. The incidence of RD following capsulotomy has been reported to be from 0.17% to 3.6%,[57,59,64–68] with 69% occurring within the first six months[67] and 84.6% occurring within the first year[68] following capsulotomy. Several mechanisms have been suggested: Capsulotomy leads to changes in the vitreous, e.g., PVD, which may lead to RD;

capsulotomy induces direct retinal damage through shock waves, leading to RD; and capsulotomy is an incidental finding in patients prone to RD.[64] Significant risk factors for RD following YAG capsulotomy are axial length greater than 25 mm, lattice degeneration or other pre-existing vitreoretinal adhesions, history of RD in fellow eye, and others.[39,64,68] Capsulotomy should be delayed as long as practical if risk factors are present. A thorough peripheral retinal evaluation post-capsulotomy, as well as making the patient alert to signs and symptoms of RD, is highly recommended. Other complications of Nd:YAG capsulotomy that have been reported include endothelial cell loss,[39,40] iris hemorrhage,[58,59,61] ruptured anterior hyaloid face,[58,69] IOL displacement,[57,59] vitritios,[58,59] and macular hole.[62,70]

8.4 Nd:YAG Anterior Vitreolysis

Vitreous strands sometimes pass through the pupillary space and become attached, or incarcerated, in the corneoscleral wound following cataract extraction. This incarceration or "vitreous-tug syndrome" may lead to CME. The Nd:YAG laser is effective in cutting the vitreous bands.[41,71] Initial power settings are identical to those for capsulotomy (Table 8-7). Due to the relative difficulty of visualizing vitreous in the anterior chamber, the use of an iridotomy contact lens is recommended to increase magnification. Inducing miosis preoperatively with 2% pilocarpine is advantageous because it facilitates identification and cutting of the strand. The laser is focused on the strand at a point approximately midway between the cornea and iris (Fig. 8-15). The desired end point is a complete cutting of the vitreous strand with release of tension.

8.5 Argon Laser Trabeculoplasty

ALT is initially successful in increasing aqueous outflow in 60% to 95% of patients with primary open angle glaucoma[27,42,72–75] with most studies reporting pressure lowered 5 to 14 mm Hg.[27,42,72–75] Unfortunately, the effect of ALT tends to diminish with time so that only 30% to 60% of initially successful

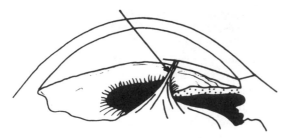

FIGURE 8-15
Diagram demonstrating vitreous incarcerated into cataract incision. Arrow represents ideal location for application of laser shots at midpoint between iris and cornea.

ALTs are still successful after 5 years. The majority of failures occur in the first 12 months.[80] The mechanism by which ALT produces its pressure-lowering effect is not well understood.[72,81,82]

Indications

Patients with primary open angle glaucoma, pseudoexfoliative glaucoma, and pigmentary glaucoma respond best to ALT,[27,76,77,83,84] especially if they are over 40 years of age.[27,42,85] ALT is not considered to be effective in cases of inflammatory glaucoma, congenital glaucoma, or glaucoma secondary to trauma,[2,76,83] although it may be effective in low-tension glaucoma.[27] Aphakia is considered to be a relative contraindication for ALT. Pseudophakic eyes with posterior chamber IOLs appear to respond to ALT as well as phakic eyes.[26] Cataract surgery after ALT does not appear to adversely affect the success of the ALT.[100] Primary angle-closure glaucoma is also a contraindication because an open, accessible angle is a prerequisite for the successful performance of ALT.

The timing of an ALT has undergone almost constant revision over the past several years. Originally, ALT was used after the failure of maximum medical therapy as an alternative to surgical intervention. Most practitioners today consider ALT before adding oral to existing topical medications, and many use ALT before adding miotics.

Controversy has been created by the Glaucoma Laser Trial, a multicenter, randomized clinical trial investigating the efficacy and safety of ALT as an alternative to *any* topical medication.[28,29] Previously untreated patients with newly diagnosed primary open angle glaucoma were randomly treated with ALT in one eye (laser first—LF) and with timolol maleate 0.5% in the other eye (medication first—MF). Medication was initiated or changed for either eye according to a specific stepped-up regimen if the IOP was not controlled. After two years of follow-up, 44% of LF eyes were controlled, compared to 30% of the MF eyes. There were no major differences between the two treatment approaches with respect to changes in visual acuity or visual field over the two years of follow-up. The authors conclude "It appears that ALT is at least as good as if not better than starting with medications, because in the short term, ALT provides good pressure control and has the advantage of postponing and/or reducing the inconvenience, nuisance, and side effects associated with taking medications."[29] Other practitioners have urged caution in evaluating the data from the Glaucoma Laser Trial.[86,87] Additional factors to consider in comparing ALT to medication include availability of adequate follow-up, patient compliance, and side effects of medications.

General Techniques

Above-average skill with the gonio lens and knowledge of anterior chamber anatomy are prerequisites for successful completion of an ALT. The entire 360° of the angle should be viewed carefully prior to the ALT to ensure proper orientation and adequate visualization of angle structures. Angle vessels and peripheral anterior synechiae should be noted and avoided during treatment.

Wise and Witter[72] recommended 100 laser applications at 1000 to 1500 mW of power applied to 360° of the trabecular meshwork at one sitting. A number of variations on this original protocol have been proposed.[27,73,88–92] The generally recommended protocol distilled from these various reports is given in Table 8-8. Individual practitioner preference, along with patient parameters such as type of glaucoma, amount of pigment, and response to initial settings, play a role in determining the approach in a particular patient.

Most practitioners recommend treating 180° at a time. The inferior 180° is treated first because it is

Spot size	50 microns
Duration	0.1 seconds
Energy level	300–1000 mW

Note: Initial power is set low and increased until endpoint of slight blanching is reached. Heavily pigmented eyes require less energy and should be started at 300 mW. In eyes with little to no pigment, it may be difficult to ascertain the blanching endpoint. Generally 1000 mW remains the upper power limit, even if no visible response is noted. Large bubble formation, shower of pigment, or rupture of the meshwork indicates excessive power. The beam is aimed at the junction of the pigmented and nonpigmented trabecular meshwork. Treat the inferior 180 degrees with 35–50 equally spaced burns. The superior 180 degrees is usually treated 4–6 weeks later if necessary.

Pre-op: 1 gtt apraclonidine one hour before ALT
Post-op: 1 gtt apraclonidine immediately after ALT
   1 gtt topical steroid QID × 7 d
   Maintain all pre-op glaucoma meds

TABLE 8-8
Argon Laser Trabeculoplasty Technique

generally the widest and the most heavily pigmented. It is helpful to begin treatment at an angle landmark to prevent overlapping of laser burns when the additional 180° is treated. The beam spot should be maintained as a circle because this represents the most precise focus, and proper placement of the burns is crucial. The aiming beam should be focused on the junction of the pigmented and nonpigmented trabecular meshwork (Fig. 8-16). Treating too close to the scleral spur increases the risk of developing inflammation and synechiae,[93] whereas treating too close to Schwalbe's line has been associated with pain, lessened effect, and overgrowth of endothelium over the meshwork.[94] The proper end point is slight blanching of the tissue or small bubble formation. Applications should be spaced 3° to 4° apart so that 35 to 50 applications will be placed in 180°. The remaining superior 180° can be treated in 4 to 6 wk if the IOP drop is insufficient.

Narrow angles are more difficult to treat because visualization of angle structures is vital to the success of ALT. Having the patient look in the direction of the mirror being used will often result in improved visualization. If this approach fails, a peripheral gonioplasty can be performed to flatten the iris in front of the angle and thereby improve the view.

Because initially successful ALTs have been shown to fail with time,[78-80] many authors have investi-

gated the efficacy of retreatments. At this time the status of repeat argon laser trabeculoplasty (RALT) is controversial.

Complications

The most serious complications following ALT is a pressure spike. This transient elevation in IOP is similar to that seen following LPI and capsulotomy. However, pressure spikes are usually more serious in ALT patients because they tend to have greater compromise of their optic nerves and thus are often unable to tolerate even a transient elevation.[26-30] Pretreatment and posttreatment as described earlier in this chapter help reduce or prevent the spike, but careful monitoring of IOP in the immediate postoperative period is mandatory. Treating only 180° of trabeculum at one sitting rather than 360° also tends to reduce the chance of a pressure spike.[26,27,31,32] A sustained pressure spike occurs in 1.5% to 3% of patients undergoing ALT.[26,27]

Iritis can occur following ALT but is usually suppressed by the topical steroids administered postoperatively. Occasionally a trabeculitis is produced

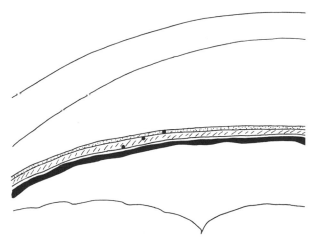

FIGURE 8-16
Diagram demonstrating proper placement of ALT burns. The two anterior-most dots represent adequate placement (at or near the junction of pigmented and nonpigmented meshwork). The third dot lies near the scleral spur and burns this far posterior should be avoided.

postoperatively. The appearance of keratic precipitates on the trabecular meshwork is the hallmark sign of trabeculitis. The aggressive use of topical steroids usually produces a rapid resolution.

Hemorrhaging is an uncommon complication of ALT.[30] It is readily stopped by applying slight pressure on the gonio lens. It can then be prevented by further photocoagulation at a lower power setting.[32]

The formation of peripheral anterior synechiae is a relatively common occurrence following ALT but is usually of no serious consequence.[30,95] Positioning the burns properly and avoiding posterior placement near the scleral spur helps to reduce their incidence.[95]

Other reported complications include corneal burns,[26,32,42] CME,[37] pupillary distortion,[2] decreased vision,[37] and syncope.[37]

8.6 Argon Peripheral Gonioplasty (Iridoplasty)

Argon peripheral gonioplasty (or iridoplasty) is a technique by which the peripheral iris is contracted or flattened to pull it away from the angle. The argon laser can produce significant contour changes in the iris because of the heat and coagulative effect. This technique can be used to "open" sections of the angle and may be effective as a treatment in cases of acute angle closure that are not responsive to medical management. Such nonresponsive cases are not amenable to LPI because of the extreme corneal edema that renders precise focusing impossible. Gonioplasty, however, is performed using a large spot size (300–500 μm versus 25–50 μm for LPI), which makes precise focusing less critical. Whereas this technique may be used to break an attack of acute angle closure, it is not a cure, and LPI will still need to be performed when the corneal edema resolves. Gonioplasty is also useful as an adjunct to ALT in patients with narrow angles. Pulling the peripheral iris away from the angle by performing a gonioplasty increases visualization of the anterior chamber anatomy, and the ALT is performed more effectively.

Technique

The technique consists of placing large, low-power burns to the peripheral iris just inside the limbus

(Table 8-9). Topical anesthetic is sufficient, and most practitioners do not use a contact lens. Pilocarpine (2%) used one hour prior to treatment will put the iris on stretch and make shrinking of tissue more easily visible. If gonioplasty is being used to break an attack of acute angle closure, generally all 360° are treated at one sitting (Fig. 8-17). If gonioplasty is to serve as an adjunct to ALT, just the 180° undergoing ALT receives the gonioplasty. Most practitioners will place their patients on a short course of topical steroids after a gonioplasty. Complications are uncommon and mirror those of the other anterior segment laser procedures discussed in this chapter.

8.7 Photorefractive Keratectomy (PRK)

The use of the excimer laser is the latest in many procedures that have been considered for refractive surgery. The excimer photoablates tissue in very precise and discrete steps (Chapter 7). Although many wavelengths are available, the current technology uses 193 nm. Because of the precision of the beam and delivery system used for PRK, the procedure must be done under computer control. The optimal details for PRK are being investigated in phase III clinical trials.

General Techniques

After examination of the patient and determination of the patient's visual needs, the parameters

Spot size	300–500 microns
Duration	0.2–0.5 seconds
Energy level	200–400 mW

Note: Visible contraction of iris tissue is the desired endpoint. Use the lowest energy level that accomplishes this. Avoid charring of tissue. The author generally uses the 500 micron spot size—only reducing spot size if the patient reports pain. Burns should be equally spaced with a frequency of 4–8 per quadrant.
    Pre-op: 1 gtt pilocarpine 2% one hour before gonioplasty
    Post-op: 1 gtt topical steroid BID–QID × 4 d

TABLE 8-9
Argon Laser Gonioplasty

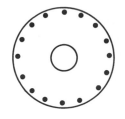

FIGURE 8-17
Diagram representing proper placement of peripheral gonioplasty burns.

for the laser are set for the desired visual outcome. One current approach is to debride the central corneal epithelium after instillation of a topical anesthetic. Following this the patient is aligned under the laser and the computer guided procedure is initiated. After 10–15 seconds the procedure is concluded and the patient is placed on topical antibiotics and steroids. The steroids are continued for 3–4 months. The laser commonly delivers 180 mJ/cm^2 at 10 Hertz and uses 70–250 pulses. The initial clinical results appear to have a reasonable rate of success, where success is defined as ± 1.00 D.

Complications

The short-term side effects include ocular pain, corneal haze, and in some patients regression of the refractive error. The long term side effects of the procedure are currently being studied, including the long-term health of the cornea. The excimer procedure usually removes about 40 microns of tissue including Bowman's membrane. Although the cornea reepithelializes in a few days to a week, Bowman's membrane does not regenerate. The absence of this membrane may make the cornea more vulnerable to future insults and infections. In addition, the use of high levels of ultraviolet radiation (about 180 J/cm^2) have the potential to cause radiation damage, mutagenesis and carcinogenesis (see Chapter 6).

Protection of the eyes against all laser procedures is necessary (see Chapters 7 and 9).

References

1. L'Esperance FA. Introduction. In L'Esperance FH (ed): Ophthalmic Lasers, pp 1–10. St. Louis, CV Mosby, 1989.
2. Ritch R, Solomol IS. Laser treatment of glaucoma. In L'Esperance FA (ed): Ophthalmic Lasers, pp 650–748. St. Louis, CV Mosby, 1989.
3. Alward WLM. Laser iridotomy. In Weingeist TA, Sneed SR (eds): Laser Surgery in Ophthalmology, pp 139–147. Norwalk, CT, Appleton and Lange, 1992.
4. Hoskins HD, Kass MA. Laser treatment for internal flow block. In Hoskins HD, Kass MA (eds): Becker-Shaffer's Diagnosis and Therapy of the Glaucomas, pp 499–510. St. Louis, CV Mosby, 1989.
5. Diekert JP, Mainster MA, Ho PC: Contact lenses for laser applications. Ophthalmology (Instrument and Book Suppl.), 1984; 79–87.
6. Quigley HA. Surgery of the glaucomas. In Rice TA, Michels RG, Stark WJ (eds): Ophthalmic Surgery, pp 177–208. St. Louis, CV Mosby, 1984.
7. Robin AL. Medical management of acute postoperative intraocular pressure rise associated with anterior segment ophthalmic laser surgery. Int Ophthalmol Clin 1990; 30:102–110.
8. Robin AL, Pollack IP, deFaller JM. Effects of topical ALO 2145 (p-aminoclonidine hydrochloride) on acute intraocular pressure rise after argon iridectomy. Arch Ophthalmol 1987; 105:1208–1211.
9. Krupin T, Stone RA, Cohen BH, Koller AE, Kass MA. Acute intraocular pressure response to argon laser iridotomy. Ophthalmology 1985; 92:922–926.
10. Schrems W, Eichelbronner O, Krieghtein GK. The immediate IOP response of Nd:YAG laser iridotomy and its prophylactic treatability. Acta Ophthalmol (Copenh) 1984; 62:673–680.
11. Liv PF, Hung PT. Effect of timolol on intraocular pressure elevation following argon laser iridotomy. J Ocul Pharmacol 1987; 3:249 255.
12. King MH, Richards DW. Near syncope and chest tightness after administration of apraclonidine before argon laser iridotomy. Letter to the Editor. Am J Ophthalmol 1990; 110:308–309.
13. Richter CU, Arzeno G, Pappas HR, Arrigg CA, Wasson P, Steinert RF. Prevention of intraocular pressure elevation following neodymium-YAG laser posterior capsulotomy. Arch Ophthalmol 1985; 103:912–915.
14. Brown SV, Thomas JV, Belsher CD, Simmons RJ. Effect of pilocarpine in treatment of intraocular pressure elevation following Nd:YAG laser posterior capsulotomy. Ophthalmology 1985; 92:354–359.
15. Baen-Tan TN, Stilma JS. Prevention of IOP rise following Nd:YAG laser capsulotomy with pre-operative timolol eye drops and 1 tablet acetazolamide 250 mg. Doc Ophthalmol 1986; 64:59–67.

16. Fleck BW, Dhillon B, Khanna V, et al. A randomized, prospective comparison of Nd:YAG laser iridotomy and operative peripheral iridectomy in fellow eyes. Eye 1991; 5:315–321.

17. Iwata K, Abe H, Sugiyama J. Argon laser iridotomy in primary angle-closure glaucoma. Glaucoma 1985; 7:103–106.

18. Robin AL, Pollack IP. A comparison of neodymium:YAG and argon laser iridotomies. Ophthalmology 1984; 91:1011–1016.

19. Wise JB. Low-energy linear-incision neodymium:YAG laser iridotomy versus linear-incision argon laser iridotomy. A prospective clinical investigation. Ophthalmology 1987; 94:1531–1537.

20. Del Prioro LV, Robin AL, Pollack IP. Neodymium:YAG and argon laser iridotomy. Long-term follow-up in a prospective, randomized clinical trial. Ophthalmology 1988; 95:1207–1211.

21. Gray RH, Honre Nairn J, Ayliffe WHR. Efficacy of Nd:YAG laser iridotomies in acute angle-closure glaucoma. Br J Ophthalmol 1989; 73:182–185.

22. Assaf AA. Argon laser iridectomies. Glaucoma 1985; 7:75–83.

23. Moster MR, Schwartz LW, Spaeth GL, et al. Laser iridectomy: A controlled study comparing argon and neodymium:YAG. Ophthalmology 1986; 93:20–24.

24. Fourman S, Apisson J. Late-onset elevation in intraocular pressure after neodymium-YAG laser posterior capsulotomy. Arch Ophthalmol 1991; 109:511–513.

25. Flohr MJ, Robin AL, Kelly JS. Early complications following Q-switched neodymium:YAG laser posterior capsulotomy. Ophthalmology 1985; 92:360–363.

26. Hoskins HO, Kass MA. Laser treatment for outflow block. In Hoskins HD, Kass MA (eds): Becker-Shaffer's Diagnosis and Therapy of the Glaucomas, pp 511–518. St. Louis, CV Mosby, 1989.

27. Thomas JV, Simmons RJ, Belcher CD, III. Argon laser trabeculoplasty in the presurgical glaucoma patient. Ophthalmology 1982; 89:187–197.

28. Glaucoma Laser Trial Research Group. The Glaucoma Laser Trial 1. Acute effects of argon laser trabeculoplasty on intraocular pressure. Arch Ophthalmol 1989; 107:1135–1142.

29. The Glaucoma Laser Trial Research Group. The Glaucoma Laser Trial (GLT) 2. Results of argon laser trabeculoplasty versus topical medicines. Ophthalmology 1990; 97:1403–1413.

30. Weinrebh RN, Wilensky JT. Clinical aspects of argon laser trabeculoplasty. Int Ophthalmol Clin 1984; 24:79–95.

31. Weinreb RN, Ruderman J, Juster R, Wilensky JT. Influence of the number of laser burns administered on the early results of argon laser trabeculoplasty. Am J Ophthalmol 1983; 95:287–292.

32. Watson AP, Rosenthal AR. Complications following argon laser trabeculoplasty. Glaucoma 1986; 8:60–63.

33. Schwartz LW, Moster MR, Spaeth GK, Wilson RP, Poryzees E. Am J Ophthalmol 1986; 102:41–44.

34. Fankhauser F, Roussel P, Steffen J, Van Der Zypen E, Chrenkova A. Clinical studies on the efficiency of high power laser radiation upon some structures of the anterior segment of the eye. Int Ophthalmol 1981; 3:129–139.

35. Kolder HE. YAG laser capsulotomy. In Weingeist TA, Sneed SR (eds): Laser Surgery in Ophthalmology, pp 167–174. Norwalk, CT, Appleton and Lange, 1992.

36. Murphy PH, Trope GE. Monocular blurring: A complication of YAG laser iridotomy. Ophthalmology 1991; 98:1539–1542.

37. Hoskins HD, Hetherington J, Minckler DS, Leiberman MF, Shaffer RN. Complications of laser trabeculoplasty. Ophthalmology 1983; 90:796–799.

38. Schwartz AL, Martin NF, Weber PA. Corneal decompensation after argon laser iridectomy. Arch Ophthalmol 1988; 106:1572–1574.

39. Axt JC. Nd:YAG laser posterior capsulotomy: A clinical study. Am J Optometry Physiol Opt 1985; 62:173–187.

40. Slomovic AR, Parish RK, II, Forster RK, Cubillas A. Neodymium:YAG laser posterior capsulotomy: Central corneal endothelial cell density. Arch Ophthalmol 1986; 104:536–538.

41. Katzen LE, Fleishman JA, Trokel S. YAG laser treatment of cystoid macular edema. Am J Ophthalmol 1983; 95:589–592.

42. Wilensky JT, Jampol LM. Laser therapy for open-angle glaucoma. Ophthalmology 1981; 88:213–217.

43. Higginbotham EJ, Ogura Y. Lens clarity after argon and neodymium:YAG laser iridotomy in the rabbit. Arch Ophthalmol 1987; 105:540–541.

44. Robin AL, Pollack IP. Argon laser peripheral iridotomies in the treatment of primary angle-closure glaucoma: Long-term follow-up. Arch Ophthalmol 1982; 100:919–922.

45. Prum BE, Shields SR, Shields MB, Hickingbotham D, Chandler DB. In vitro videographic comparison of argon and Nd:YAG laser iridotomy. Am J Ophthalmol 1991; 111:589–594.

46. Hodes BL, Bentivegna JF, Weyer NJ. Hyphema complicating laser iridotomy. Arch Ophthalmol 1982; 100:924.

47. Welch RN, Apple DJ, Mendelsohn AD, Reid JJ, Chalkley THF, Wilensky JT. Lens injury following iridotomy with a Q-switched neodymium:YAG laser. Arch Ophthalmol 1986; 104:123–125.

48. March WF. Ophthalmic lasers: Current clinical uses. Thorofare, NJ, Slack Inc, 1984.

49. Abraham RK, Miller GL. Outpatient argon laser iridectomy for angle-closure glaucoma: A two-year study. Trans Am Acad Ophthalmol Otolaryngol 1975; 79:529–538.

50. Pollack IP, Patz A. Argon laser iridotomy: An experimental and clinical study. Ophthalmic Surg 1976; 7:22–30.

51. Mandelkorn RM, Mendelsohn AD, Olander KW, Zimmerman TJ. Short exposure times in argon laser iridotomy. Ophthalmic Surg 1981; 12:805–809.

52. Aron-Rosa D, Abitol Y: Laser capsulotomy. Ophthalmology Clinics of North America 1989; 2:549–554.

53. Nishi O. Incidence of posterior capsule opacification of eyes with and without posterior chamber intraocular lenses. J Cataract Refract Surg 1986; 12:519–522.

54. Sawuch MR, McDonnell PJ. Posterior capsule opacification. Current Opinion in Ophthalmology 1990; 1:28–33.

55. Moisseive J, Bartov E, Schochat A, Blumenthal M. Long-term study of the prevalence of capsular opacification following extracapsular cataract extraction. J Cataract Refract Surg 1989; 15:531–533.

56. Emery JM, Wilhemus KR, Rosberg S. Complications of phacoemulsification. Ophthalmology 1978; 85:141–150.

57. Shah GR, Fills JP, Durham DG, Ausmus WH. Three thousand YAG lasers in posterior capsulotomies: An analysis of complications and comparisons to polishing and surgical discission. Ophthalmic Surg 1986; 17:473–477.

58. Stark WJ, Worthen D, Holladay JT, Murray G. Neodymium:YAG lasers, an FDA report. Ophthalmology 1985; 92:209–212.

59. Keates RH, Steinert RF, Puliafito CA, Mazwell SK. Long-term follow-up of Nd:YAG laser posterior capsulotomy. Am Intraocular Implant Soc J 1984; 10:164–168.

60. Trokel SL, Katzen LD. The mode-locked laser: Principles and clinical results. In Trokel SL (ed): YAG Laser Ophthalmic Microsurgery, pp 147–179. Norwalk, Appleton-Century-Crofts, 1983.

61. Aron-Rosa DS, Aron JJ, Cohn HC. Use of a pulsed picosecond Nd:YAG laser in 6,664 cases. Am Intraocular Implant Soc J 1984; 10:35–39.

62. Chambliss WS. Neodymium:YAG laser posterior capsulotomy results and complications. Am Intraocular Implant Soc J 1985; 11:31–32.

63. Lewis H, Singer TR, Hanscom TA, Straatsma BR. A prospective study of cystoid macular edema after neodymium:YAG laser posterior capsulotomy. Ophthalmology 1987; 94:478–482.

64. Salvesen S, Eide N, Syrdalen P. Retinal detachment after YAG-laser capsulotomy. Acta Ophthalmol (Copenh) 1991; 69:61–64.

65. Leff SR, Welch JC, Tasman W. Rhegmatagenous retinal detachment after YAG laser posterior capsulotomy. Ophthalmology 1987; 94:1222–1225.

66. Winslow RL, Taylor BC. Retinal complications following YAG laser capsulotomy. Ophthalmology 1985; 92:785–789.

67. Ambler JS, Constable IJ. Retinal detachment following Nd:YAG capsulotomy. Aust N Z J Ophthalmol 1988; 16:337–341.

68. Rickman-Barger L, Florine CW, Larson RS, Lindstrom RL. Retinal detachment after neodymium:YAG laser posterior capsulotomy. Am J Ophthalmol 1989; 107:531–536.

69. Terry AC, Stark WJ, Maumenee AE, Fagadau W. Neodymium:YAG laser for posterior capsulotomy. Am J Ophthalmol 1983; 96:716–720.

70. Blacharsk PA, Newsome DA. Bilateral macular holes after Nd:YAG posterior capsulotomy. Am J Ophthalmol 1988; 105:417–418.

71. Iliff CE. Treatment of vitreous tug syndrome. Am J Ophthalmol 1986; 62:856–859.

72. Wise JB, Witter SL. Argon laser therapy for open-angle glaucoma: A pilot study. Arch Ophthalmol 1979; 97:319–324.

73. Shirakashi M, Iwata K, Nakayama T, Fukuchi T. Long-term efficacy of low power argon laser trabeculoplasty. Acta Ophthalmologica 1990; 68:23–28.

74. Wise JB. Long-term control of adult open-angle glaucoma by argon laser treatment. Ophthalmology 1981; 88:197–202.

75. Ponjanpelto P. Argon laser treatment of the anterior chamber angle for increased intraocular pressure. Acta Ophthalmol (Copenh) 1981; 59:211–220.

76. Gross BR, McCole CE. Argon laser trabecular photocoagulation in the treatment of chronic open-angle glaucoma: A preliminary report. Glaucoma 1981; 3:283.

77. Wise JB. Status of laser treatment of open-angle glaucoma. Ann Ophthalmol 1981; 13:149–150.

78. Sherwood MB, Lattimer J, Hitchings RA. Laser trabeculoplasty as supplementary treatment for primary open-angle glaucoma. Br J Ophthalmol 1987; 71:188–191.

79. Moulin F, Haut J, Rached JA. Late failures of trabeculoplasty. Int Ophthalmol 1987; 10:61–66.

80. Shingleton BJ, Richter CV, Bellows AR, Hutchinson BT, Glynn RJ. Long-term efficacy of argon laser trabeculoplasty. Ophthalmology 1987; 94:1513–1518.

81. Melamed S, Pei J, Epstein DL. Short-term effect of argon laser trabeculoplasty in monkeys. Arch Ophthalmol 1985; 103:1546–1552.

82. Van Buskirk EM, Pond V, Rosenquist RC, Acott TS. Argon laser trabeculoplasty: Studies of mechanisms of action. Ophthalmology 1984; 91:1005–1010.

83. Robin AL, Pollack IP. Argon laser trabeculoplasty in secondary forms of open-angle glaucoma. Arch Ophthalmol 1985; 103:793–795.

84. Higginbotham EJ, Richardson TM. Response of exfoliation glaucoma to laser trabeculoplasty. Br J Ophthalmol 1986; 70:837–839.

85. Forbes M, Bansal RK. Argon laser goniophotocoagulation of the trabecular meshwork in open-angle glaucoma. Trans Am Ophthalmol Soc 1981; 79:257–275.

86. Lichter PR. Practice implications of the glaucoma laser trial. Ophthalmology 1990; 97:1401–1402.

87. Van Buskirk EM. The laser step in early glaucoma therapy. Am J Ophthalmol 1991; 112:87–89.

88. Wilensky JT, Weinreb RN. Low-dose trabeculoplasty. Am J Ophthalmol 1983; 95:423–426.

89. Schwartz IW, Spaeth GL, Traverso G, Greenridge KC. Variation of technique on the results of argon laser trabeculoplasty. Ophthalmology 1983; 90:781–784.

90. Wickham MG, Worthen DM. Argon laser trabeculoplasty. Long-term follow-up. Ophthalmology 1979; 86:495–503.

91. Rouhiainen H, Terasuirta M. The laser power needed for optimum results in argon laser trabeculoplasty. Acta Ophthalmol (Copenh) 1986; 64:254–257.

92. Blondeau P, Roberg JF, Asselin Y. Long-term results of low power, long duration laser trabeculoplasty. Am J Ophthalmol 1987; 104:339–342.

93. Rouhiainen JG, Terasvirta ME, Tuorinen EJ. Peripheral anterior synechia formation after trabeculoplasty. Arch Ophthalmol 1988; 106:189–191.

94. Rodriguez MM, Spaeth GL, Donohoo P. Electron microscopy of argon therapy in phakic open-angle glaucoma. Ophthalmology 1982; 89:198–210.

95. Traverso CE, Greenridge KC, Spaeth GK. Formation of peripheral anterior synechia following argon laser trabeculoplasty. Arch Ophthalmol 1984; 102:861–863.

Additional Readings

Gass JDM. Stereoscopic Atlas of Macular Disease: Diagnosis and Treatment (3rd ed). St. Louis, MO, CV Mosby, 1987.

L'Esperance FA (ed). Current Diagnosis and Management of Chorioretinal Diseases. St. Louis, CV Mosby, 1977.

March WF (ed). Ophthalmic Lasers. A Second Generation. Thorofare, NJ, Slack Inc, 1990.

March WF (ed). Ophthalmology Clinics of North America, Vol 2, Practical Laser Surgery. Philadelphia: Saunders, 1989.

Shields MB. Textbook of Glaucoma (2nd ed). Baltimore, Williams & Wilkens, 1987.

Sigelmann J. Retinal Diseases: Pathogenesis, Laser Therapy and Surgery. Boston, Little, Brown, 1984.

Sliney D, Wolbarsht M. Safety with Lasers and Other Optical Sources—A Comprehensive Handbook. New York, Plenum Press, 1980.

SECTION THREE

OCULAR PROTECTION AGAINST OPTICAL RADIATION HAZARDS

Section III will develop the methodology required to determine the protection needed by the eye against damage from exposure to the harmful radiation described in the previous section. Four different areas must be considered in developing an optical protective system for the eye: (1) a knowledge of ocular damage caused by exposure to the radiation, (2) the optical radiation of the source, (3) the optical characteristics of the material, and (4) the physical characteristics of the protective device. Ocular protection shall consider each of these parameters in detail and the concepts can then be used in determining the ideal optical material for a particular protective system.

CHAPTER NINE

Principles in Ocular Protection

Donald G. Pitts, O.D., Ph.D.

9.1 Optical Radiation of the Source

A complete description of the source is necessary to establish the potential damage to the eye from exposure to the source. The description should include the irradiance, area of the source at the site of exposure, spectral irradiance, divergence or convergence of the beam of the source, and whether the beam is continuous or flashing. The duration of the exposure is required for a continuous source, and an intermittent or flashing source requires the duration of "off" and "on" cycles in addition to the duration of the total exposure. The spectral irradiance of a number of commonly used sources has been presented in Section II.

9.2 Optical Protection

There are three major considerations in providing optical protection for the visual system: the optical characteristics of the material, the transmittance of the material, and the physical characteristics of the optical material.

Optical characteristics refer to the ability of the optical manufacturing process to shape the material into the desired optical system. A certain material may possess excellent transmittance and physical characteristics but may not be adaptable to the manufacturing process. Until these shortcomings are overcome, the material has little value as an ocular protective material.

Transmittance characteristics refer to the ability of an optical material to absorb, reflect, or polarize incident radiation to provide the optimum spectral transmittance for the best possible vision. Selective absorption and transmittance characteristics allow proper protection against a multitude of sources, such as lasers, arc welding, mercury vapor, and other industrial sources.

Physical characteristics refer to the ability of the optical material to withstand thermal, mechanical, and acoustic stress without breaking. In the optical industry very little attention is paid to thermal or acoustic stress because most lenses are not exposed beyond their limits; however, mechanical stress in the form of impact resistance has received considerable attention. Care must be taken to ensure that certain physical characteristics of the optical material are not exceeded. For example, laser protective lenses must possess a thermal expansion that exceeds the absorbed energy or the lens will break, shatter, or explode.

Critical to the concept of protection is a knowledge of the ocular damage caused by the radiation in question. We have discussed the damage to the ocular system that is caused by the exposure to the optical radiations; however, the use of data in establishing protection criteria was not covered. Now the ocular damage data will be used to establish the need for and level of the protection required to allow normal visual performance.

Transmittance

Radiant flux incident on the first and second surfaces of a lens is lost due to reflectance and absorption by the lens media. The losses by reflection are related to the index of refraction of the optical medium, the index of refraction of the surrounding medium, and the angle of incidence of the light beam. The absorption of the radiant flux by the optical glass is about 2% per centimeter thickness.

The total transmittance of a lens is equal to the radiant flux incident on the lens reduced by the losses due to reflectance ρ and the absorption A by the optical material ($\tau_t = \tau_1 - (\rho + A)$). The transmittance of an optical device is usually measured by a spectrophotometer and the values obtained take into account the losses by absorption and reflection. Corrections for losses due to reflection and absorp-

tion must be made if the true transmittance is required. The total transmittance of a series of lenses can be determined by multiplying the individual transmittances

$$\tau_t = \tau_1 \times \tau_2 \times \tau_3 \times \ldots \tau_n \qquad (9\text{-}1)$$

where τ_t is the total transmittance, τ, transmittance of lens 1, and so on until the last lens t_n is considered.

Optical Density

Optical density (OD) is a second term used to describe the passage of light through a lens. OD is related to transmittance by the expression

$$D = \log_{10} \frac{1}{T} \text{ or } -\log_{10} T \qquad (9\text{-}2)$$

The most common use of OD is in identifying neutral density filters (ND). ND filters are specified with a number determined by the optical density of the material; for example, ND1 = 10% τ, ND2 = 1% τ, ND3 = 0.1% τ, ND0.5 = 32% τ, and ND0.3 = 50% τ. In using Fresnel's expression (equation 9-5) 4.4% of the light is lost due to reflection at the first and second optical interfaces of a common glass lens, leaving a 91.2% transmittance. These losses calculate to an optical density of

$$D = \log_{10} \frac{1}{\tau} = \frac{1}{0.912} = 0.04 \qquad (9\text{-}3)$$

To determine the total density of a series of optical lenses, the OD for each component must be added.

Shade Number

Filters used for welding are designated by shade numbers that are related to luminous transmittance by the relation

$$SN = \frac{7}{3} \log_{10} \frac{1}{T_L} + 1 \qquad (9\text{-}4)$$

It is convenient to relate the welder's protective lens system to either optical transmittance or optical density, topics that will be covered more fully in Chapter 15 on welding.

Fresnel's Expression

Fresnel has shown that the losses of radiation incident on an optical surface are related to the index of refraction of the media:

$$\rho = \frac{(n_1 - n_2)^2}{(n_1 + n_2)^2} \qquad (9\text{-}5)$$

where ρ is the reflected light, n_1 the index of refraction of the first medium, and n_2 the index of refraction for the second medium. The loss at the first surface of an ophthalmic crown glass lens with an n = 1.532 would be 4.4%, or 8.8% for both surfaces in air. The index of refraction n of an optical medium varies with the wavelength; therefore, losses due to reflection will also vary with wavelength. The error resulting from changes in the index of refraction with wavelength will not be too great for the visible (VIS) spectrum if a single index value based on sodium D line at 589.9 nm is used. Fresnel's expression assumes that the incident ray is normal to the optical surface.

Fresnel's expression is important in establishing the index of refraction for single layer antireflection coatings. To establish equal light intensities reflected from each surface of the antireflection coating, the refractive index of the film should be equal to the square root of the refractive index of the glass in air or a vacuum.[1] The beams reflected from the two surfaces of the coating will be the value expressed above unless the thickness of the coating is made an odd number of quarter wavelengths in thickness. The thickness of the coating can be determined by the formula

$$nt = (k + \tfrac{1}{2}\tfrac{\lambda}{2}) = (k + \tfrac{\lambda}{4}) \qquad (9\text{-}6)$$

where nt is the optical thickness and must be an odd number of quarter wavelengths, k is the odd integer, and λ the wavelength. The reflectance of light normal to the lens surface is reduced materially when these expressions are applied.

Validity of Relating Animal Data to Man

An important consideration in using the ocular damage data to establish criteria for protection lies in the fact that most ocular data have been derived from animal experimentation. There are two re-

search efforts that can be used to validate the use of animal data in the solution of human problems.

Data on the comparison of retinal burn thresholds for the human, the primate, and the rabbit are given in Table 9-1.[2] The exposure conditions for each species were identical using a retinal image diameter of 1 mm, an exposure duration of 135 ms, and a spectrum from 400 to 800 nm. The area of retinal exposure was the paramacula for all species but included the fovea centralis for the human and monkey. Using the retinal burn data, the radiant threshold exposure levels are in ratio from 12 (human): 6 (monkey): 4 (rabbit); therefore, the human retina requires twice the radiant exposure of the monkey and three times the radiant exposure of the rabbit to produce a threshold retinal lesion. Blumthaler et al[3] reconstructed human solar exposures that produced photokeratitis in snow skiers when their UVB data of 1200 to 5600 J/m² (0.12–0.56 J/cm²) are compared to the laboratory data of 3500 J/m² (0.35 J/cm²). The results are not significantly different.[4]

	Area Exposed		
Species	Paramacula	Fovea	Comments
Human (A.E.G.)	9.0–12.2	13.8	Only temporary afterimage
Human (M.Y.)	9.5–9.9	9.7	Absolute central scotoma
Human (M.V.)	9.7		Foveal detachment
Human (White)	9.3 ± 1.56		18 patients
Human (Black)	7.9 ± 1.86		10 patients
Monkey	5.9 + 1.5	5.7 ± 0.35	22 rhesus eyes
Rabbit	4.1 ± 0.4		100 rabbits

The optical source was a filtered Osram lamp (XBO 2500 W) producing a spectrum of 400 to 800 nm. Radiant exposure is given on the retina in J/cm².

From Ham WT, Jr, Mueller HA, Williams RC, Geeraets WJ. Ocular hazard from viewing the sun unprotected through various windows and filters. Appl Opt 1973; 12:2122–2129. © The Optical Society of America; with permission.

TABLE 9-1
Comparison of Retinal Burn Thresholds in the Human, Monkey, and Rabbit

These research efforts demonstrate that animal-generated laboratory data can, indeed, be applied to the solution of human radiant exposure problems and, when the data are extrapolated with caution, the result is satisfactory. If the animal data are applied directly without extrapolation a protective factor would be automatically built into the calculations because human exposures are always a higher value than the comparable animal data. The data from the rhesus monkey have been accepted as a model for safety standards for the human.[2] Incidentally, the rabbit UVC and UVB laboratory data have been used in the development of safe ultraviolet (UV) filtering for the Gemini, Apollo, and Shuttle space programs.[4]

9.3 Calculation Methods for Ocular Protection

Methods to determine safe exposure from optical radiation includes the safe exposure duration (SED), the protection factor (PF), and the relative effectiveness (RE) methods. Protection against laser exposure uses the maximum permissible exposure (MPE) concept that was discussed in Chapter 7, Lasers in Industry and the Clinic. Each of the ocular protection calculation methods will be presented in detail, with example calculations followed by recommendations on the preferred method for particular safe calculation situations.

Safe Exposure Duration

The SED can be used when the threshold radiant exposure H in J/cm^2 and the source irradiance E_e in W/cm^2 are known ($1\ W \cdot s/cm^2 = 1\ J/cm^2$). The safe exposure duration t in seconds may be calculated by

$$t[s] = \frac{H(J/cm^2)}{E_e(W/cm^2)} \qquad (9\text{-}7)$$

Care must be taken to ensure that the threshold determination and the source used for exposure are for the same spectral waveband for the SED calculation to be valid. This formula may be used for all divisions of the optical radiation spectrum. For example, assume that the retinal threshold for the 441-nm wavelength is 30 J/cm^2 and that a worker is exposed to a source that provides an irradiance of 0.01 W/cm^2 at 441 nm. The SED would be

$$t = \frac{30\ J/cm^2}{0.01\ W/cm^2} = \frac{30\ W \cdot s/cm^2}{0.01\ W/cm^2} = 3000\ s$$
$$= 60\ min \qquad (9\text{-}8)$$
$$= 1\ hr$$

Protection Factor Method

The thresholds for ocular damage are often expressed in terms of irradiance (W/cm^2) rather than radiant exposure (J/cm^2), and an evaluation of safety can be accomplished quickly:

$$PF = \frac{E_e\lambda\ \text{for Damage}\ (W/cm^2)}{E_e\lambda\ \text{of Source}\ (W/cm^2)} \qquad (9\text{-}9)$$

A PF of 1 would indicate that the eye is protected but without a margin of safety. A PF greater than 1 would indicate adequate protection and assure a margin of safety. A PF less than 1 would indicate that the eye was unsafe when exposed to the source and additional protection would be required.

The PF method is a quick evaluation of the safety of ocular exposure, but certain precautions must be observed. The irradiance for ocular damage and the irradiance of the source must be in the same spectral waveband because the eye demonstrates a spectral response to damage in certain wavebands. If the radiant exposure H (J/cm^2) is provided, the duration of the exposure in seconds is usually also provided, and the irradiance of the source can be calculated.

Assume that the source irradiance is 0.125 W/cm^2 and the threshold for damage to the eye for the same waveband was found to be 0.75 W/cm^2, the PF could be calculated:

$$PF = \frac{0.75\ W/cm^2}{0.125\ W/cm^2} = 6 \qquad (9\text{-}10)$$

A PF of 6 means that the eye can be exposed to the source environment with a safety factor of 5; i.e., the source could be increased five times before ocular damage would occur.

Relative Effectiveness Method

ULTRAVIOLET RADIATION IN THE PHOTOKERATITIS AND CATARACT WAVELENGTH RANGE (200–320 NM)
The information required to calculate the safe UV ocular exposure to prevent photokeratitis in the 200- to 320-nm wavelength range must include the

spectral irradiance of the source, the spectral transmittance τ_λ of the protective device, and the relative efficiency S_λ of UVR to produce photokeratitis.[5] The threshold data for corneal damage H_c and lens damage H_L are used to calculate the relative efficiency S_λ of the UV by normalizing the data in Figure 6-16 to the 270-nm wavelength value for the cornea and the 300-nm wavelength value for the lens. The results are found in Table 9-2. The relative spectral efficiency S_λ is a weighting factor that allows the calculation of the effective irradiance E_{euv} for the production of photokeratitis, cataracts, or for any action spectrum. The relative efficiency S_λ for photokeratitis given in Table 9-3 is from the National Institute of Occupational Safety and Health (NIOSH) recommended standard[6] and the threshold limit values used by the American Conference of Governmental Industrial Hygienists (ACGIH).[7] All known action spectra data for the skin and the eye were plotted and then a hazard envelope drawn to encompass the data as shown in Figure 9-1.[8] The values for the relative spectral effectiveness in Table 9-3 were extrapolated from Figure 9-1.[7] The relative effectiveness values in Table 9-2, which were taken directly from experimental data presented in Chapter 6, differ somewhat from the envelope concept relative effectiveness data. In calculations, either set of S_λ data will provide adequate protective criteria. The effective irradiance of source to produce minimal corneal damage or photokeratitis may be calculated as follows:

$$E_{euv} = \sum_{210}^{320} E_\lambda \tau_\lambda S_\lambda \Delta\lambda \qquad (9\text{-}11)$$

where E_{euv} is the effective irradiance of UV producing minimal damage to the cornea (photokeratitis) in W/cm^2; E_λ the source power per wavelength interval in $W/cm^2 \cdot nm$; T_λ the transmittance of the protective device in decimal form, i.e., for protective goggles or glasses; S_λ the relative spectral effectiveness from Table 9-2; and $\Delta\lambda$ the bandwidth of the wavelength in nanometers. The effective irradiance for the cornea relates the ability of the UV from the source to produce photokeratitis after being transmitted through a protective device. The effective irradiance formula can also be used to calculate the effective irradiance of the source to produce cataracts by using the lens data in the 290- to 320-nm wavelength range from Figure 6-24 and the lens S_λ data from Table 9-2.

Wavelength (nm)	Human	Primate	Rabbit	Lens Rabbit
210	—	0.012	0.007	—
220	0.40	0.19	0.11	—
230	0.31	0.18	0.17	—
240	0.53	0.33	0.15	—
250	0.50	0.20	0.12	—
260	0.53	0.36	0.28	—
270	1.00	1.00	1.00	—
280	0.68	0.67	0.45	—
290	0.57	0.57	0.42	0.05
295	—	—	—	0.20
300	0.57	0.36	0.10	1.00
305	—	—	—	0.50
310	0.29	0.20	0.09	0.20
315	—	—	—	0.30
320	—	0.0004	0.0005	0.01
325	—	—	—	0.003

The dashes indicate that data are not available.
From Pitts DG, Cullen AP. Ocular Ultraviolet Effects from 295 nm to 400 nm in the Rabbit. Publication 77-175. Dept. Health, Education and Welfare, Natl Inst Occup Safety Health, 1977.

TABLE 9-2
The Relative Efficiency S_λ in Producing Corneal Ocular Damage and Lenticular Ocular Damage for the Human, Rabbit, and Primate

The effective irradiance E_{euv} may now be used to calculate the SED t allowable before photokeratitis or cataracts are induced. The duration of SED t in seconds is given by

For the cornea

$$t = \frac{H_c 270}{E_{euv}(200\text{-}320)}$$

t = safe duration in seconds
H_{C270} = radiant exposure threshold for photokeratitis at 270 nm or 3×10^{-3} J/cm^2
$E_{euv}(200\text{-}320)$ = the effective irradiance for photokeratitis

$$(9\text{-}12)$$

For the lens

$$t = \frac{H_L 300}{E_{euv}(295\text{-}320)}$$

t = safe duration in seconds

Wavelength (nm)	Permissible Eight-hour dose (mJ/cm^2)	Relative spectral effectiveness (S_λ)
200	100.0	0.03
210	40.0	0.075
220	25.0	0.12
230	16.0	0.19
240	10.0	0.30
250	7.0	0.43
254	6.0	0.50
260	4.6	0.65
270	3.0	1.00
280	3.4	0.88
290	4.7	0.64
300	10.0	0.30
305	50.0	0.05
310	200.0	0.015
315	1000.0	0.003

From Sliney DH. The merits of an envelope action spectrum for ultraviolet exposure criteria. Am Ind Hyg Assoc J 1972; 33:644–653. Reprinted by permission of the American Industrial Hygiene Association.

TABLE 9-3
Total Permissible 8-h Doses and Relative Spectral Effectiveness of Some Selected Monochromatic Wavelengths

H_{L300} = radiant exposure threshold for cataracts at 300 nm or 0.15 J/cm^2

$E_{euv}(295–320)$ = the effective irradiance for cataracts

The RE procedure can be used also to calculate the transmittance of a protective device. If the total transmittance of the device does not exceed the calculated mean transmittance, τ_λ may be removed from the right of the summation sign in the formula and placed to the left of the summation sign as follows:

$$E_{euv} = \sum_{210}^{315} E_\lambda\, \tau_\lambda\, S_\lambda\, \Delta_\lambda \text{ and } E_{euv} = \tau \sum_{210}^{315} E_\lambda\, S_\lambda\, \Delta_\lambda$$

Therefore

$$t = \frac{H_{c270}J/cm^{-2}}{\tau \sum_{200}^{315} E_\lambda\, S_\lambda \Delta_\lambda [W/cm^{-2}]} \text{ and}$$

$$\tau = \frac{H_{c270}[J/cm^{-2}]}{t \sum_{210}^{315} E_\lambda\, S_\lambda \Delta_\lambda [W \cdot S/cm^{-2}]} \tag{9-13}$$

The total transmittance of a protective device must not exceed τ_λ or the calculated mean transmittance of the system.

An example calculation for photokeratitis is provided in Table 9-4, where column 1 presents the waveband in nanometers (nm), column 2 the spectral irradiance $E_{e\lambda}$ of the source, column 3 the spectral transmittance T_λ of a protective device, column 4 presents the relative spectral effectiveness S_λ from Table 9-2, and column 5 presents the relative irradiance $E_{e\lambda}$ of the source. The effective irradiance E_{euv} of the source is obtained by summing column 5 and multiplying by the wavelength interval, 10 nm. In this example, the effective irradiance is equal to 76.2 × 10^{-7} W/cm^2. The SED t allows an exposure equal to 394 s, 6.5 min, or 0.1 h. If the total transmittance

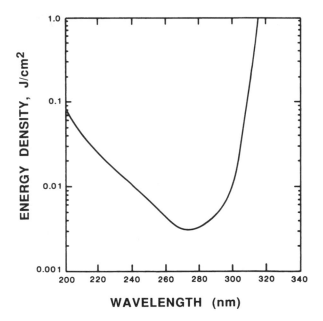

FIGURE 9-1
Recommended UVR exposure standard. Adapted from a figure developed and published by the American Conference of Governmental Industrial Hygienists in "*Threshold Limit Values for Chemical Substances and Physical Agents in the Workroom Environment with Intended Changes for 1972." From* Sliney DH. The merits of an envelope action spectrum for ultraviolet exposure criteria. Am Ind Hyg Assoc J 1972; 33:644–653. Reprinted by permission of the American Industrial Hygiene Association.

of a protective device does not exceed the limit for the mean calculated transmittance, the maximum allowable transmittance can be determined for varying durations of exposure. The example from Table 9-4 assumes an 8-h exposure duration (2.8×10^4 s), for which the mean integrated transmittance of 0.003 or 0.3% would provide protection for 2.8×10^4 s or 8 h exposure to the source.

The potential hazards to the cornea from exposure to UVA in the 320- to 400-nm wavelength range are difficult to evaluate because calculations for protection should be based on the RE method. The radiant exposures necessary to cause damage to the cornea are extremely high when compared to the defined action spectrum from 200 to 315 nm. The corneal exposure levels adopted by the ACGIH and recommended as a standard by NIOSH are an irradiance of 1 mW/cm^2 for exposure durations greater than 1000 s and a total radiant exposure of 1 J/cm^2 for durations less than 100 s. Recent biologic data[9] indicate that a reevaluation of these exposure levels may be indicated because the exposure level of sunlight in the 320- to 400-nm wavelength range on a sunny day is on the order of 2 mW/cm^2. However, comparison of the irradiance in W/cm^2 from a source with the ACGIH- and NIOSH-recommended exposure limits will provide information about the potential hazard of the source.

The retinal data do not provide sufficient information in the UV wavelength range to establish a retinal action spectrum for hazard evaluation by the RE method.[10,11] However, the retinal radiant exposures (J/cm^2) and retinal irradiance (W/cm^2) may be used to determine efficacy of exposure using the individual wavebands with either the SED or PF methods.

Wavelength in nm (10 nm)	Source Spectral Irradiance (W/cm$^2 \cdot$ nm) $E_{e\lambda} \times 10^{-7}$	Spectral Transmittance Protective τ_λ in Decimal	Relative Efficiency S_λ	Irradiance ($E_\lambda \cdot T_\lambda \cdot S_\lambda$) (W/cm$^2 \cdot$ nm) $E_\lambda \times 10^{-9}$
210	3.0	0.01	0.075	0.23
220	4.4	0.02	0.12	1.06
230	5.9	0.02	0.19	2.24
240	5.9	0.03	0.30	5.31
250	6.8	0.04	0.43	11.69
260	13.2	0.05	0.65	42.90
270	25.6	0.05	1.00	128.00
280	21.0	0.07	0.88	129.36
290	53.8	0.07	0.64	241.02
300	61.0	0.10	0.30	183.00
310	76.0	0.12	0.015	13.68
320	85.0	0.15	0.003	3.83

$$E_{euv} = \sum_{210}^{320} E_\lambda \, \tau_\lambda \, S_\lambda \, \Delta\lambda = 762.02 \times 10^{-9} \text{ W/cm}^2 \cdot \text{nm} \times 10 \text{ nm} = 76.2 \times 10^{-7} \text{ W/cm}^2$$

$$t = \frac{H_{c270}}{E_{euv}} = \frac{3 \times 10^{-3} \text{ [J/cm}^2\text{]}}{76.2 \times 10^{-7} \text{ [W/cm}^2\text{]}} = 3.94 \times 10^2 \text{ [s] safe duration}$$
$$= 6.5 \text{ min}$$
$$= 0.1 \text{ h}$$
$$\tau = \frac{H_{c270}}{t \, E_{euv}} = \frac{3 \times 10^{-3} \text{ [J/cm}^2\text{]}}{2.8 \times 10^4 \text{ s} \cdot 3.64 \times 10^{-5} \text{ W/cm}^2} = 0.003 \text{ transmittance for eight hours' safe exposure}$$

TABLE 9-4
Example Calculation for Safe Exposure Duration for the Cornea Against UVR in the 210- to 320-nm Wavelength Range

VIS RADIATION IN THE 380- TO 760-NM WAVELENGTH RANGE

The early research on retinal lesions interpreted them as being thermal in nature; however, in the recent years, it has become increasingly evident that there is a photochemical element from the blue portion of the VIS spectrum that causes part of the retinal injury when exposure durations are greater than 10 s. The hazard evaluation of a source must consider both the thermal and the blue-hazard components of the source.[12]

The data from Ham et al[1] bear directly on the VIS spectrum problem because the data were obtained with broadband exposures and provide a practical approach to protection criteria against the solar irradiance levels of radiation. For the 180 s exposure, 4.8 ± 0.8 mW entered the eye and required a retinal irradiance of 18.9 ± 3.5 W/cm^2 to produce a threshold retinal lesion with an image diameter of 158 μm. The data may be analyzed in terms of radiant exposure (J/cm^2) to establish retinal lesion thresholds because radiant exposure is time-related.

For hazard analysis, it is best to relate retinal irradiance to the radiance (W/cm^2-sr) of the source. The radiance of the source L_s may be calculated from the irradiance of the source at the cornea E_c by the projected solid angle Ω[13]: $L_c = E_c/\Omega$ [W/cm^2-sr]. The projected solid angle Ω at distance r may be calculated as $\Omega = A/r^2$, and the retinal irradiance can be found by using

$$E_r = 0.27 \, L_c \, \tau \, d_p^2 \qquad (9\text{-}14)$$

where E_r is the retinal irradiance (W/cm^2), L_c the source irradiance (W/cm$^2 \cdot$ sr) at the plane of the cornea, τ the integrated or mean transmittance (0.77), and d_p the diameter of the pupil (in centimeters). Note that this formula is independent of the distance of the eye from the source.

When the retinal irradiance for damage is provided and it is preferable for the corneal irradiance to be used for a hazard evaluation, the corneal irradiance may be found:

$$\begin{aligned} E_r &= E_c \times \tau \times A_c/A_r \text{ and} \\ E_c &= E_r \times A_\tau/\tau \times A_c \end{aligned} \qquad (9\text{-}15)$$

where E_r is the retinal irradiance (W/cm^2), τ the integrated transmittance of the ocular media (0.77), E_c the corneal irradiance (W/cm^2), A_c the area of the

image at the corneal plane (mm^2), and A_r the area of the image at the retinal plane (mm^2).

Thermal Hazard Evaluation

An evaluation of the thermal injury of the eye from exposures to a source requires that the spectral irradiance of the lamp L_λ be weighted against the burn hazard function R_λ provided in Table 9-5:

Wavelength (nm)	Blue-Light Hazard Function B_λ	Burn Hazard Function R_λ
400	0.10	1.0
405	0.20	2.0
410	0.40	4.0
415	0.80	8.0
420	0.90	9.0
425	0.95	9.5
430	0.98	9.8
435	1.0	10.0
440	1.0	10.0
445	0.97	9.7
450	0.94	9.4
455	0.90	9.0
460	0.80	8.0
465	0.70	7.0
470	0.62	6.2
475	0.55	5.5
480	0.45	4.5
485	0.40	4.0
490	0.22	2.2
495	0.16	1.6
500–600	$10^{[450-\lambda/50]}$	1.0
600–700	0.001	1.0
700–1060	0.001	$10^{[(\lambda-700)/515]}$
1060–1400	0.001	0.2

From Sliney DH, Marshall WJ, Carothers ML, Kaste RC.[17] Hazard Analysis of Broad-band Optics Sources. Aberdeen Proving Ground, MD, US Army Environmental Hygiene Agency, 1980.

TABLE 9-5
Spectral Weighing Functions for Assessing Retinal Hazards from Broadband Optical Sources

$$L_{HAZ} = \sum_{400}^{1400} L_\lambda R_\lambda \Delta\lambda \leq 1/\omega \cdot t^{\frac{1}{2}} \qquad (9\text{-}16)$$

where L_{HAZ} is the radiance of the source, L_λ the spectral radiance of the source W/cm^2-sr, R_λ the spectral burn hazard function, $\Delta\lambda$ the wavelength interval in nanometers, ω the solid angle of the source in radians, and t the duration of the exposure in seconds. If the source is pulsed, t is limited from 1 μs to 10 s.[17]

Extended-Source VIS Spectrum Retinal MPE

An additional evaluation of retinal hazard can be made using the extended-source laser MPE for the VIS spectrum (Table 9-5). The ocular parameters suggested by Calkins and Hochheimer[15] include a 7-mm pupillary diameter, a posterior focal point of 2.15 cm, an index for the vitreous of 1.333, and an ocular transmittance of 0.90, which results in an MPE of 2.92 J/cm^2. Substituting a more realistic transmittance of 0.77^2 provides an MPE for the 400- to 700-nm wavelength range of 2.40 J/cm^2. The SED t in seconds would be

$$t(s) = \frac{MPE~(2.40~J/cm^2)}{E_e~(W/cm^2)} \qquad (9\text{-}17)$$

The ocular transmittance of 0.90 used by Calkins and Hochheimer results in a greater radiant exposure of 2.92 J/cm^2 and a built-in safety factor of 17.8%. The 2.40 J/cm^2 MPE is two magnitudes below the LD 50 threshold for producing an ophthalmoscopically visible lesion in the primate retina. Actually, the safety factor for the human is greater because the human retina requires twice the radiant exposure of the primate to produce a retinal lesion (see Table 9-1). Using an MPE of 2.40 J/cm^2 simplifies the evaluation process for broadband, extended sources commonly encountered in most industries and some ophthalmic instruments.

Blue Hazard Effects

Blue VIS radiation near 440 nm appears to be the most hazardous wavelengths in the VIS spectrum for the production of retinal injury, and the threshold value was found to be 0.3 mW/cm^2 for a 1000-s exposure using the HeCd laser.[16] The U.S. Army Environmental Hygiene Agency (USAEHA)[17] devel-

oped a blue-light hazard function B_λ (Table 9-5) from the data of Ham et al[11] for the purpose of evaluating noncoherent, broadband sources. Excessive retinal pigment damage resulted from exposure to blue light (463 nm) on the order of 0.01 to 0.1 mW/cm^2 for 3600 s or about 0.36 J/cm^2 when measured at the cornea.[18] Blue-light hazard formula for the evaluation of retinal damage is

$$E_{Bef} = \sum_{400}^{500} E_\lambda \cdot B_\lambda \cdot \Delta\lambda \qquad (9\text{-}18)$$

where E_λ is the source irradiance (W/cm^2), B_λ the blue-light hazard function (Table 9-5), and $\Delta\lambda$ the wavelength interval (10 nm). To protect against retinal damage from blue-light exposure, the integrated spectral radiance of the source L_S weighted with the blue-light hazard function B_λ should not exceed

$$\sum_{400}^{1400} L_\lambda B_\lambda \Delta\lambda~t = 100~J/cm^2\text{-sr} \qquad (9\text{-}19)$$
$$\text{for } t < 10^4~s$$

$$\sum_{400}^{1400} L_\lambda B_\lambda \Delta\lambda = 10^{-2}~W/cm^2\text{-sr} \qquad (9\text{-}20)$$
$$\text{for } t > 10^4$$

where L_λ is the spectral radiance of the source ($W/cm^2 \cdot sr$), B_λ the blue-light hazard function, $\Delta\lambda$ the wavelength interval, and t the exposure duration.

The weighted product of L_λ and B_λ is designated as L (blue) and, if the weighted source radiance exceeds 2 $mW/cm^2 \cdot sr$ in the blue portion of the VIS spectrum, the MPE duration in seconds may be determined by

$$t(max) = \frac{100~J/cm^2\text{-sr}}{L(blue)(W/cm^2\text{-sr})} \qquad (9\text{-}21)$$

If the weighted blue-light irradiance of the source (E_{blue} in W/cm^2) exceeds 1 $\mu W/cm^2$, the maximum exposure duration is calculated

$$t(max) = 10~mJ/cm^2/E(blue) \qquad (9\text{-}22)$$

The research demonstrating that the blue portion of the VIS spectrum is more effective in creating a retinal lesion than the remainder of the VIS spectrum has created undue concern. Under normal situations, sunlight does not create a blue hazard from the blue end of the VIS spectrum and need not concern us. The blue-light hazard does play a role in lesions obtained from observing a solar eclipse without ocular protection or when observations are made near the solar disk using binoculars. The major hazard from blue light is from man-made sources where chronic blue-light exposure may result in photochemical damage to the retina. The eye needs protection against blue hazard photochemical injury when hazard evaluation of a particular environment determines that exposure of the eye is unsafe.

Hazard Evaluation of IRA (770–1400 nm)

There are no presently adopted standards that establish permissible levels of infrared (IR) exposure. The ACGIH has proposed threshold limit values for IR, but they have not been formally adopted. The standards for IR are tentative because of the lack of sufficient quantified biologic data from which definitive standards can be established. The values calculated from IR exposure cannot be taken to establish a narrow border between a safe exposure level and a dangerous exposure level. In fact, the IR data clearly demonstrate that acute retinal exposure to IR in the 700- to 1400-nm wavelength range required to produce a retinal lesion varies from 1500 to 17,532 Jcm^{-2} for both the rabbit and primate animal models.[2,19,20] The fact that the IR threshold is related to the power of the source and to the exposure duration is demonstrated by shorter exposure durations requiring higher power levels to achieve threshold.[2] The IR threshold exposure is also related to the rate of delivery, which is illustrated by data showing that exposures at 4 W/cm^2 and below require more than twice the radiant exposure than when the IR irradiance is greater than 4 W/cm^2.[20]

Research data indicate that the cornea, iris, and lens are almost equally sensitive to IR damage, but a much higher exposure is required to induce an IR retinal lesion. The IR threshold for the retina varies between 1500 and 17,532 J/cm^2.[2,20] It appears that the cornea should protect the retina, but the concept fails when the irradiance is below threshold and the effects are cumulative. In addition, when the irradiance is very high and delivered in a short period of time, the retina and lens may be severely damaged, but minimal damage occurs to the cornea. This condition has been demonstrated by the laser. The additive effects of UV, VIS, and IR spectra in pro-

ducing ocular damage is illustrated in Figure 6-26, where the straight line indicates that IR-induced ocular damage is a single process and that the UV, VIS, and IR spectra are added in producing the damage. The data of Pitts et al[19] are important from a different aspect. When a 50-nm waveband at 1050 nm and an irradiance of 0.048 W/cm^2 with exposure durations up to 29,000 s was used, a radiant exposure of 1323 J/cm^2 did not result in ocular damage. Identical 8-h exposures for 5 d (28,800 s per day) also failed to induce ocular damage to the cornea, lens, or retina.

If the cataract is used as the ocular damage criterion, the level of hazardous exposure may be determined from the data of Lydahl et al.[21-25] Glassworker data for age 70 using a waveband of 760 to 1400 nm results in a mean exposure duration of 49.4 y, which yields a median lifetime radiant exposure of 9.5×10^5 J/cm^2. If the average work year were taken to be 240 d, the 49.4-y exposure would equate to an irradiance of 2.9×10^{-3} W/cm^2. Matelsky[26] has suggested that U.S. glassworkers and steelworkers exposed to IR irradiances of 0.08 to 0.4 W/cm^2 develop lenticular opacities within 10 to 15 y. These exposure irradiances are 28 to 140 times higher than the measurements in the Swedish data of Lydahl. The corneal IR irradiance from sunlight is about 0.001 W/cm^2,[13] and it has been argued that a corneal IR irradiance of 0.1 W/cm^2 is too low to cause acute damage to the anterior ocular structures.[27] Thus, the IR contained in sunlight should not be sufficient to produce damage to the eye. An IRA irradiance of 0.01 W/cm^2 has been claimed to be safe, and 0.1 W/cm^2 for continuous wave (CW) lasers or 0.1 J/cm^2 for pulsed wave (PW) lasers allows a safe exposure for the IRB and IRC wavebands. The IR exposure data from a number of researchers have been placed in Table 9-6 for comparison.

Sidney and Conover[28] used ACGIH (threshold limit values, or TLVs) and ANSI Z136.1 (MPEs) to establish laser protection standard exposure levels. The laser standard for eye exposure for the 800- to 1060-nm wavelength range when viewing extended or diffuse reflections can be calculated

$$\text{Exposure level} = 0.2 \, C_A \, [\text{W/cm}^2], \quad (9\text{-}23)$$

where $C_A = e(\lambda - 700)/224$ and for 880 nm $C_A = 2.2$; therefore

Wavelength Range (nm)	Type of Source	Exposure Duration	Exposure Threshold W/cm²	Portion of Eye	Authors
IR	Diffuse	—	0.1	Cornea	27,29
IRA, IRB, and IRC	Extended	10–15 y	0.08–0.4	Lens	26
IRA	Extended	Chronic	0.01	Anterior segment	13
IRB and IRC	Intrabeam viewing		0.1 (CW laser) 0.1 J/cm⁻² (PW laser)	Retina	13
800–1060	Extended	$100-10^4$ s	1.38	Anterior segment	28
IRA	Extended	49.4 y	2.9×10^{-3}	Lens	22

TABLE 9-6
Comparison of the IR Thresholds for Different Wavelength Ranges and Sources

$$\text{Exposure level} = 0.2 \times 3.1416 \times 2.2$$
$$= 1.38 \text{ W/cm}^2 \qquad (9\text{-}24)$$

This calculation is for a 7-mm pupil, and the irradiance cannot be modified for smaller pupil sizes. The allowable exposure duration for a 1.38 W/cm⁻², 7-mm pupil for an 880-nm IR source is 100 s to 10^4 s (2–8 h).

The IR threshold data show a lowest irradiance value of 0.01 W/cm², and the highest value is 1.38 W/cm². It is proposed that 20 mW/cm² be defined as the MPE for the IRA waveband using a 7-mm diameter pupil and an indefinite or chronic exposure.

The ACGIH[7] has recommended that the 400- to 1400-nm IRA waveband viewed by the eye be limited to

$$\sum_{770}^{1400} L_\lambda \cdot R_\lambda \cdot \Delta\lambda \leq 1/\omega t^{1/2} \qquad (9\text{-}25)$$

where the pupillary diameter is 7 mm and ω is the steradian of the source (A/r²).

9.4 When Should a Particular Safe Protection Concept Be Used?

The most important consideration in evaluations of visual protection is that the person performing the evaluation be cautious and prudent because, in some instances, the future visual welfare of the worker is at stake.

The SED concept requires that the irradiance of the source and the threshold radiant exposure be known. SED can be used for UV, VIS, and IRA portions of the electromagnetic spectrum (EMS). The formula can be used for both broad waveband or narrow waveband sources as long as the source irradiance and the threshold value are within the same wavebands. SED may also be used to evaluate the protection afforded by a filter. If the irradiance of the source is known, multiply the irradiance of the source by the integrated transmittance of the protective filter, then use the safe exposure calculation to determine the allowable duration of exposure to the eye. The SED method is used also with the RE method to calculate the duration of safe exposure.

The PF concept requires that the irradiance to produce threshold ocular damage and the irradiance of the source are known. It can be used for the UV, VIS, and IRA portions of the EMS. Laser damage to the retina is often reported in retinal irradiance for a given exposure duration, and the PF method allows a quick evaluation for safe exposure from the source. Caution must be used to ensure that the same spectral wavebands are being compared and that the calculated value is below published laser safety criteria.

The RE method requires that the spectral irradiance of the source $E_{e\lambda}$, the relative effectiveness of ocular damage S_λ, and the transmittance of the protective system τ_λ be known. This method requires that the action spectrum for the wavelength band must be established. The RE is the method of choice, but its utility is presently limited to the UV spectrum because the action spectra for the VIS and IR portions of the optical spectrum are not established.

9.5 Protection Devices

Ocular protection has commonly taken the form of spectacles, goggles, face shields, and helmets, with each of these devices being developed for a particular task. Figure 9-2 illustrates most of the modern ocular protective devices, and a description of each will follow.

Safety spectacles are manufactured in both metal and plastic materials and are provided with or without sideshields. Sideshields protect the eye against objects flying from the side. Some versions of the sideshields are made from wiremesh to allow greater ventilation. Safety spectacles may be supplied with plano lenses or with the worker's prescription, but all the lenses must conform to safety standards.

Tasks involving grinding and chipping may introduce foreign particles capable of striking the eye from any direction, the sides, top, or bottom. The chipping goggle or impact cup goggle is a coverspectype design that fulfills this need. Impact or dust

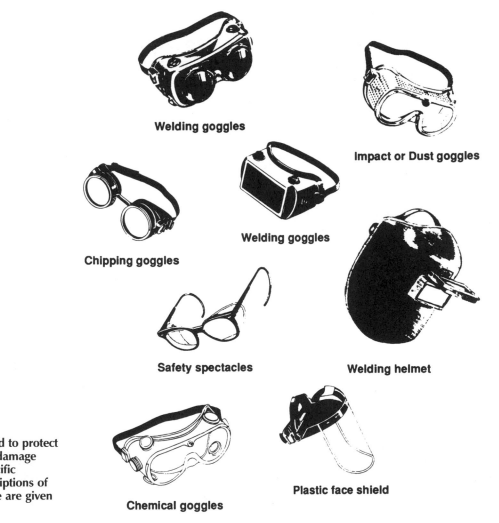

Welding goggles

Impact or Dust goggles

Chipping goggles

Welding goggles

Safety spectacles

Welding helmet

Chemical goggles

Plastic face shield

FIGURE 9-2
Optical devices developed to protect the eye against possible damage while accomplishing specific occupational tasks. Descriptions of each and its intended use are given in the text.

goggles are made from a soft, flexible plastic material that is molded in a single front to fit snug to facial contours. Lenses are inserted into the frame of the eye cup to provide rigidity to the goggle. The lenses are usually made from flat, 0.05-inch (1.27 mm) thick polycarbonate material capable of withstanding extremely high impacts without shattering. The lenses may also be tinted to provide the necessary filtering of optical radiation. These goggles are designed to be worn over a pair of spectacles. Ventilation is important to prevent the lenses from fogging. The sides of the eye cup extending from the mask to the facial area are usually perforated with holes to allow excellent ventilation. In dusty environments, the sides of the goggle should have ventilation holes that are constructed to prevent the passage of dust into the eye while allowing maximum flow of air through the goggle.

Chemical goggles are constructed the same as impact goggles except for the ventilation system. The chemical ventilation system consists of a series of plastic louvers designed to provide indirect ventilation while preventing chemical splashes, flying particles, and dust from entering the system. Chemical goggles may also be worn with dress and safety glasses.

Welding goggles are designed to protect the welder's eyes from impact and harmful radiation. They are designed for use with the acetylene-oxygen welding systems in welding, brazing, cutting, burning, and scarfing operations. There is a choice between the lens-type welding goggle and the wide-view, faceplate-type goggle. The welding helmet provides the required protection for the head, neck, and eyes during electric arc welding operations. The welding helmet is made from fiberglass with the inside of the helmet shell coated to eliminate reflections. The helmet is equipped with a headgear that allows the helmet to be raised when not welding. There is a window through which the welder can view the welding process. The window is actually a filter holder designed to hold a series of flat filter plates 5.1 × 10.8 cm (2 × 4½ inches) for protection of the eyes against UVR, IR, and the VIS spectrum radiation generated by the welding arc. The filter holder is integrally molded into the helmet or a flip-front configuration combined with a molded window as shown. The filter holder usually contains five flat plates, 1.5-mm thick, for the protection of the welder's eyes. The cover lens is an exterior clear

polycarbonate filter plate and serves for impact and spatter resistance. The spatter from the weld will pit and scar glass lenses but do little harm to a hardened polycarbonate lens. The second filter is a gold metallic filter designed to eliminate IR. The intermediate filter plate eliminates the UV, while the fourth filter plate reduces the VIS spectrum light of the welding plasma to a comfortable level for the welder. The inside filter plate is a clear polycarbonate lens. The flip-front filterplate holder can be raised to allow the welder to view the work through the clear plastic plate in the stationary portion of the holder. Thus, the welder can pause and view the work without raising the helmet or moving the helmet from the welding position.

The face shield is worn to protect the head, neck, face, and eyes from flying particles and chemical and molten metal splash. Eye protection can be worn underneath to allow control of possible hazards from optical radiation. The newest addition to the optical protection inventory is the high impact personal protector goggles. These goggles are molded from UV-absorbing polycarbonate and incoporate a variety of tints from clear to neutral grey to yellow that can be selected to provide protection against most optical radiation. They can be worn over most personal spectacles with comfort. The temples provide protection against objects flying from the side. Such spectacles provide excellent ocular protection for the average person doing those "thought to be safe" but often-dangerous weekend tasks.

9.6 Protection and Transmittance of Ophthalmic Materials

Ocular protection has commonly taken the form of spectacles, goggles, helmets, or shields that use absorptive, polarizing, or interference filters to control the undesirable optical radiation. Filtering of optical radiation by absorption is accomplished by incorporating metallic oxides within the lens; for example, iron oxides incorporated into the glass melt absorb about 95% of the UV and IR radiation. Cerium incorporated into an ophthalmic crown glass lens absorbs UV and remains clear. Figure 9-3 illustrates blue, green, and cyan absorptive filters that incorporate into the melt cobalt oxide for blue, chromium for green, and copper for cyan. In addition, cut-off

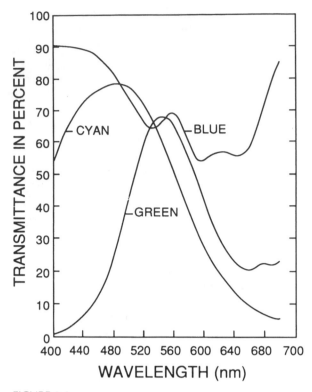

FIGURE 9-3
Broad-bandpass glass filters for blue, green, and cyan portions of the visible spectrum. Cobalt has been incorporated into the melt to produce a blue broadband filter. A combination of chromium, copper, and iron is necessary to produce a bell-shaped green filter. Copper oxide alone will produce a cyan-colored filter. *From Kriedl NJ, Rood JL. Filters. In Kingslake R (ed). Applied Optics and Optical Engineering, Vol I, pp 111–115. New York, Academic Press, 1965.*

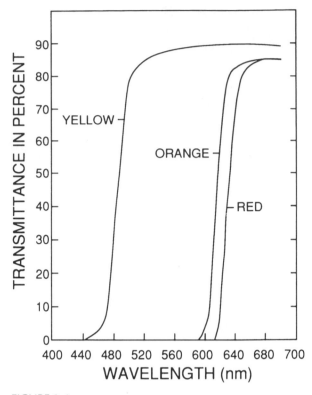

FIGURE 9-4
Cut-off filters may be used to eliminate the wavelengths of undesirable radiation. The yellow, orange, and red cut-off filters are made by adding progressively greater amounts of cadmium sulfide and cadmium selenide to the glass melt. *From Kriedl NJ, Rood JL. Filters. In Kingslake R (ed). Applied Optics and Optical Engineering, Vol I, pp 111–115. New York, Academic Press, 1965.*

filters may be used to eliminate undesired portions of the spectrum (Fig. 9-4).[35] Silica or boric acid are added to glass to increase transmittance of UV.

Reflective filters are usually metallic coatings that are vacuum-applied to the front surface of the lens. Reflective filters can provide very effective protection when properly chosen to transmit the VIS spectrum and reflect the unwanted IR radiation, but unless carefully selected, they do not absorb UV. It is dangerous to assume the protective characteristics of a lens from its color or tint because the tint may or may not provide protection.[30–32] For example, the grey or neutral glass lens usually transmits both UV and IR radiation in sufficient amounts that it should not be used for industrial protection against UV and

IR, but it has been used as a sunglass lens because its grey color does not affect color perception.[33,34] Photochromatic filters do not provide full UVB and UVA protection (Fig. 9-5). Plastic lenses are made absorptive by incorporating organic dyes into the lens during manufacturing or adding them after the lens has been surfaced and edged.

Color filters may be used to optimize visual performance under a variety of environmental conditions. For example, if a target or object is white or red and seen against a clear blue sky, a red filter placed before the eye will make the sky appear relatively dark and the objects more visible. Conversely, a dark object that is not red in color may be seen but, if the object is colored, a filter that darkens the object relative

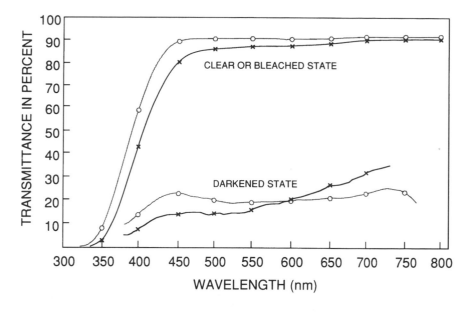

FIGURE 9-5
Photochromic filters in the bleached or clear state and the dark state do not absorb sufficient UV for use in the industrial environment in the clear state. In the darkened state UV transmittance decreases, but extrapolation of the curve to zero allows too much UVB to be considered adequate for protection.

to the blue sky must be selected for visual enhancement. The filter changes the relative contrast between the object and the sky, thereby improving visibility. The same principle is used in developing ocular protection against lasers. Ensure maximum transmittance of the VIS spectrum while making the optical density at the wavelength of the laser as high as possible. Careful selection will allow the absorption of the damaging laser beam while maintaining excellent luminous transmittance for vision.

Polaroid filters provide plane polarized light and may be the method of choice for protection in certain environmental situations. Part of the light incident on smooth, nonmetallic surfaces such as blackboards, glass windows, polished tables, smooth concrete surfaces of streets and sidewalks, glazed pottery, automobile hoods, automobile windshields, and water is reflected in the form of polarized sunlight. A polaroid filter oriented with its plane of polarization perpendicular to the reflected polarized light eliminates the annoying glare and allows comfortable vision. The polarized light transmitted by a polaroid lens is only about 32% of the incident light, and this reduction should be considered when polaroid lenses are used as protective filters.

Robertson[36] states that the glare from automobile headlights could be eliminated if the headlight were polarized and viewed through an appropriate polaroid lens. Care would need be taken to ensure that the plane of polarization of the headlights and the viewing polaroid are at right angles to each other. A difficulty would be that the angle of polarization shifts as the plane of the roadway changes relative to the headlights.

Interference filters consist of multiple layers of vacuum-deposited dielectric coatings that provide spectral transmittance in the desired wavebands. The transmitted wavelengths are controlled by using the appropriate coatings of different materials that possess the proper index of refraction. The combinations of the different layers of dielectric materials are usually proprietary to the company manufacturing the filter. Interference filters suffer from being sensitive to the angle of incidence of the light beam and to temperature. As the angle of incidence from normal changes, the spectral wavelength of the filter changes. Increases or decreases in temperature result in the same response by the dielectric coating and, because the interference depends on coating thickness, the spectral characteristics would change. These two obstacles make the use of interference filters in an uncontrolled environment very difficult; therefore, further discussion will not be pursued.

For assistance in understanding some of the principles of using filters for ocular protection, study some of the UVR transmittance curves of selected optical materials.[37] Figure 9-6 shows the UV transmittance of three different commonly used optical

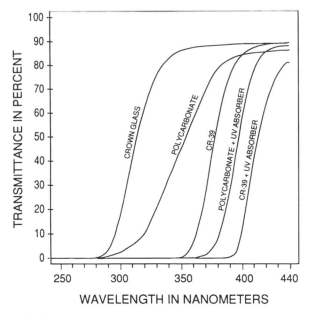

FIGURE 9-6
UV spectral transmittance of selected ophthalmic lens materials. The ophthalmic crown glass lens is clear and provides minimal UVB and UVA protection. The polycarbonate lens in curve 2 transmits less than 10% UVR to 330 nm but still provides limited UVR protection. The CR-39 lens provides full protection against UVB and partial protection against UVA. The polycarbonate and CR-39 lens with UV absorbers provide excellent UV protection. All lenses are 2.5 mm in thickness.

materials including ophthalmic crown, CR-39, and polycarbonate. Most optical glass lenses are manufactured from crown glass that begins to transmit UV at about 280 nm and quickly increases to about 90% at 340 nm. Ophthalmic crown glass is not acceptable for use as a UV protector unless a UV absorber is incorporated into the melt. The CR-39 curve is a polymer that has been used in spectacle lenses for many years. The CR-39 lens presented in the third curve contains a UV inhibitor that begins transmittance at 350 nm and achieves maximum transmittance around 400 nm. This is the transmittance curve of the ordinary CR-39 lens from the ophthalmic laboratory. The UV-400 curve is a CR-39 lens that contains UV absorbers and provides excellent protection against UVC, UVB, and UVA. Adding more UV-absorbing monomer to the CR-39 polymer can move the curve along the wavelength axis up to 450 nm. Such a lens is not preferable for

two reasons: first, the lens becomes yellowish or orangish-yellow in appearance; second, absorbing the blue wavelengths creates a pseudotritanopia that eliminates the blue color in normal vision. Shifts in color perception are unacceptable in an ophthalmic device unless the absorption characteristics are required for protection. CR-39 lenses require a scratch-resistant coating to maintain the life of the optical surfaces for extended periods of time.

Polycarbonate is a polymer with excellent temperature and impact physical characteristics, but it tends to scratch easily and transmits UV radiation readily (Fig. 9-6). The clear polycarbonate lens absorbs UV minimally and transmits UV beginning at 290 nm, attaining an 86% transmittance at about 380 nm. The polycarbonate UV absorption lens has been coated with a scratch-resistant chemical that shows amazing resistance to abrasion, excellent absorption of UVR, and an increased transmittance in the VIS wavelengths of the spectrum. The small amount of UV transmitted in the 380- to 400-nm waveband should not pose a hazard to the eye because the cut-off wavelength of the human crystalline lens is nearly identical to the polycarbonate curve.

UV-absorbing contact lenses have been used in empiric studies to determine if these materials would provide protection against UVR exposure. In recent experiments, pigmented rabbits were fitted with a soft UV-absorbing contact lens on one eye and a clear nonabsorbing soft contact lens on the other eye; their transmittance curves are shown in Figure 9-7. The UV-absorbing lens afforded full protection, whereas the normal soft contact lens showed similar or slightly more damage than an eye not wearing a contact lens.[38–40] The enhanced effect was probably due to a reduced availability of oxygen through the contact lens. Figure 9-8 compares the UV transmittance of three soft contact lenses and indicates that some lenses do not provide full UV protection. The transmittance of the Equalens-Blue* gas permeable contact lens for 0.1 mm and 0.2 mm thicknesses (Fig. 9-9) illustrates that transmittance characteristics vary with lens thickness. When a UV-absorbing contact lens is prescribed, care must be taken to explain that full ocular protection may not be provided because of the lens size. All aphakes and pseudophakes should be provided with protection against UVR when contact lenses are prescribed. Figure 9-10 presents the UV spectral transmittance of a non–UV-absorbing PMMA intraocular lens (IOL) and a

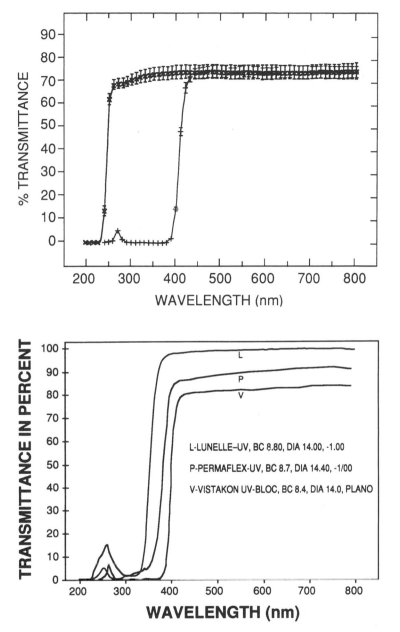

FIGURE 9-7

UV spectrum transmittance of a normal and a UV-absorbing 58% water content soft contact lens. The normal soft contact lens begins transmittance at 225 nm and achieves maximum transmittance at 250 nm. The UV contact lens absorbs almost all UVR to 400 nm. The small 5%, 20-nm bandwidth curve centered at 270 nm is of little concern because it is outside the wavelengths of sunlight reaching the Earth. Transmittance measurements were made with the lenses in air.

L-LUNELLE–UV, BC 8.80, DIA 14.00, -1.00

P-PERMAFLEX–UV, BC 8.7, DIA 14.40, -1/00

V-VISTAKON UV-BLOC, BC 8.4, DIA 14.0, PLANO

FIGURE 9-8

Transmittance of three soft contact lenses that are claimed to be UV-absorbing. Sunlight on the Earth begins at 288 nm, and the portions of the curves below 288 nm can be ignored. The Lunelle lens is a very poor UV protector because it transmits more than 30% of the UVB and about 70% of the UVA. The Permaflex lens transmits about 4% of the UVB and 40% of the UVA. The Vistakon lens transmits no UVB and only 5% of the UVA above 380 nm.

UV-absorbing IOL, compared with the transmittance of the human.[41,42] These transmittance curves demonstrate that the UV-absorbing IOL would protect the retina against UVC, UVB, and UVA as well as the normal human crystalline lens.

An ophthalmic material with the transmittance characteristics that reduces UVR to a minimum such as the UV-absorbing CR-39, polycarbonate, soft contact lenses, and IOLs should be used for a number of different types of people. Such a lens for aphakic and pseudophakic patients will prevent a retinitis from overexposure to sunlight by preventing UVA and UVB radiation from reaching the retina.[41,43–47] People with cataracts often experience excessive glare when driving or when they are in sunlight for fishing, golfing, and gardening. A UV-absorbing lens would eliminate the UVR that causes scatter and fluorescence in the cataractous lens and would

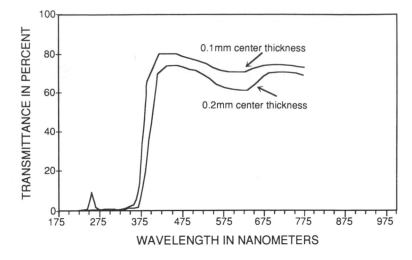

FIGURE 9-9

UV transmittance of the Equalens-Blue gas permeable contact lens for 0.1-mm and 0.2-mm center thickness. At 0.1-mm center thickness, there is about 1% UV transmittance to 380 nm that is essentially eliminated by the 0.2-mm center thickness lens.

FIGURE 9-10

UV transmittance of IOLs and the human eye. Normal PMMA begins transmitting UVR at 320 nm and quickly increases to maximum transmittance in the UVA. It affords retinal protection against UVB but transmits the UVA that is very damaging to the pseudophakic retina. The UV-PMMA absorbs essentially all of the UVB and UVA. The phakic human eye also absorbs most of the UV, but the transmittance of 2.7% centered at 320 nm and below 1% until 370 nm is still capable of causing cumulative retinal damage. *From Werner JS et al: Loss of human photoreceptor sensitivity associated with chronic exposure to ultraviolet radiation. Ophthalmology 1981; 96:1552–1553; with permission.*

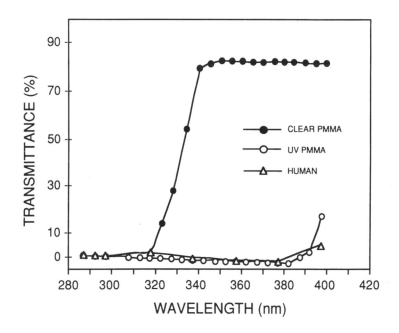

result in more comfortable vision. Corneal changes from exposure to UV involve the endothelium, stroma, and epithelium.[3,48–53] People who are prescribed photosensitizing drugs that cause a number of ocular problems triggered by UVR should be provided UV-absorbing lenses.[54,55] People who sunbathe, participate in activities in the snow such as skiing, sledding, and skating, or climb mountains expose themselves to the harshest solar UV environments and require full UVR protection. Finally, UV-

absorbing lenses should be used for any person who has a vocation or avocation that requires excess exposure to UVR to eliminate or reduce the threat of UV-induced corneal, lenticular, or retinal damage.

Control of the VIS spectrum will be covered in detail in Chapter 11, Sunglasses for Ocular Protection; however, an abbreviated discussion is necessary here. The type of filtration needed depends on the environment in which the eyes are used, but most VIS spectrum filters are absorptive. The optimum level of light for good, comfortable vision is about 1370 cd/m² (400 ft L). This is the intensity of light found under a shade tree in full sunlight, and the transmittance of an ophthalmic lens needed to arrive at the proper luminance may be found by the following formula:

$$\tau = \frac{1400 \ [cd/m^2]}{L_v \ [cd/m^2]} \quad (9\text{-}26)$$

where τ is the transmittance of the ophthalmic lens in the VIS spectrum and L_v the luminance of the sun or other source.

The method of choice in controlling IR is by mirror-type metallic, vacuum-deposited coatings. Absorptive filters re-radiate IR as heat at a lower wavelength that easily penetrates the ocular media to the retina and affords little protection. The most common metallic coatings used to control IR are silver (Ag), gold (Au), aluminum (Al), and more recently, copper (Cu). Figure 9-11 presents percent-reflectance curves in the 220- to 5000-nm waveband

for vacuum-deposited coatings.[56] Vacuum deposition is the method of choice because it provides the highest IR reflection.

Table 9-7 presents data from six different, commonly used optical coatings for the UV, VIS, and IR portions of the EMS. Aluminum possesses a high reflectance across the entire optical spectrum. Silver, gold, and copper transmit about 60% of the UV and reflect greater than 98% of the IR wavelengths. Silver would be the metallic coating of choice to transmit UV while reflecting both VIS spectrum light and IR. Gold and copper transmit close to 30% of VIS spectrum light, over 60% of UV, and reflect all but about 2% of the IR. A mirror coating should be applied to a UV-absorbing substrate to provide full protection against UVR.

Care must be taken to keep the thickness of the protective film small compared to the wavelength of the radiation. Reflectance decreases when thicker protective layers are used. Pairs of dielectric films can be used by alternating low and high

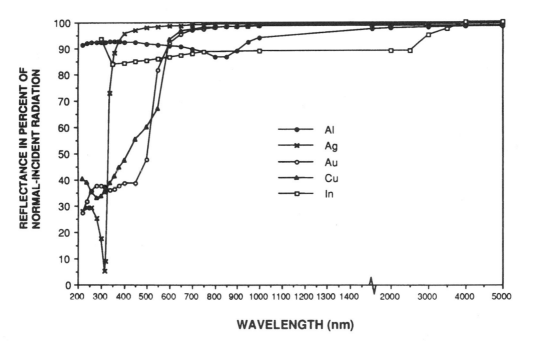

FIGURE 9-11
Percent reflectance of normal incident radiation for aluminum (Al), silver (Ag), gold (Au), and copper (Cu) in the wavelength range from 0.22 to 5.0 µm (200–5000 nm). Note the change in scale of the x-axis prior to 0.4 µm and 2.0 µm. *Data from* Hass.[56]

Metallic Coating	Ultraviolet (220–380 nm)		Visible (380–750 nm)		Infrared (750–5000 nm)	
	% R	% τ	% R	% τ	% R	% τ
Aluminum	92.5	7.5	911	8.9	93.4	6.6
Silver	39.8	60.2	97.5	2.5	99.3	0.7
Gold	35.5	64.5	69.5	30.4	98.7	1.3
Copper	37.8	62.2	73.3	26.7	98.4	2.6
Rhodium	71.6	28.4	79.1	20.9	87.9	12.1
Platinum	56.1	43.9	72.4	27.6	83.7	16.3

These data are from freshly deposited coatings without scratch resistance protective layers.

TABLE 9-7

Percent Reflectance and Transmittance of the Most Commonly Used, Vacuum-Deposited Metallic Coatings in the Optical Industry

indices of refraction to protect the mirror and enhance reflectance. Thus, an ocular protective system that must control IR and allow vision would use gold as a reflecting filter deposited on a UV-absorbing substrate for protection against UVR. If IR control were needed without the necessity of vision, silver would be the metal of choice. If cost is a consideration, copper transmits slightly less of the VIS spectrum than gold but performs quite well in eliminating the IR; however, copper should be deposited on a UV-absorbing substrate to eliminate undesirable UVR.

The subject of interference and mirror filters is very involved and complex. It is not the intent of this tentative summary to cover the detailed mathematic and theoretic aspects of the subject but, instead, to provide practical information that may be used in the solution of everyday visual problems. Jenkins and White,[57] Fincham and Freeman,[58] and other standard texts on the subject should be useful. In addition, recent developments in the literature should be reviewed in the *Journal of the Optical Society of America* and *Applied Optics*.

9.7 Recommended Standards for the Optical Spectrum

The recommended standards for ocular exposure may be used in determining adequate protection against UVR, the VIS spectrum, and IR radiation.

Recommended Standards

Spectrum	Waveband	Standard
UVC or UVB	290–315 nm	0.1 μW/cm^2
UVA	320–400 nm	1 mW/cm^2
VIS	380–760 nm	1 cd/cm^2
IRA	700–1400 nm	10 mW/cm^2

The formula for calculating the maximum transmittance of an ophthalmic protective lens would be

$$\tau = \frac{\text{Recommended std [W/cm}^2]}{\text{Radiation incident on eye [W/cm}^2]} \qquad (9\text{-}27)$$

For sunlight, the radiation incident on the Earth has been shown to be 0.727 W/cm^2 with 14% UV, 43% VIS, and 43% IR. This is equivalent to 1.02×10^{-2} W/cm^2 in the UV, 3.14×10^{-2} W/cm^2 in the VIS spectrum, and 3.14×10^{-2} W/cm^2 in the IR portions of sunlight. Sunlight on the Earth for air mass 1 produces an illuminance of about 30,000 cd/m^2 or 3 cd/cm^2, an irradiance for UVB of 0.0265×10^{-2} W/cm^2, and an irradiance for UVA of 0.5222×10^{-2} W/cm^2. The allowable or maximum permissible transmittance of a protective filter would be 33% for the VIS spectrum light, 0.02% for UVC in sunlight, 0.038% for UVB in sunlight, 18% for UVA in sunlight, and 31.8% for the IR. This type of evaluation may be made for any source as long as the spectral irradiance is known. The transmittances illustrate that sunlight does not contain harmful levels of IR and that the UVR in sunlight reaching the Earth does require protective measures.

9.8 Binoculars and High Intensity Sources

Viewing high intensity sources such as the sun or laser beam through binoculars or the telescope is not recommended. A laser beam is usually sufficiently small in diameter to pass through the pupillary aperture and be focused on the retina, resulting in a small retinal burn or lesion. With binoculars or the telescope, the energy of the source is reduced by the transmittance of the binocular, but there is an increase in the hazard to the retina. The exit pupil of the binoculars is larger than the pupil of the eye;

consequently, the pupillary diameter is completely filled with the emergent parallel beam from the eyepiece. The result is a larger image on the retina, which requires a lower threshold exposure to produce a retinal burn. When a laser beam is viewed, the actual damage depends on whether the exit pupil of the eyepiece is larger or smaller than the pupil and the transmittance of the eyepiece for the wavelength of the laser. The rule is that binoculars lower the threshold when the sun, HID source, or a laser beam is viewed and should never be used.

References

1. Fincham WHA, Freeman MH. Optics (9th ed). London, Butterworths, 1980.

2. Ham WT, Jr, Mueller HA, Williams RC, Geeraets WJ. Ocular hazards from viewing the sun unprotected and through various windows and filters. Appl Opt 1973; 12:2122–2129.

3. Blumthaler M, Ambach W, Daxecker F. On the threshold radiant exposure for keratitis solaris. Invest Ophthalmol Vis Sci 1987; 28:1713–1716.

4. Pitts DG. Photokeratitis: Laboratory versus solar exposure. Invest Ophthalmol Vis Sci 1988; 29:1759.

5. Pitts DG. The ocular ultraviolet action spectrum and protection criteria. Health Phys 1973; 25:559–556.

6. Criteria for a Recommended Standard—Occupational Exposure to Ultraviolet Radiation. HSM-73-11009. U.S. Department of Health, Education and Welfare, Public Health Service, National Institute of Occupational Safety and Health, 1972.

7. American Conference of Governmental Industrial Hygienists. TLVs: Threshold Limit Values for Chemical Substances and Physical Agents in the Work Environment with Intended Changes for 1991–92. Cincinnati, OH, 1992.

8. Sliney DH. The merits of an envelope action spectrum for ultraviolet radiation exposure criteria. Am Ind Hyg Assoc J 1972; 33:644–653.

9. Pitts DG, Cullen AP. Ocular ultraviolet effects from 295 nm to 400 nm in the rabbit. Publication 77-175. U.S. Department of Health, Education and Welfare. National Institute of Occupational Safety and Health, 1977.

10. Schmidt RE, Zuclich JA. Retinal lesions due to ultraviolet laser exposure. Invest Ophthalmol Vis Sci 1980; 19:1166–1175.

11. Ham WT, Jr, Mueller HA, Ruffolo JS, Jr, Guerry D III, Guerry RK. Action spectrum for retinal injury from near ultraviolet radiation in the aphakic monkey. Am J Ophthalmol 1982; 93:299–306.

12. Ham WT, Jr, Mueller HA. The photopathology and nature of bluelight and near-UV retinal lesions produced by laser and other optical sources. In Wolbarsht ML (ed): Laser Applications in Medicine and Biology, pp 227–228. New York, Plenum Press, 1989.

13. Sliney DH, Freasier BC. Evaluation of optical radiation hazards. Appl Opt 1973; 12:1–24.

14. American National Standard for the Safe Use of Lasers. ANSI Z136.1-1986. New York, American National Standards Institute, Inc., 1986.

15. Calkins JL, Hochheimer BF. Retinal light exposure from ophthalmoscopes, slit lamps, and overhead surgical lamps: An analysis of potential hazards. Invest Ophthalmol Vis Sci 1980; 19:1009–1015.

16. Ham WT, Jr, Sliney DH. Retinal sensitivity for short wavelength light. Nature 1976; 260:153–155.

17. Sliney DH, Marshall WJ, Carothers ML, Kaste RC. Hazard analysis of broad-band optics sources. Aberdeen Proving Ground, MD, U.S. Army Environmental Hygiene Agency, 1980.

18. Harwerth RS, Sperling HG. Prolonged color blindness induced by intense spectral lights in rhesus monkeys. Science 1971; 174:520–523.

19. Pitts DG, Cullen AP, Dayhaw-Barker P. Determination of ocular threshold levels for infrared radiation cataractogenesis. Publication No. 80-121. Washington, DC, U.S. Department of Health, Education and Welfare, National Institute of Occupational Safety and Health, 1980.

20. Pitts DG, Cullen AP. Determination of infrared radiation levels for acute ocular cataractogenesis. Graefes Arch Clin Exp Ophthalmol 1981; 217:285–297.

21. Lydahl E, Glansholm A, Levin M. Ocular exposure to infrared radiation in the Swedish iron and steel industry. Health Phys 1984; 46:529–536.

22. Lydahl E. Infrared radiation and cataract. Acta Ophthalmol (Suppl) 1984; 166:1–63.

23. Lydahl E, Philipson B. Infrared radiation and cataract, I. Epidemiological investigation of iron- and steel-workers. Acta Ophthalmol (Copenh) 1984; 62:961–975.

24. Lydahl E, Philipson B. Infrared radiation and catarct, II. Epidemiological investigation of glass-workers. Acta Ophthalmol (Copenh) 1984; 62:976–992.

25. Lydahl E, Glansholm A. Infrared radiation and cataract: III. Differences between the two eyes of glass workers. Acta Ophthalmol 1985; 63:39–44.

26. Matelsky I. The non-ionizing radiations. In: Industrial Hygiene Highlights. Industrial Hygiene Foundation of America, Pittsburgh 1968; 1:140.

27. Jacobson JH, Cooper B, Najac HW. Effects of thermal energy on retinal function. Technical Document Report No. AMRL-TDR-62-96. Life Support System Laboratory. Wright-Patterson Air Force Base, Ohio, 1962.

28. Sliney DH, Conover DL. Nonionizing radiation. In: Indust Environmental Health, The Worker and the

Community, 2d ed. New York: Academic Press Inc, 157–177, 1975.

29. Peppers NA, Vassidialis A, Dedrick LG, Chang H, Peabody PR, Rose H, Zweng HC. Corneal damage thresholds for CO_2 laser radiations. Appl Opti 1969; 8:337–381.

30. Anderson WJ, Gebel RKH. Ultraviolet windows in commercial sunglasses. Appl Opti 1977; 16:515–517.

31. Rosenthal FS, Bakalian AE, Taylor HR. The effect of prescription eyewear on ocular exposure to ultraviolet radiation. Am J Pub Health 1986; 76:1216–1220.

32. Rosenthal FS, Bakalian AE, Lou C, Taylor HR. The effect of sunglasses on ocular exposure to ultraviolet radiation. Am J Pub Health 1988; 78:72–74.

33. Maslovitz B, Pitts DG. Transmittance of ophthalmic materials. St. Cloud, MN: Vision-Ease Corp, 1–119, 1984.

34. Cotnam MP, Chou BR, Cullen AP. Optical protection factors of selected safety lenses. Occupat Health in Ontario 1988 Fall; 9:197–201.

35. Kreidl NJ, Rood JL. Filters. In: Kingslake R, ed. Applied optics and optical engineering, Vol I. New York: Academic Press, 5:111–115, 1965.

36. Robertson JK. Introduction to physical optics. 3rd ed., New York: D. Van Nostrand Co, pp 340–341, 1948.

37. Pitts DG. Threat of ultraviolet radiation to the eye—how to protect against it. J Am Optom Assn 1981; 52:949–957.

38. Pitts DG, Lattimore MR, Jr. Protection against UVR using the Vistakon UV-BLOC soft contact lens. International Contact Lens Clinic 1987; 14:22–30.

39. Bergmanson JPG, Pitts DG, Chu L W-F. The efficacy of a UV-blocking soft contact lens in protecting the cornea against UV radiation. Acta Ophthalmol (Copenh) 1987; 65:279–286.

40. Ahmedbhai N, Cullen AP. The influence of contact lens wear on the corneal response to ultraviolet radiation. Ophthalmic Physiol Opt 1988; 8:183–189.

41. Werner JS, Steale VG, Pfoff DS. Loss of human photoreceptor sensitivity associated with chronic exposure to ultraviolet radiation. Ophthalmology 1989; 96:1552–1558.

42. Boettner EA, Wolter JR. Transmittance of the ocular media. Invest Ophthalmol 1962; 1:776–783.

43. Schmidt RE, Zuclich JA. Retinal lesions due to ultraviolet laser exposure. Invest Ophthalmol Vis Sci 1980; 19:1166–1175.

44. Ham WT, Mueller WA, Ruffolo JJ, Jr, Guerry D III, Guerry RK. Action spectrum for retinal injury from near ultraviolet radiation in the aphakic monkey. Am J Ophthalmol 1982; 93:299–306.

45. Kamel ID, Parker JA. Protection from ultraviolet exposure in aphakic erythopsia. Can J Ophthalmol 1973; 8:563–565.

46. Saraux H, Manuet LP, LaRoche L. Erythopsie chez ur porteur d'implant. Etude physiologique et electrophysiologique. J Fr Ophthalmol 1984; 7:557–562.

47. Goodeve CF. Vision on the ultraviolet. Nature (London) 1934; 134:416–417.

48. Good GW, Schoessler JP. Chronic solar radiation exposure and endothelial polymegethism. Curr Eye Res 1988; 8:157–162.

49. Yee RW, Matsuda M, Schultz RO, Edelhauser HF. Changes in the normal corneal endothelial cellular pattern as a function of age. Curr Eye Res 1985; 4:671–678.

50. Karai I, Matsumura S, Takise S, Horiguchi S, Matsuda M. Morphological change in the corneal endothelium due to ultraviolet radiation in welders. Br J Ophthalmol 1984; 68:544–548.

51. Pitts DG, Bergmanson JPG, Chu L W-F, Waxler M, Hitchins VM. Ultrastructural analysis of corneal exposure to UV radiation. Acta Ophthalmol (Copenh) 1987; 65:263–273.

52. Cullen AP, Chou BR, Hall MG, Janey SE. Ultraviolet-B damages corneal endothelium. Am J Optom Physiol Opti 1984; 61:473–478.

53. Doughty MJ, Cullen AP. Long term effects of a single dose ultraviolet-B on albino rabbit cornea, I. In vivo analyses. Photochem Photobiol 1989; 49:175–180.

54. Lerman S. Radiant Energy and the Eye, Vol I. Functional Ophthalmology Series. New York, MacMillan, 1980.

55. Fraunfelder FT. Drug Induced Ocular Side Effects and Drug Interactions. Philadelphia, Lea & Febiger, 1976.

56. Hass G. Mirror coatings. In Kingslake R (ed): Applied Optics and Optical Engineering, Vol IV, pp 309–330. New York, Academic Press, 1965.

57. Jenkins FA, White FE. Fundamentals of Optics (4th ed). St. Louis, McGraw-Hill Book Co, 1965.

CHAPTER TEN

Ophthalmic Materials for Ocular Protection

Gregory L. Stephens, O.D., Ph.D.

In recent years, there has been increased concern for eye protection, impact resistance of spectacle lenses, and liability for broken eyeglasses. The introduction of new lens materials, especially polycarbonate, requires that materials be carefully chosen to best meet a patient's visual and eye safety needs. The upsurge in interest in sports has also increased awareness by the general public of the protective eyewear worn by professional athletes, as well as impact resistance. It is the purpose of this chapter to describe available lens materials and to compare their impact resistance, to describe the principles of eye protection in industry and sports, and to discuss briefly the relevant legal issues.

10.1 Choice of Materials

The ophthalmic lens market is rapidly changing, and one goal is the development of materials with higher indices of refraction but less dispersion. A higher index of refraction allows the thickness of high power lenses to be reduced, while lower levels of dispersion result in fewer problems with chromatic aberration. Lens materials available at this time are presented in Table 10-1. Many of these materials, especially the high index plastics, are available in different chemical formulations from a number of manufacturers, with slightly different indices of refraction, Abbé numbers (optical "nu" values), and densities.

Three types of high index glass are available: flint, titanium oxide, and photochromic. Flint glass, the original high index glass, is used today only for x-ray protective lenses and the segments of Kryptok bifocals. Because flint glass cannot be tempered to significantly increase impact resistance, patients must sign a waiver when it is used. The titanium oxide and photochromic high index glasses have replaced flint glass primarily because they can be tempered. These materials are also less dense than flint glass but may still be very heavy in high powers. It is best to keep

Material (Manufacturer)	n_D	Abbé number	Density (g/cm^3)	Comments
Glass				
Ophthalmic crown	1.523	58.6	2.54	
Photogrey Extra (Corning)	1.523	57	2.41	Photochromic glass
Photobrown Extra (Corning)	1.523	56.3	2.41	Photochromic glass
LHI-II (Hoya)	1.600	40.2	2.59	
1.60 Crown (Schott)	1.601	40.7	2.62	
Photogrey Extra 1.6 (Corning)	1.600	42.2	2.73	Photochromic glass
Photobrown Extra 1.6 (Corning)	1.600	42.2	2.73	Photochromic glass
HC-Photosolar (Schott)	1.601	42.5	2.75	Photochromic glass
LHI (Hoya)	1.702	40.2	2.99	
High-Lite (Schott)	1.706	31	2.99	
Index 8 (Ohara)	1.805	25.4	3.37	
1.80 High Index (Schott)	1.805	25.4	3.39	
Thin-Lite (Schott)	1.701	25	4.05	Flint glass, cannot be tempered
X-Ray (Vision-Ease)	1.806	25.4	5.18	Flint glass, cannot be tempered
Plastic				
CR-39 (PPG)	1.4985	58	1.32	
Transitions Plus (Transitions)	1.500	57	1.28	Photochromic plastic
Spectralite (Sola)	1.537	47	1.21	
Polycarbonate (Gentex)	1.586	31	1.20	
Hi-Lux II Hard (Hoya)	1.556	40	1.27	
Hi-Ri (PPG)	1.556	37.7	1.221	
Diacoat Thin (Seiko)	1.556	40	1.27	
1.56 High Index (Signet Armorlite)	1.555	36	1.23	
Cristyl Hi Index 1.56 (Titmus)	1.562	38	1.42	
Youngerlite (Younger)	1.556	37.7	1.216	
Cristyl Hi Index 1.58 (Titmus)	1.577	35	1.47	
True Lite (Truesight)	1.577	37.5	1.40	
Hi-Lux Exc (Hoya)	1.600	36	1.35	
Hyper Index 1.60 (Optima)	1.597	37	1.34	
HIX 1.60 (Pentax)	1.594	36	1.34	
1.60 High Index (Signet Armorlite)	1.600	36	1.45	
Thin & Lite (Silor)	1.595	36	1.36	
Cristyl Hi Index 1.60 (Titmus)	1.592	36	1.43	
Truelite 1.60 (Truesight)	1.600	35	1.39	
Hyperindex (Optima)	1.660	32	1.35	

TABLE 10-1
Glass and Plastic Lens Materials

lens eyesizes small when using high index glasses and ensure that a good frame bridge fit is achieved.

High index plastic lens materials are usually divided into indices of 1.54 (actually 1.537), 1.56 (actually 1.555–1.562), 1.58 (actually 1.577), 1.60 (actually 1.592–1.600), and 1.66, with polycarbonate (1.586) as a separate category. The primary advantage of these materials over high index glass is decreased lens weight. However, some plastics tend to have a slight inherent coloration, which is most noticeable in thicker, higher power lenses. To avoid complaints, it is always best to show sample lenses to a patient before ordering. All high index materials tend to be more expensive than other lens materials, have more internal and external reflections, may take longer for the optical laboratory to process, and except for polycarbonate, may be available in only limited lens types.

Proper base curve selection and proper positioning of the lenses in the frame are especially important for high index lens materials. All of these materials produce more chromatic aberration than either CR-39 allyl resin plastic or ophthalmic crown glass. A patient may notice color fringes when looking through the lens periphery and experience decreased peripheral visual acuity.[1-3] These effects will be more noticeable the lower the Abbé number and the higher the power of the patient's lenses, especially for lens powers above five to six diopters.[3] (The Abbé number is defined as $(n_D - 1)/(n_F - n_C)$, where n_C, n_D, and n_F are the indices of refraction for the Fraunhofer wavelengths of 656.3 nm, 589 nm, and 486.1 nm, respectively.) Lateral chromatic aberration may interact with radial astigmatism to further decrease a patient's visual acuity through the lens periphery, especially when a lens manufacturer does not use the optimum base curve.[1-4] To decrease chromatic aberration problems, lenses should be fit at short vertex distances, with the use of monocular (split) PDs, and with vertical positioning of the major reference point (MRP) 3 to 5 mm below the center of the pupil. Whenever possible, the base curve should be chosen to match the eyewire distance of the spectacles.[3]

10.2 Impact Resistance

Standards

Ophthalmic lenses may be divided into two types for purposes of impact resistance: dress safety lenses worn every day and industrial safety lenses worn for occupational or educational eye protection. Impact considerations for dress safety lenses will be discussed in this section. The standards for dress lenses are regulated in the United States by the Food and Drug Administration (FDA).

Effective January 1, 1972, the FDA made it illegal for ophthalmic practitioners to prescribe dress safety lenses that are not impact resistant. The most recent version of this ruling is provided in the Federal Register[5] and is also available from the FDA.[6] The impact resistance standard or "referee" test is the dress safety "drop-ball" test in which a lens must be able to withstand the impact of a ⅝-inch (15.875-mm) steel ball weighing approximately 0.56 oz (15.88 g) dropped 50 inches (1.27 m) onto the front surface of the lens. Exact specifications for the drop-ball test equipment are described in the FDA ruling, although methods of testing impact resistance that are equal or superior to the drop-ball test are allowed. The test method is similar to that described for dress safety lenses in ANSI Z80.1-1987.[7]

All prescription lenses must be tested, with the exception of those lenses that could be damaged by drop-ball testing, such as plastic lenses and raised ledge multifocals (e.g., executive-style multifocals). However, statistically significant batches of these lens types also must be tested by the lens manufacturer (before the lenses are sent to the optical laboratory) to demonstrate that the lenses will pass the drop-ball test if surfaced to the proper thickness and edged properly. The FDA allows the impact resistance of both glass and plastic nonprescription sunglass lenses to be tested by statistical testing of batches. Special or unusual lens designs such as eikonic lenses, biconcave lenses, and prism segment multifocals are exempted from testing.

In addition to drop-ball testing, the FDA requires that all parties in the chain of distribution of prescription ophthalmic lenses—the manufacturer, optical laboratory, and optometrist—maintain records of impact resistance testing, copies of invoices, shipping documents, and bills of sale for at least 3 years. Records of those purchasing nonprescription sunglasses and nonprescription eyeglasses (i.e., over-the-counter reading glasses) at the retail level need not be maintained. The ophthalmic practitioner may waive the impact resistance requirement if such lenses will not fulfill a patient's visual requirements, but the patient must be notified in writing. Because of problems with liability, it is difficult to justify waiving the impact resistance requirement. One possible situation might be the use of flint glass for X-ray protection. Another would be the need for replacement spectacles in an emergency when there is insufficient time to temper the lenses properly.

The FDA has no minimum thickness requirement for dress safety lenses. However, lenses made from most materials will not reliably pass the drop-ball test unless they are at least 1.5 to 2 mm thick, so these values are often used as informal standards.

Methods of Measurement

The drop-ball test and the so-called "ballistic" tests, in which a small, high velocity projectile is fired at a lens, have become the standards for impact resistance testing and research in the U.S. Testing can be performed using one of two procedures. Either the impact energy can be increased until a given lens breaks on repeated testing, or a sample of identical lenses can be tested consecutively. The consecutive method tests each lens once with the energy of impact increased or decreased from lens to lens to determine the threshold required for breakage. The impact resistance of a lens as measured by the repeated impact method depends on the initial drop-ball height and the height increment used in subsequent drops.[8] It is not possible to impact exactly the same point on a lens repeatedly, so the lens is stressed in a different manner with each impact. Because of these problems, consecutive testing has become the procedure of choice.

Two parameters may be varied to change the impact energy when conducting drop-ball or ballistic testing: projectile size and drop height or projectile velocity. For a given drop height, drop-ball size can be increased until a lens breaks. The drop-ball size that results in breakage or the energy of the ball at impact is the measure of impact resistance. The principal problems with changing drop-ball size are that the size of the impact zone changes with drop-ball size, as does the duration of the impact. These factors change the distribution of stresses on the lens and confuse interpretation of the results.[9] Different mechanisms of breakage may occur with different drop-ball sizes,[10] and the effects of changes in drop-ball size on impact resistance are different for different lens materials.

Varying drop-ball height or projectile velocity is preferred over varying projectile size for measurement of the impact resistance of ophthalmic lenses. The measure of impact resistance is either drop height, projectile velocity at impact, or energy of impact. An important consideration is that the test object be spherical or always present the same impacting surface to the lens. Some early studies of impact resistance[11,12] utilized irregular objects (e.g., cubes, screw caps and nuts), which complicated the analysis of the data because the energy transferred to the lens on impact varied as the area of impacting surface changed.

Three major concerns expressed about the drop-ball test have stimulated a search for alternatives. First, drop-ball testing may decrease the impact resistance of a patient's spectacle lens, as is demonstrated by lens failure after repeated drop-ball testing.[13] However, an alternative explanation for this effect may be that the repeated impacts occur at slightly different points on the lens and eventually find a preexisting weak spot on the lens surface, resulting in breakage.[14] Second, the drop-ball tests the impact resistance of just a small portion of a lens, with high stresses occurring only in a limited area surrounding the point of impact.[9,14,15] Lens defects that are not directly under the impact point may not be tested. Third, because much of the energy of impact is absorbed by the lens mount in the impact resistance test equipment, it has been argued that the drop-ball test is more a test of the lens mount than of the lens itself.[16] In fact, measured impact resistance varies considerably with the type of lens mount used.[8,9,16,17] Because the drop-ball test does not take much time to perform, needs few performance skills, and does not require expensive equipment, it is unlikely that a different test will be developed and accepted as a standard in the foreseeable future.

A second method for testing impact resistance is static testing, the application of a gradually increasing load to the lens front surface, with the energy resulting in lens fracture the measure of impact resistance. The advantage of static testing is that the energy applied to the lens can be measured with greater accuracy than for drop-ball testing.[16,18] Disadvantages include that the test does not simulate the process of lens breakage under conditions of use and that the equipment is more expensive than a drop-ball tester.[16,18] Research suggests that drop-ball and static testing methods provide equivalent results for glass lenses[16,17] but the two methods are not comparable for plastic lenses.[19] The difference is the result of the slow increase in pressure of static testing, which allows plastic lenses to flex more than during drop-ball testing. Static testing may not be appropriate for plastic lenses.

Mechanics of Lens Fracture
and Impact Resistance Testing

The strength of a spectacle lens can be expressed as the amount of tensile stress that must be applied to the lens before the lens fractures or breaks.[20] Tensile stress is the force per unit area to which a material is subjected when the atoms or molecules of the material are being separated. Compressive stress is the force per unit area which pushes the atoms or molecules of a material together. One commonly applied theory of lens fracture, the "flaw" theory, states that fracture occurs when the tensile stress acting on the lens exceeds a critical value at a flaw or defect in one small area of the lens surface.[14,20–24] At this tensile stress value, a crack will then propagate through the lens, starting at the flaw. The flaw may be a small crack created during the surfacing and polishing operations or by rough handling.[14,20,21] Poor edging of a lens, especially poor safety beveling or pin beveling where chips are left on the lens edges, will result in flaws. All types of glass also contain submicroscopic surface defects termed "Griffith flaws" that may be created by contact of the surfaces with dust particles, by inhomogeneities at the lens surfaces, or by formation of surface oxide layers.[21] Etching a glass surface with acid eliminates surface flaws and greatly increases the strength of a glass, but handling or exposure to the atmosphere immediately recreates the flaws and decreases impact resistance.[21,25,26]

Since increasing impact resistance by elimination of surface flaws is not practical, a better approach is to increase the compressive stress on the lens. A tensile stress must then overcome this extra compressive stress before the lens can fracture. Compressive stresses are applied by treating or tempering a lens with heat or chemicals. Heat tempering increases the impact resistance of a lens but a heat tempered lens is not as impact resistant as a chemically tempered lens,[27] so heat tempering is not recommended.

Chemical tempering increases impact resistance of a glass lens by creating a compressed surface layer using a process of ion exchange.[28,29] Crown glass lenses are immersed in a molten (approximately 450°C) potassium nitrate bath for 16 hours. Different chemical mixtures, bath temperatures, and immersion times are required for lens materials such as photochromics and high index glasses.[30] Sodium ions diffuse out of the glass and are replaced by larger potassium ions from the bath. This crowding of the lens matrix with larger ions creates surface compression, and a compensating zone of internal tension also develops. The maximum surface compression achieved with chemical tempering is much higher than that of heat tempering, resulting in greater impact resistance.[27,28] Chemical tempering is the preferred process for glass lenses.

The different distributions of compressive and tensile stresses developed in heat tempered and chemically tempered lenses are shown in Figure 10-1. Although the compressive stresses developed at the surfaces of a chemically tempered lens are higher, the surface compression layer is thinner, 50 to 100 microns for a 2 mm thick lens versus 200–600 microns for a heat tempered lens.[10,25,31] A flaw or scratch that penetrates the compression zone severely weakens a lens,[32–34] so the impact resistance of a chemically tempered lens is more susceptible to compromise from a deep scratch. When a scratch is deep enough to reach the area of tension, the tensile stress may cause the defect to continue to propagate. This so-called "spontaneous breakage" has been

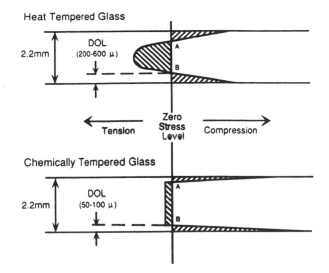

FIGURE 10-1
Stress distributions in heat tempered and chemically tempered glass lenses. Compressive stress in both lens types is a maximum at the lens surfaces. At points A and B the compressive stress has decreased to zero. Inside these points the lenses are under tension. DOL marks the depth (thickness) of the surface compression layer. Modified from Horne[31] and Chase.[25]

shown to occur after mechanical or thermal shock to a heat tempered lens.[35,36]

Improvements in the original method of chemical tempering have been developed. Agitation of the chemical bath with ultrasound can increase the impact resistance of a crown glass lens to values better than that obtained with standard chemical tempering in only 4 hours rather than the normal 16 hours.[37] A new chemical tempering process for photochromic lenses that reduces the immersion time to 2 hours has been developed.[38]

An important problem with chemical tempering is the difficulty of identifying a chemically tempered lens. Heat tempered lenses show a birefringence pattern when held between the crossed polarizing filters of a polariscope. However, a chemically tempered lens and an untempered annealed glass lens do not show a pattern. Chemical tempering can be verified by immersing the edge of the lens in glycerine or a liquid similar in index to that of the lens while viewing the lens edge through crossed polarizers.[39,40] If the lens has been chemically tempered, the edge glows.

Evaluation of large numbers of glass lenses broken by impact suggests that breakage occurs by at least four different mechanisms.[10,14] The first is simple fracture of the lens front surface, originating at a surface flaw (Fig. 10-2A) and occurring most commonly from the impact of small, high velocity projectiles. The cone-shaped glass fragments (Hertzian fracture) are very sharp. This type of fracture is not considered to be common with the standard drop-ball test.[14]

The second mechanism is rear surface fracture initiated by flexure of the lens, which transfers the stress from a front surface impact to the back surface of the lens (Fig. 10-2B). Back surface fracture is commonly found with impacts from moderate velocity, moderate mass projectiles on minus power lenses and is believed to be the most common type of breakage found with the drop-ball test. This suggests that the quality of the back surface may be a significant determinant of the measured impact resistance of a lens.[15,25] Rear surface fracture occurs less commonly in plus power lenses because a thicker lens is less likely to flex.[25]

The third mechanism of fracture is edge fracture from simple flexure or flattening of the lens (Fig. 10-2C). Edge fracture is found primarily with large,

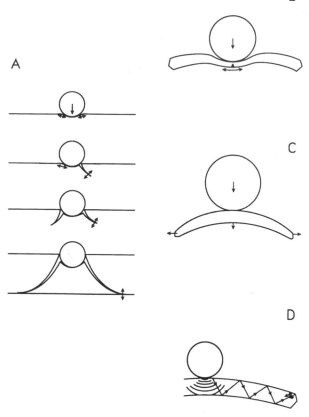

FIGURE 10-2
Mechanisms of glass lens fracture. A. Front surface deformation fracture initiated by a small, high velocity projectile. ***B.*** Rear surface fracture caused by lens flexure, transferring stress to the back surface. ***C.*** Edge fracture as a result of flexure or flattening of the lens. ***D.*** Edge fracture as a result of an elastic wave. *From* **Brandt RJ: The anatomy and autopsy of an impact resistant lens. American Journal of Optometry and Physiological Optics 1974; 51(12):982–986. Copyright The American Academy of Optometry, 1991; with permission.**

slow projectiles impacting plus power lenses. The fourth mechanism, edge fracture due to elastic wave reflection (Fig. 10-2D), occurs rarely when a high velocity, low mass object impacts a lens but does not cause breakage at the point of impact. The stress of the impact initiates fracture at a peripheral flaw.

CR-39 plastic lenses and polycarbonate lenses behave somewhat differently from glass lenses under impact or stress. CR-39 plastic can crack or fracture in a manner similar to glass, but it can also flex or deform under impact, decreasing the likelihood that a crack will form.[41] CR-39 breakage often begins at the lens edge,[19] suggesting that the mechanism of breakage for larger projectiles (e.g., ⅝″ drop-balls) is the transfer of stress to the edge as the lens flexes and that the impact resistance of CR-39 may be highly dependent on the quality of the lens bevel.[42]

Polycarbonate shows large amounts of plastic deformation before breakage occurs,[41,42] and this ability to deform probably gives the material its incredible impact resistance. The difference in impact resistance between CR-39 and polycarbonate has been attributed to the increased number of molecular cross-links of the CR-39 polymer, which increases hardness but decreases flexibility relative to polycarbonate.[41]

Comparisons of Impact Resistance for Ophthalmic Materials

When a spectacle lens is impacted by a projectile, the projectile imparts some of its energy to the lens, which causes the lens and its mount to recoil, the lens to flex, or the lens to fracture (Fig. 10-2). The energy of impact depends primarily upon the projectile mass and its velocity, although unusual projectile shapes may result in impacts that do not effectively transfer the missile energy to the lens.

Impact resistance may be expressed as projectile drop height, velocity of impact, or as impact energy. The most general expression for energy of the projectile at impact is[20]

$$E = m \times g \times h, \qquad (10\text{-}1)$$

where E is the energy of the projectile in newton-meters (N-m) or joules, m is the projectile mass in kilograms, g is the gravitational constant (9.8 m/s^2), and h is the projectile drop height in meters. (Energy may also be expressed in foot-pounds, where 1 ft-lb = 1.356 N-m.) If the velocity at impact is known, the energy at impact is[43]

$$E = \tfrac{1}{2} \times m \times v^2 \qquad (10\text{-}2)$$

where v is the projectile velocity in meters/s. Impact energy is also sometimes expressed as[27]

$$E = m \times h \qquad (10\text{-}3)$$

where E is expressed in kilogram-meters (kg-m). Although not a rigorous unit of energy, the kg-m is directly related to projectile energy by the gravitational constant, so the unit can be a useful and convenient measure for comparisons of impact resistance.

A comparison of the impact resistance of ophthalmic materials begins at 2-mm thickness, which is the minimum usually used for dress safety lenses. The impact resistances of heat-tempered glass, chemically tempered glass, and CR-39 plastic have been compiled from a number of studies[27] and are given in Figure 10-3. Projectile size was generally ⅝ inch (15.875 mm), although some higher impact energies were obtained with a ¾-inch (19.05-mm) drop-ball. The most important conclusion that can be drawn from this data is that glass lenses show a much larger range of impact resistance values than CR-39 lenses. This variability is most likely related to variations in quality of the lens surfaces and edges as a result of the surfacing and edging processes. In addition, environmental factors such as temperature and humidity affect impact resistance and may contribute to the variability.[8,20,41,44–46] This difference between glass and plastic demonstrates that it is more difficult to predict the impact resistance of a glass lens. On average, chemically tempered lenses are more impact resistant to a ⅝-inch steel ball than CR-39 plastic lenses, and CR-39 plastic lenses are more impact resistant than heat-tempered lenses, but a given heat-tempered lens can be more impact resistant than a chemically tempered lens or CR-39 lens, and a chemically tempered lens can be much less impact resistant than a CR-39 lens. Approximately 0.5% of all chemically tempered prescription lenses will fail the drop-ball test,[38] whereas less than 0.05% of CR-39 prescription lenses may be expected to fail,[47] a difference in performance that is related to the inherent variability of glass lens impact resistance.

The relative impact resistance of lens materials varies with projectile size (Fig. 10-4). In general, both heat-tempered and chemically tempered glass perform poorly relative to CR-39 plastic for small projectiles (less than ¼ inch or 6.35 mm diameter), but chemically tempered glass is superior for larger projectiles. As previously mentioned, the differences reflect in part changes in the mechanisms of breakage as projectile size changes.

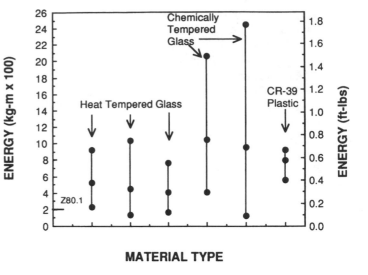

FIGURE 10-3
Mean impact energies and range of energies that result in fracture of 2-mm spectacle lenses. Z80.1 indicates the impact energy of a ⅝-inch steel ball dropped 50 inches, the FDA dress safety standard. *Modified from* **Davis JK: Perspectives on impact resistance and polycarbonate lenses. Int Ophthalmol Clin 28:215–218, 1988; with permission.**

The impact resistance of polycarbonate is shown by two data points (open triangles) in Figure 10-4. These data were obtained for 1.9-mm thick polycarbonate goggles impacted with ⅛-inch (3.175-mm) and ¼-inch steel balls fired at high velocity.[48] These values are roughly 21 times the impact resistance of CR-39 for the same projectile sizes, and similar results have been reported.[45,49] Data do not exist giving the energy required to break polycarbonate for larger projectiles. Polycarbonate is extremely impact resistant for larger projectiles, and the projectile velocity required to break a lens is difficult to achieve. The most striking demonstration of the impact resistance of polycarbonate for large objects is that a 40-lb (89.6-kg) steel plate dropped 3 ft (0.91 m) onto a lens bridging two timbers did not break the lens.[27] Polycarbonate is much superior in impact resistance to CR-39 plastic and crown glass at all projectile sizes, with the advantage increasing as projectile size increases.

The size, shape, and sharpness of the fragments formed when a lens breaks are important for eye safety. CR-39 plastic breaks into larger, duller pieces than heat-tempered glass when impacted by large (⅞-inch or 22.2-mm) steel balls.[50,51] CR-39 plastic also breaks into fewer, duller pieces than glass when impacted by 0.172-inch (4.37-mm) diameter steel and lead BBs.[52,53] When a plastic lens breaks, the pieces tend to remain in the frame. However, a heat-tempered glass lens tends to become a source of secondary missiles, which are sprayed toward the eye. This occurs even when the impacting projectile does not reach the eye, and it can happen whether or not the lens fractures.[11,53] These breakage characteristics suggest that CR-39 may be a better lens material than tempered glass, although neither is equal or superior to polycarbonate.

It has been claimed that tempering a glass lens changes its pattern of breakage. An untempered lens is supposed to break into large numbers of sharp, pointed splinters, whereas the tempered lens crumbles into fewer, larger, duller pieces.[2,25] Such a pattern of breakage has been demonstrated for heat-tempered lenses broken by large, low velocity projectiles,[48,50] although 25 of 30 heat-tempered lenses broken by a ⅝-inch steel ball formed long, sharp slivers.[54] Untempered, heat-tempered, and chemically tempered lenses have been reported to form sharp, pie-shaped fragments when they are broken by a static test procedure.[55] Impact from small, high velocity projectiles breaks both untempered and heat-tempered lenses into small triangular pieces or small, sharp splinters.[11,48,51–53] Thus tempering appears to have little effect on the breakage pattern of lenses.

Data on the impact resistance of 3-mm thick (industrial safety) materials for steel balls of various diameters are shown in Figure 10-5. The data mirror that for 2-mm thick materials. CR-39 has impact resistance superior to glass when projectiles are of

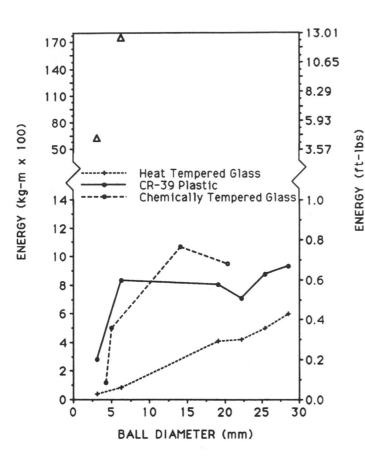

FIGURE 10-4
Average impact energies resulting in fracture of 2-mm lenses as a function of projectile size. For a given energy level, increases in projectile size require a decrease in projectile velocity or drop height. Two kg-m × 100 is the Z80.1 standard. The open triangles represent the impact resistance of 1.9-mm polycarbonate for ⅛-inch (3.175-mm) and ¼-inch (6.35-mm) steel balls, as determined by Wigglesworth.[48] *Modified from Davis JK: Perspectives on impact resistance and polycarbonate lenses. Int Ophthalmol Clin 28:215–218, 1988; with permission.*

small size, whereas the reverse is true when projectiles are large. Data concerning the impact required to break polycarbonate with a 1-inch (25.4-mm) steel ball are not available. However, a 12.2 N-m (9 ft-lb) impact of a 1-inch steel ball on 3-mm polycarbonate resulted in no breakage of any lens tested.[57] This value for polycarbonate is approximately 6.2 times that of glass and 8.2 times that of CR-39 for the same ball size.

Figure 10-6 presents the impact resistance of 3-mm thick industrial safety lens materials for a ¼-inch steel ball.[58] The ANSI Z87.1-1989 test procedure for nonprescription lenses was used.[59] A velocity of 45.72 m/s (150 ft/s) is the minimum that any lens less than 3-mm thick must be able to withstand. The impact resistance of polycarbonate is superior to other materials, and only polycarbonate will meet the standard when less than 3-mm thick.

Lens materials may also lose considerable impact resistance when coated (Fig. 10-6), which is an im-

portant consideration for plastic lenses because they are generally impact-tested only by the manufacturer. An optical laboratory that applies coatings to plastic lens materials must follow the coating procedures approved by the lens manufacturer to ensure that a coated lens will meet impact standards. A coating applied by a lens manufacturer is not generally of concern because the impact resistance of the coated lenses will be tested by appropriate statistical procedures before being sent to the optical laboratory for edging.

The new high index plastics can have increased impact resistance relative to CR-39. For example, the 1.60 polyurethane plastics at their standard thickness of 1.5 mm are roughly two times more impact resistant than 2-mm CR-39 to a ⅝-inch steel ball.[60] The advantage is lost when a coating is applied to the lens back surface, but the lenses can still pass the drop-ball test at 1.5-mm thickness with a comfortable reserve strength.[60]

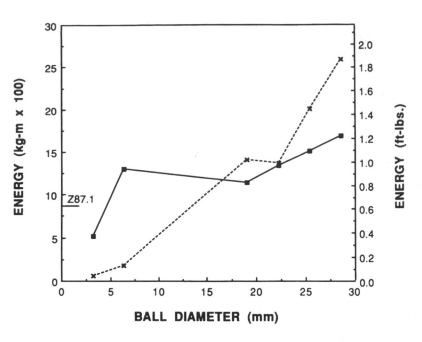

FIGURE 10-5
Average impact energies resulting in fracture of 3-mm heat-tempered (*dotted line*) and CR-39 plastic (*solid line*) lenses as a function of drop-ball size. Z87.1 indicates the impact energy of a 1-inch steel ball dropped 50 inches, the ANSI Z87.1 standard. *Data from* **Wigglesworth.**[56] *Modified from* **Davis JK: Perspectives on impact resistance and polycarbonate lenses. Int Ophthalmol Clin 1988; 28:215–218, with permission.**

Eye Injuries

What types of objects are responsible for eye injuries in spectacle lens wearers? A large study of eye injuries occurring as a result of spectacle lens breakage in nonindustrial situations found that most broken lenses were caused by the impact of large, relatively slow moving objects (Table 10-2).[61] Other smaller studies of spectacle lens breakage have found sim-

ilar results.[62,63] Studies of the incidence of eye injuries in children and in the general population (with or without spectacle wear) show that a wide variety of object sizes and velocities cause injury, with a substantial percentage of the injuries related to sports.[64–66]

Some of the causes of lens breakage that result in litigation have been identified.[27] Large objects of low velocity result in high energy impacts far beyond

FIGURE 10-6
Average impact velocities of ¼-inch steel balls resulting in the fracture of 3-mm lens materials. The cross-hatched portions of the histogram bars of the 3-mm heat-tempered glass and 3-mm CR-39 plastic indicate the range of lens breakage velocities normally encountered: 21.3–27.4 m/s (70–90 ft/s) and 38.1–53.3 m/s (125–175 ft/s), respectively. The standard deviation of impact velocities required to break 3-mm polycarbonate is approximately 15.2 m/s (50 ft/s). According to the ANSI Z87.1-1989 standard, all nonprescription lenses less than 3-mm thick must be able to withstand an impact velocity of 45.7 m/s (150 ft/s). *Modified from* **Greenberg I, Chase G, LaMarre D: Statistical protocol for impact testing prescription polycarbonate safety lenses. Optical World 14:7–8, 1985; with permission.**

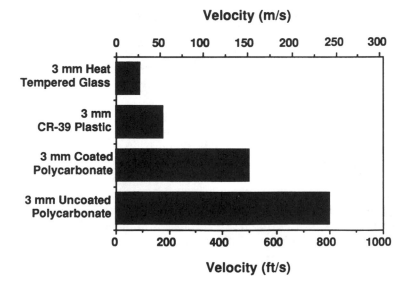

Cause	Number	Percentage
Rocks	73	24.5
Sports	53	17.8
Baseball	(22)	
Basketball	(8)	
Golf ball	(5)	
Other balls	(8)	
Fishing weights	(4)	
Hockey stick	(1)	
Archery bow	(1)	
Plastic hockey puck	(1)	
Spinning top	(1)	
Boomerang	(1)	
Golf club	(1)	
Auto crashes	28	9.4
Falls	25	8.4
Flying objects	20	6.7
Assaults	18	6.0
BB pellets	16	5.4
Running collisions	12	4.0
Tree branches	7	2.3
Nails	6	2.0
Exploding objects	4	1.3
Tools (screwdriver, pliers, etc.)	4	1.3
Auto and truck springs	2	0.7
Corks	2	0.7
Wrestling	2	0.7
Miscellaneous (one each)	11	3.7
Unknown	15	5.0
Total	298	100%

Note: Eye injuries occurred in 157 of the 298 cases.

Modified from Keeney AH, Fintelman E, Renaldo D. Clinical mechanisms in nonindustrial eye trauma. Am J Ophthalmol 74:662–665, 1972. Published with permission from the American Journal of Ophthalmology. Copyright The Ophthalmic Publishing Company.

TABLE 10-2
Causes of Broken Spectacle Lenses

Projectile	Potential Impact Energy	
	N-m	Ft-lbs
Pitched baseball	28.5	21
Softball	23	17
Volleyball	4.1–8.1	3–6
Average apple, tossed 6 ft	1	0.75
Human fist	2.7–5.4	2–4
Fall (head striking object from 1–3 ft)	6.8–20.3	5–15
Automobile crash at 20 mph; head striking dashboard	91.1	67.2
3-lb hammer dropped 10 ft	40.7	30
BB	0.7–2	0.5–1.5
22-caliber slug	13.6	10
Flying gravel (⅛ in.) @ 30 mph	0.4	0.3
Flying gravel (⅛ in.) @ 50 mph	1.1	0.8
Stone 1¾ in. × ¾ in. × ½ in. thrown 30 ft	10.7	7.9
Stone 2 in. × 1½ in. × 1 in. thrown 30 ft	12.1	8.9
Lawnmower blade throwing small stone 30 ft	8.1–31.2	6–23
Grinding wheel throwing chips 2 ft	0.9–38	0.7–28
FDA test: ⅝ in. steel ball dropped 50 in.	0.2	0.15
ANSI Z87.1-OSHA: 1 in. steel ball dropped 50 in.	0.8	0.60

Data supplied by J. Davis of the Gentex Corporation.

TABLE 10-3
Impact Energies of Selected Projectiles

that which can be withstood by crown glass or CR-39 plastic. Table 10-3 presents impact energies of selected projectiles. The average value for the impact resistance of crown glass and CR-39 plastic, obtained from Figure 10-3, is roughly 1 N-m or 0.75 ft-lb and below the impact energy of most of the projectiles listed in this table.

Eye injuries in industry have been reported to be caused by both large, low velocity and small, high velocity projectiles.[8,61] A recent study of industrial accidents involving eye injury found that roughly 90% of the injuries were the result of objects estimated to be 6 mm or less in size, and most were estimated to be traveling at fairly high velocities.[67] Military eye injuries are usually caused by small, high velocity projectiles.[49]

The wide variety of projectile sizes, velocities, and energies associated with broken spectacle lenses and eye injuries in both the industrial and nonindustrial situation demonstrates that neither crown glass nor CR-39 plastic can provide reliable protection against all impacting objects. Polycarbonate is the only material that can adequately resist the high energy impact of both large and small objects. Whenever eye protection is a major concern, as, for example, in industry, in sports, for children, for the elderly, and for the monocular or amblyopic patient,[27,68] only polycarbonate provides adequate protection.

10.3 Industrial Safety Eye Protection

The U.S. Occupational Safety and Health Administration (OSHA) requires that all industrial eye and face protectors meet the requirements of the ANSI Z87.1 standard. At present the 1968 standard is still the required version,[69,70] but OSHA is revising its general industry safety standards and plans to eventually adopt the most recent version, ANSI Z87.1-1989.[59,71,72] The ANSI Z87.1-1989 standard reflects a change in philosophy from the "design" standard of earlier versions to a "performance" standard. Emphasis has been shifted away from precise descriptions of the manufacturing requirements for each individual component of a protector. Instead, the entire protector must meet standards for such performance properties as impact resistance, corrosion resistance, and flammability. Because the methods used to meet these requirements are not specified, a manufacturer may take advantage of new lens and frame materials and new manufacturing processes. OSHA also prefers performance standards, with the anticipation that this type of standard will result in new types of protectors and better employee acceptance of the protectors.[71]

Prescription industrial safety eyewear requires that both lenses and frames meet the ANSI Z87.1-1989 standard. Industrial safety lenses in a dress safety frame or dress safety lenses in an industrial safety frame do not meet the standard and should never be prescribed. The following is a summary of the requirements for all industrial safety prescription lenses:

1. All lenses must be able to withstand the impact of a 1-inch steel ball dropped 50 inches onto the lens front surface (the industrial safety drop-ball test). The lenses are removed from the frame for testing, and the test apparatus is described in the standard. Lenses that might be damaged by the test (e.g., plastic lenses) are tested by an appropriate statistical testing protocol.

2. All lenses must have a minimum thickness of 3 mm. Lenses of power greater than +3.00 diopters (D) in the most plus meridian can have a minimum thickness of 2.5 mm.

3. All lenses must be permanently marked with the monogram or trademark of the optical laboratory that edges the lenses. This provides proof to a manager or supervisor in the workplace that an employee's lenses are truly industrial safety lenses.

4. In general, the standard does not prohibit the use of tints for industrial safety lenses. This would include, for example, sunglass tints and light tints for comfort or cosmetic purposes. However, tints must be prescribed with knowledge of the patient's lighting and working conditions. For example, lenses of low transmittance (sunglasses) should not be worn indoors, and lightly tinted lenses for indoor use should be prescribed only if the workplace has adequate lighting or if glare is a problem. Sunglasses should not be worn by the operator of a vehicle with a tinted windshield, nor should sunglasses be worn by those driving at night. Older patients with decreased media transmittance may also be poor candidates for any type of tint in the workplace. Tints should be prescribed only with extreme caution.

A tinted lens is classified as a protective filter (for use in welding and other potentially hazardous situations) only if the tint meets the ANSI Z87.1 standards for minimum and maximum visible light transmittance and maximum ultraviolet (UV) and infrared (IR) radiation transmittance. The tints used for dress safety prescription lenses or sunglasses usually will not meet these standards. Protective filters must be marked with the shade number. When "special purpose" lenses, such as those used for glass blowing or for working around glass furnaces, are prescribed, the lenses must be marked with a letter "S." These lenses do not need to meet the transmittance requirements for protective filters.

The use of photochromic lenses in industry has long been a source of confusion. The 1968 version of the ANSI Z87.1 standard prohibited the use of photochromic lenses.[70] The 1979 version of the standard allowed the use of photochromics outdoors,[73] but this version was never adopted by OSHA. OSHA now considers the use of photochromics under conditions in which a violation of the standard has no direct or immediate relationship to safety or health to be a "de minimis" violation.[74] This means that if a violation is found upon inspection of a facility, it is not necessary for the violation to be corrected, nor is a fine imposed. However, photochromic lenses would be prohibited in situations where use of the lenses could present a hazard. The best example is a fork lift operator. When this employee passes from outdoors to indoors, the lenses would not lighten immediately, and the employee would be at risk for accident or injury because vision would be reduced. The use of photochromics indoors by older patients with decreased media transmittance may also be a problem because the lenses have a slight tint even in the lightened state. Photochromic lenses (glass or plastic) are also not as impact resistant as polycarbonate. The ANSI Z87.1-1989 standard does not prohibit the use of photochromics but recommends that the lenses be used with care when critical vision is needed and when workers pass from outdoors to indoors.[59] OSHA's final decision on its new general industry standards should eliminate the confusion.

5. Requirements for prescription power accuracy are those of ANSI Z80.1-1987.[7] Note that the Z80.1 standards are voluntary for dress safety lenses but are required for prescription industrial safety eyewear.

Industrial safety spectacle frames for use in prescription eyewear must meet a number of performance standards, including high mass–low velocity and low mass–high velocity impact resistance standards, flammability standards, and corrosion standards. In addition, all industrial safety frames for prescription use must be marked with the frame "A," "DBL," and overall temple length measurements, and all frames must be marked "Z87" to indicate compliance with the standard.

Polycarbonate is obviously the best lens material to use in prescription industrial safety eyewear. The decreased scratch resistance of coated polycarbonate relative to crown glass should not be considered reason for prescribing glass unless the work environment provides very severe conditions. Polycarbonate can be a problem in cold, dusty work environments because static charges cause dust to cling to the lenses.

OSHA is considering a revision of its general industry standards for eye and face protectors to include issues not specifically addressed by the ANSI Z87.1 standard.[71,72] One important potential revision is a requirement for sideshields on all safety spectacles. This revision is based upon a report by the Bureau of Labor Statistics[67] that 94% of occupational eye injuries studied were the result of projectiles reaching the eye from the unprotected sides, tops, or bottoms of the protector. OSHA is also considering changes in the way eye and face protectors are labeled and a requirement for third-party certification of protectors. OSHA's final decision on the new standards is still pending.

The ANSI Z87.1 standards for nonprescription eyewear have changed considerably from previous versions of the standard. In general, protectors of all types must meet high mass and low mass impact resistance standards, penetration resistance standards, lens and filter minimum thickness requirements, and standards for prism and refractive power error, haze, definition, transmittance, corrosion resistance, and flammability resistance. The lenses of protectors with removable lenses are drop-ball tested separately from the protector, but all protectors must be able to pass the impact and penetration standards with the lenses mounted in the protector. The high velocity impact test provides a good example. Protectors are mounted on an anthropomorphic headform and ¼-inch diameter steel balls are fired at the protector straight-on and from a number of angles to the side. The ball velocity used depends upon the type of protector being tested. A protector fails the test if the eye of the headform is contacted by any part of the protector or by the impacting ball. This type of integrated testing is probably a better index of eye protection than individual component testing.

10.4 Ophthalmic Lenses in Sports

Sports-related eye injuries account for roughly 10% of all ocular injuries treated at hospitals.[61,62,64,65,75,76] Significant numbers of eye injuries have been documented in a variety of sports, especially baseball, ice hockey, basketball, football, golf, and racquet sports.[64–66,75,76] BB guns and air rifles have been reported to be the cause of a large number of severe eye injuries.[77-81] The use of proper eye protection has decreased substantially the number of eye injuries in ice hockey and racquet sports,[75,82,83] but injuries are still a problem in other sports.

The only appropriate lens material for sports protection is polycarbonate. The high velocities and high impact energies of racquet sports balls, for example, far exceed the impact resistance of all lens materials except polycarbonate (Table 10-4). Polycarbonate is superior to all other materials for impacts from large objects and also provides superior protection from small, high velocity projectiles such as BBs.

The frame or protector chosen for eye protection in sports is just as important as the lenses. Not all frames are adequate. For example, the lensless protectors recommended at one time for use in racquet sports have been shown to allow racquetballs and squash balls to deform and penetrate the protector, resulting in eye injury.[75] Frames with temple hinges can be a source of injury if the hinge area breaks and allows the frame front or temple hinge to contact the eye.[84] The best recommendation is to use only frames or protectors that meet consensus standards such as those provided by the American Society for Testing and Materials (ASTM) or the Canadian Standards Association (CSA).[75,85] Racquet sports and ice hockey have received the most attention in this regard. Most often, sports frames and protectors are made from clear, injection-molded polycarbonate.[75] The best summaries of the sports vision field and excellent discussions of frame and protector needs for a wide variety of specific sports are provided by Vinger[75] and Gregg.[84]

10.5 Legal Considerations

Liability from breakage of ophthalmic lenses has become an important issue in optometry because of the development of new lens materials and because of the development of national standards that have become the basis for legal decisions.[86] The topic of liability from ophthalmic materials has been covered in considerable detail elsewhere[86-90] and will be summarized only briefly, with recommendations for minimizing liability.

The most common cause of ophthalmic materials liability is failure to prescribe the proper lens material when protection may be of considerable concern. Whenever necessary, polycarbonate should be prescribed and the lens material written on the prescription form. Patients should be carefully questioned concerning their lifestyle, and the types of lens materials available should be discussed when it becomes obvious that polycarbonate is a consideration. Special eye protectors for specific sports should also be recommended. If the proper materials are prescribed, liability from breakage of lenses or damage to the eye should be minimized.

A patient should not be provided with guarantees that cannot be met. The most obvious problem is use of the terms "unbreakable" or "shatterproof." These terms imply extreme lens safety, and a patient may wear the lenses under conditions for which the spectacles were not designed, resulting in lens breakage and eye injury. The term "impact resistant" is preferred to describe the characteristics of lenses, and it may be necessary to specifically warn a patient not to

Sport	Mass (g)	Weight (oz)	Velocity (m/s)	Range (ft/s)	Impact (N-m)	Energy (ft-lb)
Racketball	39.7	1.4	38–49	125–161	28–49	21–36
Squash	19.8	0.7	58–63	191–205	34–39	25–29
Handball	62.4	2.2	25–31	81–103	19–31	14–23
Tennis	56.7	2.0	38–49	125–161	42–70	31–52

Calculated from experimental data developed at Pennsylvania State University by Professor C.R. Morehouse for the ASTM Racket Sport Standard Committee. *Modified from* Davis J: Lenses for sports vision. *In* Pizzarello LD, Haik BG (eds): Sports Ophthalmology. Springfield, IL, Charles C. Thomas, 1987; with permission.

TABLE 10-4
Ball Velocity and Impact Energy for Certain Sports

wear the spectacles in certain situations. For example, racquetball and squash players should be warned that their everyday glasses are inadequate for sports eye protection.

Another problem that may lead to liability claims for spectacles is failure to verify that spectacle prescriptions meet applicable standards. If industrial safety lenses were ordered but 2-mm thick dress safety lenses were provided, the patient is not adequately protected. If workmanship on a spectacle prescription is defective, it might lead to decreased impact resistance. To prevent these problems, it is necessary that all finished spectacles be inspected and verified when received from the optical laboratory. A measurement of the center thickness of all lenses might also be useful because impact resistance will be related to lens thickness.

In summary, the following suggestions to minimize or prevent materials liability are provided.[86-90]

1. Be familiar with the current ANSI Z80.1 (dress safety) and ANSI Z87.1 (industrial safety) standards and the FDA and OSHA requirements. A copy or summary of the Z80.1 standards should be posted in the dispensary area for reference. Note that both prescription and nonprescription sunglasses must meet the relevant FDA impact resistance standard.

2. Recommend polycarbonate to:
   Athletes
   Monocular patients
   Amblyopes
   Patients with hazardous occupations or
     avocations
   Children

3. Take careful case histories to determine if patients have special needs for eye protection. Discuss the properties of the different lens materials with these patients. Consider special eye and face protectors for sports.

4. When prescribing specially designed protectors for sports, especially racquet sports, be sure that the protectors meet applicable standards.

5. Maintain good records. When prescribing special lens materials, always write the lens material on the prescription form. If a patient refuses your advice, be sure to document this in your records as well.

6. Avoid the terms "unbreakable" and "shatterproof." Always use the term "impact resistant." Do not guarantee that lenses are unbreakable.

7. Be certain that ancillary personnel are aware of impact resistance considerations. Optometric assistants and technicians are often in a position to recommend lens materials and sports protectors to patients.

8. Always verify all spectacles before dispensing them to a patient. This includes not just measurement of power and prism but a determination of the quality of the lens surfaces and bevels, verification of the lens material, verification that impact resistance testing was performed, and measurement of lens center thickness.

9. If a manufacturer of frames or lenses supplies a warning about the product, be sure to pass this warning along to the patient.

10. Never place industrial safety lenses in a dress safety frame or dress safety lenses in an industrial safety frame.

References

1. Young JM. In search of the right high index lens. Optical World 1989; 18(124):10–20.
2. Merigold PA. Developments in glass materials. Aust J Optom 1982; 65:107–115.
3. Davis JK. Prescribing for visibility. Probl Optom 1990; 2:131–155.
4. Loshin DS, Fannin T. Ophthalmic lens design for high index materials. Paper presented at the American Academy of Optometry, 1983.
5. Use of Impact Resistant Lenses in Eyeglasses and Sunglasses. Code of Federal Regulations 21 CFR 801.410. Washington, DC, Office of the Federal Register, April 1, 1990.
6. Impact Resistant Lenses. Questions and Answers. Rockville, MD, U.S. Department of Health and Human Services, Food and Drug Administration, Bureau of Medical Devices, 1987.
7. American National Standards Institute. American National Standard for Ophthalmics-Prescription Ophthalmic Lenses—Recommendations, ANSI Z80.1-1987. New York, American National Standards Institute, 1987.
8. Wigglesworth EC. The impact resistance of eye protector lens materials. Am J Optom Arch Am Acad Optom 1971; 48:245–261.
9. Fields JM, Goldsmith W. Impact resistance of variously mounted ophthalmic lenses. Am J Optom Physiol Opt 1983; 60:725–738.
10. Brandt NM. The anatomy and autopsy of an impact resistant lens. Am J Optom Physiol Opt 1974; 51:982–986.

11. Stewart GM. Eye protection against small high-speed missiles. Am J Ophthalmol 1961; 51:80–87.

12. Bryant RJ. Ballistic testing of spectacle lenses. Am J Optom Arch Am Acad Optom 1969; 46:84–95.

13. Duckworth WH, Rosenfield AR, Gulati ST, Rieger RA, Hoekstra KE. Strength of thin chemtempered lenses: Drop-ball testing. Am J Optom Physiol Opt 1978; 55:801–806.

14. Berger RE. Impact testing of ophthalmic lenses: Stress distribution and the "search" theory. J Am Optom Assoc 1976; 47:86–92.

15. Berger RE. Dynamic strain gage measurements on ophthalmic lenses impacted by low energy missiles. Am J Optom Physiol Opt 1976; 53:279–286.

16. Scaief AL. An alternative to the drop ball test for the measurement of ophthalmic glass fracture resistance. Am J Optom Physiol Opt 1975; 52:765–773.

17. Goldsmith W, Taylor RL. Impact on ophthalmic lenses. Exp Mechanics 1976; 16:81–87.

18. Duckworth WH, Rosenfield AR, Gulati ST, Rieger RA, Hoekstra KE. Strength of thin chemtempered lenses: Static load testing. Am J Optom Physiol Opt 1979; 56:39–47.

19. Dain SJ. Pressure testing of ophthalmic safety lenses. The effects of different materials. Am J Optom Physiol Opt 1988; 65:585–590.

20. Duckworth WH, Rosenfield AR, Gulati ST, Rieger RA, Hoekstra KE. Basic principles of lens fracture testing. Am J Optom Physiol Opt 1978; 55:751–759.

21. Lawn BR, Wilshaw TR. Fracture of Brittle Solids. Cambridge, University Press, 1975.

22. Phillips CJ. The strength and weakness of brittle materials. Am Sci 1965; 53:20–49.

23. Ernsberger FM. Origin and detection of microflaws in glass. In Bradt RC, Hasselman DPH, Lange FF (eds): Fracture Mechanics of Ceramics, Vol. 1, Concepts, Flaws, and Fractography, pp. 161–173. New York, Plenum, 1974.

24. Rawson H. Properties and Applications of Glass. Amsterdam, Elsevier, 1980.

25. Chase GA. Impact-resistant ophthalmic lenses. Manufacturing Opt Int 1972; 25(16):683–686.

26. Proctor B. The effects of hydrofluoric acid etching on the strength of glasses. Phys Chem Glasses 1962; 3:7–27.

27. Davis JK. Perspectives on impact resistance and polycarbonate lenses. Int Ophthalmol Clin 1988; 28:215–218.

28. Chase GA, Kozlowski TR, Krause RP. Chemical strengthening of ophthalmic lenses. Am J Optom Arch Am Acad Optom 1973; 50:470–476.

29. Kozlowski TR, Chase GA. Parameters of chemical strengthening and impact performance of Corning code 8361 (white crown) and Corning code 8097 (Photogray) lenses. Am J Optom Arch Am Acad Optom 1973; 50:273–282.

30. Fannin TE, Grosvenor T. Clinical Optics. Boston, Butterworths, 1987.

31. Horne DF. Spectacle Lens Technology. New York, Crane, Russack and Co., 1978.

32. Lueck IB. Toughened Safety Lenses. Scientific and Technical Publication Number 23, Bausch and Lomb, Rochester, New York, 1961.

33. Peters HB. The fracture resistance of industrially damaged safety glass lenses. Am J Optom Arch Am Acad Optom 1962; 39:33–35.

34. Silberstein IW. The fracture resistance of industrially damaged safety glass lenses, plano and prescription—An expanded study. Am J Optom Arch Am Acad Optom 1964; 41:199–221.

35. Moss HL. Safety lens legislation—the need for a closer look. Opt J Rev Optom 1970; 107(19):19–21.

36. Moss HL. The spontaneous breakage of heat-treated lenses. Opt J Rev Optom 1973; 110(2):49–52.

37. Duckworth WH, Rosenfield AR. Strength of glass lenses processed in an ultrasonically stimulated chemtempering bath. Am J Optom Physiol Opt 1984; 61:48–53.

38. Two-hour Chemtempering of Corning Photochromic Glasses. Corning Technical Bulletin. December, 1990.

39. Kirschen M. Verifying impact resistance. Optom Management 1977; 13(9):55–59.

40. Pomeranz RB. Checking your chemtemp lenses. Opt J Rev Optom 1977; 114(1):86.

41. Howes VR, Goldsmid JM, Silk RK, Were AV. Impact testing of a thermosetting polymer (allyl diglycol carbonate-CR-39). J Appl Polymer Sci 1981; 26:3623–3631.

42. Goldsmith W. Projectile impact on glass and polymeric ophthalmic lenses and circular plates. Am J Optom Physiol Opt 1974; 51:807–831.

43. Sears FW, Zemansky MW, Young HD. College Physics (4th ed). Reading, MA, Addison-Wesley, 1977.

44. Rieke JK. Instrumented impact measurements on some polymers. In Evans RE (ed): Physical Testing of Plastics—Correlation with End-Use Performance, pp 59–76. ASTM STP 736. Philadelphia, American Society for Testing and Materials, 1981.

45. Simmons ST, Krohel GB, Hay PB. Prevention of ocular gunshot injuries using polycarbonate lenses. Ophthalmology 1984; 91:977–983.

46. Kors K, St. Helen R. Base line fracture resistance studies of tempered and non-tempered glass ophthalmic lenses. Am J Optom Arch Am Acad Optom 1973; 50:632–640.

47. LaMarre D. Personal communication, Gentex Corporation, January, 1991.

48. Wigglesworth EC. A comparative assessment of eye protective devices and a proposed system of acceptance testing and grading. Am J Optom Arch Am Acad Optom 1972; 49:287–304.

49. Hornblass A. Eye injuries in the military. Int Ophthalmol Clin 1981; 21(4):121–138.

50. Keeney AH. Lens Materials in the Prevention of Eye Injuries. Springfield, IL, Charles C. Thomas, 1957.

51. Wigglesworth EC. Evaluation of eye protector lens materials. Aust J Optom 1967; 50:343–352.

52. Williams RL, Stewart GM. Ballistic studies in eye protection. Am J Ophthalmol 1964; 58:453–464.

53. Newton AW. Industrial eye protection—an appraisal of some current safety lens materials. J Inst Eng Aust 1967; 39:163–170.

54. Dowaliby M, Griffin J, Palmer B, Voorhees L. A study involving glass safety lenses. Am J Optom Arch Am Acad Optom 1972; 49:128–136.

55. Scaief AL. Analysis of glass fragments as a function of fracture resistance. Optom Weekly 1976; 67:110–1111.

56. Wigglesworth EC. A ballistic assessment of eye protector lens materials. Invest Ophthalmol 1971; 10:985–991.

57. LaMarre D. Development of Criteria and Test Methods for Eye and Face Protective Devices. Publication No. 78-110. Washington, DC, Department of Health, Education, and Welfare (National Institutes for Occupational Safety and Health), August 1977.

58. Greenberg I, Chase G, LaMarre D. Statistical protocol for impact testing prescription polycarbonate safety lenses. Optical World 1985; 14(Mar/Apr):7–8.

59. American National Standards Institute. American National Standard Practice for Occupational and Educational Eye and Face Protection, ANSI Z87.1-1989. New York, American National Standards Institute, 1989.

60. Young JM. Personal communication, Essilor of America, Inc, December 1990.

61. Keeney AH, Fintelmann E, Renaldo D. Clinical mechanisms in non-industrial eye trauma. Am J Ophthalmol 1972; 74:662–665.

62. Scrivener AB. Impact-resistant spectacle lenses. Br J Physiol Opt 1973; 28:26–33.

63. Schutten G, Reim M. Augenverletzungen durch Brillenglaser. Klin Monatsbl Augenheilkd 1987; 191:237–239.

64. Karlson TA, Klein BEK. The incidence of acute hospital-treated eye injuries. Arch Ophthalmol 1986; 104:1473–1476.

65. Grin TR, Nelson LB, Jeffers JB. Eye injuries in childhood. Pediatrics 1987; 80:13–17.

66. Nelson LB, Wilson TW, Jeffers JB. Eye injuries in childhood: Demography, etiology, and prevention. Pediatrics 1989; 84:438–441.

67. Accidents Involving Eye Injuries. Report 597. Washington, DC, U.S. Department of Labor, Bureau of Labor Statistics, April 1980.

68. Tommila V, Tarkkanen A. Incidence of loss of vision in the healthy eye in amblyopia. Br J Ophthalmol 1981; 65:575–577.

69. OSHA Safety and Health Standards (29 CFR 1910). Section 1910.133. Washington, DC, U.S. Department of Labor, OSHA 2206, 1983.

70. American National Standards Institute. American National Standard Practice for Occupational and Educational Eye and Face Protection, ANSI Z87.1-1968. New York, American National Standards Institute, 1968.

71. Federal Register 1989; 54(157):33832–33844.

72. Federal Register 1990; 55(22):3412–3415.

73. American National Standards Institute. American National Standard Practice for Occupational and Educational Eye and Face Protection, ANSI Z87.1-1979. New York, American National Standards Institute, 1979.

74. Auchter T. Letter to Senator David L. Boren, Occupational Safety and Health Administration, July 29, 1981.

75. Vinger PF. The eye and sports medicine, Chap 45. In Tasman W, Jaeger EA (eds): Duane's Clinical Ophthalmology, Vol 5. Philadelphia, JB Lippincott, 1989.

76. Elman MJ. Racket-sports ocular injuries. Arch Ophthalmol 1986; 104:1453–1454.

77. Strahlman E, Sommer A. The epidemiology of sports-related ocular trauma. Int Ophthalmol Clin 1988; 28:199–202.

78. Sheets W, Vinger P. Ocular injuries from air guns. Int Ophthalmol Clin 1988; 28:225–227.

79. Sternberg P, De Juan E, Green WR, et al. Ocular BB injuries. Ophthalmology 1984; 91:1269–1277.

80. Bowen DI, Magauran DM. Ocular injuries caused by airgun pellets: An analysis of 105 cases. Br Med J 1973; 1:333–337.

81. Parver LM. The National Eye Trauma System. Int Ophthalmol Clin 1988; 28:203–205.

82. Pashby TJ. Ocular injuries in hockey. Int Ophthalmol Clin 1988; 28:228–231.

83. Easterbrook M. Ocular injuries in racquet sports. Int Ophthalmol Clin 1988; 28:232–237.

84. Gregg JR. Vision and Sports: An Introduction. Boston, Butterworths, 1987.

85. Davis JK. Lenses for sports vision. In Pizzarello LD, Haik BG (eds): Sports Ophthalmology, pp 9–43. Springfield, IL, Charles C. Thomas, 1987.

86. Classe JG. Clinicolegal aspects of practice. South J Optom 1986; 4:36–43.

87. Classe JG. Legal Aspects of Optometry. Boston, Butterworths, 1989.

88. Classe JG. Legal aspects of sports-related ocular injuries. Int Ophthalmol Clin 1988; 28:211–214.

89. Classe JG, Scholles J. Liability for ophthalmic lenses. J Am Optom Assoc 1986; 57:470–477.

90. Young JM. Liability in ophthalmic lenses. Optical World 1989; 18(118):16–24.

CHAPTER ELEVEN

Sunglasses for Ocular Protection

Donald G. Pitts, O.D., Ph.D.

11.1 Are Sunglasses Fashion or Protection?

The sunglass industry sold $1.3 billion of their products during 1988.[1] A record number of publications on sunglasses have appeared that cite quality control,[2] how to select a "perfect" pair of sunglasses,[3] how to select sunglasses for speed,[4] why sunglasses should be worn for "all seasons,"[3] the need for ultraviolet (UV) protection,[5] and how to "prescribe" nonprescription eyewear.[6] Fashion has been the emphasis of these articles in spite of the fact that the major need for sunglasses is to protect the eyes. Protection of the eyes is necessary regardless of whether corrective, prescription sunglasses or plano, noncorrective sunglasses are worn. Protection must include maintaining night vision, eliminating undesirable wavelengths of radiation, reducing excessive luminances, and for comfort and maximum visual performance.

A number of misconceptions related to sunglasses need to be discussed. Sunglasses, except for polaroid lenses, do not eliminate glare, nor do they usually change contrast. The sunglass lens reduces the excessive luminance called glare to an intensity level tolerated by the eye. Sunglasses ordinarily absorb the reflected luminance from objects and their background in the same proportions, which ensures that contrast remains constant. Special purpose sunglasses may be designed to alter the luminance reflected between the background and target to enhance apparent contrast. An ophthalmic lens that possesses 40% or greater transmittance is useless as a protective sunglass. Colored sunglasses may alter color discrimination and serve to render red and green traffic lights indistinguishable. There is no sunglass for night driving because all sunglasses remove light and the eye needs all available light at night. Unequal transmittance between the two lenses may disrupt the perception of depth.

Poorly prepared optical surfaces produce visual distortions that may cause headaches, eyestrain, and other subjective symptoms. The surface quality of a lens may be checked by projecting a light on the surface of the lens and looking for waves or grey areas that indicate poor polishing of the surface. The mires of the lensometer will appear distorted when a poorly polished lens is moved up or down across the exit port. An easy method to check for dioptric power and quality is to select a door with vertical and horizontal straight edges. Hold the lens at about one half arm's length and observe the vertical edge of the door while moving the lens from side to side a short distance. Now move the lens up and down while observing the horizontal edge. Movements, waving, or jumping of either edge indicates distortion and waves in the lens and the lens should be rejected, whereas movements with or against the motion of the lens indicates dioptric power. Place a plano lens in front of the projector while observing the effect on the smallest letters. Blurred letters indicate poor optical quality, and the lens should be rejected.

11.2 The Optimum Sunglass Lens

The ideal or optimum sunglass lens should provide the following:

1. Reduce the solar ambient luminance for optimum visual comfort and visual performance.
2. Elimination of the optical spectrum not required for vision that serves as a hazard to the eye.
3. Maintenance of optimum dark adaptation or night vision.
4. Maintenance of normal color vision. Traffic signal lights must be able to be seen quickly and correctly.
5. Minimum care and increased resistance against impact and scratching.

Each of these attributes will be briefly discussed to validate the scientific need for sunglasses of people who are exposed to prolonged periods of sunlight. Discussions on impact resistance of ophthalmic materials, optical transmittance, optical density,

Fresnel's equation, and methods of calculating protection have been presented in Chapters 9 and 10 and need not be repeated here.

Controlling Levels of Ambient Luminance

Sunglass lenses are usually classified by their color and their percent transmittance. The dominant wavelength of the broad-band transmitted and reflected light usually determines the color. The saturation of the color is related to the intensity of the transmittance of the lens. There are four types of filter lenses commonly used for sunglasses: (1) absorptive colored lenses, (2) neutral lenses, (3) polarizing lenses, and (4) metallic reflecting lenses, including interference filters.

ABSORPTIVE LENSES. Absorptive lenses selectively transmit portions of the optical spectrum with the transmittance and reflectance characteristics providing the hue or color of the lens. A red lens transmits maximally in the red region of the spectrum and absorbs in the blue region of the spectrum. A green lens transmits maximally in the green region of the spectrum while absorbing both the blue and red portions of the spectrum. Absorptive lenses do not add light but subtract the absorbed wavelengths from the total light available. Photochromic lenses are a special type of absorptive lens and may be chromatic or grey in color (Fig. 9-5). The spectral transmittance of commercially available glass sunglass lenses (Fig. 11-1), CR-39 plastic sunglass lenses (Fig. 11-2), and polycarbonate sunglass lenses (Fig. 11-3) are provided for comparison.

Green-colored sunlenses such as Ray-ban or Calobar offer UV protection and absorb some infrared (IR) but usually demonstrate broadband transmittance. Yellow lenses such as the Hazemaster or Kalichrome eliminate all of the blue end of the visible (VIS) spectrum but transmit the long wavelengths. Blue-green lenses such as the Therminon or Unisol absorb IR, but care must be used in prescribing for IR protection because the lenses become secondary emitters and place the IR source closer to the eye.

NEUTRAL LENSES. Neutral lenses absorb almost equally across the VIS spectrum and appear grey in color. Neutral filters made from ophthalmic crown glass usually transmit both UV and IR (Fig. 11-4).

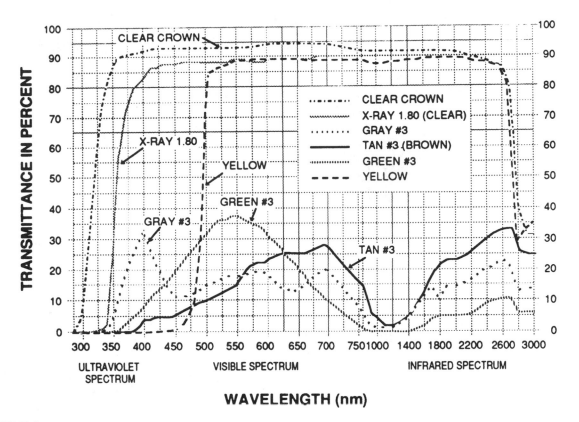

FIGURE 11-1

Spectral transmittance of commercially available clear ophthalmic crown and tinted ophthalmic crown lenses commonly used for sunglasses. The X-RAY1.80 is used to protect the eyes of technicians working in X-ray facilities. The descriptive titles indicate the color of the lens.

Neutral lenses made from plastic will transmit both UV and IR unless the lens material is manufactured or dyed to absorb these undesirable wavebands. Neutral or grey lenses prevent color distortion because they transmit almost evenly across the VIS spectrum.

POLARIZED FILTER LENSES. Polarized filter lenses are constructed by stretching a thin polyvinyl film that contains iodine and quinine compounds or herapathite crystals between two thin glass or plastic lenses. The color of the lens is derived from the glass or plastic. The transmittance of polarizing lenses is variable and depends on the degree and the plane of polarization of the incident light. When a beam of plane-polarized light is analyzed by a second polarizing lens, the intensity of the beam changes from a minimum to a maximum as the analyzer is rotated through 90° (law of Malus). When light is reflected from a surface, it is partially or completely plane polarized with the plane of polarization of the reflected ray perpendicular to the plane of incidence of the light. Light incident on smooth surfaces such as glass, concrete, automobile windshields, asphalt, water, and glazed pottery produce polarized reflected light that may be removed by viewing the surface through a polarizing lens oriented with its vibration plane perpendicular to the reflected light. Care must be taken when polarizing lenses are used because of the possible transmittance of undesirable UVR.[7]

REFLECTING FILTERS. Reflecting filters are manufactured by the vacuum deposition of metallic coatings on a glass or plastic substrate. Metallic filters are the preferred method to control IR. Gold, silver, and copper reflect greater than 95% of the infrared. Aluminum reflects greater than 90% of the UV, about

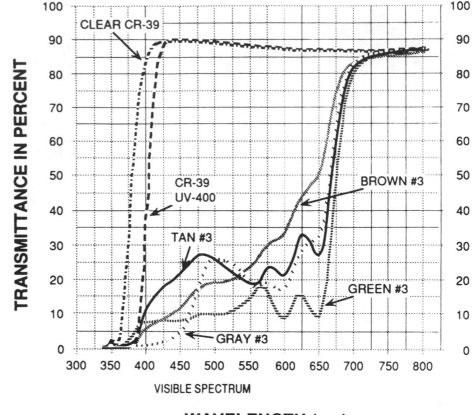

FIGURE 11-2
Transmittance of CR-39 lenses. The clear CR-39 lens contains a UV inhibitor to maintain clarity of the lens. The CR-39 UV-400 absorbs UVR up to 400 nm. The remaining sunglass lens colors are indicated by descriptive titles. Note that sunglass lenses often transmit a small amount of UVR to 350 nm.

85% of the VIS spectrum, and about 95% of the IR. Silver and copper transmit greater than 60% of the UV and about 50% of the VIS spectrum. Inconel, a mixture of iron, nickel, and cobalt is commonly used for sunglasses (Fig. 11-5). Inconel is neutral grey in appearance for the VIS spectrum while transmitting both UV and IR spectra. The proper combination of metallic thin film coatings and lens substrates allow excellent control of optical radiation. The major difficulty with metallic coatings is the ease with which they scratch. A protective coating overlay must be used to protect the thin, metallic film surface.

Other film coatings that are used to alter the optical properties of lenses include antireflection coatings (ARC), scratch resistant coatings (SRC), interference filters, semitransparent mirrors, beam splitters, and heat control filters. The coatings are vacuum deposited, except for the SRC coating, and are not commonly used for spectacle optics. The ARCs reduces unwanted reflections from the lens surface and increases the transmittance of the visible spectrum. ARC coatings are necessary for people who work in movies, television, and occupations where the reflection pattern is not acceptable. SRCs increase plastic lens resistance to scratching.

Determining Adequate Levels of Sunlight

The levels of sunlight on a clear day may be as high as 70,000 cd/m^2 (Table 11-1), which is uncomfortable for normal vision. The optimum level of lighting for good, comfortable vision is about 1400 cd/m^2 (425 fL), which is equivalent to the intensity of full sunlight under a shade tree.[8] Studies have shown that sunglasses in the 9% to 25% transmittance range are preferred by all but older people.[9–12] The measurements of a number of different outdoor scenes range from 300 cd/m^2 (86 fL) to 70,000 cd/m^2 (11,500 fL), with an average of about 9000 cd/m^2

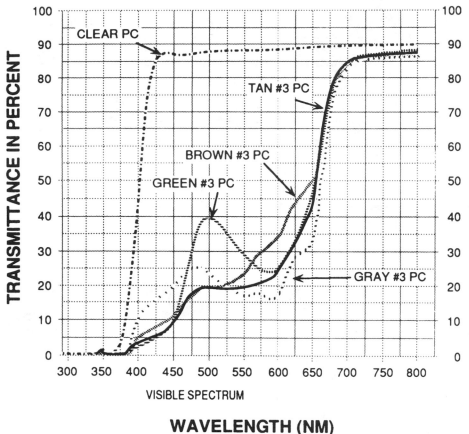

FIGURE 11-3
Transmittance of polycarbonate ophthalmic lenses. Clear polycarbonate lenses absorb UVR to about 380 mm. The colors of the remaining lenses are designated by descriptive titles and are used for sunglass lenses. Note that their transmittance below about 390 nm is zero.

(2600 fL) (Table 11-1). Concrete freeways provide a luminance after reflection from the roadway surface of about 6000 cd/m^2 (1735 fL) on overcast days that increases to 9000 cd/m^2 (2600 fL) on bright sunny days. The visual albedo or reflectance from different surfaces is provided in Table 11-2.[13,14] The levels of sunlight, skylight, and total sunlight at the Earth's surface are given in Table 4-5.

These data may be used to establish the proper transmittance of an ophthalmic lens in providing optimum visual performance:

$$\tau = \frac{1400 \text{ cd/m}^2}{L_V \cdot \rho} \qquad (11\text{-}1)$$

where τ is the transmittance of the sunglass lens for optimum visual performance, L_V the luminance of the source reaching the eye, and ρ the reflectance of the light from the visual task or visual scene. For example, assume that on a bright sunny day a lumi-

nance of 30,000 cd/m^2 falls on a tennis court with a 35% reflectance. What is the optimum sunglass transmittance?

$$\tau = \frac{1400 \text{ cd/m}^2}{30,000 \text{ cd/m}^2 \cdot 0.35} = 0.13 \text{ or } 15\% \qquad (11\text{-}2)$$

A sunglass with 15% transmittance would provide optimum vision and protect the eye against excessive sunlight. These same data may be used to determine the contrast of the tennis ball against the sky or tennis court surface. Assume that a tennis ball with a reflectance of 0.65 is seen against the tennis court by a player wearing 15% transmittance grey sunglasses; what is the contrast of the tennis ball? The luminance of the ball would be $L_B = 30,000 \text{ cd/m}^2 \times 0.65 \times 0.15 = 2925 \text{ cd/m}^2$. The luminance of the concrete would be $30,000 \text{ cd/m}^2 \times 0.65 = 10,500 \text{ cd/m}^2$. The contrast of the tennis ball would be

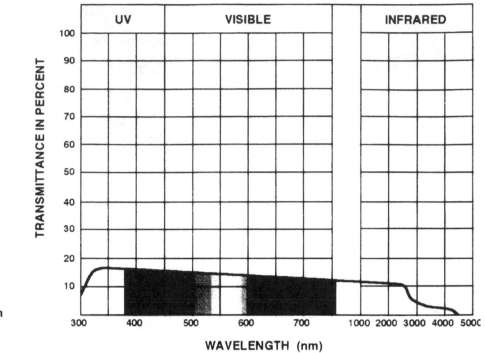

FIGURE 11-4
Crown glass neutral or grey filters. Such filters appear grey in color because equal amounts of the VIS spectrum are transmitted at all wavelengths. Note that UVR and IR are transmitted.

$$C = \frac{2925 \text{ cd/m}^2 - 10{,}500 \text{ cd/m}^2}{2925 \text{ cd/m}^2 + 10{,}500 \text{ cd/m}^2}$$

$$= \frac{-7575}{13{,}425} = -0.56 \qquad (11\text{-}3)$$

The minus ($-$) sign indicates that the tennis ball is darker than its background.

Sunglass transmittance requirements for UV and IR may also be calculated based on the occupational radiation exposure guidelines (Table 11-3):

$$\tau = \frac{\text{recommended standard [W/cm}^2]}{\text{incident radiation [W/cm}^2]} \qquad (11\text{-}4)$$

Radiation incident from the sun at the Earth's surface has an irradiance of 726.6×10^{-4} W/cm^2, and the irradiance for various portions of the spectrum may be determined by using the percentages of each waveband:

14% UV or 0.0102 W/cm^2
   4.8% of the UVB (300–320 nm) or (0.0035 W/cm^2)
   9.2% of the UVA (320–400 nm) or (0.0067 W/cm^2)
43% IR or 0.0313 W/cm^2

The maximum permissible transmittance of sunglass lenses would be

$$\tau \text{ UVA} = \frac{1 \text{ mW/cm}^2}{0.0067 \text{ W/cm}^2} = 0.149 \text{ or } 14.9\%$$

$$\tau \text{ UVB} = \frac{1 \times 10^{-6} \text{ W/cm}^2}{0.0035 \text{ W/cm}^2} = 2.86 \times 10^{-4}$$

$$\text{or } 0.0286\% \qquad (11\text{-}5)$$

$$\tau \text{ IR} = \frac{10 \text{ mW/cm}^2}{0.0313 \text{ W/cm}^2} = 0.319 \text{ or } 31.9\%$$

The transmittances calculated establish the maximum allowable transmittance for each waveband to protect the eye against solar damage.

*Eliminating the Optical Spectrum
Not Required for Vision*

Chapter 6 discussed the effects of exposure to UV, VIS, and IR portions of the optical spectrum. It seems practical and prudent to exclude UVR in sunglasses to eliminate any risk of eye damage

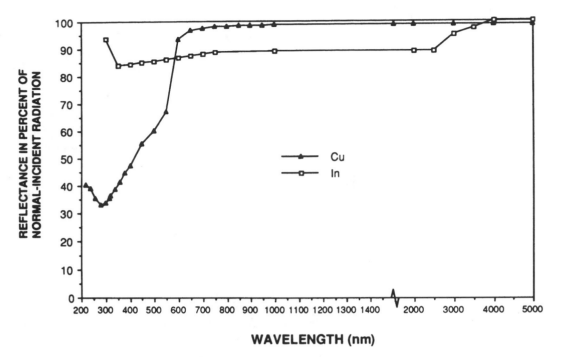

FIGURE 11-5
Reflectance of inconel (In) and copper (Cu) vacuum deposited metallic coatings. Inconel is essentially neutral or grey, whereas copper-transmitted light appears almost tan. Inconel is an excellent protector against IR but transmits UVR.

from long-term and short-term exposure. IR requires massive amounts of exposure to cause acute ocular damage, but exposure to IR lowers the threshold for the photochemical damage from UVR and should be reduced to a minimum when possible.

Excessive radiation in the VIS spectrum should be reduced to maintain optimum visual performance. Increased visual acuity with ND filters with a 10% transmittance as a sunglass lens has been reported.[15] People above the age of 40 were able to improve vision outdoors in bright sun with a 10% filter, but vision became worse as the transmittance decreased below 10%. The visibility of lines and squares seen against the sky as a background improved as the background luminance increased from 400 to 3000 cd/m^2 when a 12% neutral filter was used.[16] A rule of thumb is that for ambient luminances in the visual field above 1000 cd/m^2 sunglasses with 10% and greater luminous transmittance do not produce losses in visual acuity.[11,17]

Outdoor Scene	Luminance (cd/m^2)
Bright hazy sky under the sun	40,000–70,000
Sun on snow	15,000–30,000
Sun on clouds	15,000–30,000
Bright beaches	6000–15,000
Concrete pavement	3000–9000
Sunlit fields and foliage	3000–7000
Shade beside trees	300–600
Backlighted signs	300–600
Shady side of buildings	300–600
Deep blue sky away from sun	300–3000
Comfortable viewing	350–2000
Required for adequate seeing	350

Data from Davis JK.[36]

TABLE 11-1
Luminance of Selected Commonly Experienced Outside Scenes

Type of Surface	Albedo or Reflectance
Fresh water	0.03–0.13
Salt water	0.03–0.08
Sea surf, white	0.25–0.30
Soil, dry	0.07–0.15
Soil, wet	0.05–0.08
Sand, dry	0.15–0.18
Sand, wet	0.07
Forest	0.03–0.10
Grass	0.03–0.05
Snow, fresh-fallen	0.88–0.95
Concrete, sidewalk, fresh	0.10–0.12
Concrete, sidewalk, aged	0.07–0.08
Roadway, asphalt, fresh	0.04–0.05
Roadway, asphalt, aged	0.05–0.09

Data from Handbook of Geophysics for Air Force Designers and Sliney DH.[14]

TABLE 11-2
Reflectance of UV from Different Types of Commonly Encountered Surfaces

Spectrum	Wavelength	Recommended Standard
UVC and UVB	200–315	0.1 W/cm^2
UVA	320–400	1 mW/cm^2
VIS	400–760	1 cd/cm^2
IRA	770–1400	10 mW/cm^2

TABLE 11-3
Recommended Occupational Radiation Exposure Limits

Maintaining Optimum Retinal Adaptation for Night Vision

Exposure of the eye to sunlight produces both a temporary and cumulative effect on the subsequent ability to see at night.[18,19] A 2- or 3-h exposure to sunlight delays the initial phase of dark adaptation as much as 10 min and elevates the final level of adaptation 0.5 log unit, and after 10 daily exposures visual acuity and contrast discrimination show a 50%

elevated threshold.[19–21] The effects of sunlight on the sensitivity of the eye are related to the duration of exposure,[22] hue,[23] size, brightness, and retinal location.[24,25] Solar exposures result in a decrease in the ability to see at night, as well as a decrease in visual acuity, contrast discrimination, and retinal sensitivity. The reduction in oxygen with altitude also has been shown to elevate night vision,[26] which may be of interest to skiers and mountain climbers.

The visual decrements experienced from excessive sunlight exposure usually return to normal after a 24 h period of protection against sunlight,[19] but prolonged periods of time away from sunlight do not improve night vision abilities beyond the normal seasonal peak.[27] Sunglasses with a luminous transmittance of 12% to 15% were effective in preventing the loss of night vision, contrast discrimination, and visual acuity.[11,28–30] Sunglass lenses with a transmittance from 35% to 50% were not effective in maintaining normal visual performance in sunlight or after dark.

The conclusion from this research is that a person who is engaged in any task where night vision is critical such as driving or flying, or in occupations such as the police, military personnel, sailors, ship captains, and harbor pilots, must wear sunglasses to maintain maximum visual performance on the job. Astronomers who make their observations at night are particularly susceptible to exposure to sunlight. People who perform tasks that require critical night vision should always wear sunglasses of less than 20% luminous transmittance when undertaking activities of a 2 h or greater duration in sunlight. Daytime outdoor exposure should be assessed for people with complaints of poor night vision.

Maintaining Normal Color Vision

One common task performed by people who wear sunglasses is to observe and obey traffic signal lights. It is imperative that colored sunglasses allow the wearer to recognize and react to traffic lights. This requirement is made more stringent when it is recognized that approximately 8.5% of the male population possess defective color vision.

Using the Nagel anomaloscope, we can see certain trends in color perception by those wearing filters. Rose smoke and yellow lenses impair color vision significantly and may be dangerous as sunglass lenses for drivers.[31,32] Green and brownish lenses result in a number of errors on red, green, and white colors due to the selective shift in the spectral transmittance of the lenses. Greenish filters absorb red and shift the color vision of the normal observer toward protanomaly, whereas brownish filters absorb blue and green while shifting color normals toward the deuteranomal direction. The deuteranomalous individual is shifted toward the normal by greenish filters and away from normal by brownish lenses. The protanomalous color defective is shifted toward normal by the brownish tint but away from normal by the greenish tints.[32,33]

These results appear to justify recommending brownish filters to protanomals and greenish lenses to the deuteranomal to assist in color discrimination, but care must be taken. The deuteranomal will lose brightness in the red traffic light, which may be more serious than the loss in intensity of the green traffic light. Brownish lenses are a distinct advantage for the protanomal when traffic lights are viewed. If colored lenses are prescribed as an aid for color defectives, it is important that the proper diagnosis of the defect be made prior to applying a filter. Any lens used with color-defective people should be checked against a very practical test—the traffic light—prior to dismissing the patient.

The prolonged wearing of chromatic filters results in distortions of color perception that persist as long as 36 d.[34] These phenomena were postulated to be the result of a modification in cellular function at the level of the visual cortex. Evidence for the conclusion was an "interocular" transfer of the effect from the eye behind the sunglass lens to the contralateral control eye. Further studies are warranted to determine the cause of such effects.

The elimination of color distortion was a major consideration in the U.S. military selection of a neutral grey lens.[35] The ANSI Z80.3-1986 American National Standard for ophthalmic nonprescription sunglasses color requirements was based on the recognition of traffic signals.[36] Empiric studies using color normals and color defectives demonstrate that the apparent color shift and the apparent luminosity of the traffic signals are important in establishing standards.[37–39] These findings resulted in the conclusion that all colored filters change the color vision of military pilots to such an extent as to endanger the recognition of color signals[32] and that only grey sunglasses were recommended for use by the pilot.

The safest sunglass lens worn by both color normals and color defectives maintains normal color perception. Color recognition tasks clearly demonstrate that the neutral grey is the color of choice, with the brown tints being next. Green tints create serious color shifts in some color defectives and should be used with caution. It is recognized that special colored filters are required for particular situations; the wearers of the special color filters should be warned that the special filters should not be worn as a general purpose sunglass lens.

CORRECTION OF COLOR VISION DEFECTS WITH FILTERS

Maxwell[40] was the first to suggest that the use of colored filters by dichromats would assist in the perception of colored objects. The red and green filters were mounted as spectacle lenses, and colored objects were alternately viewed through the lenses. The suggested mechanism is a changing of the brightness of the colored object or a shift in the color of the object.[41,42] The red-green filter combination was suggested to be less than ideal for the dichromat and was replaced by a magenta and cyan filter. Such filters produce a perceptible binocular stereoscopic luster[43] and a color shift for both the protanope and deuteranope; however, these lenses produced only marginal improvement in color discrimination.[44] The X-chrom contact lens has also been reported to correct dichromats,[45,46] but its deep red color produces poor depth perception because it is worn on one eye.

More recently, a computer-graphics quantitative program has been developed to classify, describe, and design additional filters to aid the dichromat.[47,48] The concept was experimentally tested using the X-chrom lens on deuteranopes and protanopes. The protanope was shown to gain less luminous information than the deuteranope, which is intuitively correct, because a red filter before a protanopic eye should reduce the remaining spectrum while further reducing the luminous intensity information available. Deuteranopes demonstrated an increase in hue discrimination for the blues and purples.

Colored filters potentially provide additional luminous or chromatic information for the dichromat, but care in the selection of specific filters must be used.[47] A filter having minimal middle wavelength transmittance and optimal transmittance to provide monocular color discrimination for the confused colors provides maximum discrimination for tasks.[48] Analysis of a rose-colored filter that suppresses mid-wavelength transmittance of the greens, similar to a Wratten #30 filter, has been made. When used monocularly by the dichromat, such a filter aids in providing chromaticity information for tasks requiring color discrimination but does not assist the anomalous trichromat in color perception.[43,48]

11.3 Night Driving Sunglasses? Or Yellow Filters?

Yellow filters with a spectral transmittance similar to that shown in Figure 11-1 have been advertised for night driving for many years. The luminances encountered during night driving are on the order of 3 cd/m^2 at twilight and 0.3 cd/m^2 at night. The rods and cones are both operating at these levels of luminance. A person wearing a 50% transmittance filter has been shown to suffer up to 60% loss in visibility when driving at night.[49–51] Tinted lenses in association with the green windshield result in losses in visual acuity, stereopsis, and the discrimination of angular velocity.[52] Combine these losses with the decrement from exposure to sunlight, and it would be dangerous to drive at night. Filters have been related to the cause of a nighttime aircraft accident.[53] Research indicates that any sunglass lens worn before the eyes reduces the amount of light available for vision and must not be worn at night for driving or flying.

Considerable research has been expended in demonstrating the visual effects of the yellow-tinted lens. The lens has been claimed to be useful to the hunter,[54] target shooter,[55] skiers, mountain climbers, arctic explorers, and aviators.[10,11] The experimental evidence available demonstrates that the yellow filter does not enhance night driving, nor does it improve visual acuity,[11,16] contrast sensitivity,[56,57] or stereopsis.[58]

Contrast and Apparent Brightness

How are the yellow filters supposed to work? For the shooter, skier, and outdoorsman, it has been claimed that the short wavelengths that are scattered by haze

and atmospheric moisture are removed by the filter. The result is an apparent increase in contrast for long wavelength objects viewed against a short wavelength background. It has also been suggested that the absorption of the short wavelengths of the spectrum reduces lenticular fluorescence and thereby enhances contrast. The exact mechanism of the yellow filter has not been demonstrated definitively.

There are two visual attributes that show improvement when yellow lenses are worn: reaction time and the increase in apparent brightness. Reaction time to low contrast targets with low spatial frequencies is statistically shorter in duration with a yellow filter than with a neutral filter equated for luminances.[59] This result may explain why pilots and air crew feel that target detection is improved when the yellow filter is worn.

The brightness of light viewed through a yellow filter shows an enhancement over a one-log range from 7 to 70 cd/m^2 when compared to a matched luminance neutral filter using large field targets. The enhancement at 7 cd/m^2 appears simultaneously with the chromatic perception of yellow.[60] This indicates that the fovea shows a threshold for yellow light about 10 times the absolute foveal threshold.[61] The yellow light appears 40% brighter when its chromatic content is above threshold and the peripheral retina is stimulated. The rod receptors are the mediators of the enhancement effect, and the stimulation of the chromatic channels does not produce the brightness enhancement.[60] This interpretation is strengthened because the brightness enhancement effect was not found when the rods were saturated by bleaching and the cones were fully operative.[60]

Snowscapes and the Yellow Filter

The yellow lens has been recommended for use as ocular protection in snow, during white-out and to improve the perception of depth and contours under poor visibility conditions.[10] Attempts have been made to suggest possible mechanisms whereby the yellow filter may aid these visibility conditions.[62,63] A comparison of neutral and yellow filters was made by requesting skiers to determine which was the deeper of two depressions on either side of a snow track. The skiers judged the correct depth more accurately when wearing the yellow goggles. Kinney[64] suggested that the yellow filter reduces the shorter wavelengths that allow the chromatic opponents channels to become more sensitive, which results in an enhanced visual performance.

Corth[62] maintains that the ability of the yellow goggle to enhance the perception of contours is simply an apparent contrast enhancement of the "bluer" shadows when compared to the unshadowed surface. Troscianko[65] requested skiers to describe sunlight at the bottom of holes 20 to 40 cm deep in the snow. The surface snow was described as white, but the bottoms of the hole became blue or greenish-blue. The change of color is due to the absorption of the longer wavelengths by the water in the snow and the transmittance of the shorter blue wavelengths.[66]

11.4 Short Wavelength Visible Spectrum Absorbing Filters

The short wavelength VIS spectrum absorbing filters became popular during the 1980s, including the NoIR Amber (40% transmittance—τ); the Corning CPF 511, 527, and 550 series (about 23.5% τ); and the Blu-Blocker and the Vuarnet 4006 (7% τ). Advertisements often claim that such lenses are beneficial for people with developing cataracts, aphakia, pseudoaphakia, macular degeneration, diabetic retinopathy, glaucoma, corneal dystrophy, optic atrophy, albinism, retinitis pigmentosa, and aniridia.[67] These claims are based on the assumption that blue light from the blue portion of the visible spectrum is more hazardous than the remainder of the visible spectrum in producing ocular damage. However, little scientific information is available that demonstrates the efficacy of such lenses,[68] because most of the research is subjective and must be evaluated carefully. These lenses are reported to be preferred; however, 30% of the subjects in one study rejected their use.[69] No statistical difference in acuity was found in comparing a plano lens, CPF 527, and an equivalent neutral density filter.[70] Contrast sensitivity was also not found to be statistically different when the CPF 550, a 20% ND filter, and unaided vision were compared.[71]

In a comparison of the CPF 550, NoIR Amber 405, Blu-Blocker, and Vuarnet 4006, with an ND filter as the control, the Farnsworth D-15 color test showed color abnormalities for the Blu-Blocker and Vuarnet lenses. The errors for the Blu-Blocker were variable, but the Vuarnet 4006 showed tritan-type errors that were classified as moderate to severe in color confusion.[72] Comparison of the data may be somewhat misleading because the lens groups showed large differences in transmittance of the VIS spectrum. The Blu-Blocker and Vuarnet were reported to have visible transmittance of less than 10%, whereas the remaining lenses were in the 20% to 30% transmittance levels. These differences may account for some of the color errors; however, the lenses are manufactured with the transmittances used in the test.

The influence of the Blu-Blocker lens (Fig. 11-6) on several aspects of human performance has been assessed recently.[73] An ND filter of equivalent luminance was used for control. The Blu-Blocker and the ND filters showed an increase in the contrast sensitivity for the low spatial frequencies, no change at intermediate frequencies, and a decrease at high spatial frequencies. The threshold for stereopsis was unchanged at 12 s of arc. The FM-100 hue test was used to check color vision, and normal subjects showed an induced tritan color defect, reduced color discrimination, and an increase in the mean error score from 24 to 205, which indicates a loss in color discrimination when the Blu-Blocker lens was worn. Protanopes showed an increase in error score from 21 with their normal correction to an error score of 721 when the Blu-Blocker lens was worn. Deuteranopes had an error score of 219 with their habitual lenses but an error score of 599 when wearing Blu-Blocker lenses. These color discrimination losses may seriously affect the ability of people with normal or color-defective vision to detect the proper traffic light. The green traffic signal becomes dimmer, which increases the difficulty of the deuteranope in detecting it. Color defectives have been shown to have slower reaction times to traffic lights and occasionally, to confuse the colors of the traffic signals.[39] Subjects in an evaluation of the CPF 550 lens reported difficulty in identifying traffic signals.[71]

The errors induced in the Farnsworth Munsell 100 hue test and in color discrimination tasks using the CPF 500, Vuarnet 4007, NoIR Amber 40%, and the Blu-Blocker raised the concern about proper labeling of these lenses.[74] Errors induced in people who are color defective serve to aggravate an already

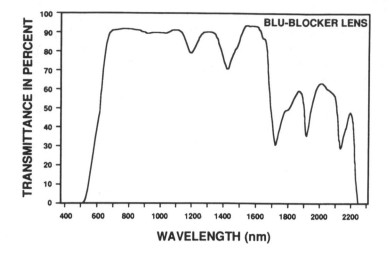

FIGURE 11-6
Spectral transmittance for the Blu-Blocker lens. Note the spectral cut-off at about 510 nm, which eliminates all of the blue VIS spectrum and part of the green VIS spectrum, resulting in a reddish-orange appearance of the filter.

difficult problem and may result in traffic light color discrimination losses. These lenses do not fulfill the coloration requirements of Z80.3-1986.

A basic question is, Does the blue portion of the VIS spectrum need to be blocked? Under normal circumstances, the blue portion of the VIS spectrum from the sun is not a hazard to the eye.[75] The effective blue hazard irradiance for solar radiation, air mass 1, is 90.19×10^{-4} W/cm^2, and with a reflectance from the surrounds of 10%, the duration of safe exposure before reaching the 30 J/cm^2 blue hazard damage threshold at 441 nm would be 9.2 h. The 9.2 h would increase to 46 h when 20% transmittance grey sunlenses are worn; therefore, sunlight should not pose a hazard to the eye. Clinical trials are needed to demonstrate if the Blu-Blocker–type lenses are beneficial in protecting the diseased retina from the short wavelength VIS radiation.

11.5 Standards for Sunglasses

A number of publications have set forth the transmittance, refractive, and color requirements for nonprescription sunglasses.[76–79] Suggested standards for general purpose sunglasses and the spectral transmittance properties of eye-protective lenses have been discussed.[80–82] The ANSI Z80.3-1986 Requirements for Nonprescription Sunglasses and Fashion Eyewear provides transmittance, impact resistance, and color requirements for sunglasses.[83]

Davis[36] reviewed the development and rationale of the Z80.3-1986 standard. The standard contains the mathematics and data required to evaluate the ability to recognize a traffic signal when a filter is being used from its spectrophotometric transmittance curve. He reviewed the UVR requirements and demonstrated that if the proper class of sunglasses is worn, protection is adequate when compared to the 1980 American Conference of Industrial Hygienists (ACGIH) recommended tolerance levels. He also claims that protection against UVA and the "blue hazard" risk seems adequate.

Data on spectral transmittance requirements and transmittance curves for nonprescription sunglass lenses,[84,85] sports and occupational tinted lenses,[86] and safety lenses[87] are given here and in Chapter 9. Intraocular lenses, aphakic contact lenses, and contact lenses with UV absorption have not always been available. UV absorption for aphakes is required to provide adequate to the protection retina.[88–90]

11.6 Summary

Sunglasses should serve to protect the eye from excess ambient luminance, to maintain optimum night vision, to eliminate those portions of the optical spectrum that are hazardous to the eye, and to provide normal color vision while maintaining optimum visual performance. To accomplish these goals the ambient luminance from the sun should be about

1400 cd/m^2. A sunlens with a luminous transmittance of about 15% will maintain adequate luminance for most daylight conditions. UVR should be absorbed to 380 nm and IR should be reduced where practical.

References

1. Lauren L. How safe are your sunglasses? Conde Nast Traveler. June 1988; pp 78–81, 145–149.
2. Shades of greatness: Picking the perfect sunglasses. Better Homes and Gardens. June 1988, p 58.
3. Vives JR, Vaughn B. Shades for all seasons. Mariah/Outside. April-May, 1979.
4. Jordan M. Sunglasses for speed. Car & Driver. July 1986, pp 81–91.
5. Drew R. A guide to UV sunglass protection. Optom Manag. Jan 1989, pp 87–90.
6. Runninger J. How to 'prescribe' plano sunwear. Optom Manag. Jan 1981, pp 113–121.
7. Clark BAJ. Polarizing sunglasses and possible eye hazards of transmitted radiation. Am J Optom Arch Am Acad Optom 1969; 46:499–509.
8. Richards OW. Sunglasses for eye protection. Am J Optom Arch Am Acad Optom 1971; 48:197–200.
9. Logan HL. Specification points of brightness. Trans Illum Eng Soc 1939; 4:881–906.
10. Hedbloom EE. Snowscape eye protection. Development of a sunglass for useful vision with comfort from Anartic snowblindness, glare and calorophthalgia. Arch Environ Health 1961; 2:685–704.
11. Clark BAJ. The luminous transmittance factor of sunglasses. Am J Optom Arch Am Acad Optom 1969; 46:362–378.
12. Luria SM. Preferred density of sunglasses. Am J Optom Physiol Opt 1984; 61:397–402.
13. Handbook of Geophysics for Air Force Designers. U.S. Air Force, Air Research and Development Command, Air Force Cambridge Research Center, Massachusetts, 1957.
14. Sliney DH. Physical factors in cataractogenesis. Ambient radiation and temperature. Invest Ophthalmol Vis Sci 1986; 27:781–790.
15. Peckham RH, Harley RD. Reduction in visual acuity due to excessive sunlight. Arch Ophthalmol 1950; 44:625–627.
16. Hecht S, Ross S, Mueller CG. The visibility of lines and squares at high brightnesses. J Opt Soc Am 1947; 37:500–507.
17. Farnsworth D. The luminous transmission factor of sunglasses. Am J Optom Arch Am Acad Optom 1969; 46:362–378.
18. Effect of Bright Sunlight on Subsequent Dark Adaptation, ARL/N.1/84.11/0. Teddington, Middlesex, England, Admiralty Research Laboratory, August 1943.
19. Hecht S, Hendley CD, Ross S, Richmond PN. The effect of exposure to sunlight on night vision. Am J Ophthalmol 1948; 31:1573.
20. Clark B, Johnson ML, Dreher RE. The effect of sunlight on dark adaptation. Am J Ophthalmol 1946; 29:828–836.
21. Kinney JAS. Night vision sensitivity during prolonged restriction from sunlight. J Appl Psychol 1963; 47:65–67.
22. Diamond AL, Gilinsky AS. Luminance Thresholds for the Resolution of Visual Detail During Dark Adaptation Following Different Durations of Light Adaptation. Technical Report 52-257. Wright Air Development Command, Wright-Patterson Air Force Base, Ohio, April 1952.
23. Lowry EM. The effect of hue on dark adaptation. J Opt Soc Am [A] 1943; 33:619–620.
24. De Groot SG, Doge JM, Smith JA. Factors in night vision sensitivity, II. The interrelationships of size, brightness and location. NRL Report No. 234. Washington, DC, Naval Research Laboratory, Sept 14, 1953.
25. Hecht S, Haig C, Wald G. The dark adaptation of retinal fields of different size and location. J Gen Physiol 1935; 19:321–339.
26. Pinson EA. Effect of Altitude on Dark Adaptation. U.S. Army Air Forces, Material Division, Exp Eng Sect, Oct 7, 1941.
27. Sweeney EJ, Kinney JAS, Ryan A. Seasonal changes in scotopic sensitivity. J Opt Soc Am [A] 1960; 50:237–240.
28. Peckham RH, Harley RD. Reduction in visual acuity due to excessive sunlight. Arch Ophthalmol 1950; 44:624–627.
29. Peckham RH, Arner WJ. Visual acuity, contrast and flicker, as measures of retinal sensitivity. J Opt Soc Am [A] 1952; 42:621–625.
30. Peckham RH, Harley RD. The effect of sunglasses in protecting retinal sensitivity. Am J Ophthalmol 1951; 34:1499–1507.
31. Farnsworth D. The effect of colored lenses upon color discrimination. J Opt Soc Am [A] 1946; 36:365–366.
32. Rose HW, Schmidt I. Physiological Effect of Reflective, Colored and Polarizing Ophthalmic Filters, II. Effect of Ophthalmic Filters on Color Vision. Project No. 21-02-040. Report No. 2. U.S. Air Force School of Aviation Medicine, Randolph Field, Texas, March 1950.
33. Polizzotto L. Effects of using an orange filter on the color perception of dichromats. Am J Optom Physiol Opt 1984; 532–537.
34. Hill AR, Stevenson RWW. Long-term adaptation to ophthalmic tinted lenses. Mod Probl Ophthalmol 1976; 17:264–272.
35. Factors to be Considered in the Selection of Smoke, Rose or Neutral Glass to Be Used in the USAF Standard Flying Sunglasses. Aero-Medical Laboratory, MCREXD-690-1D. Air Materiel Command, Wright-Patterson Air Force Base, Ohio, August 1950.

36. Davis JK. The sunglass and its rationale. Optom Vis Sci 1990; 67:414–430.

37. Phillips RA, Kondig W. Recognition of traffic signals viewed through colored filters. J Opt Soc Am [A] 1975; 65:1106–1113.

38. Cole BL, Brown R. Optimum intensity of red traffic signal lights for normal and protanopic observers. J Opt Soc Am [A] 1966; 56:516–522.

39. Clark BAJ. Effects of tinted ophthalmic media on the detection and recognition of red signal lights. Aerospace Med 1968; 39:1198–1205.

40. Maxwell JC. Experiments on color, as perceived by the eye. Trans Roy Soc Edinburgh 1885; 21:275–298.

41. Schmidt I. Visual aids for correction of red-green color deficiencies. Can J Optom 1976; 38:38–47.

42. Richer S, Adams AJ. Development of qualitative tools for filter-aided dichromats. Am J Optom Physiol Opt 1984; 61:246–255.

43. Sheedy JE, Stocker EG. Surrogate color vision by luster discrimination. Am J Optom Physiol Optics 1984; 61:499–505.

44. Wilson JA, Robinson JO. Binocular filters as an aid to color discrimination by dichromats. Am J Optom Physiol Opt 1980; 57:893–901.

45. Zeltzer HI. A typical case study correcting color deficiency. J Am Optom Assoc 1975; 46:622–626.

46. Zeltzer HI. The X-chrom contact lens and color deficiency. Opt J Rev Optom 1973; 110:15–19.

47. Richer S, Adams AJ. An experimental test of filter-aided dichromatic color discrimination. Am J Optom Physiol Opt 1984; 61:256–264.

48. Richer SP, Adams AJ, Little AC. Toward the design of an optimal filter for enhancement of dichromat monocular chromatic discrimination. J Am Optom Physiol Opt 1985; 105–110.

49. Blackwell HR. Visual detection at a low luminance through optical filters. Highway Research Board Bull 1954; 89:34.

50. Blackwell HR. The Influence of Yellow-Tinted Glasses on Visibility at Low Luminance. Minutes and Proceedings of the Thirty-first Meeting of the Armed Forces NRC-Committee on Vision, pp 302–311. Wright-Patterson Air Force Base, Ohio, Nov 20–22, 1952.

51. Haber H. Safety hazard of tinted automobile windshields at night. J Opt Soc Am [A] 1955; 45:413–419.

52. Miles PW. Alleged effects of tinted lenses to aid vision in night driving by reducing ultraviolet light. Am J Ophthalmol 1953; 36:404–405.

53. Clark BAJ. Vision loss from windshield tinting in a night visual flying accident. Aerospace Med 1971; 42:190–195.

54. Clark BAJ. Color in sunglasses. Am J Optom Arch Am Acad Optom 1969; 46:825–840.

55. Bierman EO. Tinted lenses in shooting. Am J Ophthalmol 1952; 35:859–860.

56. Kelly SA, Goldberg SE, Banton TA. Effect of yellow-tinted lenses on contrast sensitivity. Am J Optom Physiol Opt 1984; 61:657–662.

57. Yap M. The effect of a yellow filter on contrast sensitivity. Ophthal Physiol Opt 1984; 4:227–232.

58. Pokorny J, Graham CH, Lanson RN. Effect of wavelength on foveal grating acuity. J Opt Soc Am [A] 1968; 58:1410–1414.

59. Kinney JAS, Schlichting CL, Neri DF, Kindness SW. Reaction time to spatial frequencies using yellow and luminance-matched neutral goggles. Am J Optom Physiol Opt 1983; 60:132–138.

60. Kelly SA. Effect of yellow-tinted lenses on brightness. J Opt Soc Am [A] 1990; 7:1905–1911.

61. Graham CH, Hsia Y. Saturation and foveal achromatic interval. J Opt Soc Am [A] 1969; 59:993–997.

62. Corth R. The perception of depth contours with yellow goggles—An alternative explanation. Perception 1985; 14:377–378.

63. Kinney JAS, Luria SM, Schlichting CL, Neri DF. The perception of depth contours with yellow goggles. Perception 1983; 12:363–366.

64. Kinney JAS. The perception of depth contours with yellow goggles—comments on letter by Richard Corth. Perception 1985; 14:378–379.

65. Troscianko T. Snowhole blues: Comments on Kinney and Corth. Perception 1986; 15:219–221.

66. Bohren CF. Colors of snow, frozen waterfalls, and icebergs. J Opt Soc Am [A] 1983; 73:1646–1652.

67. Corning CPF lenses were first to filter blue light precisely, while providing photochromic comfort. Corning OPM-39-10M-12/85 IMP. Corning, NY, 1985.

68. Megla GK. Selectively absorbing glasses for the potential prevention of ocular disorders. Appl Opt 1983; 22:1216–1220.

69. Morrissette DL, Mehr EB, Keswick CW. Users' and non-users' evaluations of the CPF 550 lenses. Am J Optom Physiol Optics 1984; 61:704–710.

70. Barron C, Waiss B. An evaluation of visual acuity with Corning CPF527 lens. J Am Optom Assoc 1987; 58:50–54.

71. Lynch DM, Brilliant R. An evaluation of the Corning CPF 550 lens. Optom Monogr 1984; 75:36–42.

72. Thomas SR, Kuyk TK. D-15 performance with short wavelength absorbing filters in normals. Am J Optom Physiol Opt 1988; 65:697–702.

73. Hovis JK, Lovasik JV, Cullen AP. Physical characteristics and perceptual effects of "blue-blocking" lenses. Optom Vis Sci 1989; 66:682–689.

74. Kuyk TK, Thomas SR. Effect of short wavelength absorbing filters on Farnsworth-Munsell 100 hue test and hue identification task performance. Optom Vis Sci 1990; 67:522–531.

75. Sunglasses. Consumer Reports. August 1988; pp 504–509.

76. Requirements for General Purpose Sunglasses for Over-the-Counter Sale. Report 52-6. U.S. Navy Medical Research Laboratory, New London, Connecticut, 1956.

77. Garner LF. A guide to the selection of ophthalmic tinted lenses. Aust J Optom 1974; 57:346–350.

78. Miller D. Effect of sunglasses on the visual mechanism. Surv Ophthalmol 1974; 19:38–44.

79. Clark BAJ. A survey of optical properties of sunglasses. Aust J Optom 1968; 51:150–162.

80. Farnsworth D. Standards for General Purpose Sunglasses. Color Vision Report No. 17. U.S. Navy Medical Research Laboratory, New London, Connecticut, 1948.

81. Farnsworth D. Standards for sunglasses. Sight Saving Review 1950; 20:81–87.

82. Stair R. Spectral-transmissive properties and use of eye-protective glasses. Circular 471. Washington, DC, National Bureau of Standards, 1948.

83. American National Standards Institute. ANSI Z80.3-1986, Requirements for Nonprescription Sunglasses and Fashion Eyewear. New York, American National Standards Institute, 1986.

84. Chou BR, Cullen AP. Spectral transmittance of selected tinted ophthalmic lenses. Can J Optom 1983; 45:192–198.

85. Chou BR, Cullen AP. Optical radiation protection by nonprescription sunglasses. Can J Optom 1986; 48:17–23.

86. Chou BR, Cullen AP. Spectral characteristics of sports and occupational tinted lenses. Can J Optom 1985; 47:77–112.

87. Cotnam MP, Chou BR, Cullen AP. Optical protection factors of selected safety lenses. Occupational Health in Ontario 1988; 9:197–207.

88. Thoms M, Fishman GA, Meulen DV. Spectral transmission characteristics of intraocular and aphakic contact lenses. Arch Ophthalmol 1983; 101:92–93.

89. Bruce AS, Dain SJ, Holden BA. Spectral transmittance of tinted hydrogel contact lenses. Am J Optom Physiol Opt 1986; 63:941–947.

90. Werner JS, Spillmann L. UV-absorbing intraocular lenses: Safety, efficacy, and consequences for the cataract patient. Graefes Arch Clin Exp Ophthalmol 1989; 227:248–256.

CHAPTER TWELVE

Contact Lenses in the Work Environment

Anthony P. Cullen, O.D., Ph.D.

Much of the controversy concerning the use of contact lenses in the workplace has been generated by a few inaccurately and inappropriately cited anecdotes. Although these have been investigated and refuted, restrictive policies have been introduced in many industries with limited enforcement and probably even less compliance by the workers. To expect compliance would be naive when the majority of recent epidemiologic and scientific research efforts, as well as the worker's own experience, fail to support these policies. A survey conducted by the National Safety Council(US) in conjunction with its Industrial Division's Chemical Section Executive Committee revealed that only 53% of members replying had formal policies concerning contact lenses in their companies.[1] The variability of policies from one company to the next emphasizes the arbitrary manner in which contact lens policies are generated and enforced.

Contact lenses are prosthetic devices that offer a number of advantages over spectacle lenses for many occupations, including

- Improved performance in rain or mist
- Fewer broken or lost spectacles
- No fogging with changing temperatures or humidity
- Elimination of spectacle lens reflection

12.1. Material contained in this Chapter was previously published in Bennett ES, Weissman BA: Clinical Contact Lens Practice, Philadelphia, J.B. Lippincott, 1991.

- No mechanical interference with instruments such as microscopes
- Elimination of the broken spectacle lens hazard
- No spectacle lens greasing or smearing or dust accumulation when tasks are performed in unclean environments
- Reduction of perspiration problems
- Increases compatibility with gas masks and other safety equipment
- Increased visual field
- No "jack-in-the-box" effect
- No ring scotomata
- Improved visual acuity in some cases, e.g., high myopes/keratoconics
- Reduced cost and easier repair of plano safety lenses

In a study of police officers, it was found that 52% who routinely wore prescription spectacles while on duty had had their glasses dislodged while performing police duties,[2] whereas fewer of those who wore contact lenses on duty had their lenses dislodged: hard lens wearers, 31%; RGP, 10.5%, and hydrogel, 19%. It was also noted that 56% needed to remove their glasses in order to see due to fogging and rain or snow, respectively, whereas 56% of hard lens wearers, 58% of RGP wearers, and 47% hydrogel wearers had removed their lenses while on duty because of irritation due to such environmental factors as dust, smoke, or wind. Extended wear contact lenses have been found to be ideal for firefighters.[3] All subjects in this study commented that the self-contained breathing apparatus was much easier to use while they were wearing the contact lenses.

The increasing numbers of successful contact lens wearers wish to wear their lenses constantly in all aspects of their lives, including the workplace. Occupational health and safety personnel find themselves in a dilemma due to conflicting and sometimes controversial information circulated by various agencies concerning the advisability of contact lens wear in the workplace. Contact lenses add a complicating factor to eye safety considerations. When contact lens wear policy in particular environments is the responsibility of those with little knowledge of how that wear may affect the level of risk for eye injury or how contact lens removal may adversely affect the wearer, then policies may be unreasonable and discriminatory.

12.1 Potential Hazards and Contact Lens Wear

In risk management it is necessary to balance risk with benefits and to differentiate a perceived risk from the actual risk. Obsessive and unrealistic risk avoidance with its accompanying overregulation and bans may reduce quality of life and productivity while contributing little to safety. Because both contact lenses and certain environments or situations may produce adverse ocular effects, it is tempting to assume that a contact lens wearer is at greater risk in a hazardous environment because of presumed additive or synergistic effects. A simplistic approach has been to ban contact lenses in any situation in which there is a perceived or actual risk to the eye without regard to all factors involved.

There are many reasons why individuals choose not to remove their contact lenses in the workplace or in an environment perceived to contraindicate contact lens wear (Table 12-1). These may be optical, therapeutic, hygienic, or cosmetic, or it may be simply that they do not accept or recognize the potential risk.

Optical	Cosmetic
No alternate spectacle correction	Prosthesis
Spectacle blur with long-term wear of PMMA lenses	Cosmetic shells
	Scars
Oblique astigmatism	**Hygiene**
Irregular astigmatism	No access to clean facilities
Change in depth perception	No care
	No solutions
Change in spatial adaptation	**Other**
Therapeutic	Rigid adherence to wearing schedule
Albinism	Lens used to aid color discrimination
Anirida	Unable to remove lens due to poor instruction
Aphakia—monocular and binocular	Ignorance of hazard
Keratoconus	
Nystagmus	
Bandage lens	
Ptosis	

TABLE 12-1
Reasons Why Contact Lens Wearers Choose Not to Remove Their Lenses Temporarily in a Hazardous Environment

When considering the advisability of wearing contact lenses in a given work environment, a number of questions must be addressed:

1. Is there an actual ocular hazard?
2. Does the wearing of a contact lens place the eye at greater risk than a naked eye?
3. Does the removal of a contact lens increase the risk to the eye or increase its susceptibility to insult?
4. Is the risk different for various contact lens designs and materials?
5. Are there associated risks for the contact lens wearer who removes lenses?
6. Do contact lenses decrease other safety strategies?

If a potential hazard in wearing contact lenses in a specific workplace is identified, it is essential to consider the effects of the various risk factors encountered, both on the eye and on the individual who is not wearing contact lenses. Once these are determined, the situation may be evaluated theoretically using the known physical parameters and physiologic effects of the contact lens. There may or may not be laboratory studies, epidemiologic data, or well-documented case reports to support or refute the theoretical conclusions.

Ocular hazards are greater in some occupations than others. Clearly, optometrists and ophthalmologists who prescribe contact lenses for industrial workers should be concerned as to the advisability of wearing the lenses in a given environment. The type of work involved may influence the selection of lens type. In making the decision *if* and *what* to prescribe, an expansion of the case history may be useful in determining

- Toxic chemicals and physical agents that may be encountered
- Raw material and by-products involved
- Potential for exposure
- Protective equipment available and used
- Other protective measures available
- Hygiene facilities available
- Presence or absence of health personnel
- Factors that may influence compliance with cleaning and wearing schedules

When an incident involving contact lens wear is assessed, the pitfall is to assume that because the victim was wearing contact lenses, they were the causative or a contributive factor. For objectivity, it is essential to be familiar with the signs of trauma and/or toxicity, the mechanisms by which they occur, and the divers alternatives to the claimed cause of the injury or toxic response. It is important to obtain a copy of the original report as well, preferably with any clinical records that may be available. There is a tendency for terms such as "presumed," "perhaps," "possibly," and "maybe" to be lost in the recounting. Knowing the response of the noncontact lens wearer when exposed to similar circumstances also would be of value, as would access to materials that provide physical, chemical, toxicologic, and other data pertinent to the actual or perceived environmental hazard. Additionally, because the signs and symptoms may be unrelated to either the circumstances described or to contact lens wear, a knowledge of other possible causes of the general and ocular responses described is essential. If we are not willing to evaluate carefully a particular patient with a problem with contact lenses in a particular work situation, it would be better for all concerned for the response to the question, "Could it be due to my work?" to be, "I don't know," rather than a vague, "Possibly."

12.2 Chemical Hazards

There is a perception that chemicals may become trapped behind hard contact lenses or may be absorbed, concentrated, and released by hydrogel contact lenses onto an already compromised cornea. Some safety bulletins actually claim, without providing documented evidence in support of their assertions, that contact lenses cause worse than normal burns from chemicals by holding the agent against the eye. In addition, it has been suggested that the presence of a lens in the eye would prevent adequate irrigation following a chemical injury. The basis for this appears to be a case report by Hedwig Kuhn (cited in Novak and Saul[4] without a reference) in which a process engineer was conducting an experiment in an eye-hazard area wearing both contact lenses and safety goggles. An unidentified 50% caustic substance splashed into his "eyes and face." The emergency bath was reported to have flushed the chemical from his face and partially from his eyes. It was claimed that some of the chemical pooled beneath the contact lens, causing "severe burns of the eye" before the contact lenses could be removed. The possibility of such an occurrence in a person wearing safety goggles is highly questionable, yet cases such as this form the basis for claims that contact lenses have no place in any chemical laboratory.

Fumes and Vapors

Some noxious gases, vapors, fumes, aerosols, and smoke have the ability to seep behind inappropriate protective devices and directly affect the outer coats of the eye. The ocular response, as with other types of chemical injury, varies with the concentration and the physical and chemical properties of the agent. Highly toxic substances stimulate the protective mechanisms of blepharospasm and lacrimation, which limit access to the eye and dilute the concentration of the chemical, respectively. Avoidance may be initiated by a characteristic odor or stimulation of other parts of the respiratory tract. Insidious long-term exposure may produce a chronic conjunctivitis, possibly with a mild superficial keratitis, and it is unlikely that individuals subjected to such environments would wear contact lenses comfortably or even have them prescribed. A number of chemicals that are inert to ocular tissues may act as lacrimogens while producing little or no detectable changes in the cornea or conjunctiva. Other vapors may produce a delayed response that manifests several hours after a symptomless exposure; the clinical signs include loss of epithelial cells, edema, and epithelial vacuoles. The ocular nasolacrimal route is insignificant relative to the respiratory route when considering systemic absorption of airborne-toxins.

Many hydrogel contact lens wearers have reported that they are able to peel onions without the usual excessive tearing, thus demonstrating protection by the lenses against the lacrimonogenic actions of the allyl disulfides present in onions. Tear gases also tend to be insoluble in water, and hydrogel contact lenses have been found to be effective in protecting the eye from the tear gas CS (ortho chlorobenzylidine malonitrile).[5] Kok-van Alphen et al,[6] reported, following their studies of the protection provided by soft lenses against tear gas, that the Dutch Police (who are no longer required to wear gas masks) permitted the wearing of hydrogel contact lenses during action with tear gas involvement.

It is improbable that the corneal response to volatile substances would be affected significantly by the wearing of a rigid contact lens, because these substances would be eliminated rapidly by tear flow; however, water-soluble gases and fumes and substances capable of binding to or being absorbed into hydrogel lens materials would be expected to produce prolonged exposure with the resulting more severe or chronic response. This view is supported by Dennis et al,[7] who have demonstrated that a hydrogel lens acts as a reservoir for chemical agents for about 1 hour and then may act as a sink, prolonging corneal exposure after the original risk had abated.

The uptake by high plus hydrogel lenses of trichlorethylene and xylene when suspended in 640 ppm and 700 ppm, respectively, was found to be up to 90 times the uptake of physiologic saline.[8] The release of the solvents into simulated tears was far less than the release into the air, however. It was concluded that the absorption of these solvents by hydrogel contact lenses is not as dangerous as previously thought and that the "vacuum cleaner" effect of the lenses would result in a lower concentration at the corneal surface than if exposed directly.

The effects of isopropanol and ethanol vapor, at the maximum levels recommended by the ACGIH, on 38% water content HEMA lenses has been studied.[9] From the results it was extrapolated that these two vapors could pass through or bind to the contact lens surface to be released later into the tear film. This was not confirmed *in situ*. It was suggested that workers should "take care" when wearing hydrophilic contact lenses in such environments.

It has been found in human subjects wearing "impermeable" contact lenses that exposure to 50 ppm of sulfur dioxide (SO_2) produced no significant change in the level of tear production, whereas the production in unshielded control subjects increased by 83%.[10] It was re-emphasized that, while the results did not contraindicate the wearing of contact lenses in certain occupations, the necessity for stringent restrictions is less important if protective eyewear is worn.

Oily mist in the air can be adsorbed onto hydrogel contact lenses, causing them permanent damage, but it can be washed off hard lenses.[11] Actual chemical reaction of fumes with contact lens does not appear to be a major problem. One case has been reported of an operating room nurse exposed to methylmethacrylate polymerization materials while wearing hydrogel contact lenses who experienced discomfort and watering that necessitated the removal of her lenses.[12] Some time after removal, the lenses had become hard, and one was so brittle that it cracked; it was assumed that the lenses had undergone a "chemical reaction." No mention was made of whether or not the lenses were placed in solution or left to dry out. Of more importance in this report is the fact that the discomfort, presumably caused by the fumes, forced the nurse to remove her lenses, and no injury was suffered. Similarly, contact-lens-wearing beauticians and hairdressers, when exposed to ammonia fumes and hairsprays that may adhere to the surface of a contact lens, will discontinue lens wear if ocular irritation occurs.

Chemical Splash

The accidental splashing of toxic chemicals into the eye is one of the most frequent causes of serious eye injury in the workplace and in other environments. In 1966 Wesley[13] studied the effect of corrosive substances on eyes wearing PMMA lenses. The technique involved spraying and squirting 0.25 mL of varying percentages of sulfuric acid (H_2SO_4), sodium hydroxide (NaOH), and creosol into the eyes of rabbits. The animals had been injected with an analgesic that spared the protective reflexes in order to permit protection by blinking. The results indicated that an eye without a contact lens was 1.8 times more likely to suffer total corneal opacity than an eye with a contact lens and that the eye with a contact lens is more likely to be damaged if the lens is dislodged during the splash or subsequent irrigation. Similar protection by PMMA lenses against splashed 5% acetic acid, 0.5% n-butylamine, and 50% acetone was reported by Guthrie and Seitz.[14] They found that the chemicals were not trapped behind the lenses but rather the blepharospasm induced by the chemical irritation acted to tighten the lens against the cornea, creating a "barrier" effect.

The effect of strong alkalis and acids on the corneas of anesthetized rabbits wearing hydrogel contact lenses has been evaluated.[15] Neither type of hydrogel lens used provided any protection against 20% or 40% NaOH, nor did this worsen the condition. Leaving the lens on the eye for a minute or two did not make any significant difference. The protection provided by high plus lenses against the effects

of 20% and 40% hydrochloric acid (HCl) was definite, reducing the corneal damage to about 75%. A case has been reported in which splashed boiling acid from a test tube produced a punctate burn on the cheek and presumably "pit-marked" a corneal lens with no effects on the cornea.[16]

These results do not suggest that contact lenses may be used as a substitute for protective eyewear where there is a chemical hazard, but they do emphasize that a contact lens wearer with appropriate protection is at no greater risk than a non–contact-lens-wearing colleague. It is also essential that workers in such situations be reminded that even the most seemingly trivial eye injury has the potential for disastrous results and that emergency procedures must be followed. An unfortunate incident has been reported in which a worker did not irrigate his eyes after a chemical splash for fear of losing his contact lenses.[17]

12.3 Mechanical Hazards

Mechanical injuries to the eye result from contusion and concussion, foreign bodies (which may be superficial or perforating), exposure to atmospheric dust and particles, and wounds (which include abrasions, cuts, and lacerations). These may occur as isolated incidents or in combination.

It is reasonable to speculate that a haptic (scleral) contact lens would provide considerable protection from both contusion and concussion injury, whereas a thin high-water-content hydrogel lens would offer little protection. There are numerous cases in the literature describing the protection from blunt trauma provided by contact lenses.

Foreign Bodies

A superficial corneal foreign body is one of the most common minor ocular injuries. The symptoms of pain, foreign body sensation, and lacrimation are readily alleviated by simple removal of the offending particle. If a foreign body of suitable size, shape, and velocity impinges on the eye, it may penetrate into the cornea or sclera or actually perforate the globe. The protection of the cornea by a contact lens would depend on the thickness and rigidity of the lens.

Whereas foreign bodies may be trapped beneath rigid lenses, this rarely happens with hydrogel lenses unless the speck is inserted with the lens.

Nilsson et al[18] exposed the eyes of anesthetized contact-lens-wearing rabbits to showers of burning grit particles. They found that all particles rebounded from the surface of hard lenses, effectively protecting the covered part of the cornea. High- and low-water-content hydrogel lenses also offered some protection, but the lenses themselves were severely damaged. An occasional particle perforated a hydrogel lens to damage the epithelium superficially. Because their study simulated the use of a grinding wheel, the operation of which is usually brief, the researchers felt that with normal eye protection, the use of contact lenses hardly involved any additional risk; indeed, the wearing of contact lenses under these conditions provided additional protection for the cornea. We have confirmed that both rigid and hydrogel lenses provide protection from airborne metal particles (Fig. 12-1). In order to approximate the condition of an eye hit by a larger sharp projec-

tile, Nilsson et al[18] fired a 22-mm long, 1-mm diameter metal projectile from an air gun. Their results for high-water-content lenses confirmed the opinion of Highgate[19] that a hydrogel lens offers little protection. Surprisingly, low-water-content lenses significantly increased the energy required for corneal perforation (32 mJ compared with 21 mJ for an eye without a contact lens). Hard lenses shattered when energy levels reached 8.3 mJ, with splinters of plastic entering the cornea, thereby introducing a complicating factor.

A case where a corneal lens patient was attempting to reduce the length of a screw using a hammer and chisel has also been described.[20] The screw broke and flew into his right eye. The lens was badly fractured, but the eye sustained only a slight central abrasion; had the lens not been present, the eye probably would have been perforated. In a similar accident, when an aircraft riveter was struck in the eye with a rivet, the lens was gouged but there was no damage to the eye.[21]

Atmospheric Particles

Subjects wearing hydrogel contact lenses who worked in an environment moderately contaminated with metal particles and oil droplets were followed for a period of two years.[22] At no time were there any signs of damage to the eye, and there were no subjective complaints. It is evident that hydrogel contact lenses can be worn safely in environments that may appear hazardous on cursory inspection and that may contraindicate the use of hard lenses.

Abrasions and Lacerations

The presence of a contact lens can be expected to provide some protection against abrasion and lacerations, depending upon the direction of the offending impact, with a hydrogel lens offering less resistance to a sharp object. A road traffic accident has been described that resulted in an incision by broken windshield across the brow and cheek.[23] Corneal lenses were removed in the emergency department. It was speculated that spectacles would have increased the risk to the eye in this case.

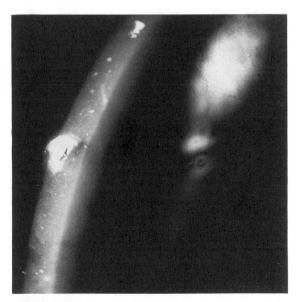

FIGURE 12-1
An airborne metal foreign body embedded in a hydrogel contact lens. The underlying porcine cornea was undamaged. *Photo courtesy of* **Karen Ritzman, University of Waterloo School of Optometry.**

12.4 Physical Hazards

The range of hazards that are neither chemical nor mechanical is wide, including those due to temperature, ionizing and nonionizing radiation, and stress.

Hyperthermia

It is evident that no type of contact lens would have a significant effect on the severity of high temperature burns; haptic or hydrogel lenses may offer slight protection to the critical limbal region in moderate burns. The air temperature in a sauna may rise as high as 80 to 100 C without affecting contact lens wear.[24] If the sauna is the dry type, evaporation of the tear film and drying of hydrogel contact lenses may be partially avoided by increasing the blink rate.

Hypothermia

There is an anecdotal report that Zeiss contact lenses (glass) used by German pilots during World War I did not become iced.[25] A Royal Air Force test pilot, exposed to wind and a temperature of − 20 C noticed no visual impairment when wearing haptic contact lenses. Modern contact lenses, which are much thinner and in closer proximity to the cornea, would be expected to provide less protection than sealed haptic lenses. Socks[26] fitted rabbits with hard (PMMA) contact lenses and exposed them to temperatures of − 28.9 C with winds up to 125 km/h (78 mph) for 3-h periods. He found no effects of cold on contact lenses in 85% of the eyes, and the remainder showed only a mild keratitis, which cleared within a few hours. No histologic abnormalities attributable to the cold were detected. It was concluded that rabbits wearing contact lenses in extreme cold suffered no acute deleterious effects to the eye and that contact lenses may be acceptable in and even offer protection from wind-driven ice and snow in cold environments.

Radiation

The absorption characteristics of a contact lens will determine whether the lens will provide any protection against a particular form of radiation. These characteristics have been thoroughly examined for the optical wavebands,[27–30] and it has been assumed that contact lens materials are radiotransparent outside of these and immediately adjacent (extra high frequency [EHF] and soft X-ray) bands. There is no scientific rationale to support the notion that a contact lens is capable of concentrating any waveband of electromagnetic radiation (EMR) onto the cornea.[31]

IR

Infrared (IR) heaters used in the automobile and other industries for drying paint produce very little or no visible light. It has been found that the unanesthetized eye of a conscious rabbit shut or partially closed when exposed to an IR heater.[32] If the eye was kept open, the temperature of the corneal surface rose to approximately 44 C, whether or not a soft HEMA-type lens was worn. In experiments in which the eyes were kept open, it was found that the lenses dried completely, became deformed, and fell from the eye. We have observed the same phenomenon. No epithelial lesions resulted in contact lens wearers from exposure to the IR heater. In other studies involving welding arcs,[33] similar results were found; complete protection from this effect was provided by the use of an appropriate welding filter.

Welders and other workers in environments rich in IR (and ultraviolet radiation [UVR]) are often exposed to arcs while not using protective equipment. If hydrogel contact lenses are worn, they dry and become more adherent to the cornea. Instillation of a few drops of wetting solution will accelerate rehydration. This must occur before any attempt is made to remove the lenses.

VIS LIGHT

Contact lens wearers frequently complain of increased photophobia when wearing their lenses. The reasons for this are evasive. The light incident on the cornea can be calculated, using Fesnel's equation, to be approximately 8% higher than with spectacle lenses. This increase is insignificant when the dynamics of retinal adaptations are considered, and it is unlikely to be the causative factor. Most contact lens wearers suffer from a slight increase in corneal thickness, presumably due to edema. Is this edema sufficient to create enough scatter to degrade the retinal image sufficiently to produce veiling glare? Contrast sensitivity function studies are inconclusive.[34–41] Dumbleton and Cullen[42] found no significant differences in contrast sensitivity among spectacle lens wearers, UV-absorbing, and non–UV-absorbing contact lens wearers under laboratory conditions. Subjects wearing UV-absorbing lenses reported a significant (p < 0.05) increase in visual comfort and a decrease in glare from snow on sunny days, however. This suggests that when the ratio of ambient UVA to visible (VIS) spectrum light is high, ocular lenticular fluorescence will be sufficient to produce veiling glare and photophobia.

UVR

The need to protect ocular tissues from excessive exposure to UV using appropriate ophthalmic and industrial absorptive glass and plastic materials is generally accepted and well understood.[43-45] The recurrent warning of the hazard of wearing contact lenses in the workplace prompted evaluation of the absorptive properties of contact lenses,[27,28,31] and it was found that most contact lens materials provided little protection from UV. In recent years, a number of rigid and hydrogel contact lenses have been released that offer various levels of protection from UV according to the absorption characteristics of the incorporated UV absorber and the thickness of the lens.[46] Chou et al[46] derived protection factors for a number of UV-absorbing contact lenses that exhibited transmittance windows within the UV spectrum.

It has been shown empirically that when a hydrogel contact lens, which absorbed all incident radiation of the experimental waveband, was placed on the eye, it provided complete protection of the cornea.[47] These clinical findings were confirmed histologically.[48] Cullen et al[49] confirmed that the optical absorption characteristics of a given lens, and the related protection factors, may be used to predict the protection offered by a given lens. They also found that UV-transmitting hydrogel lens increased the UVB threshold of the rabbit cornea minimally, but at suprathreshold radiant exposures there was no difference in the clinical response between a cornea wearing the lens and one without a lens. This strongly suggests that an individual who is accidentally exposed to UV while wearing hydrogel contact lenses is at no greater risk than the non–contact lens wearer. Evaluation of the protection afforded by a UV-absorbing RGP lens revealed that the area of the cornea covered by the lens during irradiation was spared, whereas the exposed areas of the cornea and conjunctiva were damaged (Fig. 12-2).[50]

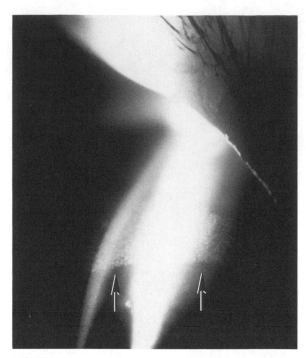

FIGURE 12.2
A cornea exposed to suprathreshold levels of UVB while wearing a UV-absorbing RGP contact lens. A clear arc of demarcation (*arrows*) indicates the position of the edge of the lens during irradiation. The unprotected superior cornea is hazy, and the epithelium contains large coalescing granules.

A dramatic difference in the nature of the response to UVB between eyes adapted to RGP lenses and control eyes has been demonstrated.[51] The adapted eyes showed less superficial damage and more "granules." It was argued that as adapted eyes lost fragile superficial squamous epithelial cells,[52,53] the deeper wing cells were subjected to more radiant exposure. It was also found that corneal swelling was less following irradiation in eyes that had been wearing contact lenses. Despite these differences the rates of recovery and recovery times were similar for both groups, suggesting that a worker exposed to UV irradiation after removing contact lenses would be incapacitated no longer than a similarly exposed noncontact lens wearer.

MW RADIATION

The principal effects of microwaves (MWs) on ocular tissues *in situ* are vibrational and rotational at the molecular level, thereby producing a thermal response. Distribution and absorption of microwave radiation is dependent on its wavelength, the size and shape of the total structure (or subject), and the chemical nature of the tissue irradiated. EHF and super high frequency (SHF) produce superficial injury to the cornea and adnexa, and even ultrahigh frequency (UHF) damage is confined to the anterior segment. No MW damage to the eye has been reported in workers wearing contact lenses. One may reasonably speculate that the superficial heating effect on high-water-content contact lenses would result in drying similar to that produced by IR. Also, theoretic considerations negate the possibility of MWs welding a contact lens to the cornea or selectively evaporating the precorneal/sublens tear layer.

LASERS

Elkington and Watts[54] demonstrated that the transmittance of laser light by ocular media corresponds to the transmittance of incoherent light of the same wavelength. Thus transmittance (absorptance) studies of the human eye may be used to predict the action of a laser on a given ocular tissue, or if it will even reach the structure. Similarly, the absorptance data for contact lenses may be employed to determine whether a given lens contributes to eye protection.

The high absorption by the anterior corneal structure of UV shorter than 290 nm and IR beyond 1400 nm results in lasers of sufficient power (e.g., excimers, CO and CO_2) photoablating or burning the cornea. YAG and argon lasers have the ability to damage intraocular structures, intentionally or unintentionally. Argon, krypton, HeNe, and ruby laser light will reach the retina, and some are used for laser coagulation of the retina and other structures. Intraocular lenses (IOLs) have been damaged during laser capsulotomy. Most contact lens materials will absorb some incident excimer, CO, or CO_2 laser radiation, but the power would probably disintegrate the lens.

IONIZING RADIATION

Soft X-rays and α-particles have low penetrance, producing damage to the superficial corneal and conjunctival epithelia with associated hypoesthesia, hyperemia, and edema similar to the response to UVC but with a longer latent period. Any contact lens would provide some protection against such ir-

radiation and also against low energy β-radiation.

Higher energy β-radiation may damage corneal epithelium and endothelium, resulting in corneal edema. This radiation requires more than 1 cm of Lucite* or 1.5 mm of lead for protection. The presence of a contact lens on the eye would not influence the ionizing response. Therapeutic gamma rays and X-rays used in and around the eye require appropriate protection for the lens; this may be in the form of a lead haptic lens or a molded shell with a lead button glued to the front surface. Although at 25 keV only 1-mm thickness of lead is adequate, a button of 5 mm is usually employed.

ULTRASOUND

Clinical ophthalmic ultrasound, in the frequency range of 8 to 10 MHz, produces a power level of approximately 5 mW cm^{-2}; the presence of a contact lens on the eye will affect the ultrasonogram in accordance with the acoustic impedance and absorption of the lens material. No increased risk is created. There have been no reports of corneal damage resulting from airborne ultrasound.[55]

Barometric Pressure

The interest in the effects of hypobaric, hyperbaric, and rapidly changing atmospheric pressure environments has increased with the desire of many to wear their contact lenses at high altitudes, when flying, and during a variety of underwater activities.

It has been suggested that the reason for discomfort among some contact-lens-wearing air travelers is due to the effect of low atmospheric pressure resulting in relative hypoxia,[56-58] although the pressure in a modern commercial aircraft corresponds to a modest 2000 to 3000 m of altitude. In decompression chamber experiments Castrén[59] noted corneal changes in hydrogel contact lens wearers that were not observed in control subjects after 3 h. Habitual (haptic type) contact lens wearers have been reported to consistently develop bubbles under their lenses when subjected to simulated altitudes in excess of 5400 m.[60]

Flynn et al[61] and Strath[62] have verified that the physiologic responses of the cornea to hydrogel contact lens wear (e.g., corneal thickening) are greater at

12.2. *Dupont, Wilmington, DE.

high altitudes. Despite this, researchers have concluded that hydrogel contact lenses may be worn while flying military aircraft, thus supporting the 13 y or more of experience of pilots in the Swedish and other air forces.[63]

Five climbers on the British 1975 assault on Mount Everest were fitted with continuous wear hydrogel lenses.[64] Two wore their lenses for over 50 d up to an altitude of 7925 m with no observed corneal problems. The other three reverted to their glasses for reasons other than discomfort or corneal problems. It should be noted that in an avocation such as mountain climbing, the rate of decompression is, of necessity, slow. Conversely, despite adherence to standard decompression schedules, it is not unusual for hard-contact-lens-wearing divers to complain of ocular discomfort, halos, and decreased acuity immediately after decompression. These symptoms may persist for several hours. The effects of decompression on two PMMA-wearing divers exposed to a depth of 45.5 m (150 ft) in a hyperbaric chamber for 30 min has been evaluated.[65] The formation of small bubbles was noted beneath the hard lenses at 21 m (70 ft) en route to the 9 m (30 ft) stop point; these coalesced as the "surface" was approached. No bubbles formed in the precorneal tear film if no contact lenses were worn, if hydrogel lenses were worn, or if the PMMA lenses were fenestrated centrally. The bubbles disappeared after 30 min at sea level, leaving "nummular patches of corneal epithelial edema." These lesions, presumed secondary to the trapping of nitrogen between the epithelium and the hard lens, persisted for up to 2 h. In a subsequent study of the effect of altitude, no bubble formation in an ascent to a simulated 11,277 m (37,000 ft) was noted.[66] At this altitude a few minute bubbles appeared in the tear layer, they did not coalesce, and they disappeared within 10 min without inducing any symptoms.

Similar studies have shown that bubbles also occur under hydrogel lenses and RGP lenses during decompression in a hyperbaric environment.[66–68] The degree of bubble formation and subsequent corneal insult was less than the PMMA lenses. Some subjects reported that the lenses were more comfortable after they reached the bottom and during decompression than on the surface. Socks et al[68] found that no type of lens was displaced during dives and suggested that it is relatively safe for military and sport divers to wear contact lenses in lieu of the cumbersome modifications otherwise necessary to the diving mask.

It has been found that rapid decompression of subjects (2438 m–11,582 m) produced no bubble formation in either hydrogel contact lenses or the cornea.[69] While recognizing the potential hazards for aircrews, it was felt that hydrogel contact lenses would be beneficial to young myopes flying fast jet aircraft. This opinion is supported by the results of a study in which tests were performed at simulated altitudes of 6096 m and 9144 m and used supplementary oxygen.[70] No lenses were dislodged. No bubbles formed in or under the soft lenses. Some subjects did report that their eyes were dry and tired. These findings are contradicted by Castrén et al,[71] who concluded that the additive effect of hypoxia and low atmospheric pressure produced ocular symptoms. Although the latter studies were conducted at a simulated altitude of 4000 m, the hydrogel contact lens subjects suffered from corneal erosions and stromal opacities. It is interesting and perhaps relevant that these experiments were carried out at a relatively high humidity.

It has been concluded that hydrogel lenses were preferable for divers and that they may be used "with care" by experienced divers for sports and commercial diving; due to the potential hazard from *Pseudomonas aeruginosa*, which apparently thrives on the inside walls of pressure chambers, contact lenses should not be permitted for saturation diving.[72]

Vibrational Stress

One can encounter vibrational stress while operating machinery, such as pneumatic drills or chain saws, or while traveling in or on modes of transportation ranging from low capacity motorcycles to aerospace vehicles. Whereas the symptoms associated with low frequency oscillation are usually attributed to vestibular disturbance, more rapid vibration will reduce visual acuity, depending on frequency and compensatory or associated involuntary head and eye movements. Considering the relative stability of a contact lens and its closer proximity to the nodal points of the eye, one might anticipate less visual disturbance for the contact lens wearer than the spectacle lens wearer, especially for higher refractive corrections. In one study, subjects wearing conventional flying spectacles or hydrogel contact lenses were vibrated sinusoidally at frequencies from 2 to 32 Hz.[69] Snellen visual acuity was impaired at 6 and 8 Hz, but no significant difference between the two methods of correction occurred. No contact lens was dislodged during these experiments.

Acceleration Stress

It has been speculated that high gravity (G) forces would cause a contact lens to dislodge from the cornea. In order to evaluate this hypothesis Brennan and Girvin[69] subjected volunteer Royal Air Force (RAF) aircrew wearing two types of hydrogel lenses (50% and 75% water content) to +4 Gz and +6 Gz for 20-s periods. They found that the maximum downward displacement of any lens was only 1.5 mm at +4 Gz and 1.75 mm at +6 Gz; tightly fitted lenses remained central regardless of the G forces. Any reduction in vision during these studies was due to retinal ischemia rather than displacement of the contact lenses. Similar results for RGP lenses have been reported.[73] Positive G forces of +3, +4, +6, and +9 caused all lenses to decenter downward along the z-axis, with a maximum decentration of 2 to 3 mm at the highest G force. Visual acuity was not affected adversely. Jet fighter pilots may be exposed to acceleration forces of up to +12 Gz for brief periods during combat maneuvers, yet hydrogel contact lenses have been worn successfully under these circumstances. Hart[74] speculated that the zero gravity of space flight would have little negative effect on the cornea-contact lens relationship and proposed that continuous wear contact lenses would be suitable for ametropic mission specialists. During long-term flight on Solyut-7 and on the Mir orbital stations, an ametropic crew member wore a hydrogel contact lens for 5-h periods without problems, confirming that contact lenses can be employed during space flight.[75]

Humidity

Based on climatic chamber experiments, Lovsund et al[76] concluded that there are no risks for contact lens users in environments with high relative humidity. They also found no differences in adhesion for either hard or hydrogel lenses among environments with relative humidities of 21% and 97%, respec-

tively. Other studies indicate that temperature and humidity are not important factors for contact lens wearers except in situations in which the environment is very dry.[77,78] An exception is that the comfort and performance of very thin high-water-content contact lenses are susceptible to changes in humidity. This type of lens dries and distorts, thereby contributing to corneal desiccation in conditions of low relative humidity.[79] However, a recent report showed that a new high-water-content (67.5%) lens was not as affected by high altitude and low humidity as other high-water-content lenses.[80] It should not be overlooked that noncontact lens wearers, especially those with dry eye syndromes, also experience increased discomfort under conditions of low humidity.

The optimum humidity range for comfort is between 40% and 60%, and it has been suggested that in air travel, where cabin humidity may drop to 11% within 30 min of takeoff, low humidity is possibly more significant than other environmental factors in contributing to the discomfort of hydrogel contact lenses.[81]

A relationship between discomfort, tear break-up time (BUT), lens deposits, and low relative humidity has been noted.[82] It was concluded that discomfort was more prominent in relative humidity less than 25% or when lens deposits were present in relative humidity of greater than 40%. Subjects with lens deposits and a short BUT on a hydrogel contact lens were particularly sensitive to low relative humidities. Factors that may be responsible for the discomfort include decreased hydration of the surface of the lens, which decreases oxygen transmissibility[83]; an increase in lens deposits; and a tightening of the lens with decreased movement. Useful strategies in improving comfort in dry environments are frequent lens replacement, "loose" fitting techniques, and the use of enzymatic cleaners.[3]

Wind

Wind can be expected to have two effects in the eye, drying and stimulation of tearing. Following a study of military helicopter pilots, it was found that 61% of the subjects experienced a drying effect of direct air currents on their hydrogel contact lenses.[84] Similarly, some firefighters have experienced no drying of their extended wear contact lenses while riding the tailboard at speeds up to 80 km/h, whereas others noticed that their lenses dried out.[3] Wind and other air currents may also exaggerate problems with dust.

12.5 Visual Display Terminals

The visual display terminal (VDT) user who wears contact lenses has less reflections and perhaps less of certain spectacle lens aberrations; these advantages are offset by a number of potential disadvantages. Myopic wearers require a presbyopic addition earlier. Some practitioners are willing to ignore residual refractive errors, especially low levels of astigmatism, despite findings that these may contribute to VDT-user discomfort.[85–89] Similarly, problems of binocularity may be conveniently considered insignificant. VDT tasks requiring concentration may reduce the blink rate, which in turn will reduce lens movement and increase drying effects. In offices where the poor quality of the air is contributing to what is termed the *sick building syndrome* it is logical to anticipate that factors involved, e.g., temperature, relative humidity, air movement, CO_2 levels, and airborne pollutants, would adversely affect contact lens wear.

12.6 Should Contact Lenses Be Banned in the Workplace?

The question of whether or not contact lenses cause a greater risk of more severe ocular trauma in the event of an accident involving the eyes has been posed since contact lenses became available for general use. It is a common misconception that if a patient is injured while wearing contact lenses, the lens will contribute to the extent of the injury. Actually, the evidence confirms that contact lenses in many cases are far safer than spectacles. Over the years surveys of optometrists and ophthalmologists have been conducted by a variety of organizations including the National Eye Research Foundation, the Z-80 Sub-committee on Contact Lenses of the American National Standards Institute (ANSI), and the College and University Safety Council of Ontario. None

of these surveys provide evidence to support the claim that wearing contact lenses increases the risks of eye damage.

When contact lenses are worn, the natural defenses of the periorbital structures are always in effect. When ordinary spectacles are worn, these defenses are rendered less effective by the fact that the spectacles extend beyond the defenses. Any blow to the face is liable to strike the spectacles and break the frame and/or lenses, which may, in turn, injure the eye. This is particularly true of missles flying toward the eye.

There are few well-documented cases in which a contact lens has increased severity of an injury when compared with the numerous instances in which a contact lens provided protection (Table 12-2). This disproportion is supported by laboratory research.

A number of review articles[90–92] and reports[93–102] in addition to those already cited confirm that in most instances contact lenses provide some degree of protection. The extent of the protection is governed by the nature of the injury and the type of contact lens worn.

In 1962, after evaluating employees successfully wearing rigid contact lenses in a heavy industry, Silberstein concluded

(a) That contact lens wearers in industry should not be permitted to work in certain jobs and particular environments that are specifically and peculiarly hazardous to them. (b) That in the field of visual rehabilitation, contact lenses have unique advantages to the industrially employed as well as to others and they can be successfully used in full time unrestricted industrial employment providing administrative, medical and safety supervision is exercised. (c) That contact lens wearers can be employed in a wide variety of industrial positions safely and efficiently provided they are adequately trained in the use of their lenses and they observe normal industrial eye-safety practices.[98]

Since that time, numerous industries, educational authorities, and other organizations have arbitrarily restricted the use of contact lens within their administrative domains. Others are opposed to a universal ban of contact lenses in the workplace.[99] The wearing of eye protection in eye hazardous areas is self-evident, and this should be enforced in accordance with regulations. It has been stated that the answer to industrial eye safety is to enforce safety regulations in

Acetone	Metal clip	Screw
Acid	Metal particles	Screwdriver
Acid fumes	Metal piece	Shell casing
Baton tip	Metal shaving	Ski pole
Bleach	Metal sliver	Solvents
Broomstick	Metal splinter	Squash ball
Bullwhip	Molten slag	Stairs
Cardboard box	Nail	Staple
Caustic soda	Needle	Steel-tipped dart
Cleaning fluid	Orange	Steel pellet
Electric plug	Oven cleaner	Stick
End mill	Paint	Stone
Field hockey stick	Paint fumes	Sulfur vapors
Fingernail	Pea	Sulfuric acid
Fist	Pencil point	Sun visor
Fist with ring	Plastic	Tear gas (CS)
Flame	Plastic comb	Thumb
Flour	Popgun	Tip of fishing pole
Football shoe	Radiator	Toy rocket
Foreign body	contents	Tree
Glass	Rattail comb	Tree limb
Grease	Rear view	Truck wheel
Hair spray	mirror	Ultraviolet
Hot metal	Religious medal	radiation
Hydrochloric acid	(star)	Umbrella rib
Hypothermia	Rivet	Varnish
Kitchen knife	Rope	Varnish remover
Lacrosse stick	Rosin	Wind
Metal buckle	Rugby boot	Windshield glass
Metal chip	Scissors	Wood chip

TABLE 12.2
Eye Hazards against which Contact Lenses Have Provided Protection

the workplace rather than ban indiscriminately the wearing of contact lenses on the job.[100] Energy would be better spent in ensuring that facilities are available at the workplace, that include clean areas with sink, soap, towels, and mirror where workers can wash their hands and remove/replace their lenses. Education and voluntary action tend to be more effective than a regulation that is perceived to be unjustified or unreasonable. The fact that those formulating regulations may be unfamiliar with the nature and performance of contact lenses in different environments is not an indictment of contact lenses; rather it indicates a need for additional education for all involved.

12.7 Contact Lens Emergencies and First Aid

The management of any industrial injury involving contact lenses is enhanced by the existence of proactive policies and operating procedures that involve responsibilities for both employer and employee.

Contact lens wearers in the workplace should ensure that appropriate management and health personnel are aware that they are wearing contact lenses in case emergency removal is required. Contact lenses should be removed by the wearer when the situation warrants. A spare pair of contact lenses, alternate spectacles, and appropriate cleaning solutions should be available on site. Adherence to existing policies governing the wearing of personal protective equipment is presumed.

Health and safety personnel should record on the employee's health record the type of lenses worn (rigid or hydrophilic) and the name, address, and telephone number of the prescribing optometrist. Ocular first aid procedures for the contact lens wearer are essentially the same as those for any similar incident not involving contact lenses. All personnel should be familiar with the procedures likely to be encountered in a given workplace. Emergency removal of contact lenses by other than the wearer is rarely indicated, the exception being when the victim is unconscious and a chemical or other foreign material has entered the eye. Another contact lens wearer is typically the best qualified to carry out this procedure.

Suggested first aid management, by wearer or safety personnel, for emergency and other contact lens–related problems is given in Table 12-3.

12.8 Conclusions

Most authorities have concluded that contact lenses may be worn safely under a variety of environmental situations including those that, from a superficial evaluation, might appear hazardous. Indeed, some types of contact lenses may give added protection to spectacle lens and non–spectacle lens wearers in instances of chemical splash, dust, flying particles, and nonionizing radiation. The evidence also refutes claims that contact lenses negate the protection provided by safety equipment or make the cornea more susceptible to damage by nonionizing radiation, in

Exposure to Fumes or Vapors

Remove lenses for cleaning and rinsing. If no irritation is experienced, the lenses may be reinserted.

Chemical Splash

Copiously irrigate the eye with water while holding the lids apart. Do not worry about losing the contact lens. If the lens remains after initial flushing, remove it or slide it onto the conjunctiva and re-irrigate, then seek emergency professional management. For caustic splash, irrigation should be continued during transportation.

Foreign Bodies

Remove the lens and irrigate the eye if indicated. If the eye remains uncomfortable—if it seems that the foreign body has remained in the eye or vision is blurred, the eye should be examined by an eye care practitioner prior to reinserting lenses. All cases of high speed flying particles should be evaluated professionally.

Dust in Eyes

Remove the contact lenses and irrigate eyes. Clean lenses and reinsert if eyes are not red or uncomfortable, otherwise consult practitioner before reinserting lenses.

Blunt Trauma

Swelling or lacerations may make lens (or pieces of lens) removal difficult. Professional evaluation of whole eye is indicated.

Uncomfortable Lenses, Red or Sore Eyes

Do not wear the lenses. Seek advice from prescribing practitioner.

Adherent Lenses

If due to drying of hydrogel material by hyperthermia, infrared radiation, wind, or low humidity environment, do not attempt to remove the lenses until they have rehydrated. This may be accelerated by appropriate eye drops.

Dry Eyes or Environments

Increase humidity if possible. Request practitioner to prescribe suitable lubricating eye drops.

Exposure to Welding or Other Arc

If protective filters were not in place, remove lenses prior to the onset of photokeratitis. If there are no symptoms, resume contact lens wear in 24 hours; otherwise consult practitioner before wearing lenses again.

Blurred Vision

Remove and clean the lenses. If on reinsertion (ensuring that lenses are in the appropriate eyes) vision remains blurred, consult prescribing practitioner.

Lost Lens(es)

Check that lens is not displaced onto the conjunctiva. If it is, carefully recentre the lens. Check clothing and surrounding floor. If the lens is found, clean and evaluate it for damage. If undamaged, reinsert. If this causes discomfort or if the lens is damaged, consult practitioner.

TABLE 12-3
First Aid for Contact Lens Emergencies and Problems

particular arc flashes.[31,101,102] Thus a universal ban of contact lenses in the workplace or other environments is unwarranted. Regulations limiting the wearing of contact lenses in any given circumstance must be scientifically defensible and effectively enforceable; they should not be based on perceived hazards, random experience, isolated unverified case histories, or unsubstantiated personal opinions.

Conversely, it would be imprudent for a practitioner to prescribe contact lenses in order to circumvent uncorrected visual acuity standards in those occupations in which individuals may be required to function without correction on some occasions or in environments contraindicated for the type of lens prescribed. In conclusion, optometrists and ophthalmologists who prescribe contact lenses ought to be concerned as to the advisability of their patients' wearing lenses in a particular work environment. Practitioners must continue to stress that personal protective equipment, including safety eyewear, is not replaced by contact lenses. Where circumstances create the necessity, eye protection must be worn.

References

1. Nejmeh G, Jr. To keep them in or keep them out, on the job—that is the question. National Safety News 1982; June:58–61.

2. Good GW, Augsberger AR. Uncorrected visual acuity standards for police applicants. J Police Sci Admin 1987; 15:18–23.

3. Kartchner MN. Fight fires with contacts? Contact Lens Forum 1985; 10:13, 21, 23–25, 27–30.

4. Novak JF, Saul RW. Contact lenses in industry. J Occup Med 1971; 13:175–81.

5. Rengstorff RH. The effects of riot control agent CS on visual acuity. Military Medicine 1969; 134:219–221.

6. Kok-van Alphen CC, van der Linden JW, Visser R, Bol AH. Protection of the police against tear gas with soft contact lenses. Military Medicine 1985; 150:451–454.

7. Dennis RJ, Flynn WJ, Oakley CJ, Block MG. Soft Contact Lenses: Sink of Barrier to Chemical Warfare Agents. USAFSAM-TR-89-2. USAF School of Aerospace Medicine, 1989.

8. Nilsson SEG, Andersson L. The use of contact lenses in environments with organic solvents, acids or alkalis. Acta Ophthalmol 1982; 60:599–608.

9. Cerulli L, Tria M, Bacaloni A, Palmieri N. Lenti a contatto idrofile ed inquinamento in ambiente di lavoro. Boll di Oculistce 1985; 64:299–305.

10. Coe JE, Douglas RB. The effect of contact lenses of ocular responses to sulphur dioxide. J Soc Occup Med 1982; 32:92–94.

11. Mäkitie J. Contact lenses in the work environment. Acta Ophthalmol 1984; Suppl 161:151–152.

12. Jenks C, Jr. Letter to the editor. J Am Assn Nurse Anesth 1984; 52(3):262.

13. Wesley NK. Chemical injury and contact lenses. Contacto 1966; 10(3):15–20.

14. Guthrie JW, Seitz G. An investigation of the contact lens problem. J Occup Med 1975; 17(3):163–166.

15. Nilsson SEG, Andersson L. The use of contact lenses in environments with organic solvents, acids or alkalis. Acta Ophthalmol 1982; 60:599–608.

16. Dickinson F. Contact lenses: The safety factor. Optician 1969; 158:355.

17. Kingston DW. Contact lenses in the laboratory. J Chem Ed 1981; 58:A289–A290, A293.

18. Nilsson SEG, Lövsund P, Öberg PA. Contact lenses and mechanical trauma to the eye: An experimental study. Acta Ophthalmol (Copenh) 1981; 59.

19. Highgate DJ. Contact lenses at work. Occup Health Saf 1974; 3:8–11.

20. Cohen JM. Corneal protection through contact lenses. Optom Weekly 1964; 55:30–31.

21. Fisher EJ. Personal communication, 1989.

22. Nilsson SEG, Lindh H, Andersson L. Contact lens wear in an environment contaminated with metal particles. Acta Ophthalmol (Copenh) 1983; 61:882–888.

23. Dickinson F. Contact lenses: The safety factor. Optician 1969; 157:355.

24. Mäkitie J. Contact lenses and the work environment. Presented at the Ergophthalmology Symposium, Tampere, Finland, August 6–7, 1983.

25. Mercier A, Dugnet J, United States Air Force (trans). Physiopathology of the Flyer's Eye, p. 83. 1950.

26. Socks JF. Contact lenses in extreme cold environments: Response of rabbit corneas. Am J Optom Physiol Opt 1982; 59:297–300.

27. Nilsson SEG, Lovsund P, Öberg PA, Flordahl LE. The transmittance and absorption properties of contact lenses. Scand J Work Environ Health 1979, 5:262–270.

28. Chou BR, Cullen AP, Egan DJ. Spectral transmittance of contact lens materials. Int Contact Lens Clin 1982; 11:106–114.

29. Chou BR, Cullen AP, Dumbleton KA. Protection factors of ultraviolet-blocking contact lenses. Int Contact Lens Clin 1988; 15:244–250.

30. Parker JH. A qualitative evaluation of some commercially available UV filtering soft contact lenses. Int Contact Lens J 1988; 16:61–63.

31. Cullen AP, Chou BR, Egan DJ. Industrial non-ionizing radiation and contact lenses. Can J Public Health 1982; 73:251–254.

32. Lövsund P, Nilsson SEG, Lindh H, Öberg PA. Temperature changes in contact lenses in connection with radiation from infrared heaters. Scand J Work Environ Health 1979; 5:280–285.

33. Lövsund P, Nilsson SEG, Lindh H, Öberg PA. Temperature changes in contact lenses in connection with radiation from welding arcs. Scand J Work Environ Health 1979; 5:271–279.

34. Applegate RA, Massoff RW. Changes in contrast sensitivity function induced by contact lens wear. Am J Optom Physiol Opt 1975; 52:840–846.

35. Hess RF, Garner LF. The effect of corneal edema on visual function. Invest Ophthalmol Vis Sci 1977; 16:5–13.

36. Woo G, Hess R. Contrast sensitivity function and soft contact lenses. Int Contact Lens Clin 1979; 6:37–42.

37. Mitra S and Lamberts DW. Contrast sensitivity in soft lens wearers. Contact Intraocular Lens Med J 1981; 7:315–322.

38. Bernstein IH, Brodrick J. Contrast sensitivity through spectacles and soft contact lenses. Am J Optom Physiol Opt 58:309–313, 1981.

39. Tomlinson A, Mann G. An analysis of visual performance with soft contact lens and spectacle correction. Ophthalmic Physiol Opt 1985; 5:53–57.

40. Kirkpatrick DL, Roggenkamp JR. Effects of soft contact lenses on contrast sensitivity. Am J Optom Physiol Opt 1985; 62:407–412.

41. Teitelbaum BA, Kelly SA, Gemoules G. Contrast sensitivity through spectacles and hydrogel lenses of different polymers. Int Contact Lens Clin 1985; 12:162–166.

42. Dumbleton KA, Cullen AP. Short term effects of wearing UV absorbing contact lenses on visual function and subjective comfort, in preparation.

43. Chou BR, Cullen AP. Spectral transmittance of selected tinted ophthalmic lenses. Can J Optom 1983; 45:192–198.

44. Pitts DG. Threat of ultraviolet radiation to the eye—how to protect against it. J Am Optom Assoc 1981; 52:949–957.

45. Gies P, Colin CR. Ocular protection from ultraviolet radiation. Clin Exp Optom 1988; 71:27.

46. Chou BR, Cullen AP, Dumbleton KA. Protection factors of ultraviolet-blocking contact lenses. Int Contact Lens Clin 1988; 15:244–550.

47. Pitts DG, Lattimore MR. Protection against UVR using the Vistakon UV-Block soft contact lens. Int Contact Lens Clin 1987; 14:22–29.

48. Bergmanson JPG, Pitts DG, Chu LWF. The efficacy of a UV-blocking soft contact lens in protecting cornea against UV radiation. Acta Ophthalmol (Copenh) 1987; 65:279–286.

49. Cullen AP, Dumbleton KA, Chou BR. Contact lenses and acute exposure to ultraviolet radiation. Optom Vis Sci 1989; 30:407–411.

50. Dumbleton KA, Cullen AP, Doughty MJ. Protection by a UV-absorbing RGP contact lens. Submitted for publication in Ophthalmic Physiol Opt, 1991.

51. Ahmedbhai N, Cullen AP. The influence of contact lens wear on the corneal response to ultraviolet radiation. Ophthalmic Physiol Opt 1988; 8:183–189.

52. Bergmanson JPG, Chu LWF. Epithelial morphological response to soft hydrogel contact lenses. Br J Ophthalmol 1985; 69:373–379.

53. Francois J. The rabbit corneal epithelium after wearing hard and soft contact lenses. CLAO J 1983; 9:267–274.

54. Elkington AR, Watts GH. Ruby laser transmission and the lens. Br J Ophthalmol 1970; 54:423–427.

55. Repacholi MH. Ultrasound: Characteristics and Biological Action. Publication No. NRCC 19244. Ottawa, Ontario: National Research Council, 1981.

56. Polse KA, Mandell RB. Critical oxygen tension at the corneal surface. Arch Ophthalmol 1970; 84:505–508.

57. Hapnes R. Soft contact lenses worn at a simulated altitude of 18,000 feet. Acta Ophthalmol (Copenh) 1980; 58:90–95.

58. Millodot M, O'Leary DJ. Effect of oxygen deprivation on corneal sensitivity. Acta Ophthalmol (Copenh), 1980; 58:434–439.

59. Castrén J. The significance of low atmospheric pressure on the eyes with reference to soft contact lenses. Acta Ophthalmol Suppl 1984; 161:123–127.

60. Jaeckle C. Practicability of the use of contact lenses at low atmospheric pressures. Arch Ophthalmol 1944; 31:326–328.

61. Flynn WJ, Miller RE, Tredici TJ, Block MG. Soft contact lens wear at altitude: Effects of hypoxia. Aviat Space Environ Med 1988, 59:44–48.

62. Strath RA. Personal communication, 1989.

63. Nilsson K, Rengstorff RH. Continuous wearing of Duragel® contact lenses by Swedish Air Force pilots. Am J Optom Physiol Opt 1979; 56:356–358.

64. Clarke C. Contact lenses at high altitude: Experience on Everest south-west face 1975. Br J Ophthalmol 1976; 60:479–480.

65. Simon DR, Bradley ME. Corneal edema in divers wearing hard contact lenses. Am J Ophthalmol 1978; 85:462–464.

66. Simon DR, Bradley ME. Adverse effects of contact lens wear during decompression. JAMA 1980; 244:1213–1214.

67. Molinari JF, Socks JF. Effects of hyperbaric conditions on cornea physiology with hydrogel contact lenses. Br Contact Lens Assoc J 1986; 9:3–7.

68. Socks JF, Molinari JF, Rowey JL. Rigid gas permeable contact lenses in hyperbaric environments. Am J Optom Physiol Opt 1988; 65:942–945.

69. Brennan DH, Girvin JK. The flight acceptability of soft contact lenses: an environmental trial. Aviat Space Environ Med 1985; 56:43–48.

70. Eng WG, Rasco JL, Marano JA. Low atmospheric pressure effects on wearing soft contact lenses. Aviat Space Environ Med 49:73–75.

71. Castrén J, Tuovinen E, Länsimies E, et al. Contact lenses in hypoxia. Acta Ophthalmol (Copenh) 1985; 63:439–442.

72. Benneyt TQM. The use of contact lenses for diving (Sport and commercial). Contact Lens J 1988; 16:171–172.

73. Dennis RJ, Woessner WM, Miller RE, Gillingham KK. The effect of fluctuating +Gz exposure on rigid gas permeable contact lens wear. Optom Vis Sci (Suppl.) 1989; 66:167.

74. Hart LG. Wearing contact lenses in space shuttle operations. Aviat Space Environ Med 1985; 56:1224–1225.

75. Plyasova-Bakunina A, Volkov VV, Kiraev A et al. Soft contact lenses in prolonged space flight: First use (in Russian). Kosm Biol Aviakosm Med 1989; 23:32–34.

76. Lövsund P, Nilsson SEG, Öberg PA. The use of contact lenses in wet or damp environments, Acta Ophthalmol (Copenh) 1980; 58:794–804.

77. Andrasko G, Schoessler JP. The effect of humidity on the dehydration of soft contact lenses on the eye. Int Contact Lens Clin 1980, 7:210–213.

78. Brennan NA, Efron N, Bruce AS et al. Dehydration of hydrogel lenses: Environmental influences during normal wear. Am J Optom Physiol Opt 1988; 65:277–281.

79. Orsborn GN, Zantos SG. Corneal desiccation staining with thin high water content contact lenses. CLAO J 1988; 14:81–85.

80. Hood DA. Sof-form 67 CL's in the high-altitude environment. Contact Lens Spectrum 1988; 3:71–72.

81. Eng WG, Harada LK, Jagerman LS. The wearing of hydrophilic contact lenses aboard a commercial jet aircraft, I. Humidity effects on fit. Aviat Space Environ Med 1982; 53 235–238.

82. Nilsson SEG, Andersson L. Contact lens wear in dry environments. Acta Ophthalmol (Copenh) 1986; 64:221–225.

83. Hill RM. Dehydration deficits. Int Contact Lens Clin 1983; 10:364–365.

84. Crosley JK, Braun EG, Bailey RW. Soft (hydrophilic) contact lenses in U.S. Army aviation: An investigative study of the Bausch and Lomb Soflens™. Am J Optom Physiol Opt 1974; 51:470–474.

85. Cakir A, Hart DJ, Stewart TFM. Visual Display Terminals, Chicester, pp 208–214. John Wiley and Sons, 1979.

86. Cole BL. VDUs—Not a new disease: A new challenge. Aust J Optom 1981; 64:24–27.

87. Dain S, Chan T, Williams L. Visual and ocular changes in VDU operators. Public Health (Lond) 1985; 99:275–287.

88. Woo GC, Strong G, Irving E, Ing B. Are there subtle changes in vision after use of VDT's. In Knave B, Widebäck PG (eds): Work with Display Units 86, North Holland, Elsevier Science Publishers, 1987.

89. Daum KM, Good G, Tijerina L. Symptoms in video display terminal operators and the presence of small refractive errors. J Am Optom Assoc 1988; 59:691–697.

90. Pearson RM. Ocular injury and contact lens wear. Contact Lens 1972; 3:6,8,19.

91. Robinson L. Contact lenses are eye savers. Contacto 1966; 10:7–14.

92. Rengstorff RH, Black CJ. Eye protection from contact lenses. J Am Optom Assoc 1974 45:270–275.

93. Györffy, Von ST. v., Das Verhalten der Kontaktschale bei Augenverletzungen. Ophthalmologica 1951; 122:344–347.

94. Ellison LB. Protection afforded corneal contact lenses. Contacto 1960; 4:101–102.

95. Schwartz A, Glatt LD. Contact lenses for children and adolescents—a survey. J Am Optom Assoc 1960; 32:143–146.

96. Samland HL. Wie eine Korneallinse eine perforierende Verletzung vierhinderte. Klin Monatsbl Augenheilkd 1966; 148:897–898.

97. Shindo S. Selective traumatic retinal damage while wearing a contact lens (in Japanese with English summary). Jpn J Clin Ophthalmol 1968; 22:1297–1299.

98. Silberstein IW. Contact lenses in industry. Am J Optom Arch Am Acad Optom 1962; 39:111–129.

99. Dixon WS. Contact lenses: Do they belong in the workplace? Occul Health Saf 1978; May:36–39.

100. Koetting R. Contact lenses and welding, myth or fact. Interview by CR Metzgar. Safety Management 1977; 3:24–29.

101. Kersley HJ. Arc flash and the contact lens wearer. Br Med J 1977; 2:639–640.

102. Cullen AP. Contact lenses and electric arcs. Can J Optom 1990; 52:100–101.

CHAPTER THIRTEEN

Visual Display Terminals:
Visual Problems and Solutions

Donald G. Pitts, O. D., Ph.D.

In a few short years the visual display terminal (VDT) has become a center of controversy in the workplace.[1,2] Why? Is it a serious controversy or one that can be ignored? Answers are necessary, and this chapter will attempt to explore the issues, but a basic background text on the subject is recommended.[3]

In 1982, it was estimated that 7 million workers were using VDTs. This figure reached 10 million in 1983, and by 1990, 40 million workers were using VDTs. The computer has been with us for over 30 y, and for most of that time very few problems were blamed on the terminal. In recent years, however, newspapers have reported fears that cataracts, clusters of abortions, clusters of miscarriages, and birth defects are related to VDT use. Over 75% of all VDT complaints are related to the visual system.[1–7]

The controversy about the VDT in the workplace has placed the unions representing labor at odds with business management. Unfortunately, the worker has not been provided with the information needed to make a rational decision. After all, when the worker hears that the VDT causes abortions, birth defects, miscarriages, cataracts, and the loss of sexual appetite, concern is understandable—if these claims are correct. The workers must rely for answers on those they trust, those who claim to have the correct information, and those who claim to guard their job, and frequently, it is difficult to determine who has the correct information.

Part of the answer to the VDT problem lies in the fact that early computer personnel were highly selected, highly motivated, and highly trained. Such people were and still are completely dedicated to the VDT and are willing to use the system regardless of the conditions, to use the computer language and to use the operating procedures they developed, after all, they were responsible for generating it. But how about the vast number of people who have literally been forced into the world of VDT magic? Most of them have interests and training in areas other than computer technology. They come from secretarial, bookkeeping, and other office jobs. These jobs included a number of subtasks to relieve the routine and boredom, such as answering the telephone, filing written material, and so on, which have played an important role in overall job satisfaction.

The generation of VDT operators who were retrained from the past are not particularly happy with their new positions. They claim that the VDT has made their jobs routine and repetitive, made office tasks highly specialized, and has reduced the number of subtasks. Because of this, most operators feel their jobs lack creativity, they are told how to do the task and what to do to accomplish the task. The repetitiveness of the tasks has greatly increased boredom, and there are indications that the highly specialized, routine jobs may create stress among some workers.[5] In the past, mistakes were thrown into the wastebasket, work monitoring was a rarity, and the duration of time to complete a task was not monitored directly. In the present day world, however, work is monitored in both the time domain and accomplishment domain, and this creates considerable stress. Examples of stress-inducing practices include establishing quotas, the positive rewarding of superior accomplishments, and the negative rewarding of poor performers.

The evolution of the VDT in the workplace has followed a natural process. The initial group of personnel who switched from the typewriter to the VDT were very apprehensive and experienced difficulties in the switchover. The result was a massive outcry that was probably deserved and should not have been totally unexpected. After all, look at what the VDT will do when compared to the typewriter! The worker who was lost in the changeover rebelled—

not without reason. As the younger generation takes its place in the workforce, the complaints related to the new technology probably will reduce to the pre-VDT levels because they have grown up with the "friendly" computer and have nothing to fear from its somewhat awesome power.

13.1 Types of VDT Tasks

There are at least five tasks routinely accomplished by using the VDT (Table 13-1). The attributes of the tasks will be identified and described while recognizing that they have been categorized into data entry, data acquisition, interactive communication, computer programming, and word processing, although the categorization is used as a convenient method for discussion, and identified tasks may overlap categories. Each of these tasks involves a certain emphasis that allows it to be separated into a single category for purposes of discussion.

If a researcher generates massive sets of data that need to be analyzed, or an insurance company suffers losses due to a hurricane or tornado and needs to handle the massive number of claims as quickly as possible, they need operators to enter their data on computers. The data entry tasks are document intensive and allow little or no independent decision-making or interaction with others. The operator must input the data as quickly and as accurately as possible. Data entry tasks are usually routine and require high work speed and strict monitoring of the

	Data Entry	Data Acquisition	Interactive Communication	Word Processing	Programming
Input Rate	High	Medium	Medium/intermittent	High/intermittent	Low/intermittent
Visual Emphasis	Document	Screen	Screen	Screen/copy	Copy/screen
Interruptions	Few	Some	Lags	Few	Frequent
Work Speed Control	Little	Varies	Varies	Some	Much
Decision Making	Little	Some	Some	Varies	Great

Note: The descriptive adjectives within the table are intended to set levels of performance for each task.
Data from Helander MG et al.[4]

TABLE 13-1
Types of VDT Tasks and the Characteristics of the Tasks Compared to the Required Level of Performance

task. Unfortunately, data entry tasks are at the low level of the job scale with comparable rewards.

When the data from the disaster or research have been entered into the computer, they must be analyzed. The researcher analyzes the data on the screen or by hard copy. Settlement of the insurance claim requires that the data be called to the screen, manipulated, and interpreted. In each case, the data acquisition phase must be instituted. Data acquisition is screen intensive because it requires searching the screen for information and accurately interpreting data from the screen. The data acquisition process may require interaction with others in order to ensure accuracy in determining the outcome needed from the data.

Interactive communication involves operation of the VDT system with some other person who needs the information. The travel agent is an excellent example of this process. The flight and fare information for different airlines are stored in the computer memory, and when a customer calls for a reservation, the VDT operator must interact with the VDT screen information and the customer to determine the preferred flight schedule and costs. Interactive communication requires independent decisions, allows freedom to set the work pace, and requires movements of the eye between the keyboard and the VDT screen. The major complaint that the interactive communication operators express is the time lag between when the information is requested and when the information appears on the screen. In spite of this problem, interactive communication enjoys the least number of complaints of all of the VDT tasks.

Word processing includes a little of all of the above and probably constitutes the greatest use of the computer in the VDT field. There is intense entry of data from copy, acquiring parts of the data, computer instructions, and interactive communication between the VDT screen, the operator, and the person who provided the hard copy. Word processing also allows independent thinking in establishing formats for tables, figures, and so on.

The final type of VDT task is computer programming. It is interesting that programmers, scientists, music composers, writers, and those who use the computer and its visual output—the VDT—as a "tool of the trade" do not usually have complaints. After all, the programmer is the person who provides all of the instructions that those who use the

system must follow; if programming is not done well, it creates problems for users.

13.2 VDT User Complaints

The area of complaints from VDT users is particularly difficult to assess. Human factors research concluded that the lack of scientific rigor and poor experimental design made the research in the VDT area difficult to generalize from a specific study to the general population.[4] At the same time, there is more research in user complaints related to the VDT than in any other single area. The remainder of this chapter will rely heavily on the best research in this area.[5-9]

Most studies indicate that VDT operators report more eye-related problems than non-VDT office workers. These problems, include eye fatigue, eye pain, burning, tearing, itching, and blurring. The major difference in the complaints from VDT users versus nonusers is that 50% of the VDT but only 33% of the non-VDT users experienced eye fatigue. These studies also show a decrease in visual problems as the complexity of the VDT task decreases. When the visual tasks are identical, groups using the VDTs reported more severe vision-related problems than non-VDT users.[8] The most severe vision complaints resulted from the most demanding VDT task—data entry.[8]

Studies suggest a greater number of visual discomfort problems with the VDT user.[10] An example includes the report that VDT jobs were more demanding than non-VDT jobs.[11] In contrast, in 15 measures of other types of discomfort, neck discomfort was the only statistically significant problem found in comparing the VDT and non-VDT personnel. Interestingly, there was no difference between spectacle wearers and contact lens wearers. In a repeat study, VDT users reported higher occurrence of nausea and headache.[7]

Neck discomfort is related to the ergonomics of the VDT work station and to improperly fitted spectacles. The location of the top of the VDT screen should be 10 to 15 cm (7–10 inches) below the horizon. If the spectacles were fitted to provide maximum utility for the VDT, the neck discomfort would disappear. Neck discomfort in data entry personnel probably results from constantly turning the head to the side of the VDT to read the copy and back again, using an unnatural elevation of the chin for long periods of time. Two suggestions can be offered to alleviate the problem. The first is to place a copy holder at both sides of the VDT and copy from each side alternately. The second suggestion is to place the copy holder in the center between the screen and keyboard so that prolonged turning of the head is eliminated.

13.3 Characteristics of the VDT Terminal

Radiation

The electronics and the phosphor of the VDT determine the types of electromagnetic radiation (EMR) that are emitted by the system (Table 13-2 and Fig. 3-1). Low energy X-rays can be generated by the cathode-ray tube (CRT) and the electronic circuits, but none have been found in measurements of the different terminals.[12-17] The phosphor determines whether the EMR emitted from the face of the screen is ultraviolet radiation (UVR) or visible (VIS) spectrum radiation. The electronics and phosphors used in the VDT system render the production of infrared (IR) radiation impossible. Electronic circuits can

Types of Radiation	Measured	Standard
Ionizing (X-rays)	Not found	2.5 mrem/y
Ultraviolet	6.5×10^{-7} W/cm^2	1.0 mW/cm^2
Visible	11.6 cd/m^2 (40 ft L)	1.0×10^4 cd/m^2 (2920 ft L)
Infrared	Not found	
Radio-frequency	Not found	
Electric field		*40,000 V/m^2
Magnetic field		*0.25 A/m^2

*Far field equivalent 10 mW/cm^2

TABLE 13-2
Radiation Measurements on the VDT Taken by a Number of Investigators and the Recommended OSHA Standards for Exposure

produce radiofrequency (RF) radiation and the AC power circuitry can introduce extra low frequency (ELF) radiation. Proper shielding reduces these frequencies below the levels experienced when the usual kitchen appliances are used.

Making radiation measurements requires special instrumentation and training to ensure that correct values have been obtained. The EMR measurements from VDTs clearly demonstrate that the emissions of harmful radiation are well within the standards of the United States and foreign countries. The only radiation found during the surveys by a number of investigators (Table 13-2) was UV radiation, and it was 1×10^4 or 10,000 times below any known standard.[12-17] The VDT does not emit sufficient EMR in X-rays, UVR, or the VIS spectrum to pose a health hazard to the user.

Character Generation

To understand some of the problems in contrast, legibility, jitter, and flicker, one must become familiar with how the VDT "paints" characters on the screen. The VDT or CRT screen is composed of a series of horizontal lines called the *raster*, which extends from the top to the bottom of the screen. The electron beam "paints" the character by turning the electron beam on and off as it scans the horizontal raster lines. The "on–off" action of the electron beam activates the phosphor on the screen in short line segments that make up the character. When the characters are produced within the raster lines they are called *in-raster* characters. Letters that are in-raster characters appear to be composed from a series of horizontal lines or oblong dots separated by a dark space. The dark spaces can be eliminated by narrowing the raster scan lines or by increasing the scan line width. A second method of character generation involves a continuous line process in which the electron beam is guided over the path that forms the character on the VDT screen. The process is like handwriting. These characters are termed *stroke characters* and are preferable to in-raster characters. In the United States, a television screen possesses 525 raster lines, but higher resolution VDT screens can contain from 680 to 1300 lines. More lines allow a higher resolution, and a more legible set of letters and numbers can be generated.

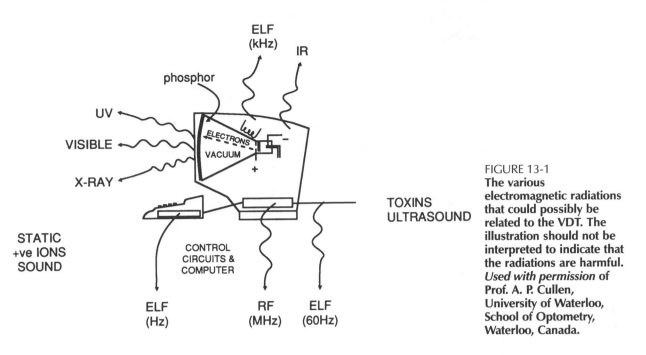

FIGURE 13-1
The various electromagnetic radiations that could possibly be related to the VDT. The illustration should not be interpreted to indicate that the radiations are harmful. *Used with permission* of Prof. A. P. Cullen, University of Waterloo, School of Optometry, Waterloo, Canada.

Each in-raster alphanumeric character on the video screen is generated within a rectangular area on the screen called a *matrix,* which is composed of rows of dots whose vertical separation is determined by the raster. The number of dots in a matrix are usually 5×7, 7×9, 9×11, or as high as 11×13 in the horizontal and vertical dimensions. The ability to generate a legible letter or number in both size and shape is related to the dot matrix of the system. A 5×7 dot matrix is the minimum acceptable matrix. The character style or font used in typing has undergone many years of research, and as the matrix of the CRT has been improved to provide more typewriter-like letters, greater acceptance in legibility and comfort has been experienced.[18]

Certain guidelines have emerged relative to the size and spacing of characters on the VDT screen (Fig. 13-2). Any raster lines that are visible are undesirable, and stroke characters are preferable to in-raster-generated characters. For the raster-generated character the minimum acceptable character height has been found to be 3 mm or 16 min of arc, but the optimum character height is 20 min of arc or 3.75 mm. The width of the character should be 70% to 80% of its height. The horizontal spacing between characters should be 20% to 30% of the height of the character. Spacing between lines should be from 100% to 150% of the character height. Thus, an optimum character for a 5×7 matrix would be 3.75 mm high and 2.6 to 3 mm in width with each character separated by 0.75 to 1.8 mm.[10,19]

Flicker and Jitter

Phosphor persistence and the color of the light emitted by the phosphor are important to visual comfort and performance. The light output of a phosphor image begins to decay immediately after the electron beam that activated it has turned off. If the image is not refreshed, it will continue to decay until the image disappears. A constant image on the VDT screen requires the phosphor to be regenerated by the electron beam. Phosphors possess different persistence characteristics, and these differences can be used to advantage.[19] For example, a television screen requires a fast decay phosphor in order to prevent "smear" as the image changes. VDTs, on the other hand, require longer persistence because the image on the screen is relatively static. If the decay and refresh rates are correct, a steady, intense image will be seen, but if not, the image will appear to increase and decrease in light intensity. Flicker is the lack of

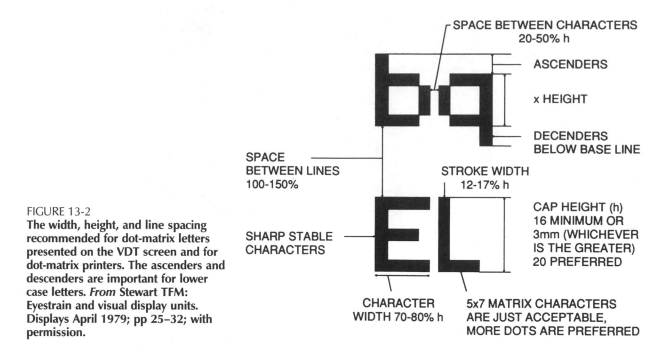

SPACE BETWEEN CHARACTERS
20-50% h

ASCENDERS

x HEIGHT

DECENDERS
BELOW BASE LINE

SPACE
BETWEEN LINES
100-150%

STROKE WIDTH
12-17% h

CAP HEIGHT (h)
16 MINIMUM OR
3mm (WHICHEVER
IS THE GREATER)
20 PREFERRED

SHARP STABLE
CHARACTERS

CHARACTER
WIDTH 70-80% h

5x7 MATRIX CHARACTERS
ARE JUST ACCEPTABLE,
MORE DOTS ARE PREFERRED

FIGURE 13-2
The width, height, and line spacing recommended for dot-matrix letters presented on the VDT screen and for dot-matrix printers. The ascenders and descenders are important for lower case letters. *From* **Stewart TFM: Eyestrain and visual display units. Displays April 1979; pp 25–32; with permission.**

stability in the brightness of the VDT screen image that results from the decay in brightness of the phosphor prior to its being refreshed by the electron beam.

Many factors affect flicker, such as size of the screen, intensity of the screen, and refresh frequency. The larger the screen, the more flicker will be seen. The brighter the luminance of the screen, the more likely that flicker will appear. Many times a VDT screen will flicker if the general lighting in the room is high, whereas lowering the general room lighting will result in the loss of flicker. The eye's sensitivity to flicker will decrease with a decrease in light falling on the retina. As the brightness of the VDT screen is raised, the eye becomes more sensitive to the flicker of the screen. For example, a VDT screen with a brightness of 10 cd/m^2 may not be perceived to flicker, but a screen brightness of 100 cd/m^2 will be seen to flicker. This is one of the disadvantages of the black on white (negative contrast) VDT display. The flicker phenomenon is not new but has been studied for years in visual science, and VDT flicker obeys the laws established by non-VDT research.[20]

Flicker can be eliminated or reduced to an acceptable rate by first ensuring that the general lighting and VDT screen lighting are maintained at a mini-

mal but comfortable level. Second, select a phosphor with a medium rate of decay and electronics with a minimum refresh rate of 65 Hz. A repetition rate of 100 Hz for negative contrast VDTs is recommended because the perceived flicker rate has been shown to increase approximately 10 Hz when the luminance of the screen is increased by a factor of 10.[21] This illustrates that the flicker rate is linearly related to the log of the intensity of the VDT screen luminance. The brightness variations caused by flicker could cause momentary changes in the adaptation of different parts of the retina and might be an important factor in visual comfort and performance.

Jitter is a term that is often confused with flicker but is an entirely different phenomenon. *Jitter* is the variation in position of the characters displayed on the VDT screen due to improper or insufficient video deflection voltages. The transients in video deflection voltages result in the phosphor being activated at a slightly different location on consecutive sweeps of the electron beam; hence, the variation in position of the displayed video symbols. The deflection voltages are time-based and result in the variation of screen brightness at different screen locations as a function of time. Unfortunately, there are no standards for the measurement of jitter, but the correction of jitter is primarily electronic.[22]

Color

The color of the video display is determined by the phosphor or combinations of phosphors used to make the CRT. VDT colors are typically not pure because the phosphors produce broadband colors incorporating a wide range of wavelengths; however, each phosphor possesses a dominant color. It is the dominant wavelength that the human eye sees by integrating all of the wavelengths of the phosphor that is perceived as the screen color. There are two major concerns in the selection of the color of the video display. The first concern is sufficient chromatic contrast between the character color and the background color to permit the characters to be visible under all conditions. The second concern is the eye's ability to focus the colors clearly on the retina.

The color of the characters on the VDT screen is one major difference between the VDT task and other office tasks. The question of color for the VDT display requires the consideration of both chromatic aberration of the eye and the stimulus to accommodation. Chromatic aberration is inherent in the optics of the human eye and results in red light being focused behind the retina and blue light being focused in front of the retina (Figs. 13-3, 13-4). Ivanoff[27] has shown that for distant objects, i.e., with accommodation relaxed, the eye prefers to focus for a wavelength in the red portion of the spectrum at about 680 nm but prefers the blue-green portion of the spectrum at about 500 nm when an accommodative demand of 2.50 Diopters (D) was required

(Fig. 13-5). There is an interval of about 0.9 D between these two wavelengths. It has been demonstrated that the defocusing of the retinal image serves as a primary stimulus to accommodation when the focal point was located behind the retina.[28] More importantly, only a moderate degree of out-of-focus served as an effective stimulus to focus the eye because, when the defocus exceeded 1.25 D, a response to accommodate was not obtained. Therefore, it was the defocus and the vergence of the rays on the retina signaling the eye to focus on and not the blur on the retina. The role of chromatic aberration as a stimulus to focus the eye is less well defined, but the retinal image for different wavelengths is focused at various locations and may well assist in the accommodative response.

COLOR AND VISUAL PERFORMANCE ACCOMMODATION. The VDT screen is placed from 50 to 70 cm from the operator's eyes, which requires 1.4 to 2.0 D of accommodation to maintain clear vision if we ignore the depth of focus from the size of the pupil. The yellow-green characters on the VDT screen vary from 550 to 570 nm from green to yellow-green and require 1 to 1.25 D of accommodation to bring the green character to a clear focus on the retina. The VDT operator must constantly use only 0.40 to 0.75 D of accommodation rather than the normal 2 D to maintain a clear focus on the retina. This means that the operator must change the normal accommodative-convergence patterns to see clearly and singularly. There could be difficulties in visual

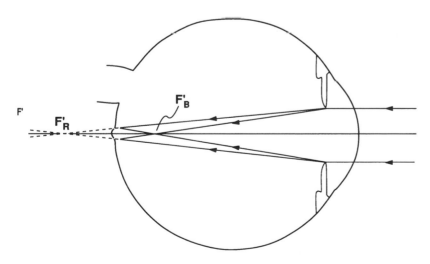

FIGURE 13-3
The longitudinal chromatic aberration of the human eye. A beam of white light is refracted by the eye and dispersed into its spectral components, with the blue rays being focused in front of the retina and the red rays being focused posterior to the retina.

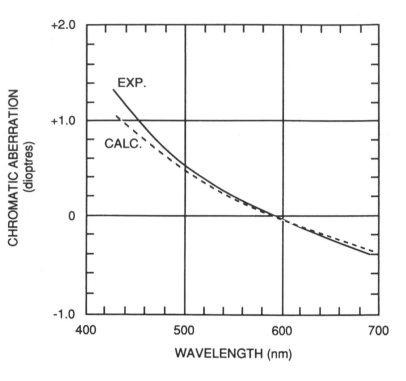

FIGURE 13-4
Chromatic aberration of the human eye. The chromatic aberration in diopters is plotted against the wavelength in nanometers. The dashed curve presents the theoretic aberration based on the schematic eye and the experimental curve gives the data found by experiment. *Data from* **Ivanoff A.**[27]

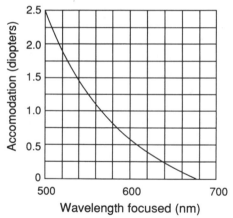

FIGURE 13-5
The wavelength of light in nanometers focused on the retina for the indicated stimulus to accommodation. The data indicate that for distant vision the red 685-nm wavelength is focused on the retina, but for 2.5 D of accommodation the blue 500-nm wavelength is in focus. *Data from* **Ivanoff A.**[27]

performance because the color of the video screen sets up conflicts between the accommodative-convergence relationships that have been habitual for the individual using normal black and white printed material.

The presbyope does not possess the accommodation required to bring the colored object into clear focus but must use ophthalmic lenses to accomplish the task. Chromatic letters in the red end of the VIS spectrum are the most difficult for the presbyope to bring into focus on the retina. If the VDT screen background differs radically in color from the characters, further difficulties may occur because of the constant conflict due to chromatic defocusing.

There have been several studies on accommodation with the VDT screen that are inconclusive because the methods used to measure accommodation were not sensitive enough. The laser optometer was used to establish some general rules relative to the VDT and printed material.[29] The eye does not focus the same for the VDT screen as it does for typed black and white material. The accommodative focus was found to be between the VDT display surface and the individual's resting point of accommodation. VDT screens do not provide optimum stimuli for accommodation, and spectacles are required to bring the display into focus on the retina.[29] Negative contrast VDT images with black on white (B/W) provide a viewable image than positive contrast images using white on black (W/B), and either B/W or W/B are superior to green, yellow-orange, blue, or red VDT characters.[29]

The visual evoked potential (VEP) and the laser optometer were used to compare retinal focus for B/W images with red, green, and blue brightness matched, video-generated displays.[30] Chromatic VDT displayed letters were found to serve as a stimulus to accommodation. W/B images produced the largest VEP amplitude, followed by green on black, red on black, and blue on black colors. Although color may serve as a stimulus to accommodation, W/B images appear to afford the best stimulus to accommodation.

There are some additional factors that affect the evaluation of accommodation. The first is that the VDT screen is curved, and images on the screen appear to originate from a position posterior to its surface. Second, the sensitivity of the laser optometer used in many studies has not been sufficient to allow valid data for the changes reported. Finally, most studies fail to take into account the vergence of the eyes. In spite of these shortcomings, it appears that accommodation-convergence and their relationships may be the major cause of complaints of tired eyes and blurred vision after prolonged VDT viewing.

A substantial body of literature exists that bears on the answer to this question of which color is best. The research was not accomplished on the VDT system but studied the interaction of printed materials and visual performance. The VDT is not so unique that a completely new body of literature must be generated, in fact, if the older research is studied, many of today's problems can be solved.

A 16% increase in visual efficiency and a 14.7% increase in legibility were found in printed material with black letters on white background when compared to red on green, green on white, blue on white, and blue on yellow.[31-33] Eye movements were much more efficient with black on white when compared to these same color combinations. Orange on black, orange on white, red on green, and black on purple produced very slow reading.[34,35] Reading speed and eye movements vary considerably with upper versus lower case letters, letter size, letter width, line width, and the separation between lines.[36,37] Optimum values have been established using printed materials and should apply to the VDT. It would be preferable, however, for this research to

be repeated using more modern electronic measurement systems.

The last problem with color is the persistent or prolonged afterimages that are experienced by some people after using VDT. The afterimages are complementary to the display color and are spatially sensitive, a condition known as *complementary chromatopsia*. Examples of pairs of colors that are complementary include blue/yellow, green/red, green/purple, and red/blue. Individuals who possess particularly sensitive color perception are usually affected. The condition is spatially sensitive because it is seen with small objects but may not be seen with large objects. People who experience chromatopsia after using the green characters report seeing reddish or pink (a desaturated red) fringes around small objects that may extend to the television screen and movies. Chromatopsia has a duration from 2 h to several hours after cessation of the VDT use. People who complain of the afterimages show errors on AO H-R-R pseudoisochromatic color vision testing plates 3 and 6, which characterize mild red-green color deficiency.[38] Subjects who do not report the chromatopsia demonstrate normal color vision after prolonged use of the VDT.

Which color or combination of colors should be adopted for CRT use? The obvious answer is that black characters on a white background is the preferred combination and color should be used only when graphics require color. The reasons for such selection include the fact that focusing of the characters on the retina is more accurate. Increase in visual efficiency, increase in letter legibility, and more efficient eye movements are noted. Complementary afterimages are reduced to a minimum or eliminated, and age-related chromatic problems are eliminated. Glare problems are reduced because the white or grayish background tends "to absorb" ambient luminances because it is brighter than the "mirror-like" dark surround or black background screen.

13.4 General and VDT Screen Lighting

General lighting and the environment are the major factors creating contrast and glare problems on the VDT screen. The reason is that the lighting in the room in which most VDTs are placed was not designed for VDT use but for typing, secretarial work, and other office tasks, which require a different layout and level of lighting. There are four major characteristics of general lighting that must be considered in any VDT area: spectral composition of the source, temporal aspects, intensity, and spatial or directional aspects. Spectral composition and temporal aspects should provide little or no difficulty for the VDT; however, intensity and directional aspects require different considerations for the VDT and non-VDT work areas. The basic information on contrast and glare were covered in Section II, Chapter 4, and should be reviewed.

The general lighting levels for non-VDT work areas usually requires between 500 to 1000 cd/m². [39] The use of windows to enhance the feeling of space is architecturally desirable but proves to be a poor choice for the VDT. [40] A room for VDT use should have between 200 and 500 cd/m² but preferably 350 cd/m² lighting luminance. [10] The VDT must be positioned within the array of lights so that minimum reflected glare is created. The VDT screen brightness should not exceed 150 cd/m² and not be less than 75 cd/m² (Table 13-3). The light immediately surrounding the VDT should not exceed the VDT average brightness and should not be less than one tenth the brightness of the visual task. It is particularly important that the general surround be free from bright lights because regional fluctuations or variations in the brightness of the visual field are uncomfortable. Such conditions demand that the visual system constantly readjust its level of adaptation, called *transient adaptation*.

The variability of the data on contrast demonstrates that it is difficult to set a standard contrast as a requirement for a visual task. Snyder and Maddox[42] have recommended a dot modulation of 75% for word type displays and 90% for graphic type displays. The dot luminance (brightness) should be greater than 20 cd/m² for word displays and 30 cd/m² for graphic displays. The character to background luminance ratios should be between 1:15 and 1:30, and the brightness contrast of the overall screen and the background in the room should be 3:1 to 4:1 (Table 13-3). The 3:1 to 4:1 task to background brightness ratios assure that transient adaptations will be kept to a minimum and that the level of the lights for a room will not exceed 3 or 4 times the luminance of the target. Shadows should be limited to a ± 10% difference from the background in order not to be annoying. [43,44] Increases in character to background contrast result in better legibility, [45,46] whereas negative contrast displays produce better legibility and are subjectively preferred. [21,47] In a survey of offices, the VDT measurements were found to lie within the recommended luminance and contrast values. [48] It appears that VDT operators are capable of setting the correct contrast and luminance values for optimum visual performance.

There are several methods of controlling the levels of luminance and reducing glare:

1. General light level should be between 300 to 500 cd/m².
2. VDT screen should be between 75 to 150 cd/m².
3. VDT screen surrounds should be equal to but not less than one tenth screen brightness.
4. Blinds, awnings, or reflective film should be installed on nearby windows.
5. Diffusers should be placed over fluorescent fixtures.
6. Fixtures should be relocated if necessary.
7. Indirect lighting should be used.
8. Dimming switches should be used to reduce background lighting.
9. The side of the VDT should be placed parallel to the fluorescent fixture to minimize its image in the screen.
10. Local lighting for documents should be used, but care should be taken to ensure that the light does not fall on the VDT screen.
11. Diffusing screen surface techniques should be used to reduce reflections.

Area	Luminance
Screen	
Maximum	150 cd/m²
Minimum	75 cd/m²
Luminance ratio for character/ background	15:30
Room	350 cd/m²
Screen average/room background	3:1–4:1

TABLE 13-3
Recommended Luminance Levels for Proper Visual Performance to Maintain Contrast Ratios and Reduce Glare

12. Filtering techniques should be used.
13. Hoods should be used.

Reflections from the VDT screen surface increase from about 4% at angles of incidence of 50° or less to about 35% at 80°. One method of reducing reflection is to etch the front surface of the CRT to diffuse the reflected light, but this treatment may cause the characters on the screen to become less defined and results in the loss of contrast.

There are four types of filters that may be used to control glare: circular polarizer, neutral density, notch or color filters, and directional or mesh filters. Each of these filters tends to enhance the contrast and increase legibility of the letters on the screen. The circular polarizing filter prevents polarized light from the room that reaches the VDT front surface from returning to the eye, and because it is neutral grey in color, it appears to enhance the contrast of the VDT image. Neutral density filters uniformly reduce the light passing through them, improving the CRT image contrast because the room light would need to pass through the filter twice to reach the eye. Notch filters work similarly and selectively remove unwanted wavelengths to reduce the glare and improve apparent contrast. Directional filters consist of wire or nylon mesh that prevents the part of the general lighting that strikes the mesh from reaching the video screen. The light passing through the mesh opening is usually reflected from the VDT surface back into the mesh. If the mesh is fine and placed relatively close to the screen, good resolution is maintained and contrast is improved. Hoods prevent unwanted general lighting from reaching the screen.

13.5 Ergonomics of the VDT Work Station

Unfortunately, the VDT is usually placed in the office at exactly the same location as the typewriter it replaced. Most people do not understand that general lighting is too high in intensity and that it is possible to orient the VDT screen to reduce or eliminate the glare. The relationship between the VDT screen and its environment is often wrong. To take advantage of the beautiful open window, the VDT screen may be placed with the operator facing the

window or facing away from the window, again resulting in wrong contrast levels and glare. The "officer furniture" was not designed for the VDT but for a typewriter.

For proper comfort and maximum productivity, the VDT requires a completely flexible furniture system (Fig. 13-6).[3,49–52] The chair must be totally adjustable in height, in anterior or posterior movement, and in the angle that the back makes with the seat so that the operator has excellent control for maximum comfort. The feet should be level on the floor. The keyboard and VDT screen also require complete flexibility. The keyboard must not be connected to the VDT screen but must be able to be moved horizontally as well as vertically to achieve the "typewriter position" for maximum comfort. Finally, the VDT screen should be placed at a comfortable viewing distance for the operator. Measurements have shown that the viewing distance varies from 50 to 70 cm (20–28 inches). The top of the VDT screen (not the overall height) should be 10° to 15° below the horizon, and the bottom of the screen should never exceed 40° below the horizon.[47] Thus, for a VDT screen located at 50 cm (20 inches) from the operator, the top of the VDT screen ideally should be 18 cm or 7 inches below the horizon to place the screen at 10°, whereas the VDT screen at 70 cm (28 inches) from the operator would be ideally located at 25 cm (10 inches) below the horizon to achieve the ideal 10° position. These recommendations place the VDT screen and keyboard as close as possible to the typing configuration that has proven successful for the officer worker over the years.

A reminder is necessary for the reading of hard copy. The early computer printers provided poor contrast hard copy that was difficult to read. Visual science has shown us that there is a wide range of contrasts and an even more expansive range of lighting that allow adequate visual performance in the reading task. It has also shown us that lighting and contrast can be interchanged to maintain good visual performance. If contrast is poor, increasing the intensity of the light can result in considerable improvement in visual performance. With poor contrast hard copy and a properly designed VDT lighting system, however, a reader of hard copy will be in trouble, because the two situations are not compatible. If we make them compatible, the VDT operator performance decreases. To solve the problem, locate a small office with increased luminance near the

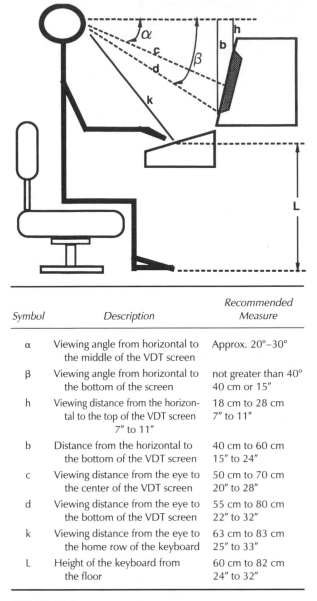

Symbol	Description	Recommended Measure
α	Viewing angle from horizontal to the middle of the VDT screen	Approx. 20°–30°
β	Viewing angle from horizontal to the bottom of the screen	not greater than 40° 40 cm or 15″
h	Viewing distance from the horizontal to the top of the VDT screen 7″ to 11″	18 cm to 28 cm 7″ to 11″
b	Distance from the horizontal to the bottom of the VDT screen	40 cm to 60 cm 15″ to 24″
c	Viewing distance from the eye to the center of the VDT screen	50 cm to 70 cm 20″ to 28″
d	Viewing distance from the eye to the bottom of the VDT screen	55 cm to 80 cm 22″ to 32″
k	Viewing distance from the eye to the home row of the keyboard	63 cm to 83 cm 25″ to 33″
L	Height of the keyboard from the floor	60 cm to 82 cm 24″ to 32″

FIGURE 13-6
Ergonomics of the VDT work station. The angles and measurements have been taken from many references in the literature and on some VDT work stations. The values are ranges that allow one to determine if the measurements are within the limits. The VDT operator must be comfortable with the workstation regardless of the measure; however, guidelines may assist in determining the cause for discomfort.

VDT area for hard copy reading and review. A second solution is to take an area, isolate it with portable walls, plants, and so on and lower light fixtures to a proper height for the office table. The light must not interfere with the VDT operator by reducing contrast or serving as a glare source.

13.6 Administration of the VDT System

The VDT area can become an administrator's nightmare if the operators have heard, believed, and passed on the myths related to the VDT. Therefore, the first task of any administrator of VDT personnel is to make certain that employees have been provided the proper information. Newspapers tend to be a very poor source of unbiased information because the material is often not checked against references to make certain the opinions expressed are indeed reflected in the data. If a document cannot be cross-checked against the sources, it is oftentimes not worth the effort to read it. A liberally referenced document provides an excellent source of potentially unbiased information. The study of Frazier and Fritz[54] provides an excellent report on work organization and worker satisfaction with the VDT.

In the administration of any work function involving the interface of man and machine, common sense must be used, and certain common rules concerning a person interacting with the VDT have evolved that are summarized here. The longer the work period, the greater the likelihood that the operator will suffer feelings of strain and tiredness. The longer the VDT operator works without interruption on materials requiring a greater degree of concentration, the more rapidly will the operator develop feelings of strain and tiredness often called fatigue in the literature.[54] The tendency toward tiredness and strain can be reduced, alleviated, or eliminated by pauses for rest or by switching the worker to another type of task. The former secretary had such tasks as filing, replacement of paper in the typewriter, correcting mistakes using an automatic system or correction fluid, and placing unusable materials in the wastebasket. The word processor accomplishes all of these tasks without a change in pace or a change in tasks. Performance has been shown to deteriorate after 4 to 6 h on the VDT. The duration of the uninterrupted work periods, the degree of concentration required in accomplishing the task, and the freedom to regulate work all enter into the VDT operator's feeling of accomplishment and job satisfaction. These statements all infer that there should be a work/rest period or a time limit on the VDT but do not explain how such time limits should be established.

Is it possible to arrive at a recommended work-rest break for the VDT operator? A system can be formulated that is related to the difficulty of the task being accomplished. Those VDT tasks with high visual demands, high work load, and repetitive work tasks, such as data entry, data acquisition, and word processing should have a more lenient work-rest period ratio, such as allowing a 15-min work break for each hour on the VDT or a supplemental task to perform occasionally during the work period. The VDT tasks that require a moderate work load or moderate visual demands and allow a great deal of independent interactions should be provided a 15-min work-rest break after 2 h of continuous VDT work. This is the same as the typist and secretarial positions enjoyed in the past.

These recommendations are not rules but suggestions. An administrator should be able to categorize work tasks, determine those workers best able to perform particular tasks, and regulate the work-rest periods accordingly. Of course, the management-worker team meetings should constantly review the tasks and work loads and recommend the work-rest break periods. During breaks, the VDT operator should not be permitted to remain at the work station but should be required to change environments to gain maximum revitalization from the rest period.

13.7 What Must the Eye Professional Do?

What corrective actions can be taken to assure a proper visual environment for the VDT operator? Please note that it is the environment that we are manipulating to ensure proper visual performance, and after the visual environment has been modified, we can begin to consider the eye and how its performance can be enhanced.

The first item to check is the workplace to ensure that the ergonomics of the work station, VDT lighting, general lighting, VDT contrast, and VDT glare are within the defined limitations. These bits of information may be obtained by providing the operator with a questionnaire that defines the required

information prior to the appointment (Fig. 13-7). One item of information that is critical is the visual working distance from the eye to the terminal, from the eye to the working document, and from the eye to the keyboard. The visual correction must combine each of these parameters into a common visual performance envelope. Do not prescribe an optical correction without knowing these distances. If you do not obtain this information from the patient by questionnaire, you or an assistant should go to the patient's office and make the measurements. You cannot rely on the patient's memory for distances; humans are terrible at estimating absolute distances from memory.

If the ergonomics of the work station are acceptable, what is the next step? Each VDT operator should be provided with an annual routine visual examination. Approximately 39% of the workforce have uncorrected or inadequately corrected visual problems that will result in the symptoms and complaints found in VDT workers if prolonged visual work at near is pursued.[55] Such data indicate that it would be prudent for the employee to have a pre-employment visual examination and an annual visual check. In fact, employer paid visual examinations would return the costs many fold in increased employee performance.

The best prescription to provide the VDT patient comfortable vision must be provided. For the younger patient, this means that the near point examination must be carefully determined and the necessary lens prescribed. Bifocals will not solve the presbyope's problem. They are usually fit too low to allow comfortable viewing of the VDT screen. The result is that the VDT operator must elevate his or her chin to see the screen, and prolonged positioning in this posture results in neck and shoulder pain as well as the classic tension headache. The normal 6-mm and 7-mm intermediate segment trifocal will likewise not solve but create problems. The vertical field of view of the 6- or 7-mm intermediate trifocal is only about 6 inches and requires constant up and down movements of the head to allow the VDT operator to visualize the entire vertical height of the screen. A 10-mm intermediate segment provides 19.5 cm (7.7 inches) vertical field if the viewing distance is 65 cm (25.6 inches). A 14-mm segment provides a 20.5-cm field of view of the VDT screen at 48-cm viewing distance. There are at least two trifocal lenses available that provide 14-mm intermediate segment heights: the Orcolite executive CRT trifocal

VDT VISION QUESTIONNAIRE

The doctor needs to know some special items about your visual display terminal (VDT) in order to prescribe the appropriate visual correction. Please complete the following and present it to the doctor at your appointment.

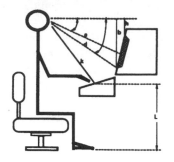

A. Measure the following distances :

    1. Distance from the top of the screen to the horizon h=_____ inches.

    2. Distance from horizon to the bottom of the screen b=_____inches.

    3. Viewing distance from the eye to the center of the VDT screen d=_____ inches.

    4. Viewing distance from the eye to the center of the keyboard k=_____ inches.

B. Locations

    1. The top of the computer screen is

        above eye level   ( )
        at eye level   ( )
        below eye level   ( )

    2. Written copy material is

        above eye level   ( )
        at eye level   ( )

      viewing distance_____inches   below eye level   ( )

C. Lighting (describe)

    1. Lighting in the work area (including windows)_____

    _____

    2. Background lighting (including windows)_____

    _____

D. General

    1. Time spent at computer:_____hours per day.

    2. Break periods:_____minutes/_____hour.

    3. Screen Color:_____background_____letters.

E. Brief job description_____

_____

Name   Date

FIGURE 13-7
VDT questionnaire covering the minimum information needed by the eye care professional to prescribe the appropriate visual correction.

and the Vision-Ease Datalite CRT 35-mm wide D trifocal. The Orcolite trifocal offers +2.25 and +2.50 D additions, with intermediate powers for either at +1.50 and +1.75 D. The Datalight CRT trifocal is available in a full range of bifocal powers with the intermediate power 66% of the bifocal power. The FD and ED trifocals provide a 14-mm intermediate with a full range of powers.

Care must be taken when fitting the CRT trifocal. It is best to set the upper edge of the trifocal at the center of the pupil. This requires the wearer to lower the chin slightly to see over the intermediate segment at distance. The usual clinical test distance for determining the near visual dioptric powers is 33 cm (13 inches) to 40 cm (16 inches) but the viewing distance from the eye to the VDT screen is usually much farther. Use the VDT viewing distance in your examination! If the segment inset to compensate for convergence for near vision is based on the normal distance for near, the patient will usually experience base-in prism. To eliminate this potentially fatiguing situation, the trifocal segments must be inset for the viewing distance of the VDT screen. A knowledge of the working distances is vital to the visual comfort of the VDT operator. Do not prescribe without knowing it!

If a VDT operator is presbyopic, does not require a correction for seeing comfortably at distance, and can tolerate blur when looking at distance, an ordinary bifocal may be used as the VDT correction. The dioptric power needed to view the VDT screen can be incorporated into the distance portion of the lens with the bifocal power being the addition necessary to allow comfortable vision at the keyboard. Normal fitting procedures may be used for the "VDT bifocal" used by VDT operators.

A small ophthalmic frame should be chosen to allow the lens to fit as close to the eye as possible because the vertex distance is an important factor in establishing the field of view. If the vertex distance for a 14-mm intermediate segment that has 20.5 cm field of view were decreased 3 mm, the field of view would increase to 24 cm.[56] A rule of thumb is that the field of view of the segment is reduced about 5% for each 2 D of power.

The patient should be counseled that the proper VDT spectacles will not be satisfactory for normal everyday tasks. The mature person will not be able to wear the VDT correction while walking within the office. This is especially true of a woman who wears high-heeled shoes in the office. The location of the bifocal and trifocal intermediate will create difficulties in mobility because viewing through either will result in an apparent displacement of the floor. The visual correction used for the VDT is a specialized prescription that is designed for the specific VDT task and will be unsatisfactory for general wear.

The same philosophy as fitting spectacle lenses should be used for the contact lens patient. It may be necessary to fit the younger patient using single-vision contact lenses with an additional pair that correct for the VDT screen distance. The presbyope should be fitted with the bifocal portion of the contact lens covering at least 75% of the pupil. Bifocal contact lenses will not translate well for the required position for the eyes to view the VDT screen, and translation is critical in orienting the bifocal segment properly for good vision at the VDT work station. Contact lens configurations using a centrally located near portion of the lens are ideal. The clinician must make certain that the keyboard and the copy mate-

rial are clear and comfortable. Monovision may be tried for those contact lens patients who can use this approach successfully. The contact lens may need more or less power for VDT use than for non-VDT tasks whether single vision, monovision, or bifocal lenses are used. The patient should be informed of this fact and told that the clinical approach with contact lenses requires a special lens for the VDT that cannot or should not be worn for extended periods of time away from the VDT. This means that the patient needs a special pair of "VDT contact lenses" to adjust the VDT environment to the desired visual comfort and performance.

Improper positioning of the material to be copied results in a multitude of complaints. Suggest that the material be held on a copy stand, located at the same distance from the eye as the print on the VDT screen and placed as near the VDT screen as possible. This suggestion requires fewer accommodation and convergence changes as the eyes switch back and forth between viewing the VDT screen and viewing the material to be copied. The copy stand should be locally lighted, but care should be taken to assure that the light does not serve as a glare source on the VDT screen.

Finally, be aware that improper optical corrections may increase the severity of the visual problem rather than solve it. It is important that the ergonomics of the work station, lighting, contrast, glare, and their remediation be a part of the overall correction of the visual problem.

13.8 Summary

The VDT terminal and the visual tasks that have been claimed to cause physical damage to health and result in a decrement in visual performance differ from the usual office tasks in two major ways: First, rather than depending upon reflected light for its stimulus effect, the VDT is self-luminous. Second, most VDTs on the market depend on a color display to perform, which requires different accommodation and convergence demands than normal tasks.

Radiation measurements have failed to find X-rays, IR, and RF radiation from VDTs. UVR was a factor of 6.5×10^4 below the recommended levels of standards. ELF and MLF radiation from normal electrical lines have not been found harmful in our homes and are not expected to be harmful in the

348   13. Visual Display Terminals: Visual Problems and Solutions

office. Therefore, we are forced to conclude that the VDT poses no radiation hazard.

The generation of characters in the VDT image fulfill accepted standards of legibility, and reading them should pose no problem as long as the proper matrix is used. A dot matrix of at least 9 × 11 is recommended, but 13 × 15 and higher provide a more acceptable letter. Flicker and jitter have been problems in the past, but the causes have been isolated and can be corrected. With proper rates of phosphor image decay and refresh, flicker should be a problem of the past. With more judicious design of the deflection beam electronics, the problem with jitter should be solved.

Color has been shown to be a problem for accommodation and results in complementary chromatopsia for some people. The problem with accommodation can be solved by using black on white for the video image. The only time different colors are needed is when graphics are required. Graphics should not be restricted to a single color in order to prevent or reduce the complementary afterimage problem. If the afterimages persist, those few people who are very sensitive to color should use only the black or white CRT for prolonged durations of use of the VDT system. The topic of color needs research in two areas. Accommodation and convergence relationships associated with the various colors and the different intensities of colors need to be defined. Second, the area of persistent afterimages needs to be pursued to delineate the colors, intensities, different saturations, and the duration of time that are required to initiate the phenomena so that corrective actions may be taken. Such research should allow the formulation of rules for those particularly color sensitive individuals to work with color VDTs.

General lighting requirements and VDT screen lighting requirements include procedures for reducing glare and keeping contrast problems to a minimum so that the environment can contribute to job satisfaction and productivity.

References

1. Bergman T. Health effects of video display terminals. Occup Health Saf 1980; (Nov/Dec):24–28, 53–55.
2. Strauch B. Video terminals spawn new phobia; Fear of computers. Houston Chronicle, July 24–25, 1984.
3. Cakir A, Hart DJ, Stewart TFM. Visual Display Terminals. New York, John Wiley & Sons, 1979.
4. Helander MG, Billingsley PA, Schurick JM. An evaluation of human factors research on visual display terminals. The Workplace, Human Factors Review: Visual Display Terminals 1984; 3:55–129.
5. Dainoff MJ. Occupational Stress Factors in VDT Operation: A Review of Empirical Research. Cincinnati, OH, National Institute for Occupational Safety and Health, 1980.
6. Starr SJ, Thompson CR, Shute SJ. Effects of video display terminals on telephone operators. Human Factors 1982; 24:699–711.
7. Starr SJ. Effects of VDTs on Service Representatives. Paper presented at the Annual Meeting of Society for Information Display, Los Angeles, CA, 1983.
8. Laubli T, Hunting W, Grandjean E. Postural and visual loads of VDT workplaces, Part 2: Lighting conditions and visual impairments. Zurich, Swiss Federal Institute of Technology, Departments of Hygiene and Economics, 1981.
9. Coe JB, Cuttle K, McClellan WC, Warden NJ. Visual Display Units: A Review of Potential Health Problems Associated with Their Use. Wellington, New Zealand Department of Health, Regional Occupational Health Unit, 1980.
10. Stewart TFM. Eyestrain and visual display units. Displays 1979; April:25–32.
11. Sauter SL, Arndt R, Gottlieb M. A Controlled Survey of Working Conditions and Health Problems of VDT Operators in the New York Times. Madison, University of Wisconsin, Department of Preventive Medicine, 1981.
12. Rupp B. Visual display standards: A review of issues. Proceedings of the Society for Information Displays 1981; 22:63–72.
13. Harlen E. Radiation: The non-hazard of VDUs. In Rading VM (ed): Proceedings of the Institute of Ophthalmology (London) Meeting on Visual Aspects and Ergonomics in VDUs. 1981.
14. Moss CE, Murray WE, Parr WH, Messite J, Karches, GI. A Report on Electromagnetic Surveys of Video Display Terminals. Department of Health, Education and Welfare Publication No. 78–129. Cincinnati OH, National Institute of Occupational Safety and Health, 1978.
15. Weiss MM, Peterson RC. Electromagnetic radiation emitted from video computer terminals. Am Ind Hyg Assoc J 1978; 30:357–362.
16. Wolbarsht ML, Sliney DH. Ocular Effects of Non-Ionizing Radiation. Paper presented at the Society of Photo-optical Instr Eng Symposium, Washington, DC, April 7, 1980.
17. Murray WE, Moss CE, Parr WH, Cox C. A radiation and industrial hygiene survey of video display terminal operations. Hum Factors 1981; 23:413–420.
18. Maddox ME. Two-dimensional spatial frequency content and confusions among dot-matrix characters. Proceedings of the Society for Information Displays 1980; 21:31–40.

19. Human Factors of Workstations with Display Terminals (2nd ed). San Jose, CA, IBM, 1984.
20. Rinalducci EJ, et al. Video Displays, Work and Vision, pp 66–110. Washington, DC, National Academy Press, 1983.
21. Bauer D, Cavonius CR. Improving the legibility of visual display units through contrast reversal. In Grandjean E, Vigiliani E (eds): Ergonomic Aspects of Visual Display Terminals, pp 137–142. London, Taylor and Francis, 1980.
22. Rosenthal S, Grundy J. Can visual display units prove a nightmare to the operator? Ind Safety 1979; Nov:8–9.
23. Donders, FC, Moore WD (trans). On the Anomalies of Accommodation and Refraction of the Eye. London, New Sydenham Society, 1864.
24. Duane A. Normal values of accommodation at all ages, Part 2: JAMA 1912, 36:299–303.
25. Hamasaki D, Ong J, Marg E. The amplitude of accommodation of presbyopia. Am J Optom Arch Am Acad Optom 1956; 33:3–14.
26. Hofstetter HW. A longitudinal study of amplitude changes in presbyopia. Am J Optom Arch Am Acad Optom, 1965; 42:3–8.
27. Ivanoff A. Les aberrations de l'oell. Revue d'Optique, Paris, 1952.
28. Fincham EF. The accommodation reflex and its stimulus. Br J Ophthalmol 1956; 35:381–393.
29. Murch G. How visible is your display? Electro-Opt Sys Design 1982; 14:43–49.
30. Kergoat H, Lovasik JV. Visual performance for chromatic displays. Can J Optom 1988; 50:181–189.
31. Patterson DG, Tinker MA. Size of type. J Appl Psychol 1929; 13:120–129.
32. Patterson DG, Tinker MA. Black versus white print. J Appl Psychol 1931; 15:248–251.
33. Holmes G. The relative legibility of black print and white print. J Appl Psychol 1931; 15:248–251.
34. Patterson DG, Tinker MA. Space between lines or reading. J Appl Psychol 1932; 16:388–397.
35. Patterson DG, Tinker MA. Influence of size of type on eye movements. J Appl Psychol 1942; 26:227–230.
36. Tinker MA, Patterson DG. Influence of type form on speed of reading. J Appl Psychol 1928; 12:359–368.
37. Tinker MA, Patterson DG. Speed of reading nine point type in relation to line width and leading. J Appl Psychol 33:81–82.
38. Khan JA, Fritz J, Psaltis P, Ide CH. Prolonged complementary chromatopsia in users of video display terminals. Am J Ophthalmol 1984; 98:756–758.
39. Simonson E, Brozek J. Effects of illumination on visual performance and fatigue. J Opt Soc Am [A] 1948; 38:384–397.
40. Hultgren GV, Knave B. Lighting considerations in positioning computer terminal screens. Appl Ergonomics 1974; 5:2–8.
41. Murray WE, Moss CE, Parr WH, Cox C, Smith MJ, Cohen BFG, Stammerjon LW, Happ A. Potential Health Hazards of Video Display Terminals. DHHS (NIOSH) 81–129. Washington, DC, Department of Health and Human Services, 1981.
42. Snyder HL, Maddox ME. Information Transfer from Computer-Generated Dot-Matrix Displays. Dept of Industrial Engineering and Operations Research, Human Factors Laboratory Report No. HFL-78-3/AR0-78-1. Blacksburg, VA, Virginia Polytechnic Institute and State University, 1978.
43. Rinalducci EJ. Early dark adaptations as a function of wavelength and pre-adapting level. J Opt Soc AM [A] 1967; 57:1270–1271.
44. Rinalducci EJ, Beare AN. Losses in night time visibility caused by transient adaptation. J Illum Eng Soc 1974; 3:336–345.
45. Snyder HL, Taylor GB. The sensitivity of response measures of alphanumeric legibility to variations in dot matrix display parameters. Hum Factors 1979; 21:457–471.
46. Shurtleff DA. How to make displays legible. Contemp Psychol 1982; 27:46.
47. Radl GW. Experimental investigations for optimal presentation—mode and colors of symbols on the CRT screen. In Grandjean E, Vigliani E (eds): Ergonomic Aspects of Visual Display Terminals, pp 127–135. London, Taylor and Francis, 1980.
48. Steffy GR. Lighting the hi-tech office. Building Operation Management, pp 40–44, June 1984.
49. Stewart T. Ergonomics and visual display units—is there a problem? In McPhee B, Howie A, (ed). Ergonomics and Visual Display Units. The Ergonomics Society of Australia and New Zealand, 1979.
50. Bandi Buti L, DeNigris F, Moratti E. Ergonomic design of a workplace for VDU operators. In Grandjean E, Vigiliani E (eds): Ergonomics Aspects of Visual Display Terminals. London, Taylor and Francis, 1980.
51. Jahn T. Ergonomics finally makes headway in computer area. Manag Inform Syst Week 1982; (March 3):35.
52. American National Standard for Human Factors Engineering of Visual Display Terminal Workstations. ANSI/HFS Standard No. 100–1988. Santa Monica, American National Standards Institute and The Human Factors Society, Inc, 1988.
53. Grandjean E. Ergonomics of VDU's: Review of the present knowledge. In Grandjean E, Vigliani E (eds): Ergonomic Aspects of Visual Display Terminals. London, Taylor and Francis, 1980.
54. Frazier TW, Fritz J. Task dependent fatigue of CRT terminal operators. Proceedings of SHARE 1978; 3:1467–1475.
55. Purdham JT. A Review of the Literature on Health Hazards of Video Display Terminals. Hamilton, Ontario, Canadian Centre for Occupational Safety and Health, 1980.
56. Stimson RL. Ophthalmic Dispensing (3rd ed). Springfield IL, Charles C. Thomas, 1979.

CHAPTER FOURTEEN

Vision and Motor Vehicle Operation

James E. Sheedy, O.D., Ph.D., and Ian L. Bailey, O.D., Ph.D.

Vision is the primary sensory input used in the operation of a motor vehicle. In order to provide for the public safety, minimal vision requirements have been established for driver licensure. This chapter examines the data which relate visual parameters to measures of driving performance, the social and economic implications of driver licensure, the current vision standards for driving, and the administration of vision standards.

14.1 Relationship Between Vision and Driving Performance

Visual Acuity

Burg[1–3] has performed the most comprehensive studies of the relationship between vision and driving performance. He studied more than 17,500 California drivers during a 3-y period. Data recorded for each driver included age, gender, and number of miles driven annually. Visual measurements on each driver included static visual acuity, horizontal heterophoria, recognition threshold in low light levels, glare recovery, horizontal visual field, and dynamic visual acuity. Correlation between these visual measures were tested with the following measures of driving performance: reported accidents, accidents recorded by the Department of Motor Vehicles (DMV), accidents excluding those caused by obvious nonvisual factors, daytime accidents, and nighttime accidents. Only very weak correlations were found between any visual factors and driving performance. A later analysis of the data[4] showed no meaningful relationships between accident rates and vision test results for people under the age of 54 years, but dynamic and static visual acuity measurement showed weak but significant relationships to accident rates for those over 54 years. The other visual measures showed no significant relationship to accident rates.

Dynamic visual acuity (DVA) was more strongly related to accidents than static visual acuity. Since DVA involves recognition of detail on a moving target, it might be expected to be more relevant to the driving task. DVA might be a more relevant measure of vision abilities, but there is no standard or accepted procedure for DVA measurement, and measures of DVA are not as repeatable as measures of static visual acuity. Therefore DVA has not gained acceptance as a visual test for driver licensure.

Hofstetter[5] compared visual acuity measurements to the self-reported accident rates of 13,786 drivers. His data show that persons whose acuity was in the lower quartile of his population were twice as likely to have had three accidents in the previous 12 m and 50% more likely to have had two accidents compared to the half of the population with better acuity. This study provides the strongest evidence yet available to show an association between poor visual acuity and driving performance. Visual acuity (and possibly other visual measures that are related to driving performance) is more strongly related to repeat accidents than to single accidents. This is presumably because a single accident could be caused by any of a variety of factors or mishaps, whereas repeat accidents probably better identify an individual who is at greater risk for accidents because of a particular factor or attribute.

Shinar[6] expanded upon some of the testing equipment developed by Burg and his co-workers. He developed an instrument called the Mark II Vision Tester, which measured the following parameters: static visual acuity, DVA, detection-acquisition-interpretation skills, low light level static visual acuity, detection threshold for movement in depth, detection threshold for central angular movement and for peripheral angular movement, horizontal extent of the visual field, and static visual acuity with glare. The test battery was administered to 890 licensed drivers whose accident history was known. Correlation coefficients for all vision parameters were determined separately for daytime and nighttime accidents and also for four different age groupings. All of the vision attributes were found to be significantly correlated with accident rates in at least one of the subtests, but none of the vision tests correlated in all of the subcategories. Poor static visual acuity under low illumination conditions was particularly related to involvement in nighttime accidents for the under-55 age groups. For the two age groups above 55, visual attributes related to motion detection were those most significantly related to accident rates. Across age groups, the low illumination static visual acuity test and DVA were the two attributes that were best related to accident rates. None of the correlations was strong, however, and the significance is diluted because of the numerous correlations that were tested.

Davison[7] also found weak but significant correlations between monocular visual acuity, binocular visual acuity, and hyperporia with the reported accident records of 1000 randomly stopped British drivers. Visual acuity was more strongly associated with accident rates in those subjects 55 years and older, and the association was stronger for the right eye visual acuity than for the left. Burg's study on U.S. drivers[8] showed the left eye visual acuity was more strongly associated with accident rates. Together, these studies seem to suggest that the road side eye visual acuity is more related to driver performance, but it is difficult to provide an explanation for this. Certainly the road side roof support pillar obstructs a different portion of the field of vision for each eye and might provide some explanation. It is also possible that lower visual acuity in the road side eye is also related to visual field loss on the road side, in which case visual field could be the more directly related visual parameter.

Most of the visual acuity testing that has been related to driving performance has been with the high contrast targets. High contrast visual acuity scores are not highly reliable predictors of the visibility of lower contrast targets.[9] A case can be made that low contrast visual acuity could be more relevant to visual tasks in driving such as detecting pedestrians, seeing the edges of the roadway, and recognizing irregularities in the road surface. Contrast sensitivity has been reported to be more related to highway sign discriminability than is high contrast visual acuity,[10] and Ginsburg[11] has recommended that tests of contrast sensitivity be used for driver vision standards instead of contrast visual acuity.

Visual Fields

Because the detection and identification of objects with peripheral vision is obviously an essential element of the driving task, it could be expected that

visual fields would be related to driving performance. Those studies already reviewed,[1-8] along
with many others, have not found significant correlations between visual field measurements and driving performance.[12] Most of these investigations used
nonstandard perimetric techniques, however, and
typically they provide inadequate control over fixation. Johnson and Keltner[13] used an automated visual field screener to test the vision of 10,000 drivers.
They found that drivers with binocular visual field
loss had accident and traffic violation rates that were
twice as high as those of drivers with normal visual
fields. Those drivers with only a monocular visual
field loss had driving records not significantly different from subjects with normal visual fields.
Johnson and Keltner's visual field measurement
procedure presented 78 static stimuli located between 50° and 60° of central fixation. For their sample, the incidence of binocular visual field loss was
3.3%, and more than one half of the subjects with
visual field losses had been unaware of them. These
results point to the possible merit of using more
extensive visual field testing for driver licensure.

Monocularity

Keeney[14] examined a group of drivers with high
accident rates and found that 8% were monocular,
which is a considerably higher proportion than the
2% incidence of one-eyed individuals found in surveys of patients from private practices. Liesmaa[15]
examined individual drivers who had exhibited
some dangerous driving behavior as judged by observers in a patrol car and a control group of good
drivers who were similarly selected. The incidence of
monocular vision was three times higher in the
group with poor observed driving behavior. Rogers
et al[16] found that heavy vehicle operators with substandard vision in one eye had significantly higher
accident rates and that within this group the more
severely impaired drivers had worse accident
records. Keeney and Carvey[17] have recommended
that monocular individuals not be licensed for commercial and professional driving. The evidence suggests that monocular individuals are at greater risk
for accidents and poor driving behavior. This is most
likely due to the field loss on one side, but it could
also be related to the loss of stereopsis. However,
stereopsis depth perception was one of the visual

parameters tested by Shinar,[6] and it was not correlated with accident rates.

Color Vision

Protanopic and deuteranopic individuals might be
expected to confuse red, yellow, and green traffic
signals and hence be at greater risk for accidents.
However, the green traffic signal has been standardized to a bluish green color which allows these dichromats to distinguish it from the red and yellow
signals. Cole[18] has argued that protanopic and protanomalous drivers may be at some driving disadvantage because they are relatively insensitive to red
light and have poorer responsiveness to red signal
lights, tail lights, and brake lights but, color vision
defects have not been shown to be associated with
higher accident rates.

Driving and Vision in the Older Driver

Older drivers are more likely to have reduced visual
function[19] due to such normal aging changes as increased light scatter, reduced pupil size, and discol-
oration of the crystalline lens or to pathologic
changes, such as maculopathy, retinopathy, glaucoma, cataract, and other age-related conditions. Accident statistics show that compared to other age
groups the elderly have fewer accidents, but their
rate of accidents per mile driven is relatively high.
When elderly drivers are involved in a accident, it is
more likely that that there will be a fatality.

Deficits of sensory, motor, and cognitive function,
often in combination, are more common in the elderly, and it becomes difficult to attribute their increased susceptibility to accidents to any particular
age-related factor or factors. It is quite probable that
reduced visual function contributes to the older
driver's increased accident rate per mile driven, but
there is no evidence to directly support or refute
such a connection.

General Considerations

Vision plays an obviously important role in driving.
Task analysis shows that numerous visual skills are

required to perform the various driving tasks. However, statistical relationships between visual parameters and driving performance measures such as accident rates and traffic violation rates have been weak. This is most likely because accidents and violations are relatively rare occurrences that usually result from a combination of many factors. The other factors include distraction, inattentiveness, other health problems, equipment failure, windshield dirt, camouflage, sunglare, obstructed signs, worn markings, and so on. It is not surprising that the correlation between visual parameters and accidents or violations are weak. Also, most individuals with more seriously impaired vision have been excluded from the driving population and are not represented in surveys and studies of vision and driving, thereby diluting the correlations in the remaining population.

14.2 Current Vision Driving Standards

Vision is obviously a requirement for driving. A person with "normal" vision has the visual skills to drive, whereas a totally blind person does not. All of the states in the United States and most of the countries in the world have established minimal vision standards that are required for driving. This usually means that somewhere between "normal" vision and blindness a line has been drawn according to visual parameters, and this criterion will separate those who will be eligible to be licensed to drive and those who will not.

As just reviewed, however, the relationships between visual measures and driving performance are weak. The evidence does not generally support a specific cut-off according to any individual parameter, such as visual acuity, to clearly distinguish good from bad drivers. Automobile driving has become a central and necessary part of the lives of most adults for occupational and recreational pursuits and many of the general activities of daily life. It is difficult to justify denial of the right to drive on the basis of a criterion, such as a 20/40 visual acuity, for example, when the measure is only weakly associated with driving performance.

On the other hand, it is necessary at the least to have some form of screening to ensure that those individuals who clearly do not possess essential vi-

sual capacities are not permitted to obtain a license. The established vision standards should be viewed primarily as screening standards, and individuals who do not meet these vision standards should be referred for a more detailed visual examination and any treatment that might allow them to pass the standard. If after appropriate treatment they are still unable to meet the vision standard, then there should be an individual determination of the suitability for licensure. These concepts are more fully described elsewhere[18] and will be discussed later in this chapter.

General Driver Licensure

All 50 states have a standard for best corrected visual acuity with both eyes open. The standards range from 20/30 to 20/60, but the most common standard is 20/40 visual acuity,[19] which is used in 41 states. Some states have less rigorous visual acuity standards if the applicant is wearing optical correction, or higher visual standards are sometimes applied if the applicant is blind in the other eye. Twenty-seven states have a visual field standard,[20] and each of these states standardizes the minimal required horizontal extent of the binocular visual field. The visual standards range from 70° to 140°.

Special Purpose Driver Licensure

Agencies responsible for licensing drivers attempt to set standards that are intended to protect the safety of the driver and the public. However, if the standards are applied to deny an individual the right or privilege to drive, there should be good evidence or a strong prima facie argument to justify the denial. For a large segment of the population, driving is essential for employment, obtaining essential goods and services, and participating in a wide range of social and recreational activities.

Some forms of driving, however, carry a higher level of responsibility or greater exposure to risk, and poor driving performance under the circumstances is more likely to result in damage, injury, or loss of life. Such forms of driving are usually occupational and include driving taxis, buses, school buses, emergency vehicles, trucks, and special purpose vehicles. For such driving special licenses may have more stringent visual requirements than those required for passenger car driving. For example, the vision standards for interstate truck drivers imposed by the U.S. Department of Transportation require that each eye be separately corrected to 20/40 visual acuity (monocular individuals and most amblyopes are thus excluded), and a color vision standard is applied (recognition of the color of traffic signals).

Screening to Meet Standards

The purpose of establishing vision standards is to improve driving safety and efficiency, particularly to reducing traffic accidents, injuries, and deaths. All driver licensing agencies (in the United States) conduct vision screening programs to test applicants against the prevailing standards. Those who pass the vision screening test are eligible for license, but the license may be restricted to driving with corrective lenses if lenses were used to pass the vision tests.

Most of those who fail the vision screening test at first attempt will be able to pass easily after an appropriate ophthalmic correction has been obtained from an eye care practitioner. Here the vision screening program is serving to improve the vision characteristics of the driving population by obliging reasonable numbers of individuals with substandard visual acuity to optimize their vision. This can reasonably be expected to contribute to driving safety and efficiency.

Most states (41 out of 50) require that applicants pass a vision screening at license renewal. The frequency of renewal ranges from 2 to 10 y, with 4 y being the most common. Refractive error and best corrected visual acuity can change during a person's lifetime for any of several reasons (most of which are associated with aging); therefore, periodic vision screening of drivers is advisable.

Failure to Meet Standards

Given the importance of driving automobiles in our society, there may be debate about whether driving is an individual's right or privilege. In either case, denial of entitlement to drive is a serious issue and the grounds for denial should be clearly justified.

Careful consideration must be given to those who, even after proper optical or medical attention for their impaired vision, cannot meet the vision standards for driving licensure. Denial of driving privileges solely because an applicant has best corrected visual acuity of just less than the common 20/40 standard cannot easily be justified. The evidence in the literature does not support the idea that a person whose visual acuity is 20/40 or better is adequately equipped for driving but that any person with poorer visual acuity is not. It is not possible to establish a single visual acuity standard that would perfectly distinguish between "visually safe" and "visually unsafe" drivers. Safe driving performance is dependent upon many nonvisual factors including attentiveness, mental state, judgment, reaction time, general health, sensory or motor disorders, and so on. To the argument that vision measurements cannot provide a distinct "black and white" criterion for driving licensure, Bailey and Sheedy[19] have brought the recommendation that a "grey zone" be established and suggested 20/40 as a criterion for referral and 20/200 for licensure denial. Applicants whose visual acuity falls within the intermediate "grey zone" would receive special screening and individual consideration. Most states already have some mechanisms for special consideration for those drivers who fail to meet the vision standards for driving.

For those individuals who cannot meet the vision standards, special consideration should be given to the following:

- Driving tests
- Driving experience
- Driving record
- Driving needs
- Anticipated driving patterns
- Other vision disabilities
- Other sensory motor disabilities
- Causative disorder and prognosis
- Variability of vision

By considering these factors along with the visual factors, a more rational and compassionate licensing decision can be made. However, just as a "black or white" decision cannot be justified upon a single vision measurement, the licensing decision itself need not be "black or white." There are several restrictions that could be placed upon a license, including

- Accident monitoring
- Violation monitoring

- Frequent license renewal
- Frequent vision reports
- Frequent driving retesting
- Time of day restrictions
- Visibility condition restrictions
- Route restrictions
- Speed restrictions
- Distance from home restrictions
- Use of bioptic telescope
- Special mirrors
- Restricted purpose

The restrictions most appropriate for each visually impaired driver should be determined on an individual basis.

As an example, take the case of a 40-year-old individual whose best corrected acuity is 20/50 due to central serous retinopathy that has resolved and who has been driving 25,000 miles per year with no accidents or violations. Given that there are no other physical limitations and an extensive driving test reveals no driving weaknesses, the DMV may decide to give this individual a license with restrictions that a vision report and an accident report be provided annually to the DMV. Significant findings in either report would trigger a new licensing decision, and in time the restrictions could be reduced.

A contrasting example could be a 70-year-old diabetic with a best corrected visual acuity of 20/120 due to retinopathy. The driving test shows this individual to be careful but methodical and slow in his driving behavior. He lives in a rural town and relies upon driving for basic shopping needs and for regular medical appointments in the town and in the nearby city. The past driving record shows no accidents or violations. The DMV might decide to allow him to drive only within a 3-mile radius of home during daylight hours and for the purposes of shopping and medical care. There could be a restriction to traveling a particular nonfreeway route only during nonrush hour daylight hours to the nearby city for medical care. Annual monitoring of vision and driving performance might also be required.

If bioptic telescope systems are to be permitted for driving, then it seems reasonable to require that the usual screening standard visual acuity (20/40) be obtainable through the bioptic telescope. However, it is also important that the conventional corrected visual acuity be within the acceptable grey zone and that the visual field be within acceptable limits. Bioptic telescopes used for driving are typically mounted superiorly in the lens so that the individual must tilt the head downward in order to "spot" through the telescope. Most driving visual tasks will be performed without the aid of the bioptic. Therefore, it is important that the individual be capable of performing most driving tasks without the bioptics. The use of the bioptic telescopes for driving usually requires training and practice that can be provided by driving instructors. Individuals intending to use bioptics for driving usually obtain extensive training and practice with private driving instructors before being tested by the state DMV.

14.3 Licensing Authority

The authority to issue a driving license clearly rests with the state DMV. The DMV sets the standards, determines and implements screening policies, and makes the inevitable borderline decisions concerning driving licensure. However, the optometrist or ophthalmologist is an expert in visual measurements and conditions, and for any particular applicant, the DMV may require visual information from the specialist to assist in making the licensing decision. It is the responsibility of the doctor to provide accurate visual measurements and assessments about the visual condition, its prognosis, and its functional limitations. The doctor also can provide opinions to the patient or to the DMV regarding the individual's visual capacity to perform the visual tasks of driving, but it should be kept in mind that the final authority rests with the DMV. The DMV considers many other parameters, many of which are not available to the eye doctor, when making the licensing decision.

References

1. Burg A. The Relationship Between Vision Test Scores and Driving Record: General Findings. Report 67–24. Los Angeles, Department of Engineering, University of California, 1967.
2. Burg A. Vision Test Scores and Driving Record: Additional Findings. Report 68–27. Los Angeles, Department of Engineering, University of California, 1968.

3. Burg A. Vision and Driving: A report on research. Hum Factors 1971; 13(1):79–87.

4. Hills BL, Burg A. A Reanalysis of California Driver Vision Data: General Findings. Crowthorne, Berkshire, England, U.K. Transport and Road Research Laboratory, 1977.

5. Hofstetter HW. Visual acuity and highway accidents. Optom Assoc 1976, 47:887–893.

6. Shinar D. Driver Visual Limitations, Diagnosis and Treatment. NHTSA, U.S. Department of Transportation, 1977. (Available from National Technical Information Service, Springfield, VA.)

7. Davison PA. Inter-relationships between British drivers' visual abilities, age and road accident histories. Ophthalmic and Physiol Opt 1985, 5:195–204.

8. Henderson RL, Burg A, Brazelton FA. Development of an Integrated Vision Testing Device: Phase I. Final Report. Santa Monica, CA, Systems Development Corporation, 1971.

9. Committee on Vision, National Research Council. Emergent Techniques for Assessment of Visual Performance. Washington, DC, National Academy Press, 1985.

10. Evans DW, Ginsburg AP. Contrast sensitivity predicts age-related differences in highway sign discriminability. Hum Factors 1985, 27(6):637–642.

11. Ginsburg AP. Contrast sensitivity, driver visibility, and vision standards. In Visibility for Highway Guidance and Hazard Protection, pp 32–39. Transportation Research Board Report 1149. Washington, DC, Transportation Research Board, National Research Council, 1987.

12. North RV. The relationship between the extent of visual field and driving performance—a review. Ophthalmic Physiol Opt 1985; 5:205–210.

13. Johnson CA, Keltner JL. Incidence of visual field loss in 20,000 eyes and its relationship to driving performance. Arch Ophthalmol 1983; 101:371–375.

14. Keeney AH. Ophthalmic pathology in driver limitation. American Academy of Ophthalmology and Otolaryngology 1968; 72:737–740.

15. Liesmaa M. The influence of a driver's vision in relation to his driving. Optician 1973; 166:10–13.

16. Rogers PN, Ratz M, Janke MK. Accident and Conviction Rates of Visually Impaired Heavy-Vehicle Operators. Department of Motor Vehicles Report RSS-87-111. California, DMV, 1987.

17. Keeney AH, Garvey J. The dilemma of the monocular driver. Am J Ophthalmol 1981, 91:801–803.

18. Cole BL. The colour blind driver. Australian Journal of Optometry 1970; 53:261–269.

19. Bailey IL, Sheedy JE. Vision screen for driver licensure. In Transportation in an Aging Society, pp 294–324. Special Report 218. Washington, Transportation Research Board, National Research Council, 1988.

20. Keltner JL, Johnson CA. Visual function, driving safety, and the elderly. Ophthalmology 1987; 94:1180–1188.

SECTION FOUR

SPECIAL PROBLEMS AND SOLUTIONS IN ENVIRONMENTAL VISION

In Section Two, the electromagnetic spectrum, light sources, lighting for vision, and the ocular effects of exposure to radiant energy were covered. Section III provides the concepts of ocular protection, ophthalmic materials, the design and use of filters, and the use of contact lenses in the workplace. Section Four uses the knowledge base of the previous sections to serve as the foundation to solve specific problems of concern in environmental vision. The problems include protection of the eyes in welding; special clinical problems including ophthalmic instruments, the dental office, and tanning parlors; and, finally, the effects of drugs on visual performance. It is intended for these examples to serve as an illustration of how the student can use the basic data contained in this book to solve environmental vision problems in a variety of environmental settings.

CHAPTER FIFTEEN

Protecting the Eye from Welding

Donald G. Pitts, O.D., Ph.D.

There are about 500,000 welders in the United States. Welding constitutes one of the most hazardous occupations to the eye because it produces the highest intensity of broad-spectrum radiation of any industrial process.[1] In addition, hot metal particles that are constantly being expelled in all directions necessitates ocular protection. Adequate welding protection for the eye requires both radiation and physical protection. For these reasons, the process, the hazard, and the protection required for the eyes need to be understood.

Welding is the process of joining two or more pieces of metal into one continuous body. The two metallic surfaces must be brought into close proximity and heated well above their melting point, allowing the atoms of one metal to intermingle with the second. A few terms need to be defined to understand the terminology of welding. *Flux* is a compound that coats a welding electrode or is contained within the electrode that, when melted, forms a gas to prevent oxygen from contacting the weld, thereby assisting in controlling unwanted metal scale and oxides. The *electrode* may be a consumable metal rod, metal wire, carbon rod, or nonconsumable metallic rod. In arc welding, the arc is struck between the electrode and the base metal being welded. The term welding rod is often confused with the term electrode. The *welding rod* is a wire or rod that may be used as a filler metal to assist in completing the weld, whereas an electrode allows completion of the electric circuit and may not be consumed. *Shielding* is a process whereby inert gases such as carbon dioxide (CO_2), argon, and helium flow through the electrode holder to prevent oxygen from reaching the weld and serves to stabilize the arc current. Shielding assists in improving the strength and appearance of the weld.

There are three types of welding used in industry: thermite, gas welding, and electric arc welding. In this chapter, the welding processes will be described, general and ocular hazards discussed, and the calculation of needed ocular protection explained.

15.1 Types of Welding Processes

Thermite Welding

Thermite welding is based on the chemical reaction between aluminum and iron oxide when external heat is applied. A mixture of iron oxide and aluminum is heated at one spot, establishing a reaction that generates a tremendous amount of heat throughout the mixture. The aluminum removes the oxygen from the iron oxide leaving free molten iron. The free molten iron is poured into a mold that encloses the base metals that are to be welded. Thermite welding is limited in use but serves an important function in industry.

Gas Welding

Gas welding is used for welding metals, cutting metals, and brazing.[2] In gas welding, a torch is used that is supplied gas from a tank of acetylene. The torch is also supplied oxygen, and the mixture of acetylene and oxygen determines the amount of heat obtained from the flame. Gas welding may not be a radiation

hazard to the eye; however, irradiances from gas welding vary with the size of the welding torch tip, type of flame filler metals, base metal, and flux.

Electric Arc Welding

Arc welding is the most widely used process because it produces the highest temperatures that can be achieved and produces the strongest welds. A short description of each type of arc welding will allow familiarization with the terminology.

Carbon arc welding (CAW) and *carbon arc cutting* (CAC) are the oldest arc welding methods. The copper-coated carbon electrode is typically the cathode and the base metal being welded serves as the anode, allowing heat to be generated between the cathode and base metal. It is the heat that melts the metal and joins them into a single system. The CAC system uses blown air to eliminate the molten metal from the cutting area. Smooth cutting can be achieved using the carbon electrode.

Shielded metal arc welding (SMAW) is the welding method most commonly used in the field, by backyard welders, and for welding requirements in

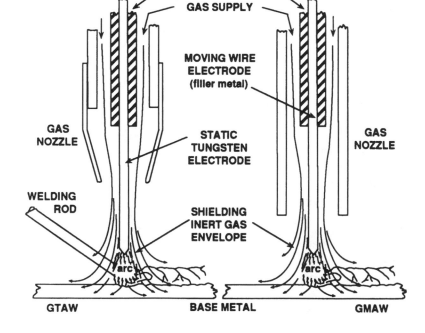

FIGURE 15-1
Welding heads used with inert gas. The inert gas flows around the electrode and over the arc to the arc-weld area. The GTAW head uses a static, nonconsumable tungsten electrode. The GMAW uses a moving wire electrode. The moving wire electrode melts at the arc-weld area and becomes part of the weld. (*from* Sliney DH, Wolbarsht, M. Safety with Lasers and Other Optical Sources. A Comprehensive Handbook: New York, Plenum Publishing Corporation, 1980; with permission.

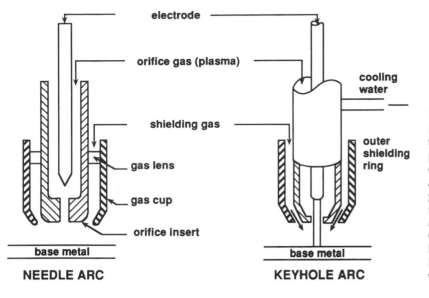

NEEDLE ARC   KEYHOLE ARC

FIGURE 15-2
Diagram of the plasma arc welding torch. The orifice gas forms the plasma, and the shielding gas eliminates the weld's contact with air. Argon is usually used as the plasma gas, and agron or helium are used for shielding. (From Sliney DH, Wolbarsht M: Safety with Lasers and Other Optical Sources. A Comprehensive Handbook. New York, Plenum Publishing Corporation, 1980; with permission.

automotive and machine shops. The electrode is a flux-coated metal rod that is consumed in the welding process. The flux serves as a shielding of the weld from air and to assist in keeping the weld clean.

The remainder of the arc welding processes use an inert gas such as argon, helium, or CO_2 to shield the weld from atmospheric oxygen and to assist in stabilizing the arc current. Some of these systems use a nonconsumed static tungsten electrode, whereas some of the systems use a consumable, moving metal electrode (Fig. 15-1 and 15-2). The plasma arc torch allows the orifice gas that creates the plasma and the shielding gas to flow through it. Argon and CO_2 produce higher levels of ultraviolet radiation (UVR) than the other welding processes.[3]

Gas tungsten arc welding (GTAW) was at one time called heliarc because helium was often used as the shielding gas. It was also termed TIG because of the use of the tungsten electrode, but its name has been appropriately changed to GTAW. This welding process was developed for the aircraft industry to be used in the welding of aluminum and magnesium. The tungsten electrode is not consumed in the welding process. The most commonly used shielding gas is argon, but helium is still used for deeper, more penetrating welds. GTAW produces a rather clean and attractive weld. Externally introduced welding rods serve as a filler for large welds.

Gas metal arc welding (GMAW) is a variation of the *metal–inert gas* (MIG) system that uses a moving metal wire as its electrode and inert gases that include argon, helium, and CO_2. Because the metal wire is consumed in the process, the GMAW is a faster method of welding. The wire electrode is often buried in the molten metal during welding, which reduces the output of optical radiation.

Flux core arc welding (FCAW) uses a consumable wire electrode that contains a flux. The flux generates the shielding gas, or externally supplied shielding gases may be used. The advantage of the flux core wire is that the complicated gas supply systems are not required. The FCAW system is used in the field for those reasons. Any of the inert gases used by the gas metal arc welding system may be used with FCAW.

The newest welding system is *plasma arc welding* (PAW) (Fig. 15-2). The tungsten electrode ionizes the argon orifice gas into a plasma that reaches extremely high temperatures. The orifice argon plasma produces a second larger plasma from the shielding gas whose heat is transferred to the base metal for welding. The keyhole arc torch permits penetrating arcs for deeper welds. The needle arc is commonly used for low currents and smaller welds. UVR is richly produced by the exposed PAW system because of the argon shielding gas.

Wiessman[4] should be consulted for additional and detailed information on welding systems.

364   15. Protecting the Eye from Welding

15.2 Optical Radiation from Welding

The mean spectral irradiance from gas welding, brazing, and cutting for four wavebands of the optical spectrum is presented in Table 15-1.[2] Spectral irradiance varies with the cathode tip, base metal, and shielding. The larger the tip size, the higher the spectral irradiance, but reducing the flame to a small, highly concentrated size produces the highest spectral irradiance. Filler metal irradiance depends on the base metal and use of stainless steel with a low carbon steel base metal produces the highest irradiance. Spectral irradiance was significantly higher for a base metal of low carbon steel when compared to a base metal of aluminum. The use of fluxes reduces the optical radiation because of the smoke and spatter that

Type of Welding	Effective Actinic UV 200–315 nm ($\mu W/cm^2$)	Near-UV 320–400 nm ($\mu W/cm^2$)	Visible Luminance 400–760 nm (cd/cm^2)	Near-IR 760–1100 nm (mW/cm^2)
Gas Welding				
Gas	5.1	0.004	8.6	0.580
Brazing	1.1	0.0002	0.1	0.008
O_2 cutting	1.9	0.001	2.1	0.039
Recommended exposure limits	1.0 $\mu W/cm^2$	1.0 $\mu W/cm^2$	1.0 cd/cm^2	10.0 mW/cm^2

NOTE: Gas welding produces the lowest values of any welding process and minimal ocular protection is required.
Data from Moss CE and Morray WE.[2]

TABLE 15-1
Optical Radiation Produced by the Gas Welding Process

Type of Welding	Effective Actinic UV 200–315 nm ($\mu W/cm^2$)	Near-UV 320–400 nm ($\mu W/cm^2$)	Visible Luminance 400–760 nm (cd/cm^2)	Near-IR 760–1100 nm (mW/cm^2)
Electric arc welding				
GTAW	100–450	—	$0.15–9 \times 10^3$	0.68–1.7
GMAW	700–2300	—	$1–3 \times 10^4$	0.68–1.7
FCAW	50–300	—	$2–3 \times 10^4$	0.68–1.7
SMAW	50–100	—	$1.3–4.1 \times 10^4$	0.68–1.7
Plasma arc welding				
PAW	7–110	—	$1.1–9.9 \times 10^4$	—
PAC/W	0.5–40	—	$1.5–8.4 \times 10^3$	—
PAC/W+ muffler	40–100	—	$0.18–1.1 \times 10^3$	—
Air carbon arc cutting				
AAC	70–2260	—	$0.11–1.0 \times 10^5$	—
Recommended exposure limits	1 $\mu W/cm^2$	1 mW/cm^2	1 cd/cm^2	10 mW/cm^2

NOTE: The gas welding figures are the maximum measured values. The electric arc welding values are ranges of measurements using different base metals, inert gas shielding, and type of welding. Measurements were made at 1 m except for PAC, PAW, and SMAW, which were measured at 2 m. The 0.68 to 1.7 mW/cm^2 for the near-IR (760–1100 nm) was calculated from Figure 15-6.
Data from Lyon TL et al[7]; *Marshall WT et al*[6]; *and Moss CE and Murray WE.*[2]

TABLE 15-2
Measurements of Spectral Outputs for Various Types of Welding Processes

is produced; however, these effects vary with the base metal, with aluminum giving the highest irradiance.

During a period from 1975 to 1977, a cooperative research program among the American Welding Society, the U.S. Army Environmental Hygiene Agency, and the National Institute of Occupational Safety and Health was conducted to characterize the optical radiation produced by various electric welding arcs.[4-7] They found that the integrated spectral irradiance for the broad-spectral bands of the optical radiation depended on the arc process used, i.e., whether the arc was GMAW, GTAW, or PAW (Table 15-2). The broad wavebands are E_{eff} for 200 to 315 nm, normalized to 270 nm; E_B for 400 to 1400 nm, normalized for 435 to 440 nm (blue-light hazard, B), and E_{IR} for 760 to 2000 nm, uniformly weighted. In each case, the integration process gives the irradiance in W/cm^2. The general form followed

$$E_{(\lambda_1 - \lambda_2)} = C \cdot I^n/r^2 \qquad (15\text{-}1)$$

Normalizing the data to provide the effective spectral irradiance changes only the constant C, with the relationship of the amperage and distance expressed as I^n/r^2 being unchanged. The exponent n equals the integer 2 for all types of welding arcs, and the constant C varies with the welding process.[8]

The effective UVR is a function of the welding arc current in amperes for most welding processes (Fig. 15-3). PAW and CAC processes are the major exceptions. Taking the highest UV output, the value for kilovolt (peak) or C for the specific welding process is 4×10^{-4} W/A^2. This value is acceptable for all welding processes using an amperage range from 20 to 700 A. The effective UV (E_{eff} in W/cm^2) for the waveband from 200 to 315 nm can easily be calculated by

$$E_{eff} < 4 \times 10^{-4} \ (W/A^2) \ I^2/r^2 \ [W/cm^2] \quad (15\text{-}2)$$

where I is in amperes and r is the distance from the welding in centimeters. This can be used for all welding processes.

The visible E_B for the blue hazard evaluation in the 400 to 1400-nm waveband can be obtained by

$$E_B < 1.1 \times 10^{-3} \ I^2/r^2 \ (W/cm^2) \qquad (15\text{-}3)$$

where kp (C) is 1.1×10^{-3} (W/A^2), I is in amperes, and r is the distance from the welding in centimeters.

This can be used for all welding processes as well. The blue hazard of the visible (VIS) radiation calculation serves for all welding processes because the constant is based on the highest welding output. The effective blue-light irradiance data using various amperes for different welding processes is shown in Figure 15-4. Additional values for constants that may be used for specific welding processes are given by Sliney et al,[8] but the blue hazard calculation given here is conservative for all processes.

The VIS spectrum is expressed in cd/cm^2 for welding hazard evaluation. The measured luminance of the GTAW exceeded all other welding processes and has been used as the base for the VIS spectrum (Fig. 15-5):

$$L_v(max) = k_2 I_a^2 \qquad (15\text{-}4)$$

where k_2 is equal to 2 $cd/cm^2 \cdot W^2$ when I_a is in amperes. The value for IR irradiance in the 760 to 2000-nm waveband is

$$E_{IR} = C_{IR} I^2/r^2 \ (W/cm^2) \qquad (15\text{-}5)$$

where C_{IR} is 9×10^{-4} W/A^2 and r is the distance in centimeters from the arc. Figure 15-6 gives the infrared (IR) spectral irradiance for three different welding processes. IR is not normally hazardous to the retina but elevates the temperature of the retina and assists the VIS and UV radiation in accomplishing their damage. Massive amounts of IR alone are required to produce a retinal lesion. Data of Lydahl et al[9] indicate that the major concern from IR exposures is anterior segment damage; however, the steelmaking process does produce measurable UV.

The previous formulas derived by Sliney et al[7] permit a hazard evaluation of any welding process when the amperes of the arc (I) and distance from the arc (r) are known. Thus, ocular hazard evaluation becomes a highly practical process. To evaluate the hazard from any welding process use the following procedure:

1. Assess the UVR using

$$E_{eff} < 4.0 \times 10^{-4} I^2/r^2 \ [W/cm^2]$$

2. Assess the blue-light hazard using

$$E_B < 1.1 \times 10^{-3} I^2/r^2 [W/cm^2]$$

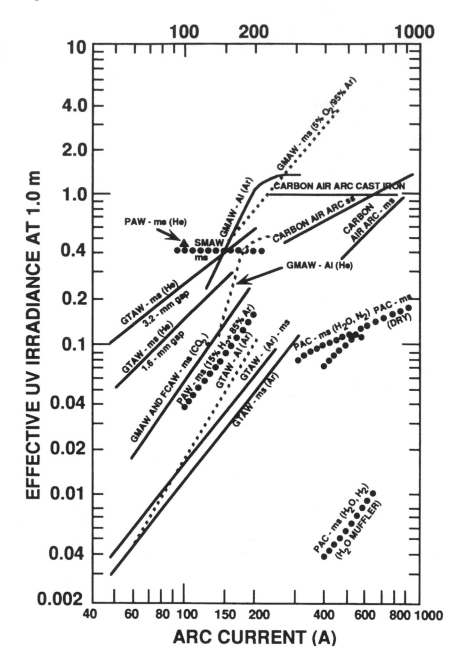

FIGURE 15-3
Effective UV irradiance from
electric arc welding as a function
of arc current in amperes for
different welding processes. The
effective UV radiation shows a
trend of $E_{eff} \propto I^2$. All data
measurements were made at
approximately 1.0 m except dotted
lines, which are extrapolated from
measurements made at 2 m. *Data
from* Lyon et al[7]; *graph taken from*
Sliney DH, Wolbarsht M: Safety
with Lasers and Other Optical
Sources. A Comprehensive
Handbook. New York, Plenum
Publishing Corporation, 1980;
with permission.

3. Assess the hazard from the VIS spectrum

$$L_v(max) = k_2 I_a^2$$

4. Assess the IR hazard using

$$E_{IR} = 9 \times 10^{-4}\ W/A^2\ I^2 r^2\ [W/cm^2]$$

5. Evaluate the results of steps 1 through 4 and use Tables 15-3 and 15-4 to select adequate protection.

The transmittance requirements for clear and filter lenses in the visible, UV, and IR spectra to be used in welding protection are presented in Table 15-3.

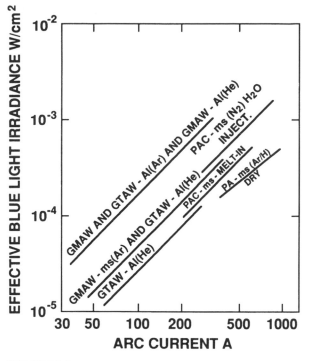

FIGURE 15.4
Effective blue-light irradiance using arc current from 30 to 1000 A for different welding processes. The GMAW and GTAW welding processes on aluminum base metal with argon or helium for a shielding gas produces the highest blue-light output. *Data from* Marshall WJ et al[5]; *from* Sliney DH, Wolbarsht M: Safety with Lasers and Other Optical Sources. A Comprehensive Handbook. New York, Plenum Publishing Corporation, 1980; with permission.

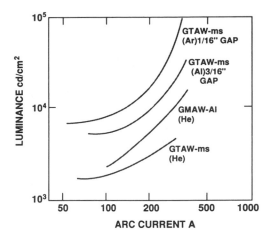

FIGURE 15-5
Luminance of the GTAW welding process. Visible spectrum output was highest for the GTAW with mild steel as the base metal, argon as the shielding gas, and a $\frac{1}{16}$-in. gap between the electrode and the base metal. As the electrode gap widens and the shielding gas changes to helium, the luminance decreases. Also note that the GMAW welding process with helium shielding and an aluminum base exceeds the luminance output of the GTAW with mild steel base and helium shielding. *Data from* Marshall WJ et al[5]; *from* Sliney DH, Wolbarsht M: Safety with Lasers and Other Optical Sources. A Comprehensive Handbook. New York, Plenum Publishing Corporation, 1980; with permission.

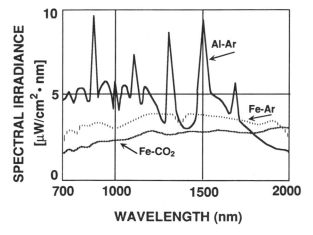

FIGURE 15-6
Spectral irradiance for infrared radiation for three welding situations. An aluminum base metal with an argon shielding gas produces the highest IR. There is a large reduction when iron becomes the base metal, indicating that the spectral output is related to base metal. Arc currents were 280 A for the iron and 200 A for aluminum. *From* Sliney DH, Wolbarsht M: Safety with Lasers and Optical Sources. A Comprehensive Handbook. New York, Plenum Publishing Corporation, 1980; with permission.

Shade Number	Luminous Transmittance			Maximum Effective Far-Ultraviolet Average Transmittance %	Maximum Infrared Average Transmittance %
	Maximum %	Nominal %	Minimum %		
CLEAR	100	—	85	—	—
1.5	67	61.5	55	0.1	25
1.7	55	50.1	43	0.1	20
2.0	43	37.3	29	0.1	15
2.5	29	22.8	18.0	0.1	12
3.0	18.0	13.9	8.50	0.07	9.0
4	8.50	5.18	3.16	0.04	5.0
5	3.16	1.93	1.18	0.02	2.5
6	1.18	0.72	0.44	0.01	1.5
7	0.44	0.27	0.164	0.007	1.3
8	0.164	0.100	0.061	0.004	1.0
9	0.061	0.037	0.023	0.002	0.8
10	0.023	0.0139	0.0085	0.001	0.6
11	0.0085	0.0052	0.0032	0.0007	0.5
12	0.0032	0.0019	0.0012	0.0004	0.5
13	0.0012	0.00072	0.00044	0.0002	0.4
14	0.00044	0.00027	0.00016	0.001	0.3

NOTE: The effective far-UV includes the waveband from 200 to 315 nm. The near-UV in the 315 to 385-nm waveband shall be less than $\frac{1}{10}$ the luminous transmittance, $\tau(NUV) < \tau_L/10$. Blue-light transmittance shall be less than the luminous transmittance, $\tau_B < \tau_L$. The infrared transmittance is for the 780 to 2000-nm wavelength range.

This material is reproduced with permission from American National Standard ANSI Z87.1-1989, copyright 1989 by the American National Standards Institute. Copies of this standard may be purchased from the American National Standards Institute at 11 West 42nd Street, New York, NY.

TABLE 15-3
Transmittance Requirements for Clear Lenses and Protective Filters Used in Occupational Eye Protection

The shade number is related to the luminous transmittance of the filter by

$$S = \frac{7}{3} \log_{10} \frac{1}{\tau} + 1 \qquad (15\text{-}6)$$

where S is the shade number and τ is the luminous transmittance. The term $\log_{10} 1/\tau$ is the optical density of the material for the VIS spectrum. The higher the shade number in welding, the more protection the filter affords and the lower the transmittance in the UV, VIS, and IR portions of the electromagnetic spectrum (EMS). The principal challenge is to eliminate all radiation hazards to the eye while allowing sufficient visible light for the welder to see comfortably. This poses a serious problem when the welder is attempting to strike the arc with the safety equipment in place because vision can be very restricted

until the arc-produced light is available. This potential hazard could be reduced or eliminated by an intense localized light. Recommended shade numbers for various welding tasks are presented in Table 15-4. Care must be taken to ensure that the filter actually provides the protection.[15–18]

15.3 Ocular Protection

Potential ocular hazards in welding include radiation, smoke, fumes, and the gaseous by-products from the iron, nickel, argon, helium, and CO_2. The gaseous by-products act as irritants to both the eyes and the lungs. In recent years, extractors have been used to remove the noxious gases from the site of the

Type of Activity	Lens Filter Shade
Electric arc welding	
Stick electrode	
30 to 75 A, up to 5/32 in. (4 mm)	10
75 to 200 A, 3/32 to 5/32 in. (4 mm)	12
200 to 400 A, 3/16 to 1/4 in. (4.8–6.4 mm)	14
Over 400 A, over 1/4 in. (6.4 mm)	14
Carbon arc	14
Atomic hydrogen	12
Gas, tungsten arc (GTAW)	12
Gas, metal arc (ferrous) (GMAW)	12
Gas, metal arc (nonferrous) (GMAW)	11
Resistance welding	
Spot welding	5
Seam welding	3 or 4
Flash welding	6 or 8
BuH welding	3 or 4
Gas welding (acetylene)	
Heavy, over 1/2 in. (12.7 mm)	11
Medium, 1/8 in. to 1/2 in. (32.–12.7 mm)	12
Light, up to 1/8 in.	4 or 5
Gas cutting (acetylene)	
Heavy, over 6 in. (150 mm)	5 or 6
Medium, 1 to 6 in. (25 to 150 mm)	4 or 5
Light, up to 1 in. (25 mm)	3 or 4
Brazing	
Torch	3 or 4
Soldering	
Torch	2
Glare	
Furnace work, bright sun, bright lights	1.5 to 3

NOTE: The welder usually selects the filter shade number based on acuity requirements. The welder should always wear corrective or plano spectacles that provide UV protection under the helmet.
Data from American National Standards Institute.[14]

TABLE 15-4
Recommended Lens Filter Shade Numbers for Various Welding Tasks

weld and circulate them through a charcoal filter prior to reintroducing the air to the workplace. Exposure of the eye to the radiation from welding can result in damage to the cornea (photokeratocon-junctivitis), cataracts, and retinal burns. The intensity of the welding arc would lead one to believe that retinal injury to welders is very common; however, Duke-Elder and MacFaul[10] state that reports of retinal injury from viewing a welding arc is "exceptional." Menton[11] described foveal lesions in two arc welders who failed to wear protective filters. Naidoff and Sliney[12] reconstructed the exposure of an 18-year-old who stared at a GTAW arc being operated at 80 A for about 10 min. The retinal exposure would have been between 25 and 70 W/cm^2, depending on the size of the pupil.

The effects of exposure to optical radiations have been discussed in Chapter 6. It should be well known that the welder's flash experienced when the arc is struck prior to lowering the helmet is painful. Arc welding requires a welding helmet to protect the face, neck, and head, as well as the eyes. A variety of acceptable eye protective devices for welding are shown in Figure 9-4 and provide good protection. Goggles are adequate for acetylene welding and cutting because the optical radiations are not severe.

The welding helmet is cylinder-shaped; of a size to protect the face, forehead, ears, and the front of the neck, and contains a window through which the wearer may see. The window is 92 mm wide × 41 mm high and is constructed to allow placement and removal of a series of filter plates. The most external and most internal filter plates are clear cover plates that provide protection for the intervening filter plates. The outermost filter plate has a golden mirror front surface designed to reflect heat from the interior of the helmet. The intervening filter plates are numbered according to their shade, and the welder generally selects the shade that provides the best visibility and comfort for the welding. A welder should wear protective spectacles under the helmet that filters out the actinic UVR for protection against inadvertent exposure.

Dynamic filter devices have been introduced into the market in recent years. These systems include photochromic filters, liquid crystal filters, electro-optic devices, and mechanically actuated shutters. The electro-optic devices can be made to close within 0.1 ms, whereas liquid crystal systems require approximately 150 ms for closure. These devices must be evaluated carefully before they are used as a welding protective system because of the different approaches used in their activation. For example, photochromics are made to darken with UVR but IR or

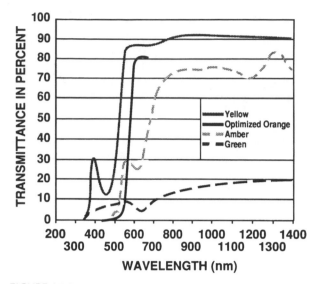

FIGURE 15-7
Transmittance of transparent welding curtains manufactured for industrial use. *Data from* Moss CE and Gawenda MC.[16]

heat converts them to the clear state. The balance between UV and IR for darkening/clearing would need to be carefully documented. A second example is the tendency of liquid crystal systems to become less dense as the temperature of the material increases. These examples indicate why the dynamic devices must be studied carefully under actual welding situations to ensure a stable protective system.

One of the difficulties experienced by welders is isolation from fellow workers because they must work behind heavy curtains or booths to prevent stray optical radiation from harming the casual passerby and other workers. A recent innovation is the transparent curtain that absorbs the harmful UVR. The requirements for these curtains have been outlined,[7] and the transmittance of different curtain materials is presented in Figure 15-7.[16] Sliney et al[17] have studied the transmittance of clothing worn by welders, and the data are available for the worker.

To prescribe the appropriate ocular protection for a welder, complete a careful case history. Determine the type of welding process used, its spectral irradiance and ocular hazards. Use Tables 14-3 and 14-4 to establish the filter needed to block the undesirable radiation. Assess all safety needs including helmet, safety lenses, curtains, supplemental lighting, and protection to the face, neck, and arms.

References

1. Horstman SW, Emmett E, Kneidielt. Field study of potential ultraviolet exposure from arc welding. Welding Research 1976; 55:121–126.
2. Moss CE, Murray WE. Optical radiation produced in gas welding, torch brazing and oxygen cutting. Welding J 1979; 58:37–46.
3. Sliney DH, Wolbarsht M. Safety with Lasers and Other Optical Sources. A Comprehensive Handbook. New York, Plenum Press, 1980.
4. Weisman C (ed). Welding Handbook, Fundamentals of Welding, Vol 1 (7th ed). Miami, American Welding Society, 1976.
5. Marshall WJ, Sliney DH, Lyon TL, Krial NP, Del Valle PF. Evaluation of Potential Retinal Hazards from Optical Radiation Generated from Electrical Welding and Cutting Arc. Report No. 4-031-77. Aberdeen Proving Ground, MD, US Environmental Hygiene Agency, 1976.
6. Marshall WJ, Sliney DH, Hoikkala M, Moss CE. Optical radiation levels produced by air carbon arc cutting processes. Welding J 1980; 59:43–46.
7. Lyon TL, Sliney DH, Marshall WJ, Krial NP, Del Valle PF. Evaluation of the Potential Hazards from Actinic Ultraviolet Radiation Generated by Electric Welding and Cutting Arcs. Report No. 42-0053-77. Aberdeen Proving Ground, MD, US Environmental Hygiene Agency, 1976.
8. Sliney DH, Moss CE, Muller CG, Stephens JB. Semitransparent curtains for control of optical radiations. Appl Opt 1981; 20:2352–2366.
9. Lydahl E, Glansholm A, Levin M. Ocular exposure to infrared radiation in the Swedish iron and steel industry. Health Phys 1984; 46:529–536.
10. Duke-Elder S, MacFaul PA. Non-mechanical injuries, Pt 2. Injuries, Vol XIV. *In* System of Ophthalmology. London, Henry Kimpton, 1972.
11. Menton J. Occupational diseases of the lens and the retina. Br Med J 1949; 1:392.
12. Naidoff MA, Sliney DH. Retinal injury from a welding arc. Am J Ophthalmol 1974; 77:663–668.
13. American National Standards Institute. American National Standard Practice for Occupational and Educational Eye and Face Protection, ANSI Z87.1-1989. New York, American National Standards Institute, 1979.
14. American National Standards Institute. American National Standard Practice for Occupational and Educational Eye and Face Protection, ANSI Z87.1-1979. New York, American National Standards Institute.

15. Horstman S, Ingram JW. A critical evaluation of protection provided by common safety glasses from ultraviolet emissions in welding operations. Am Ind Hyg Assoc J 1979; 40:770–780.

16. Moss CE, Gawenda MC. Optical radiation transmission levels through transparent welding curtains. NIOSH Report 78-176. Cincinnati, OH, National Institute of Occupational Safety and Health, 1978.

17. Sliney DH, Benton RE, Cole HM, Epstein SG, Morin CJ. Transmission of potentially hazardous actinic ultraviolet radiation through fabrics. Appl Ind Hyg 1987; 2:36–44.

18. Report on Tests of Welding Filter Plates. Publication No. NIOSH 76-198. Morgantown, WV. U.S. Department of Health, Education and Welfare, 1976.

CHAPTER SIXTEEN

Special Clinical Problems

Debra Bezan, M.Ed., O.D. and Donald G. Pitts, O.D., Ph.D.

16.1 Ocular Hazards and Protection for the Dental Office

The dental office is the site of numerous potential ocular hazards to dentists, auxiliary personnel, and patients alike. Ocular injuries may result from mechanical trauma, chemical trauma, microbial infection, or electromagnetic radiation damage. Although not all injuries are serious enough to cause loss of vision, and many are minor enough to go unreported, there appears to be a recent increase in the frequency of reported dental-related ocular injuries.

Epidemiology of Ocular Hazards

Seventeen cases of ocular injuries including contusions, foreign bodies, and infections were reported in survey by the American Dental Association's Bureau of Economic Research and Statistics. Three of the injuries cited in this report were severe enough to cause the loss of an eye.[1] It is difficult, however, to estimate the actual number of ocular injuries that occur in dental offices annually because many of these injuries are relatively minor and are not reported. The apparent rise in the frequency of ocular trauma in the dental office in recent years may be attributed, at least in part, to changes in the practice of modern dentistry that have increased the risk for ocular injuries. These include (1) the widespread use of four-handed dentistry (working with dental assistants), (2) working with the patient in a reclining rather than seated position, (3) working with the instrument tray positioned directly over the patient's chest, and (4) using high speed instruments.

Types of Ocular Injuries

The dental-related ocular injuries reported in the literature range from minor to severe, and as mentioned, can be divided into four major categories: (1) mechanical trauma, (2) chemical trauma, (3) microbial infection, and (4) visible and ionizing radiation.

Mechanical trauma is the most frequently reported type of dental-related ocular injury. A number of injuries result from particles being projected by high-speed and ultra-speed handpieces at velocities up to 50 mph.[1-3] A case of asymptomatic gold particles imbedded in the cornea of a dental student was revealed during a routine optometric examination.[4] Another source of mechanical trauma is from hand instruments. Records from ophthalmologic private practices were examined, and 10 cases of ocular injuries sustained in dental offices by dental assistants or patients were found. Most of these injuries were minor and resolved completely; however, one injury from an excavating instrument resulted in permanent vision loss in a 10-year-old child and subsequently involved a malpractice suit.[5] A similar case of a dental instrument injury resulted in the patient permanently losing vision. The patient who habitually wore spectacles was asked to remove them during the dental procedure and a lawsuit against the dentist for negligence resulted.[6]

Chemical splash is another source of ocular injury in the dental office. A number of chemicals that are potentially toxic to ocular tissues are found in most dental offices, including acetone, bleach, hydrogen peroxide, formocresol, eugenol, chloroform, ether, phosphoric acid, and gluteraldehyde. A reclining patient is particularly vulnerable to chemical trauma, and dental assistants are also at risk, both at the chairside and in the laboratory. A case has been reported in which an assistant sustained ocular damage from varnish that splashed in her eyes in the laboratory while she was not wearing protective eyewear.[5]

Ocular insult from *microbial infection* in the dental office can range from mild to sight-threatening. Bacteria that are part of the normal oral flora include species of *Streptococcus, Staphylococcus, Actinomyces, Neisseria, Treponema, Candida*, and *Lactobacillus*.[7] Viral pathogens include hepatitis and human immunodeficiency virus (HIV) may also be contacted through infected saliva and/or blood during dental procedures.[8] Water spray mists used to cool dental instruments such as high speed handpieces and ul-trasonic scalers can cause microbe-laden aerosols to contact ocular tissues. Cases of keratitis, conjunctivitis, and dacryocystitis from ocular exposure to aerosol contaminents have been reported.[3] Orbital cellulitis in an ocular complication that can result from a primary dental infection or secondary to dental procedures such as tooth extraction.[9]

The fourth potential source of ocular damage in the dental office is *electromagnetic radiation*. X-ray ionizing radiation has been found to be cataractogenic, but in the dosages and exposures typically administered for dental diagnostic X-rays, it poses minimal risk to the patient. Dentists and staff members should take precautions to avoid excessive exposure to direct and scattered X-ray radiation.[10] Ocular damage due to the ultraviolet (UV) and shorter visible (VIS) wavelengths is also possible.[11-13]. The early curing units primarily used near-UV (300–380 nm) to harden composite materials for tooth fissure sealants and esthetic restorations. Radiation from these units was implicated in damage to the skin and eyes of dentists, their staffs, and to the oral mucosa of the patients being treated.[11]

In recent years, there has been an increase in the use of visible light curing units (VCLUs), which emit light in the 465- to 525-nm range to harden composite materials.[14] (Fig. 16-1). Blue light, particularly in the 420- to 455-nm range, has been shown to cause photochemical damage to the retinal pigment epithelium in primates.[15,16] Spectral weighting functions for assessing retinal hazards from VLCUs have been recommended because the radiation from the VCLU is in the blue spectral region (Fig. 16-2).[16] There has been at least one case reported of maculopathy with loss of vision attributed to radiation from VCLU exposure in a dental setting.[17]

Prevention and Ocular Protection

The number of potential ocular hazards that exist in the dental office requires the use of appropriate protective eyewear by dentists, staff members, and patients as an essential part of an effective prevention program. A recent survey of Indian Health Service (IHS) dental clinics found that 91% of staff members reportedly wore eye protection while on duty; however, when asked how often protective eyewear was worn in the clinic, only 18% reported wearing protection all of the time (Fig. 16-3).[18] The Occupa-

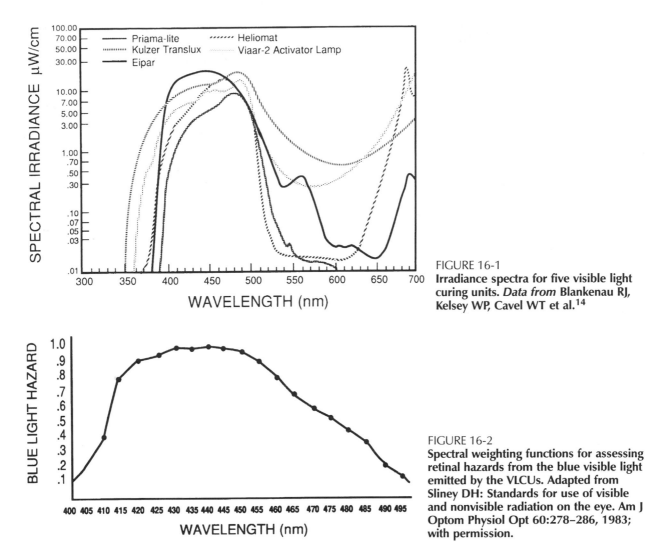

FIGURE 16-1
Irradiance spectra for five visible light curing units. *Data from* **Blankenau RJ, Kelsey WP, Cavel WT et al.**[14]

FIGURE 16-2
Spectral weighting functions for assessing retinal hazards from the blue visible light emitted by the VLCUs. Adapted from Sliney DH: Standards for use of visible and nonvisible radiation on the eye. Am J Optom Physiol Opt 60:278–286, 1983; with permission.

tional Safety and Health Administration (OSHA) is concerned about the eye safety of dental personnel to the extent that investigators evaluate the use of protective eyewear as part of a dental office hazards management inspection. OSHA recently fined a dentist $1100 for a number of citations, including removing his own eyeglasses while treating a child.[19]

The recommended lens material for safety eyewear in the dental office is polycarbonate because of its high impact resistance and ability to protect against ultraviolet radiation (UVR).[20] An incident was reported of a rubber dam clamp being ejected from the mouth with sufficient force to crack the spectacles of the dental assistant.[3] Polycarbonate

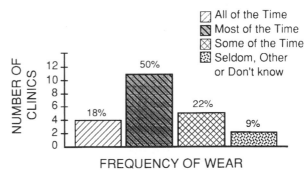

FIGURE 16-3
Frequency of use of protective eyewear in surveyed dental clinics.

lenses would have provided the required impact protection in this case. The pitting and chipping of eyeglasses of dental personnel from high velocity projectiles is quite common; therefore, polycarbonate materials should be ordered with a scratch-resistant coating applied to both surfaces.

Patients should be required to wear protective eyewear during dental procedures. Allowing patients to wear their own spectacles during all dental procedures and providing safety eyewear for those patients who do not habitually wear spectacles will assist in preventing most dental-related eye injuries.

Special filtering tints are not needed for dentists and their staffs who perform only a limited number of procedures with VLCUs. The average amount of time needed to completely cure a resin is 30 to 50 s.[13] Based on threshold limits for VIS radiation established by the American Conference of Governmental Industrial Hygienists, no more than 17 to 81 VCLU applications should be given within a 167-min time span.[21] The wide range of recommended applications is due to the varying intensities emitted by different VLCU units. When used as instructed, the VCLU is a safe instrument for use in the dental office.

Spectacle lenses with special filtering tints have been recommended for dentists and their staff members who perform a large number of restorations and sealant procedures with VLCUs (Fig. 16-4). "Blue blockers," in the form of yellow-orange tinted hand-held or instrument-mounted shields or spec-tacle lenses that block transmittance of light in the 400- to 500-nm range, have been marketed to prevent photochemical damage from prolonged exposure. These yellow-orange spectacle tints are not recommended, however, because they alter color perception and may be cosmetically unacceptable; in addition, the color perception shifts from such lenses have been shown to persist for extended periods of time (see Chapter 11). A more acceptable alternative for the VCLU user is an instrument mounted yellow-orange shield or a 20% transmittance neutral grey tinted spectacle lens that absorbs most of the potentially harmful radiation while maintaining normal color perception. Other eye safety recommendations for dentists using VCLUs include (1) not looking directly at the light and not pointing the light toward the eye of others, (2) using a delay switch whenever possible, and (3) shielding reflected light from a chairside assistant with a thumb or mirror.[18]

In addition to wearing protective eyewear and following VCLU safety precautions, dentists and their staffs should (1) always use high velocity suction when cutting on teeth or restorations to help prevent projectiles and aerosol mists from escaping the mouth, (2) never pass instruments or solutions over the patient's eyes, (3) never place sharp instruments on the patient's chest, (4) be prepared to provide first aid and then to refer to an eye care practitioner if an ocular injury should occur.[18]

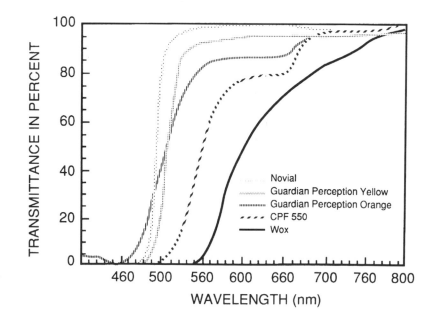

FIGURE 16-4
Transmittance spectra for five protective lenses. *Data from* Ellingson OL, Landry RJ, Bostrom RG.[21]

The key to prevention and safety is education. Many of the dentists participating in a survey of eye safety practice in the IHS dental clinics wanted more information about eye safety (Table 16-1). The study also found that disseminating information about prevention of eye injuries was an effective means of improving compliance with the eye safety policy in these dental clinics.[18] Optometrists can play a major role in preventing eye injuries in the dental office by educating dentists and their staff members about ocular hazards, by prescribing appropriate protective eyewear, and by helping the office develop guidelines for an effective eye safety policy.

16.2 Ocular Hazards from Tanning Solariums

During the 1970s when the psoralen UVA (PUVA) treatment for psoriasis evolved, fluorescent lamps were developed for exposure to the whole body. The initial research and experience with these lamps and the PUVA treatment indicated that the system was safe to the human skin.[1] This was believable because, after all, the source was UVA, and no known skin cancer had been caused by the UVA waveband. Entrepreneurs, aware that a suntan is a highly sought after commodity, especially in the colder climates of the north during the winter, established suntan par-

lors or solariums all over the world, and soon everyone was enjoying a suntan, even in the cold winter months. As time passed, it became clear that the beautiful biologic effect (the suntan) had turned into a cunning biologic hazard because the fluorescent lamps used in the PUVA treatment also produced skin cancer. The longer wavelength UVA penetrates to the deeper layers of the skin and produces a more damaging cancer. The loss in elasticity of the elastic tissue of the skin, which manifests as premature aging of the skin, remains as another of the damaging effects of UVA exposure.

The Australian Standards Association studied the sources used in solariums and the known effects of exposure to UVR because of the concerns of overexposure to UV.[2] Recommendations limited the lamp output to 200 W/cm^2 (0.02 W/m^2) and the dose to 20 J/cm^2 (200,000 J/m^2), which is about 20 min in duration. Maximum limits to UVB and UVC wavebands were set not to exceed percentages of the UVA of the source to 1% for 300 to 315 nm, 0.1% for 280 to 300 nm, and 0.01% for 100 to 280 nm. Exposure sessions were to be separated by a minimum interval of 48 h.

Occasional reports in the newspapers and the health magazines dramatize that a person can be blinded from exposure of the eye to the sun-tanning lamp. The damage to the eye is photokeratoconjunctivitis or, more simply, actinic keratoconjunctivitis. The condition usually becomes manifest 4 to 6 h after exposure, with the clinical signs of injection of the eye globes, feeling of "sand" in the eyes, redness of the adnexa, severe photophobia, and blepharospasm. Fortunately, these acute, severe symptoms can be controlled with an anesthesia for comfort and a medication to prevent secondary infection. They usually disappear within 24 h, but because UV exposures are additive over a 48-h period of time and the small doses of UV contained in sunlight may trigger a following episode. These reports require that a hazard evaluation of the solarium lamp be accomplished to determine if exposure to the eye will result in permanent damage.

	Yes	No	Don't know
Are safety glasses available to dental personnel at the nearest IHS optometry clinic?	73%	18%	9%
Are you aware that there is a PHS protective eyewear policy currently in effect?	68%	32%	0%
Do you feel that your clinic needs more information on the current policy or on eye safety in general?	64%	36%	0%

TABLE 16-1
Survey Responses About U.S. Public Health Service Policy and Availability of Protective Eyewear

Spectral Irradiance of Solarium Lamps

Table 16-2 presents various types of fluorescent lamps that are commonly used as sources in solariums. Figure 16-5 illustrates the spectral irradiance of

Manufacturer	Lamp-Ordering Abbreviation
General Electric	Sontegra F70T12/BL/S/1
Osram	L100/79
Philips	Wolff TL65/80W/09*
	TL85-100W/09
	Wolff A1.00.100W Solarium
Sylvania	Wolff RA-10-100W Relarium
	PUVA

*The only lamp in the table that produces below 100 W.

TABLE 16-2
Various Types of Fluorescent Lamps Used in the Tanning Solarium

the Philips TL65/80W lamp. The lamp output is from both the UVB and UVA regions of the optical spectrum. The spectral irradiance begins at 290 nm and extends to 400 nm, with the peak wavelength at 355 nm. The total irradiance is 0.01069 W/cm^2 with 0.000039 W/cm^2 or 0.3% being in the UVB and 99.7% being in the UVA. The log plot of the irradiance emphasizes the UVB portion of the spectrum. The remaining lamps in Table 16-2 have a radiant power of 100 W and produce considerably more UVB radiation; however, spectral irradiance data for these lamps are not readily available.

Hazard Evaluation

Table 16-3 provides the spectral irradiance for the Philips TL65/80W, the relative effectiveness S_λ for the human cornea (see Table 6-3), and the relative effectiveness for the rabbit lens (see Table 6-6). The example calculations demonstrate that, if the human cornea were exposed to the solarium lamp for greater than 22.4 min, photokeratitis will result, but lenticular cataractogenesis should not occur until 11.02 h of exposure. These data are cause for concern because the 80-W solarium lamp produces the least UVR of those listed. The remaining lamps produce 4 to 10 times the UVB as the 80-W lamp, and the allowable safe exposure duration would be shortened accordingly.

The hazard evaluation demonstrates that the lamps used in solariums are hazardous to the eye.

Nachtwey and Rundel[25] calculated that two lamps at 33 cm produce 3.94 times more sunburning irradiance than the noontime sun at 30° N latitude, which results in a minimal erythemal dose (MED) after 3 ± 1.5 min. A person who is achieving the necessary UV exposure for a tan is being exposed to UVR capable of causing cancer of the skin. The following is required to ensure safe eye exposure:

1. Protective eyewear with sideshields should be worn at all times when being exposed to the suntan lamp radiation.
2. Timers should be used that are lock protected so that the proprieter of the solarium must be present to reset time.
3. Warning notices that the lamps are hazardous to the human eye and skin should be clearly posted.
4. Exposure durations and schedule records should be maintained for each customer.
5. The maximum allowable dose should not exceed 20 J/cm^2, separated by a minimum 48-h delay.

The limitation of the maximum dose to 20 J/cm^2 still requires ocular protection because the UV irradiance to achieve the 20 J/cm^2 would exceed the corneal photokeratitis threshold before a tanning

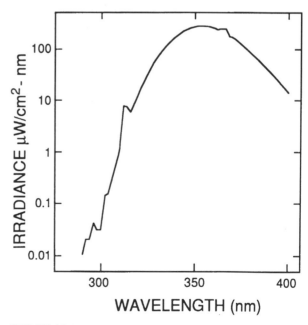

FIGURE 16-5
Spectral irradiance of a Phillips TL65/80W/09 (Wolff-type) fluorescent lamp used in a solarium. *Adapted from Perkins.*[38]

TABLE 16-3

Spectral Irradiance $E_{e\lambda}$ and Relative Effectiveness S_λ for the Human Cornea and Rabbit Lens and Effective Irradiances E_{eff} for a Wolff-type Phillips TL65/80W/09 UVA Solarium Lamp

Wavelength (nm)	Sun Tanning Lamp—Phillips TL65/80W/09—Spectral Irradiance $E_{e\lambda}$ (μW/cm²·nm)	Human Cornea Relative Effectiveness (S_λ)	Human Cornea Effective Irradiance E_{eff} (μW/cm²·nm)	Rabbit Lens Relative Effectiveness (S_λ)	Rabbit Lens Effective Irradiance E_{eff} (μW/cm²·nm)
280	0.0	0.68	—	—	—
285	0.0	—	—	—	—
290	0.01	0.57	0.0057	—	—
295	0.03	0.57	0.017	0.20	0.006
300	0.03	0.57	0.017	1.00	0.03
305	0.22	0.43	0.286	0.50	0.11
310	1.20	0.29	0.095	0.20	0.24
315	6.48	0.004	0.026	0.033	0.21
320	13.45	0.0004	—	0.012	0.16
325	33.90			—	—
330	68.80				
335	117.25				
340	174.20				
345	229.00				
350	261.00				
355	267.50				
360	248.00				
365	242.00				
370	161.30				
375	117.20				
380	80.20				
385	53.40				
390	35.00				
395	22.80				
400	14.30				

Human Cornea:
$$\Sigma = 2.23 \times 10^{-6}\ \text{W/cm}^2$$
$$*t = \frac{0.003\ \text{J/cm}^2}{2.23 \times 10^{-6}}$$
$$= 1345\ \text{s}$$
$$= 22.4\ \text{min}$$
$$= 0.37\ \text{h}$$

Rabbit Lens:
$$\Sigma = 3.78 \times 10^{-6}\ \text{W/cm}^2$$
$$*t = \frac{0.15\ \text{J/cm}^2}{3.78 \times 10^{-6}}$$
$$t = 39{,}682\ \text{s}$$
$$= 661\ \text{min}$$
$$= 11.02\ \text{h}$$

*The safe exposure duration is calculated for the human cornea and rabbit lens in the space below the effective irradiance.

session would end. Further, UV exposure is cumulative, and each exposure session increases the danger of lenticular cataracts and skin cancer.

16.3 Ocular Hazards from Clinical Instruments

During the 1960s and 1970s, five new technologies were introduced into the ophthalmic professions: fiber optics, halogen and xenon lamps, phacoemulsification, intraocular lenses (IOLs), and lasers. Each of these technologies caused an impact on the visual system independently and collectively, and the task of determining cause and effect of the ocular problems created by their use is almost impossible. These technologies will be covered in this chapter with the exception of lasers, which were treated in Chapters 7 and 8.

Halogen and xenon lamps provide high intensity sources to allow "better" visualization of the interior of the eye.[26] Excellent arguments can be made to support their need because the reflectance of light from the retina is not too great,[27] but the higher intensity sources are not without their penalties. The halogen tungsten sources operated at 3000 K and above, possessed quartz envelopes and, for the first time, produced UVR in the UVB wavelengths. The xenon lamps combined with fiber optics produced a light source called the *endoilluminator* that transported the high intensity source to the surface of the retina. These new sources provided the light source, and with fiber optics, surgical microscopes, and the phacoemulsification unit made up the technology that revolutionized ophthalmic surgery.

Cataract surgery by phacoemulsification was a surgical technique that was "tailor made" for the IOL. Phacoemulsification allowed the surgeon to retain the posterior capsule of the lens to serve as a retainer for the vitreous humor and as a "pocket" for the posterior IOL. In skilled surgical hands, phacoemulsification and IOLs became the standard for cataract surgery, but in spite of its advantages, ultrasound is a mechanical form of energy, and there was inadequate information about its effect on ocular tissue (see Chapter 6).

As soon as these new technologies were introduced into practice, ocular problems thought to be caused by their use began to appear in the literature.

The chronic or long-term effects of exposure of the human retina to light (phototoxicity) are not fully known because human epidemiologic studies are difficult and have not been done. Most of the research on the phototoxic effects of optical radiation exposure to the retina have been on acute or short-duration exposures and have been accomplished on the primate,[27-30] rabbit,[31] rat,[32] and occasionally, the pigmy pig. Only on rare occasions have human exposures been available. These human exposures were not usually under controlled laboratory conditions and include welding maculopathy,[33] eclipse blindness,[34,35] and solar retinopathy.[36] They clearly demonstrate that the human retina can suffer damage from photic exposure. Acute exposures emulate the exposures of the eye in the clinical situation and will be emphasized in the following discussion.

Macular edema was related to cataract surgery as early as 1954;[37] however, cystoid macular edema was not described until 1966.[38] A review of the records of 1000 patients who had intracapsular cataract surgery using clear corneal incisions with forceps or cryosurgery showed that less than 3% experienced macular edema.[39] Cystoid macular edema may be found in as many as 50% of the cataract patients[40] and has occurred more frequently in the 55- to 60-year-old-patient[16] since phacoemulsification and IOLs have become standard procedures.

Early experiments on the effects of light on the retina[32,42-45] supported the conclusion that the intense illumination from the indirect ophthalmoscope operating microscope, and endoilluminator was capable of causing damage to the patient's retina in the form of macular edema[46-48] and cystoid maculopathy.[49-52] Visual acuity was found reduced up to 6 mo after cataract surgery, and was related to the light in the operating microscope.[53] Visual acuity was not affected when the UVR was filtered from the lamp.[54,55] The prevalance of cystoid macular edema after cataract extraction and IOL implantation was reported to be 8.5% with intracapsular surgery, 4.35% with extracapsular surgery, and 1.69% with phacoemulsification.[56] Posterior capsulotomy was performed on 96% of the patients who underwent the extracapsular and phacoemulsification procedures.

The endoilluminator posed an additional hazard because the light is located very close to the retina, which increases the risk of phototoxicity and cumulative phototoxic effects.[57] A filter that eliminated radiation below 505 nm reduced the light intensity on the retina by 20% and increased the allowable duration of surgery.[58]

Not all experiments have claimed irreparable retinal damage from severe exposures. An indirect ophthalmoscope that produced 0.42 W at the cornea was used to expose the human eye for 45 min through a 20-Diopter lens. A dramatic decrease in visual acuity occurred 24 h postexposure and the corneal stroma remained edematous for 72 h, but the electroretinogram, electro-oculogram, and dark adaptation curves were normal 24 h after exposure. The light exposures were sufficient to cause severe anterior segment damage but failed to produce irreversible retinal damage; therefore, the clinical significance of exposure to the light of clinical instruments was questioned.[59] The recuperative powers of the eye have been documented from recovery of solar eclipse blindness[36,60] and the recovery of the photoreceptor cells of the primate retina after damage from exposure to an indirect ophthalmoscope.[61] Figure 16-6 illustrates the relationship between the retinal irradiance from clinical instruments and procedures and the ocular exposure from environmental conditions, and compares both exposure situations to the ANSI Z136.1 maximum permissible exposure (MPE) and experimental exposures for threshold damage.

Radiation Measurements for Clinical Instruments

Hazards evaluation may be accomplished when the MPE of a source in J/cm^2 and the irradiance of the source in W/cm^2 are known for equivalent wavebands. The MPE selected by Calkins and Hochheimer[62] is 2.92 J/cm^2, and if the irradiance of the source (W/cm^2) is known, calculation of the safe exposure duration can be made. The MPE can be as low as 2.40 J/cm^2 because the integrated transmittance of the human ocular media is 0.77 instead of 0.90. The MPE would be calculated as follows:

$$t[s] = \frac{MPE \text{ in } J/cm^2}{E_e \text{ in } W/cm^2} \qquad (16\text{-}1)$$

The MPE that has been selected provides a built-in safety factor because it is two magnitudes below the LD 50 threshold for producing an ophthalmoscopically visible retinal lesion. In addition, the MPE was established using the primate, and the human retina requires twice the radiant exposure as the primate retina.[29] A fuller explanation of the MPE is given in Chapter 9.

DIRECT OPHTHALMOSCOPES
An evaluation of the hand-held, direct ophthalmoscope retinal irradiance studies indicates that, with

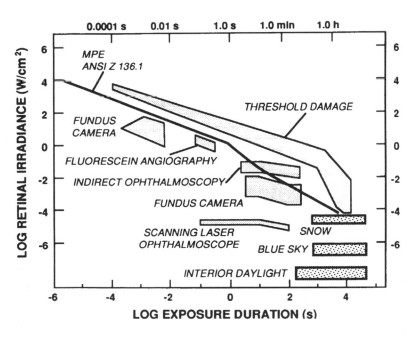

FIGURE 16-6
The relationship between the retinal irradiance of clinical instruments, clinical procedures, and environmental sources to the ANSI Z136.1 MPE and the research-established retinal threshold damage. *Data from* Mainster MA, Ham WT, Jr, and Delori FC.[48]

normal clinical use, the direct ophthalmoscope is safe.[62,63] The halogen quartz bulb of the hand-held ophthalmoscopes produce a spectral irradiance from 320 nm to greater than 1800 nm. None of the instruments measured produced radiation in the UVB and UVC spectral regions, but the mean spectral irradiance in the UVA region from 320 to 400 nm was found to vary from 2.1 to 573 $\mu W/cm^2$, with a mean value of 76.5 $\mu W/cm^2$. The infrared (IR) irradiance from 700 to 1800 nm gave a range of 2.4 to 148 mW/cm^2 and a mean value of 22.8 mW/cm^2. The VIS spectrum from 400 to 700 nm produced a range of irradiances from 1.6 to 204 mW/cm^2, with a mean value of 21.5 mW/cm^2. Table 16-4 provides a hazard evaluation of the direct ophthalmoscope that clearly demonstrates its safety. It would be very difficult to maintain the direct light from a hand-held ophthalmoscope on a single location for 75 s.

BINOCULAR INDIRECT OPHTHALMOSCOPES

Table 16-2 provides the retinal irradiance measurements for 15 individual binocular indirect ophthalmoscopes (BIOs) using the 20 D lens.[63] The retinal irradiance varies from 58.9 to 127.2 mW/cm^2 and provides a safe exposure duration from 22.9 to 49.6 s. Under normal clinical conditions the BIO may be considered safe, but care should be taken when additional clinicians view the same patient's retina repeatedly. Use caution also when viewing a diseased retina because such a retina is probably not as resistant to light damage as a healthy retina. It would be prudent to filter the UVR and IR from the light source because they are not needed to visualize the retina. Filtering UVR also eliminates concern of photochemical and cumulative damage to the cornea, lens, and retina. IR is not particularly damaging to the ocular tissues but raises the temperature,

Instrument	Number (N)	Voltage (V)	Mean Retinal Irradiance (m W/cm^2)	MPE (s)
Direct ophthalmoscope				
A-O Giantoscope and Welch-Allyn	2	Maximum	29.0	78.9
Indirect ophthalmoscope				
20d lines American Optical	10	6.5	75.3	38.8
	10	7.8–8.4	127.2	22.9
Frigi-Xonix	5	6.5	58.9	49.6
	5	7.8–8.4	121.2	24.1
Slit lamp				
Haag-Steit	4	5.0	140.0	21.0
	4	6.0	217.0	13.0
		7.5	358.0	8.0
Surgical Lamps				
Castle Model 800, 24-in.-diameter smooth reflector	2	343 cm mean distance	24.0	122.0
Castle, 18-in.-diameter ribbed reflector	4	387 cm mean distance	20.4	150.5

NOTE: The range of the indirect ophthalmoscope measurements varied from 50.9 mW/cm^2 (57.4 s MPE) to 133 mW/cm^2 (22 s MPE) at 6.5 V. With a maximum power setting at 7.8 to 8.4 V, the measured irradiance of the indirect ophthalmoscopes varied from 85 mW/cm^2 (34.4 s MPE) to 205 mW/cm^2 (14.2 s MPE). Safe exposure duration is based on an MPE of 2.92 J/cm^2 for retinal damage, with 7-mm pupils, which is two orders of magnitude below the 50% level of probability to produce a retinal lesion.

From Hochheimer BF, D'Anna SA, Calkins JL. Retinal damage from light. Am J Ophthalmol 88:1039–1044, 1979; published with permission from the American Journal of Ophthalmology. Copyright by the Ophthalmic Publishing Company.

TABLE 16-4
Mean Safe Exposure Duration from the Direct Ophthalmoscope, Indirect Ophthalmoscope, Slit Lamp, and Surgical Lamps to Achieve MPE

which lowers the threshold for UVR photochemical damage. The filter could use absorption to eliminate UVR and the inconel metallic coating to eliminate IR (Chapter 9). The BIO light is annoying to patients and should be maintained at a level as low as possible consistent with good clinical practice. The aphake and the patient who takes medications that result in increased photosensitivity must be considered.

OPHTHALMIC MICROSCOPIC SURGICAL LAMPS

Measurements for 11 ophthalmic microscopic surgical lamps showed a maximum irradiance of 96.5 mW/cm^2 and a minimum irradiance of 17.8 mW/cm^2. There was an average percent UVR below 400 nm of 0.42% and for IR above 700 nm of 27.16%. The MPE ranges from 2 min to 1 h for the phakic eye but is less than 6.5 min for the aphakic eye. These hazards evaluations indicate that the ophthalmic microscopic illuminators are safe for momentary viewing, but care should be taken by the surgeon to reduce retinal exposure to a minimum.[66]

It has been recommended that the operating microscope be directed toward the retina to miss the macular area. In addition, filtering out the UVR and IR would increase the allowable exposure duration. Care must be taken with the aphakic eye and for those patients who take medications that result in an increase in photosensitivity.

OVERHEAD SURGICAL LAMPS

Concerns about ocular exposure to overhead surgical lamps arise because surgical procedures usually require periods of time that exceed the MPE. The mean retinal irradiance of overhead surgical lamps is about 24 mW/cm^2 (Table 16-4), which is almost equivalent to the direct ophthalmoscope, about one third the irradiance of the indirect ophthalmoscope and about one tenth the irradiance of the slit lamp. Care must be taken to protect the eyes—especially the retina—when surgical lamp radiation can reach them.[62]

ENDOILLUMINATORS

The endoilluminator is of particular concern because the radiation is usually only a few millimeters from the retina and the vitreal surgical procedures are commonly long in duration. Table 16-5 provides retinal irradiance measurements for five different

		80-W Light Source		150-W Light Source	
Type of Endoilluminator	Distance from Retina	Maximum Retinal Irradiance (mW/cm^2)	Exposure Duration to Damage (min)	Maximum Retinal Irradiance (mW/cm^2)	Exposure Duration to Damage (min)
19-Gauge continuous fiber	2mm	4700	0.7	8600	0.38
	6mm	560	6.3	960	3.2
20-Gauge continuous fiber	2mm	2700	1.2	5000	3.2
	6mm	300	11.0	560	5.9
19-Gauge detachable-tip infusion needle	2mm	560	5.9	1130	2.9
	6mm	62	53.0	125	26.0
20-Gauge detachable-tip conical beam	2mm	760	4.3	1570	2.1
	6mm	84	39.0	175	19.0
20-Gauge detachable-tip membrane PIC	2mm	400	8.2	810	4.1
	6mm	44	75.0	90	37.0

From Meyers SM, Bonner RF: Retinal irradiance from vitrectomy endoilluminators. Am J Ophthalmol 94:26–29, 1982; published with permission of The American Journal of Ophthalmology. Copyright by the Ophthalmic Publishing Company.

TABLE 16-5
Measured Retinal Irradiance and Calculated Allowable Safe Exposure Durations to Achieve Ophthalmoscopic Damage Threshold for Five Endoilluminators

endoilluminators using the 80-W and the 150-W lamps, 2-mm and 6-mm distances from the retina, and the safe retinal exposure durations for each different source.[57] Depending on the configuration of the endoilluminator, the retinal irradiance varies from 8600 mW/cm^2 with a 0.38 s exposure duration to 44 mW/cm^2 with a 75 s exposure duration. The duration of time necessary for the vitrectomy surgical procedure greatly exceeds the safe allowable exposure duration, so the retina is at risk. The following suggestions are made to reduce the hazards of retinal injury when the endoilluminators are used during surgical procedures:[67]

1. Use filters to eliminate IR, UVR, and other unneeded optical radiation.
2. Plan vitreous surgery carefully to minimize the duration of the surgery.
3. Keep fiber optic light output low and at as great a distance as feasible from the retina.
4. Use intermittent lighting to allow thermal absorption to be kept to a minimum.
5. Work at different surgical sites alternately to reduce overall exposure.
6. Orient the fiber optic light in such a way to minimize direct illumination.

The risk of damage to the retina from the endoilluminator is great. Filtering UVR and IR will assist in lengthening the safe exposure durations to almost double the times in Table 16-5. An understanding of the problem and a judicious application of the previously noted suggestions will reduce the hazard and keep subsequent damage to the retina to a minimum.

References

1. Hartley JL. Eye and facial injuries resulting from dental procedures. Dent Clin North Am 1978; 22:505–15.
2. Wesson MD, Thorton JB. Eye protection and ocular complications in the dental office. Gen Dent 1989; 37:19–23.
3. Luxl F, Klopfer J. Eye injuries in the dental office. Symposium pamphlet from the annual meeting of the American Society of Dentistry for Children, October 1980.
4. Robinson E. Gold infiltrates a dentist's cornea. Rev. Optom 1981; 118:72–74.
5. Hales RH. Ocular injuries sustained in the dental office. Am J Ophthalmol 1970; 70:221–223.
6. Gregg B, Davies J. Malpractice: A case for safety glasses. J Can Dent Assoc 1986; 52:583–586.
7. Lewis ML (ed): Dental Microbiology, pp 126–134. St. Louis, Washington University, 1977.
8. Runnells RR. Practicing Infection Control Hazards Management and Dentistry in the Real World, pp 19–20. Fruit Heights, UT: IC Publications, 1989.
9. Kaban LB, McGill T. Orbital cellulitis of dental origin: differential diagnosis and the use of computerized tomography as a diagnostic aid. J Oral Surg 1980; 38:682–685.
10. Alcox RW. Biological effects and radiation protection in the dental office. Dent Clin North Am 1978; 22:517–532.
11. Mills LF. Alleged Injuries Involving Use of Ultraviolet Radiation in Dentistry, pp 1–6. Rockville, MD, U.S. Department of Health, Education and Welfare, 1973.
12. Mills LF, Lytle CD, Andersen AF, Hollman KB, Bockstahler LE. A Review of Biological Effects and Potential Risks Associated with Ultraviolet Radiation As Used in Dentistry, pp 1–27. (FDA) 76-8021. Rockville, MD, U.S. Department of Health, Education and Welfare, date.
13. Eriksen P, Moscato PM. Nonionizing Radiation Protection Study No. 25 42-0334-86: Optical Hazard Evaluation of Dental Curing Lights, August-November 1985, pp 1–5. Aberdeen Proving Ground, MD, U.S. Army Environmental Hygiene Agency, 1986.
14. Blankenau RJ, Kelsey WP, Cavel WT, et al. Wavelength and intensity of seven systems for visible light curing composite resins: a comparison study. J Am Dent Assoc 1983; 106:471–474.
15. Ham WT, Ruffolo JJ, Mueller HA, et al. The nature of retinal radiation damage: Dependence on wavelength, power level and exposure time. Vision Res 1980; 20:1105–1111.
16. Sliney DH. Standards for use of visible and nonvisible radiation on the eye. Am J Optom Physiol Opt 1983; 60:278–286.
17. Myers JS. Personal communication, April 10, 1989.
18. Bezan D, Bezan K. Prevention of eye injuries in the dental office. J Am Optom Assoc 1988; 59:929–934.
19. Jacob JA. ADA files OSHA challenge, backs dentist in test case. Am Dent Assoc News 1990; 21:1.
20. Davis JK. Perspectives on impact resistance and polycarbonate lenses. Int Ophthalmol Clin 1988; 28:215–218.
21. Ellingson OL, Landry RJ, Bostrom RG. An evaluation of optical radiation emissions from dental visible photopolymerization devices. J Am Dent Assoc 1986; 112:67–70.
22. Parrish JA, Anderson RR, Urbach F, Pitts DG. UV-A Biologic Effects of Ultraviolet Radiation with Emphasis on Human Response to Longwave Ultraviolet. New York, Plenum Press, 1978.

23. Wilkinson FJ. Recommended UV exposure limits for tanning equipment, and spectral irradiances of solarium lamps, sun lamps and daylight. Aust Phys Eng Sci Med 1983; 62:26–34.

24. Perkins RF. Personal communication.

25. Nachtwey DS, Rundel RD. A photobiological evaluation of tanning booths. Science 1981; 211:405–407.

26. Zubler EG, Mosby FA. An iodine incandescent lamp with virtually 100 per cent lumen maintenance. Illum Eng 1959; LIV:734.

27. Vos JJ, Munnick AA, Bougard J. Absolute spectral reflectance of the fundus oculi. J Opt Soc Am [A] 1965; 55:573–574.

28. Ham WT, Jr, Ruffolo JJ, Jr, Mueller HA, Clarke AM, Moon ME. Histologic analysis of photochemical lesions produced in rhesus retina by short-wave-light. Invest Ophthalmol 1978; 17:1029–1035.

29. Ham WT, Jr, Mueller, HA, Williams RC, Geeraets WJ. Ocular hazards from viewing the sun unprotected and through various windows and filters. Appl Opt 1973; 12:2122–2129.

30. Schmidt RE, Zuclich JA. Retinal lesions due to ultraviolet laser exposure. Invest Ophthalmol Vis Sci 1980; 19:1166–1175.

31. Lawwill T. Effect of prolonged exposure of the rabbit retina to low-intensity light. Invest Ophthalmol 1973; 12:45–51.

32. Noell WK, Walker VS, Kang BS, Berman BS. Retinal damage by light in rats. Invest Ophthalmol 1966; 5:450–473.

33. Naidoff MA, Sliney DH. Retinal injury from a welding arc. Am J Ophthalmol 1974; 77:663–668.

34. Flynn J. Photoretinitis in anti-aircraft lookouts. Med J Aust 1942; 2:400–401.

35. Pang HG. Eclipse retinopathy. Am J Ophthalmol 1963; 55:383–384.

36. Yannuzi LA, Fisher YL, Krueger A, Slakter J. Solar retinopathy: A photobiological and geophysical analysis. Trans Am Ophthalmol Soc 1987; LXXXV:120–158.

37. Nichols JVV. Macular edema in association cataract extraction. Am J Ophthalmol 1954; 37:665–672.

38. Gass JDM, Norton EWD. Cystoid macular edema and papilledema following cataract extraction: A fluorescein fundoscopic and angiographic study. Arch Ophthalmol 1966; 76:646–661.

39. Meredith TA, Maumenee AE. A review of one thousand cases of intracapsular cataract extraction, 1. Complications. Ophthalmic Surg 1979; 10:32–41.

40. Hitchings BA, Chisholm IH, Bird AC. Aphakic macular edema: Incidence and pathogenesis. Invest Ophthalmol 1975; 14:68–72.

41. Kraff MC, Sanders DR, Jampol DM. Prophylaxis of pseudophakic cystoid macular edema with topical indomethacin. Ophthalmology 1982; 89:885–890.

42. Vos JJ. A theory of retinal burns. Bull Math Biophys 1962; 24:115–128.

43. Gorn RA, Kuwabara T. Retinal damage by visible light. Arch Ophthalmol 1967; 77:115–118.

44. Friedman E, Kuwabara T. The retinal pigment epithelium, IV. The damaging effects of radiant energy. Arch Ophthalmol 1968; 80:265–279.

45. Hochheimer BF, D'Anna SA, Calkins JL. Retinal damage from light. Am J Ophthalmol 1979; 88:1039–1044.

46. Pomerantzeff O, Govignon J, Schepens CL. Indirect Ophthalmoscopy: Is the illumination level dangerous? Am Acad Ophthalmol Otol Trans 1969; 73:246–250.

47. Tso MOM, Shih C-Y. Experimental macular edema after lens extraction. Invest Ophthalmol Vis Sci 1977; 16:381–392.

48. Mainster MA, Ham WT, Jr, Delori FC. Potential retinal hazards: Instrument and environmental light sources. Am Acad Ophthalmol 1983; 90:927–932.

49. Tso MOM, Fine BS, Zimmerman LE. Photic maculopathy produced by the indirect microscope, 1. Clinical and histopathological study. Am J Ophthalmol 1972; 73:686–699.

50. Henry MM, Henry LM, Henry LM. A possible cause of chronic cystic maculopathy Ann Ophthalmol 1977; 9:455.

51. Hochheimer BF. A possible cause of chronic cystic maculopathy: The operating microscope. Ann Opthalmol 1981; 13:153–155.

52. McDonald HR, Irvine AR. Light-induced maculopathy from the operating microscope in extracapsular cataract extraction and intraocular lens implantation. Am Acad Ophthalmol 1983; 90:945–951.

53. Berler DK, Peyser R. Light intensity and visual acuity following cataract surgery. Am Acad Ophthalmol 1983; 90:933–936.

54. Jamopol LM, Kraff MC, Sanders DR, Alexander K, Lieberman H. Near-UV radiation from the operating microscope and pseudophakic cystoid macular edema. Arch Ophthalmol 1985; 103:28–30.

55. Parver LM, Auker CR, Fine BS. Observations on monkey eyes exposed to light from an operating microscope. Am Acad Opthalmol 1983; 90:964–972.

56. Moses L. Incidence of cystoid macular edema following cataract extraction with pseudophakes implantation: Intracapsular vs extracapsular vs phacoemulisification. Am Intra-ocular Implant Soc J 1978; IV:17.

57. Meyers SM, Bonner RF. Retinal irradiance from vitrectomy endoilluminators. Am J Ophthalmol 1982; 94:26–29.

58. Meyers SM, Bonner RF. Yellow filter to decrease the risk of light damage to the retina during vitrectomy. Am J Ophthalmol 1982; 94:677.

59. Robertson DM, Erickson GJ. The effect of prolonged indirect ophthalmoscopy on the human eye. Am J Ophthalmol 1979; 87:652–661.

60. Penner R, McNair JN. Eclipse blindness: Report of an epidemic in the military population of Hawaii. Am J Ophthalmol 1966; 61:1452–1457.

61. Tso MOM. Photic maculopathy in rhesus monkey. A light and electron microscopy study. Invest Ophthalmol 1973; 12:17–34.

62. Calkins JL, Hochheimer BF. Retinal light exposure from ophthalmoscopes, slit lamps, and overhead surgical lamps. An analysis of potential hazards. Invest Ophthalmol Vis Sci 1980; 19:1009–1015.

63. James RH, Bostrom RG, Remark D, Sliney DH. Handheld ophthalmoscopes for hazard analysis: An evaluation. Appl Opt 1988; 27:5072–5076.

64. Sliney DH, Armstrong BC. Radiometric evaluation of surgical microscope lights for hazard analysis. Appl Opt 1986; 25:1882–1889.

65. Calkins JL, Hocheimer BF. Retinal light exposure from operation microscope. Arch Ophthalmol 1979; 97:2363–2367.

66. Irvine AR, Copenhagen Dr. The focal nature of retinal illumination from the operating microscope. Arch Ophthalmol 1985; 103:549–550.

67. Kuhn F, Morris R, Massey M. Photic retinal injury from endoillumination during vitrectomy. Am J Ophthalmol 1991; 111:42–46.

CHAPTER SEVENTEEN

Vision and Drugs

Marilyn E. Schneck, O.D., Ph.D., and Anthony J. Adams, O.D., Ph.D.

Broadly speaking, drugs may be divided into therapeutic and social categories. Both classes of drugs are widely used in our society. The eye is structurally and metabolically diverse, so it is not surprising that it can be adversely affected by a wide range of substances, which results in a large number of ophthalmic disorders. Drug-induced effects may occur in the pre-retinal structures (cornea, lens, pupil); the oculomotor system; the vasculature; the retina; or the neural structures, including the optic pathways, visual cortex, or nonvisual cortex. Many of these effects can be expected to produce visual changes.

The limited space of this chapter does not permit a discussion or catalogs of all drug effects, and so we include a partial list of compendia: *The Physician's Desk Reference*; *American Drug Index* (periodical); *American Pharmaceutical Association* (periodical); *American Professional Pharmacist* (was *Pharmacy Times*); and references 2 through 13. Whereas the works by Silverman are not current, they are useful because they contain sections in which visual side effects are listed and the drugs associated with them given. A computer diskette is available that contains a very

---

The authors gratefully acknowledge the assistance of Rodger D. Hamer, MD, for medication consultation and Ken Huie for graphics.

useful program and data base, *Optometric Drug Information Summaries* (ODIS),* which provides information about many systemic drugs and their visual side effects. In this chapter we restrict ourselves to the visual effects of drugs that are so prevalent as to constitute an "environmental" factor, that is, the most common social drugs—alcohol, marijuana, and cigarettes as well as commonly used over-the-counter and prescription therapeutics. The over-the-counter and prescription therapeutics are covered in the references noted. In particular, we emphasize those effects that are likely to mimic, and therefore may be mistaken for, visual changes encountered in optometric practice.

Discussions of the adverse effects of drugs on vision should distinguish acute effects from those resulting from chronic use of the drug. In either case, a distinction must also be made between those drugs that are likely to cause visual symptoms at therapeutic dose levels from those that produce symptoms only at toxic levels. A drug may have only acute effects with no known consequences specifically attributable to chronic use, or alternatively, visual side effects may be absent with acute administration of the substance and become apparent only after prolonged exposure. Some substances, such as alcohol, produce changes in vision under both circumstances, with the pattern of disturbance differing considerably between acute and chronic cases. Information about the acute effects of drugs is typically obtained by administering a known amount of the substance to individuals of known (and usually limited) history with the drug after a specified period of abstinence from the drug. Experimentally, chronic effects are often assessed after a known period of abstinence from the drug in individuals with a prolonged and heavy usage history. However, in practice the chronic effects are most likely to come to light while the patient is currently using a drug that has been used regularly for some time. In some instances (e.g., chloroquine retinopathy), adverse effects may continue to progress after cessation of drug use. Unfortunately, many reports in the literature fail to make some of these important distinctions or provide information in interpreting reported side effects.

---

*Available from Dr. Leonard Levine, College of Optometry, Pacific University, 2043 College Way, Forest Grove, Oregon 97116. Include a $10.00 check made payable to Pacific University.

This chapter considers the visual disturbances of the social drugs, particularly alcohol and marijuana, followed by brief sections on less well studied cigarette smoking and caffeine. Where information is available, the acute and chronic effects are considered separately. Following is a consideration of the visual effects reported for some of the drugs that are most commonly prescribed, as well as drugs that are infrequently prescribed but about which much has been made of the visual side effects. A discussion of the effects of the drugs commonly used by the elderly, for whom medications present special concern[78,100] follows. Finally, within the context of drug use by the elderly, we present a discussion of common over-the-counter preparations such as anti-inflammatories, analgesics, antihistamines, and decongestants. Throughout the chapter, the intent is to emphasize the effects that social drugs have on vision, as opposed to ocular tissues per se. Such drug effects are important for the optometric practitioner to distinguish from vision changes associated with non–drug disease processes.

17.1 Alcohol

Alcohol, one of the most widely used social drugs, is generally considered a central nervous system depressant. The effect is progressive, with moderate doses affecting higher cortical centers and the fundamental body functions being disturbed at higher doses. There is evidence, however, that alcohol may act directly on the human retina, opening up the possibility for changes in the earliest stages of processing of a wide range of visual functions.[15,16] These changes are separate from and additional to changes in cognitive function, attention, and higher visual processes. Alcohol may also exert its effect on vision function by interfering with the fine control of the oculomotor system on which proper visual function critically depends.

Acute Sensory and Oculomotor Effects

SENSORY EFFECTS
Color vision changes are among the earliest alterations in vision function observed in many ocular and systemic diseases and toxicities. Acute ingestion

of alcohol, even at doses below the legal limit for driving, has also been shown to produce a characteristic pattern of color vision changes.

A loss of hue discrimination measured with the desaturated D-15 and Farnsworth Munsell 100-hue arrangement tests has been reported in observers with blood alcohol levels (BAL) of 0.07 to 0.16%.[17] Errors occurred along tritanopic and tetartanopic axes on both tests, from which the authors concluded that alcohol affected SWS (blue) cones and/or their interactions with LWS (red) cones.[18] Blue-yellow defects after alcohol ingestion but no loss of color discrimination was found using a Farnsworth 28-hue test.[19]

The results support earlier research on hue discrimination using the FM 100-hue that had shown small but significant dose-related impairments associated with alcohol ingestion.[20,21] Errors were pre-dominantly located on the blue region of the test (Fig. 17-1) indicating that alcohol consumption may lead to confusion of blues with blue-greens and blue-purples. The changes associated with acute alcohol ingestion resemble defects associated with mild acquired color vision disorders in which a tritan/deutan defect is often seen as an early sign of retinal disease.

The FM 100-hue and the anomaloscope are particularly useful in detecting and characterizing acquired color vision defects.[22] Given the similarity of alcohol-induced color discrimination loss to the early acquired color vision defects such as those associated with retinal diseases (e.g., glaucoma), anomaloscope matches can provide additional information about the nature of the color vision "loss" associated with alcohol ingestion. The anomaloscope assesses the integrity of the "red" and "green" cone systems, with little or no stimulation of the

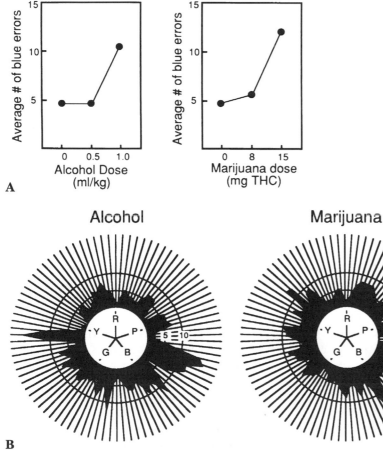

FIGURE 17-1
A. Pattern of error scores for nine subjects on the Farnsworth-Munsell 100-hue test 30 min after ingestion of 1 mL/kg ethanol (*left*) and 15 mg THC marijuana (*right*). **B.** The errors are plotted on the conventional polar coordinate score sheet and arbitrarily magnified 10 times to more clearly demonstrate differences around the color circle.

"blue" cones. The anomaloscope measures the relative amounts of red and green light in a mixture field required to match a standard yellow field. An increase in the amount of red required in a red/green mixture following ingestion of 1 mL alcohol/kg body weight has been reported.[23] A small but statistically significant change in the color mixture function as a result of acute alcohol consumption, with more red light required in the red/green mixture to match the yellow, was found.[24] Although the magnitude of the shift is small (1–2 units) and clinically insignificant (95% of the population of color normals would be included in +6 units), reflecting only subtle changes in color perception, the increased red in the mixture is just what is found in settings made by patients with early macular disease.[25,26] Other visual functions show similar patterns in early macular disease and after acute alcohol consumption.

Another visual function that is strongly dependent on the integrity of retinal structures is adaptation to changing light level. When the light level is substantially reduced, it may take the eye many seconds or minutes to achieve the readjustment processes that allow it to maintain its sensitivity to stimulus contrast. During this time, the eye is relatively blind to fine detail. Measurement of glare recovery has become an important tool for assessing retinal function in a variety of clinical situations.

Experiments show that relatively low doses of alcohol produce large, significant, dose-related increases in the time required to recover foveal contrast sensitivity following bright light exposure.[20,24] These changes in recovery time can be seen for several hours after alcohol ingestion. Using the stimulus configuration shown in Figure 17-2, researchers measured the time to recover sensitivity to a test spot of several fixed contrast levels after a 10-s exposure to a bright (5.6×10^4 cd/m^2) field. The substantial effect of the two alcohol dose levels tested (0.5 and 1 mL/kg body weight of 95% ethanol) on glare recovery time for each contrast level tested is seen in Figure 17-3 and was later confirmed.[27] Whereas there were strong parallels in the time course of blood alcohol, subjective "high rating," and glare recovery time, the peak of the recovery time function appears to be delayed slightly when compared to blood alcohol and subjective "high" or impaired rating. The significance of this result becomes apparent when one considers the similarity between the conditions of driving and the present task. The

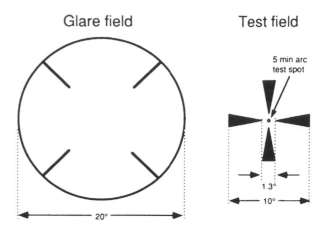

FIGURE 17-2
Stimulus configuration for foveal glare recovery test. After exposure in the bright glare field, the subject is required, over the recovery time period, to detect the successive presentation of a small test spot of decreasing contrast. Triangles in the form of a Maltese cross aid fixation.

implication is that the drunk driver's impairment from headlight glare or from the sky is likely to be prolonged beyond his feeling unsafe to drive or being measured as intoxicated.

Quite separate from the practical implications of the effect of alcohol on driving performance, these data provide additional (psychophysical) evidence that alcohol directly affects the retina. The mechanisms controlling light and dark adaptation are retinal; the electroretinogram (ERG), which is entirely a retinal response, reflects all of the changes of adaptation. Alcohol doses similar to those used in experiments by Adams et al[30] and Levett and Jaeger[28] have shown that alcohol affects the ERG. Alcohol slowed dark adaptation and the resynthesis of photopigment in albino rats.[29] It is possible that alcohol slows glare recovery by retarding photopigment regeneration.

STATIC VISUAL ACUITY.   Unlike color vision and glare recovery, static visual acuity appears to be "rather insensitive to effects of alcohol" confirm this conclusion.[19,23] Although a loss of distance visual acuity is reported, no change is evident in near visual acuity at blood alcohol levels of 0.06% to 0.075%.[14] Research also indicates that visual acuity for four-position Landolt Cs of high (49%) and low (12%)

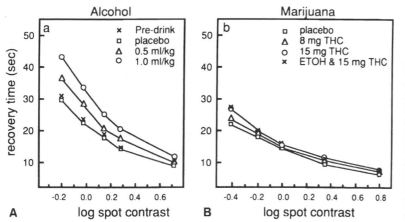

FIGURE 17-3

A. Effects of two dose levels of alcohol on glare recovery time as a function of target contrast. Alcohol produces a dose-related delay in glare recovery that is larger for low than for high contrasts. **B.** Effects of two dose levels of marijuana and combined alcohol and marijuana intake on glare recovery. Marijuana-induced delay of glare recovery is less pronounced than the alcohol-induced effect.

contrast was unaffected by low and moderate doses (0.5 and 1 mL/kg) of alcohol.[30]

DYNAMIC VISUAL ACUITY.   The results obtained were quite different when the same researchers measured acuity for these targets while they were in motion.[32] Dynamic visual acuity, the resolution of fine detail in moving targets, shows large decrements following ingestion of quantities of alcohol at levels that have little or no effect on static acuity. Figure 17-4 (*top*) shows the dose dependence of the change in dynamic acuity measured 30 min after drinking for high (49%) and low (12%) contrast targets. From Figure 17-5 (*left panel*) it can be seen that the change in dynamic visual acuity increases as drinking and target velocity increase.

Dynamic visual acuity is a complex task involving precise sensory and motor coordination. Two of the components involved in dynamic visual acuity are (1) static visual acuity and (2) ocular pursuit of the target using a combination of fast (saccadic) and slower (pursuit) eye movements. Because static visual acuity is not affected by alcohol, alcohol's effects on the oculomotor system accounts for the deficit observed in dynamic visual acuity following alcohol consumption. It might be expected that alcohol impairs the fine motor control required for visual function because it is well known to have effects on other, more gross, motor skills.

OCULOMOTOR EFFECTS

Good form and color vision require proper eye movements to achieve foveation of the visual target as well as precise binocular alignment. Conse-

quently, drug effects on the oculomotor system can alter visual perception.

TONIC EYE POSITION.   Experiments indicate that alcohol tends to cause the eyes to converge (become esophoric) under dissociated conditions with a real target at remote distances.[33] The magnitude of the esophoric shift measured was about 4 prism diopters

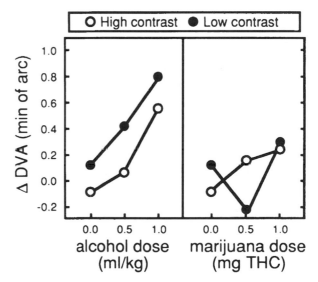

FIGURE 17-4

The change in dynamic visual acuity produced by use of two doses of alcohol (*left*) and marijuana (*right*). Alcohol produces larger changes and a more clear dose dependence than does marijuana. Dynamic visual acuity for low contrast targets is more strongly affected by alcohol than is dynamic visual acuity for high contrast targets.

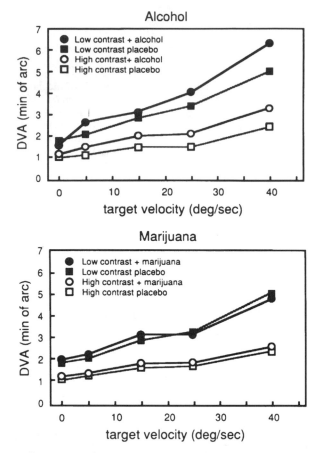

Alcohol

Marijuana

FIGURE 17-5

Effects of alcohol (*top*) and marijuana (*bottom*) on dynamic visual acuity for different target velocities. Alcohol reduces dynamic visual acuity, more so at higher velocities. Marijuana has little or no effect on dynamic visual acuity at all velocities.

ACCOMMODATION.   A loss of accommodative power has been reported,[19] as well as an increase in latency and decrease in duration of accommodative responses.[28,37,38]

PUPIL SIZE.   Brown et al. showed alcohol to have no effect on static pupil size at high and low photopic levels.[39] An increase of about 10% in pupillary diameter was found earlier with fairly high alcohol doses,[40] however. A study that measured the effects of alcohol on the frequency response of the pupil using sinusoidally modulated light reported that both the magnitude and the timing of the response were degraded by alcohol.[28]

EYE MOVEMENTS.   Ocular tracking of a smoothly moving target involves a combination of smooth pursuit movements and saccadic eye movements. The two types of movements are controlled by separate systems, which are normally well coordinated. Alcohol has significant effects on both systems, as well as on their interaction. The function of smooth pursuit movements is the tracking of objects moving in the visual field at less than 30° per second, and it is measured clinically using a pendulum.[28] Pathologic or drug-influenced pursuit is contaminated by or achieved by a series of saccades. Even at very low doses, alcohol can disturb smooth pursuit.[28] An important factor in the breakdown of smooth pursuit with alcohol is a decrease in maximum velocity. At very low frequencies, tracking is accurate but is achieved by saccades rather than smooth pursuit. Tracking ability is lost at moderate frequencies (3.5–4 Hz). The degree of saccadic contamination increases with increasing blood alcohol. Between the normal pursuit movements and the purely saccadic pursuit movements of the severely intoxicated, there exists a continuum of degraded smooth pursuit movements. These data confirm results that also showed that alcohol affects both smooth pursuit and saccadic components of tracking a target in pendular motion.[41]

Another examination of alcohol's effects on eye movements focused on the change in the eye movements required by and recorded in the dynamic visual acuity task just described. The nature of these eye movements is diagrammed in Figure 17-6.[41] The oblique line shows target position over time for the constant velocity target moved across the field. The dots represent eye position measured at regular intervals while the observer tracks this constant-velocity target. It is clear that when the target is set in

approximately 2 h after ingestion of 1 mL/kg body weight of 95% ethanol. An increase in esophoria with distant targets, with the maximum increase occurring in the first 20 min after drinking, has been reported.[14] Measured at near, an increase in exophoric deviation was found as blood alcohol level slowly fell at 40 to 60 min after drinking. A number of other researchers also have reported a decrease in convergence and a tendency for the eyes to diverge at near distances.[19,34–36] A shift of near point of convergence has been reported also.[14] Measuring ocular rotation, these researchers reported that all 10 of their subjects developed some degree of inferior oblique overaction.

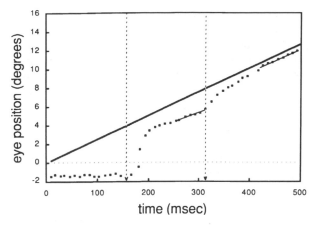

FIGURE 17-6
Eye position (degrees) as a function of time (msec) in response to a target moving at a constant velocity. The dashed vertical lines indicate the measured saccadic latencies. The slope of the lines connecting the eye position values after the saccades give an estimate of the eye velocity. The figure is an example of eye movements displayed during the experiment.

motion, eye position remains unchanged for some time, after which an abrupt saccadic eye movement toward the target is made. The latency of the saccades, shown by the vertical lines, is one of the factors of interest. The slope of the lines connecting the eye position values after the saccades give an estimate of eye velocity, the other factor of interest. The results obtained after alcohol ingestion indicate that alcohol increases saccadic latency and decreases eye velocity in the pursuit of both high and low contrast targets. These data suggest that the deficit observed in dynamic but not static visual acuity is due to deficits in eye movements caused by alcohol.

Reflex eye movements in response to regularly spaced stripes moving continuously in one direction across a fairly large portion of the visual field are referred to as optokinetic nystagmus (OKN). These eye movements become noticeably irregular after drinking 1 mL/kg alcohol, and the frequency and amplitude of the OKN saccades decreases.[21]

End-point nystagmus is the small degree of unsteadiness normally exhibited by the eyes when they are rotated maximally to one side. Alcohol exaggerates this effect, and this "peripheral gaze nystagmus" has been used by law enforcement agencies as evidence of intoxication. Adams and colleagues exam-

ined peripheral gaze nystagmus for lateral eccentric viewing at 45° in 10 subjects after alcohol consumption. Half of the subjects exhibited peripheral gaze nystagmus at moderate doses of the drug, with the effect persisting for up to 3 h after drinking. With low doses, fewer subjects showed the effect, and it disappeared within 30 min of drinking in those who did.

SUMMARY
At doses producing blood alcohol levels near the legal limit for driving, acute ingestion of alcohol deleteriously affects many but not all visual functions. Static visual acuity and stereopsis are resistant to the effects of alcohol at these dose levels. Reports of the effect of alcohol on visual fields are not conclusive. A shrinking of visual fields by about 10° in both the horizontal and vertical dimension has been reported.[19] It has been suggested that the anecdotally reported "tunnel vision" of alcohol impairment, however, it is attentional rather than sensory in origin. Subtle color vision changes occur, and the pattern of color deficit produced is similar to that seen in conditions affecting the retina, as opposed to later stages of visual processing. There is evidence that alcohol directly affects the retina,[15] and changes in the human ERG[28] and electro-oculogram (EOG)[17] have been demonstrated. The oculomotor system is also affected adversely by low to moderate effects of alcohol; accommodation, convergence, smooth pursuit, and saccadic eye movements show significant changes. The changes may have even greater impact on vision than those produced on the sensory pathways. They can result in double vision; poor tracking of moving objects, reducing their visibility by inexact fixation; and blur of near objects related to compromised accommodation.

Chronic Sensory and Oculomotor Effects

SENSORY EFFECTS
Color vision changes are among the most often described visual changes to accompany chronic use of alcohol. It is probably wise to attempt to consider separately visual changes in alcoholics from those individuals who are not alcoholics but who have regularly consumed significant amounts of alcohol for some time, but studies that have done this are rare. Color discrimination was assessed in one study by the desaturated Lanthony D-15 in 136 individuals

who were divided according to their self-report of weekly alcohol consumption. Sixteen of the subjects were undergoing treatment for alcoholism in a detoxification center. These authors report that the prevalence of dyschromatopsia, and the mean color confusion index[2] increased with alcohol intake (Figure 17-7), with all heavy drinkers (>751 g per week) showing some dyschromatopsia. Whereas in most cases blue-yellow defects were seen, 25% of the alcoholics undergoing treatment also showed a red-green defect. None of the drinkers who were not in the treatment program showed a red-green defect. The authors suggest that, whereas the blue-yellow defects represent relatively early changes involving the outer retina (by Koellner's rule), the complex dyschromatopsia reflects a more advanced phase of neural damage involving the optic nerve. They cite work showing that alcoholics undergoing prolonged treatment show an improvement in the blue-yellow loss but not the red-green loss.[43] The change in pattern of color vision loss with progression of alcohol-related damage may account for the apparent inconsistencies in the literature, with some authors reporting primarily blue-yellow defects,[44-47] while others report red-green defects[47] or generalized losses with no clear axis.

The nature of the relationship between chronic alcohol consumption and visual impairment is further complicated by the association of alcoholism with a variety of conditions. Alcohol consumption is correlated with several biochemical and hematologic disturbances (Whitehead et al, cited in Birch et al[26]). Chronic alcoholism is also associated with a variety of systemic conditions, such as malnutrition, cirrhosis, encephalopathy, and peripheral neuropathy.[26] As a result, many explanations for the association of alcoholism have been put forth, including direct damage to the visual pathways, deficits resulting from liver damage, and a genetic linkage.[42] Evidence for a genetic linkage may be found in the data that reports a significant incidence of color defects in nonalcoholic relatives of alcoholics similar to those seen in the alcoholics themselves.[47] The increased incidence of color disturbance in alcoholics with cirrhosis was attributed to a sex-linked gene that affected both. Later research by others makes this hypothesis very unlikely, however.[45,46]

Regardless of the causes, there is little doubt that alcoholism produces significant changes in color vision. Chronic alcohol consumption also produces scotomatous changes—first a central scotoma for red and green and later a caecocentral scotoma for white.[6] Alcohol amblyopia, often referred to as tobacco-alcohol amblyopia, has been described by many.[49-51] The condition is associated with symptoms such as "dimness of vision," field changes, changes in the optic disc, and color discrimination losses. Many of the changes are secondary to vitamin B deficiencies and other conditions of poor health resulting from alcoholism.

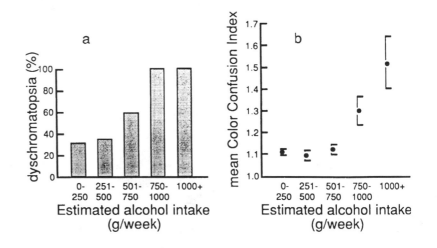

FIGURE 17-7
A. Prevalence of dyschromatopsia as it relates to weekly alcohol intake ($X^2 = 35.4$ p < 0.000). **B. Relationship between color confusion index and weekly alcohol intake. From Mergler et al, 1988.**

17.2 Marijuana

Marijuana comes from *Cannabis sativa* L., a plant that is cultivated or grows wild throughout most of the tropical and temperate regions of the world and is often called *Indian hemp*.[52] Cannabis, which is native to central Asia, is one of the oldest cultivated nonfood plants.[52] The cultivation of hemp in North America is reported to have begun in 1606 in what is now Nova Scotia, Canada; it was later planted by the Pilgrims in New England. The early colonists did not use the plant for its intoxicating effects, although certain individuals, including George Washington, may have been aware of its medicinal properties.[52] The popular, nonmedical drug use of marijuana is a phenomenon of this century. Smoking marijuana may have been introduced to this country by the migrant workers of the Southwest around 1910. It is said that the prohibition of alcohol in 1919 contributed to the spread of marijuana use in the 1920s and 1930s. Prior to World War II marijuana was predominantly used by the underprivileged. The soldiers of World War II, who were introduced to it in the army, contributed to its spread to college campuses, where it was well established by the 1960s. Marijuana is now the third most widely used social drug, after alcohol and tobacco.[53] It is the most commonly used illicit drug, with an estimated 200 to 300 million regular users worldwide.[54]

The more than 60 active ingredients of marijuana are collectively referred to as the cannabinoids. The most prevalent and pharmacologically important of these is an isomer of tetrahydrocannibinol (THC), commonly referred to as $\Delta 9$-THC, which is responsible for the major psychological, behavioral, and physiologic effects in man. Cannabis preparations can be smoked, eaten, drunk as an extract, or, rarely, injected intravenously. Smoking the drug is the most efficient way to use it; its full effects are manifest in minutes, and because up to 50% of the drug is absorbed, inhalation results in a potency as much as three times that from oral ingestion of an equivalent amount.[54] The higher potency of smoked marijuana is attributable to avoidance of first-pass metabolism in the liver and enhanced release of $\Delta 9$-THC from the pyrolysis of THC acids. Oral ingestion produces much longer lasting effects, however.

Under various conditions and doses, marijuana has been shown to have stimulant, sedative, anal-gesic, and psychedelic properties. Although it has properties common to sedative hypnotics, tranquilizers, hallucinogenics, and narcotics, it does not belong to any of these drug classes, being in a class by itself.[55,56] Paradoxically, marijuana has been shown to potentiate both the stimulant effects of amphetamines and the sedative effects of barbiturates in animals. (Truit, cited in Primo[51]). At low doses marijuana resembles alcohol in its effects. At higher doses, its hallucinogenic properties become more evident. Within 20 to 30 minutes of use, visual and auditory hallucinations develop (Walsh and Hoyt, cited in McClane et al[55]). The visual hallucinations are described as "vivid, brightly colored flashes of lights or amorphous forms that develop into shapes, faces, or complex scenes."

There are many difficulties in studying the effects of marijuana. The potency of the substance can vary by a factor of up to 2000. Regular users are affected differently than occasional users, although there is a relationship between dose and effect, on many measures it is nonlinear.

Acute Sensory and Physical Effects

The ocular side effects of acute marijuana intoxication reported include diplopia, impairment of accommodation, transient disturbances of vision, isolated instances of photophobia, nystagmus, and blepharospasm.[55,56] Despite the reports of visual hallucinations and distortions (Walsh and Hoyt, cited in McClane et al[55]), research on marijuana show that its effects on visual function in laboratory settings are relatively mild. Marijuana did not affect visual acuity or the ability to match the brightness of near targets to distant standards,[57] nor did it affect depth perception.[58]

Adams and colleagues have carried out a rather extensive investigation of the effects of marijuana on basic visual function. These studies parallel the studies with alcohol described above, permitting direct comparisons between the effects of the two drugs at social dose levels. The two drugs are often used together, and Adams and co-workers have also measured the combined effects. It is known that marijuana and alcohol can have additive effects on certain psychomotor and physiologic functions, whereas marijuana and alcohol can have antagonistic effects on some subjective variables such as visual imagery.[51] In this section, we review the findings, making comparisons between alcohol and marijuana wherever possible.

COLOR DISCRIMINATION

The effects of two dose levels (8 and 15 mg) of Δ9-THC on color discrimination was measured using the FM 100-hue test.[24,30] Like alcohol, marijuana produced an increase in total error score. The primary effect of both drugs is an increase in the errors in the blue region, with lesser effects in the red region for marijuana and in the yellow region for alcohol. The pattern and magnitude of results for the two drugs are compared in Figure 17-1, which contains standard plots of the errors on polar coordinates and a quantitative analysis of "blue" errors. The impairment of color vision has a much shorter time course for marijuana than for alcohol. The restriction of the discrimination loss to particular regions of color space indicates that the effect is not due to lapses of attention or task difficulty per se. Marijuana also causes a small shift in the color mixture settings on the anomaloscope such that more red is required in the red/green mixture than is normal. The magnitude of the shift is comparable to that seen with alcohol. The effect of the two drugs is additive: the combined dose produces about twice the shift in the setting as either drug alone. Like alcohol, marijuana produces a pattern of color vision change that resembles that seen in disease states that affect the retinal structures rather than central components of the visual system.

It was reported that recovery from glare was delayed by several seconds after marijuana smoking; later analyses of the data showed no statistically significant effect.[59] However, marijuana was found to produce significant delays in glare recovery that are of smaller magnitude to those of alcohol (Figure 17-3).[21] Interestingly, the combined effect of the drugs on glare recovery is less than for the individual drugs, despite the fact that the subjects' "high" ratings are greater. This may be explained by measurements of the subjects' blood alcohol levels, which indicated that equivalent doses of alcohol produce lower blood alcohol levels in the presence of marijuana than when ingested alone.

Static visual acuity is unaffected by marijuana as well as by alcohol. The two drugs differ in their impact on dynamic visual acuity, however (Figs. 17-3 and 17-4); the impairment is considerably smaller for marijuana than alcohol,[32] and, whereas the impairment increases with target velocity for alcohol, the small deficit produced by marijuana is rather velocity independent.

This resistance of dynamic visual acuity to degradation at high target velocities predicts that marijuana would have a relatively mild effect on the oculomotor system in comparison to alcohol. Measurements confirm this. Marijuana, even at doses higher than those typically used socially, failed to alter the maximum velocity of smooth or saccadic tracking of a target pendularly oscillating at increasing frequencies.[41] The magnitude of the esophoric shift caused by marijuana is only half that observed with alcohol.[33]

PUPIL SIZE

Changes of pupil size are reported to be one of the two major consistent signs of marijuana intoxication, with the other being injection of the conjunctiva.[60] In spite of this, the reports of the effects of marijuana on the pupil are inconsistent. Subjectively, 61% of the people interviewed reported that pupil size increased.[62] Weil et al found no effect on pupil size.[64] The results of Brown et al[39] are in agreement with those of Hepler et al,[63] who demonstrated a small, but significant, constriction of the pupil.

INTRAOCULAR PRESSURE

There are many reports that THC reduces intraocular pressure (IOP).[53,63,66] One study reports that smoking marijuana, intravenous administration of THC, or oral ingestion of marijuana decreased intraocular pressure on average 25% in non- to moderate users who experienced a substantial "high" and achieved a state of peaceful relaxation.[55] Smoking marijuana produced no change in IOP in heavy users. Other research suggests that IOP is an indirect effect resulting from the relaxed state, which can be achieved by drug or nondrug means.[65,66]

In summary, marijuana and alcohol have similar effects on some visual functions (e.g., color mixture, glare recovery), but marijuana has relatively less impact on others (e.g., dynamic visual acuity). Alcohol is more likely than marijuana to affect those functions that make a considerable demand on the oculomotor system. Finally, although subjects report that they feel more "high" on a combination of the drugs, not all vision functions show an additivity of the drug effects.

Chronic Sensory and Ocular Effects

Common ocular changes in chronic users of marijuana are abnormally low IOP,[66] congestion of the lids and conjunctiva, ciliary injection of the globe, and increased visibility of the corneal nerves.[3,67] Changes in color vision including dyschromatopsia, xanthopsia, colored flashing lights, and heightened color vision have also been reported with chronic marijuana use,[3,53,65] whereas photophobia was reported in chronic users who had used the drug recently.[65] Reductions in the total range of accommodation to between 2.50 and 5 diopters has been described in a group of chronic marijuana users.[69,70] A variety of visual functions was measured in a large group of individuals who had smoked an average of nine cigarettes per day of marijuana for at least 10 y as well as in a group of nonusers.[71] The users refrained from smoking marijuana for at least 3 h prior to testing so that the results would not be confounded by acute effects. The results may be summarized as follows: dark-adapted pupil responses to a 2.7 log ft L light were slightly, but not significantly, reduced in users compared to nonusers. IOP was slightly greater in users than nonusers. There was a small, insignificant shift in anomaloscope matches, with users requiring slightly more red; and the color and brightness match ranges of the users were significantly narrower than those made by nonusers.

17.3 Tobacco

In 1896 deSchweinitz published *Toxic Amblyopias*, including as the first chapter alcohol and tobacco amblyopias.[49] The visual characteristics of alcohol amblyopia and tobacco amblyopia are similar, the two drugs are often abused concurrently, and both are amblyopias caused by the same mechanism, specifically the result of a deficiency of vitamin B. For this reason, tobacco-alcohol amblyopia is considered a single entity,[49] whose symptomotology is described as follows:

> . . . dimness of vision is the outstanding symptom. Usually this is described as coming on gradually, but occasionally the onset is acute. Red and green often cannot be distinguished before the vision for white is materially reduced. Trouble with reading is a frequent early complaint . . . less difficulty is experienced in using the left eye than the right because the caecocentral scotoma in the left visual field does not interfere with fixation to the extent that it does with the right field. The visual acuity usually has reached a level of 20/200 or even lower before the affected individual seeks advice (p. 2613).

The often-described symptoms of tobacco-alcohol amblyopia do not reflect the actions of chronic administration of tobacco smoke or alcohol per se but rather the deficiencies (primarily B vitamins) found in individuals who abuse these substances. We therefore will not consider these issues further but, instead, report the few documented direct effects of tobacco on visual function.

Acute Oculomotor Effects

Acute inhalation of tobacco smoke affects the oculomotor system. Roberts and Adams showed that pupil size increased at least 0.75 mm during the smoking of a cigarette (Fig. 17.8A). The effect disappeared within 3 min after the cessation of smoking. All subjects also showed an immediate reduction in the amplitude of accommodation of at least 1.25 diopters and a return to normal amplitude within 5 min following cessation of smoking (Fig. 17-8B). It has also been demonstrated that tobacco smoking induced a transient primary position upbeat nystagmus in the dark that was suppressed by visual fixation.[73] Defects were found in both horizontal and vertical eye tracking during the first 5 min after smoking one cigarette.[73] The smooth pursuit defect was characterized by a reduction in the upward tracking and superposition of saccadic jerks on both horizontal and vertical tracking movements. The researchers report that the degree of the defect correlated with the amount of nystagmus in the dark. This relation led the authors to conclude that the defect during tracking is due to the addition of nystagmus to the normal smooth tracking movements, rather than breakdown in the smooth pursuit per se. The nature of the eye movement defect predicts that dynamic visual acuity would be acutely detrimentally affected by tobacco smoking. To our knowledge, this experiment has not been done.

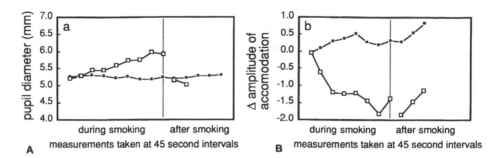

FIGURE 17-8
A. Average pupil size for 12 subjects. Open symbols indicate average pupil size during inhalation of cigarette smoke. Solid symbols indicate pupil size during inhalation of air. B. Average amplitude of accommodation for 12 subjects. Open symbols indicate average amplitude of accommodation during inhalation of cigarette smoke. Solid symbol indicates amplitude of accommodation during inhalation of air.

Chronic Sensory and Oculomotor Effects

An increase in the P2 component and an increase in the interocular difference of the latency of the transient pattern visual evoked potential (VEP) in 26 "clinically healthy smokers" has been shown.[74] It is difficult to know the precise significance of these results for visual function. A mechanism was suggested in which the increase in the VEP latency might occur.[75] Rats exposed for 5 h per day to 15 cigarettes' smoke for 52 wk showed an increase in the latency to the N1 and P2 components of the VEP. Histologic examination revealed an increase in the number of unmyelinated fibers in the optic nerve and a decrease in the thickness of the myelin sheath in the myelinated fibers. In addition, the distribution of axon diameters shifted toward smaller diameter (and hence slower) fibers. Finally, no change in the ERG recorded in these animals was found. These results suggest that chronic tobacco smoke exposure causes changes in the visual system that are primarily in the optic nerve rather than in the retina. The nature of the changes is consistent with a slowing of transmission of information and a loss of information carried in the larger fibers. These results would lead us to predict changes in visual function such as a deficit in the blue-yellow pathway, as well as a decrement in detection and flicker. An association between heavy tobacco smoking and nuclear lens opacities has been documented.[76,77] An increase in smoking dose increases the risk of nuclear opacities and the severity of opacities, and quitting smoking

decreases the risk.[77] Interestingly, it has been reported that in many cases the severity of Leber's optic atrophy is related to tobacco smoking.[78]

17.4 Caffeine

Daily caffeine use is very common in our society. Its implications for general health have been widely publicized, and scientific interest in the drug can be traced to a 1978 special committee report on drugs that were considered to be safe by the Food and Drug Administration (FDA) of the U.S. Public Health Service.[79] Yet relatively little has been studied or reported on the effects of caffeine on vision.

Caffeine has been reported to improve visual monitoring in a task of tone detection and compensator, tracking,[80] and enhanced light sensitivity.[81] Though other interpretations, based on physiology of the visual pathway, are offered, these results were attributed to the increased alertness in the subjects in the experiments. A similar attentional explanation can account for the reported effects of caffeine on perceptual structuring tasks, auditory vigilance, and reaction time improvements.[82,83] We are unaware of any reports of adverse effects on oculomotor tasks. The elimination of normally present brightness enhancement with dim surrounds associated with caffeine intake equivalent to about two cups of coffee has been reported.[84] The authors favor caffeine stimulation of the reticular formation of the medulla and the resulting changes in the excitation of "on" and "off" fibers in the visual system as the basis for the phenomenon.

The question of caffeine use or contraindication for glaucoma patients has remained in the ophthalmic literature for many years. Many practitioners advise their glaucoma patients against caffeine use,[85] yet there are studies that show little or no effect of caffeine on either flow of aqueous humor[86] or IOP.[87,88] Perhaps the uncertainty among practitioners stems from the known efffect on IOP and aqueous production of rapid ingestion of large volumes of fluid; such a procedure is known as a "provocative" test for glaucoma.

17.5 Visual Effects of Systemic Therapeutic Drugs

Americans spend billions of dollars each year on prescription and over-the-counter therapeutic drugs. In the late 1970s the average American is estimated to have received seven prescriptions per year,[89] and it is unlikely that this number has since decreased. Oculotoxicity has been reported for nearly every class of systemically administered drug.[9] It is to be expected that some ocular side effects would be common to several drug groups.[1] For example, antimuscarinics, antihistamines, tricyclics (antidepressants), and some anti-Parkinson's drugs are likely to affect the pupil and accommodation, as they are all anticholinergics.[1]

Several factors should be considered when evaluating the "importance" of visual (or other) side effects. A drug may produce visual side effects that are serious or have a high probability of occurring, but the drug may not be prescribed very often (perhaps in part because of the severity of the side effects). For example, hydroxychloroquine, an antimalarial that is also used to treat rheumatoid arthritis and systemic lupus erythematosus, may induce a retinopathy that results in severe visual loss which may be irreversible and progressive even if drug therapy is stopped.[1] On the other hand, a drug may produce only mild visual side effects, or side effects on rare occasions, but the drug might be very widely used (e.g., ibuprofen). In most cases, the effects are reversible and disappear after the drug is stopped. The frequency of occurrence of side effects might not be accurately represented in the literature because side effects are more likely to be observed and reported when they are more severe or vision-threatening. Ocular side effects are often described incompletely or ambiguously; confusion of "blurred vision" with diplopia and use of vague terms such as "visual disturbances" are examples.[89]

For the most commonly prescribed drugs, ocular side effects are rare at normal therapeutic doses; many ocular side effects occur only at toxic levels or in heavy overdosage of the drug. For example, the disturbances of color vision produced by the cardiac glycoside digoxin are usually present only when toxic doses are present.[1] Indeed, color vision changes are among the earliest signs of digoxin toxicity.[90] Since the therapeutic index of this drug is very low[89]—the toxic dose is only about twice the therapeutic dose—color vision changes are important for monitoring and maintaining proper dosages.

Many of the conditions for which the most commonly prescribed drugs are used require chronic systemic use, which would be expected to increase the frequency of a side effect. For example the incidence of chloroquine toxicity increases with the total dosage received.[1]

As Levine[89] points out, many of the reported ocular side effects for the most commonly prescribed drugs are "based on cases in which the reaction was observed when the drug was being used, and regressed when the drug was stopped. Such evidence does not meet scientific requirements to establish a causal relation, but demonstrates only an association, usually unexplained, between the period of using the preparation and the appearance of the side effect." Nevertheless, such citations are often perpetuated through the literature as "documented side effects." Finally, some side effects are idiosyncratic, and it may be that a genetic predisposition may influence their appearance.

A "systemic drug profile" of the ophthalmic practitioner's clinical population is useful in two distinct contexts. First, familiarity with the medications that are likely to be used by patients would aid the clinician in anticipating and avoiding interactions with topically or orally administered ocular agents.[10] Second, this profile and familiarity with the ocular side effects associated with these common medications assist the ophthalmic practitioner in discriminating disease from toxic drug effects and thereby help in devising treatment strategies. In the interest of developing such a profile, we begin our four-part discussion on the visual side effects of therapeutics with a discussion of some of the most commonly prescribed drugs. This is followed by a section considering the effects of prescription medications that are used less frequently but have more serious visual effects. Next, we consider the special case of the elderly patient. Within this context, we consider the effects, generally mild, of nonprescription or "over-the-counter" medications.

Visual Side Effects of Commonly Prescribed Drugs

Of all the drugs prescribed, the top 200 (published annually in the April issue of *Pharmacy Times*) represented almost 70% of the drugs prescribed in 1977; nearly 40% were accounted for by the top 50 drugs, and the top 10 accounted for nearly 15%. This list is relatively stable, with 6 of the top 10 from 1977 appearing on the list from 1986. Only one of the 1977 top 10 is now infrequently prescribed (Aldomet, known officially as methyldopa, used principally in the treatment of mild to severe arterial hypertension) and one (Dimetapp, cold remedy with three active ingredients) is now available over-the-counter, in a slightly modified formulation. Ampicillin has been replaced by Amoxil, a similar antibiotic. Found on the newer, but not the older, list are: Orthonovum, an oral contraceptive, and Tagamet, an H_2-receptor antagonist that turns off gastric acid secretion. An additional list of frequently used prescription drugs, and one that ophthalmic practitioners may find particularly useful, is that compiled by Wilcox and Bartlett[10] by surveying 502 successively seen patients in an optometric practice. They report their findings with breakdowns according to age, race, and gender, as well as citing the frequency of use for the 22 most common drugs, and present a reanalysis of the 10 most common drug groups. In Wilcox and Bartlett's sample, the most commonly used drug group were the diuretics (most frequently Dyazide), which were used by 16.6% of their sample patients. Nearly as common were the antihypertensives, with a 15.1% usage; Inderal is the most often used.

We now consider the ocular side effects of the most common drugs now prescribed, compiled from the 1977 top 10, the 1986 top 10, as well as the list of Wilcox and Bartlett.[10] The reader is referred to Levine[89] and Fraunfelder[3] from whom the following information was largely derived.

Valium, the proprietary name for diazepam, was the most often prescribed drug in 1977,[89] was in the top 10 in 1986, and is still quite common, although its use has declined.[91] It is classified as an antianxiety agent and is also used as an adjunctive in the relief of muscle spasms. Fraunfelder[4] lists 15 ocular side effects for the benzodiazepams, including decreased vision, decreased corneal reflex, effects on the extraocular muscles (oculogyric crises, decreased spontaneous movements, abnormal conjugate deviations, and jerky pursuit movements), decreased accommodation, diplopia, nystagmus, decreased intraocular pressure, subconjunctival or retinal hemorrhages secondary to drug-induced anemia, and photosensitivity. Brown lens deposits, paralysis of the extraocular muscles, and photophobia are listed as questionable effects. Fraunfelder states that these side effects are rare and reversible. The manufacturer's information carries a contraindication for use in narrow angle glaucoma, but this has been questioned and it may be used in open-angle glaucoma.[89]

Lasix is the proprietary name for furosemide, a sulfonamide that is "used principally to reduce the edema associated with congestive heart failure, renal failure, nephrotic syndrome, and hepatic insufficiency, and to treat acute pulmonary edema and "hypertensive crises."[89] Fraunfelder lists the following among the ocular side effects: decreased vision, problems with color vision (dyschromatopsia), visual hallucinations, minimal decreased intraocular pressure, decreased contact lens tolerance, and possibly decreased accommodation and photophobia. He states that ocular side effects of furosemide are rare and seldom of consequence. Levine points out that the most frequently reported of the side effects, "blurring of vision," is probably due to an osmotic mechanism involving the lens or cornea and may yet turn out to be an instance of drug-induced acute transient myopia. Other common diuretics, acetazolamide (*Diamox*) and hydrochlorothiazide (*HydroDIURIL*) have also been associated with transient myopia with perimacular edema.[92] And xanthopsia, or "yellow vision," has been associated with yet another chlorothiazide (*Diuril*).

Inderal, one of the early beta-adrenergic blocking agents, was nonselective in its action and was used to treat a number of cardiovascular diseases. The most frequently reported of the generally mild and transient side effects[89] is diplopia. Other reported side effects are decreased accommodation, "visual disturbances," visual hallucinations, and single cases of loss of vision and increased intraocular pressure. Inderal has been largely replaced by more selective agents such as *Tenormin*. Recently Tenormin has been shown to transiently reduce critical flicker fusion frequency in older hypertensives.[93] Another beta blocker, *Lopressor*, has rarely been associated with adverse ocular effects.[4]

Dyazide is a combination of two diuretics, hydrochlorothiazide and triamterene, both of which act by blocking renal absorption of sodium.[89] Although used primarily for therapy of edema in congestive heart failure and arterial hypertension, it has also been used to control the hormonally induced edema associated with pregnancy, premenstrual syndrome, and corticosteroid and estrogen therapy. The hydrochlorothiazide component is responsible for most of the ocular side effects, which are infrequent and transient. Acute transient myopia and xanthopsia have both been reported, as well as "ocular pain" and "decreased vision," "altered color vision," and blur. *HydroDIURIL* (which contains hydrochlorothiazide alone) is also a popular thiazamide diuretic.

Lanoxin is a trade name for the cardiac glycoside digoxin. Digitalis preparations have long been known for their effects on failing hearts. Digoxins are used often in the treatment of heart problems involving the myocardium, such as congestive heart failure, atrial flutter and fibrillation, and tachycardia. The therapeutic index is small, so toxicity is common, with ocular side effects being common and among the earliest signs of toxicity. The occurrence of digoxin toxicity has been estimated to be as high as 25%.[92] The visual effects reported are dose related and occur when the serum digitalis concentration exceeds 1.5 ng/ml.[1] The toxic effects of cardiac glycosides generally disappear within two weeks of cessation of drug therapy. The most common visual side effects are blurred vision and "chromatopsia," which is a sort of visual dazzle in which objects appear to be covered with colored snow or frost. These symptoms may be heightened in highly illuminated areas.[92] Other visual symptoms include reduced visual acuity, scotomas, flashes, photophobia, and, occasionally, temporary blindness and scintillating scotomas. Most common of the ocular side effects are disturbances in color vision, predominantly in the yellow and blue regions of the spectrum. There may be an alteration of color perception such that objects appear yellow or green or have haloes around them. Lyle also reports a much wider range of color vision changes in all parts of the spectrum. Robertson et al.[94] present evidence that these drugs act directly on the receptors (specifically the cones) rather than the optic nerve, but Lyle[6] suggests that the cortex may be involved too. Birch et al.[26] cite a number of sources that suggest a retinal origin for the type-I acquired red-green defect produced by digitalis. Robertson et al.[94] found an elevation of cone thresholds at digoxin levels that produced no other toxicity symptoms. It has been suggested that these effects may be due to inhibition of enzyme mechanisms responsible for cone repolarization.[95] This suggests that digoxin acts at a site at which it could affect a wide range of visual functions and that it can do so prior to any other indication of toxicity. Surprisingly, perhaps, Johnson et al.[96] failed to find any significant effects on color vision, measured with the FM-100 hue test, of the cardiac glycoside β-acetyldigoxin (*Novodigal*) in healthy subjects, although they did find an increase in the latency of one component of the visually evoked potential. Cardiac glycosides have also been known to produce palsies of the extraocular muscles.[97] Perhaps the most "famous" instance of ocular side effects from digitalis is "documented" in the paintings of Van Gogh. It has been suggested that the colored haloes and prevalence of yellow (xanthopsia) were due to digitalis.[98]

Oral contraceptives are another group of prescription medications that have been associated with a number of visual side effects. Fraunfelder[4] includes the following visual side effects of oral contraceptives: decreased vision, flashing lights, paralysis of extraocular muscles, diplopia, retrobulbar or optic neuritis; problems with color vision (dyschromatopsia, blue tinge to objects; colored haloes around lights), visual field changes (central scotomas, quadrantanopsia, or hemianopsia), exophthalmos, myopia, central serous retinopathy, macular degeneration, pupil changes, Horner's syndrome, optic atrophy, and blindness. More specifically, oral contraceptives produce "protanomaly" as well as reduced hue discrimination of blues.[26] The probability of developing a blue-yellow defect increases with the duration of drug use. The blue haloes sometimes reported are probably attributable to corneal edema. These reports date from the late 1970s and early 1980s; more recently, oral contraceptives contain lower hormone levels, so it might be expected that the side effects would be less common. Currently used contraceptive regimens are of two varieties: fixed dosage combination and triphasic. Triphasic varieties (e.g., Triphasil-28) attempt to more closely mimic the endogenous changes in hormones during the menstrual cycle, containing Levonorgestrel and ethinyl estradiol in a triphasic regimen. The fixed-dose regimen pills contain fixed doses of the same two hormones in each pill, which are taken for 21 days. As both contain the same active ingredients, it is to be expected that they will produce similar effects. Ocular side effects listed on the package insert include optic neuritis and retinal thrombosis. It is advised that the medication be discontinued if sudden or gradual onset of diplopia, papilledema, or retinal or vascular lesions occur.

Uncommon Drugs with Frequent or Severe Ocular Effects

There are several compounds that one comes across quite often in the literature on ocular side effects of drugs, although they are used infrequently. These are typically drugs that produce dramatic or irreversible visual changes. We discuss them only briefly here.

Ethambutol, an antituberculous medicine, has associated with it quite a few visual effects, many of which are reversible, but there are some well-documented irreversible changes, including blindness.[4] Davidson and Rennie's[1] description of the effects may be summarized as follows. Color vision testing, for example, with the FM-100 hue, is a suitable means for detecting early toxicity, as color vision changes (dyschromatopsia) are among the earliest changes. Field loss may be both central and peripheral, and though some cases present initially with unilateral loss, bilateral loss occurs within a month. Optic neuritis with decreased visual acuity and red-green color vision loss have been described, and Sanford[107] recommends monthly evaluation of visual acuity with losses greater than 10% considered significant. Visual effects are typically dose related; severe visual loss is rarely seen in individuals receiving less than 15 mg/kg/day. Sanford[107] suggests that color vision also be evaluated monthly at doses greater than 15 mg/kg/day. There are many cases of severe ethambutol toxic-

ity in the literature; toxicity may be associated with renal disease, as these individuals have more trouble clearing the drug.

Chloroquine and *hydroxychloroquine* are antimalarial agents that are also used to treat rheumatoid arthritis and systemic lupus erythematosis. As the incidence of toxicity increases with the total dose received, and higher doses are required to treat the chronic conditions (arthritis and lupus), the likelihood of adverse effects is higher in these conditions than in malaria. Retinal toxicity is the most important adverse effect, having been reported in 2.9% to 45% of the patients being treated for these diseases.[1] The absence of a foveal reflex is among the earliest signs and is followed by the development of a "bull's eye" maculopathy that may be accompanied by decreased visual acuity, impaired color vision, and central, paracentral, and/or peripheral scotomas. Resolution of the maculopathy may occur in the early stages, but is irreversible and may even progress after the cessation of therapy once well-developed macular lesions are present.

Iso-tretinoin, a synthetic analogue of Vitamin A that is used to treat acne, has recently received a good deal of press. Both ocular (blepharoconjunctivitis) and visual changes have been reported. For example, Weleber et al.[99] report visual changes in three of 50 patients undergoing therapy, including abnormal ERGs and changes in dark-adaptation function, characterized by elevated thresholds. These authors postulate that the drug may affect retinal function by competing with retinol.

Visual Disturbances Associated with Over-the-Counter Preparations

In some respects, over-the-counter preparations represent the greatest of the ophthalmic clinician's diagnostic drug traps. Patients often consider them so "safe" or unimportant that they fail to report them in drug histories. Also, many patients believe that since the medication is over-the-counter and therefore "safe," they can ignore dose recommendations and follow the "more-is-better" rule. In addition, since they are not monitored as prescription medications are, they are likely to be taken in combinations that increase the likelihood of adverse visual reaction through interaction effects. It is very important that the ophthalmic practitioner emphasize to patients the importance of reporting over-the-counter drug use. Drugs that are taken for long periods of time to treat chronic conditions, such as ibuprofen, are especially likely to both produce side effects and be "overlooked" by the patient on questioning. Since these drugs are commonly used by the elderly, the visual consequences of their use are discussed below in the context of general drug use in the elderly.

Visual Effects of Therapeutic Drug Use in the Elderly

The population of individuals over 65 years of age in the United States is growing. The Census Bureau predicts that by the year 2000, 12.7 million men and 19 million women will be in this age group. A number of factors contribute to make adverse reactions to medications a special concern with respect to the elderly patient. Although older individuals are not much thought to use illicit drugs, their use of legal drugs is substantial. This age group constitutes only about 11% of the population, but accounts for 25% of the drugs dispensed, both prescription and over-the-counter. Most older people take multiple prescription drugs concurrently. Older patients may be getting as many as 14–18 different drugs within a year and nursing home patients as many as 20 to 30 drugs over the course of a year.[100] Lyle and Hayhoe, citing the United States Senate's Special Committee on Aging in the mid-1970s, indicate that the average nursing home patient is given four to seven different drugs daily.[7] This tendency toward "polypharmacy" puts the older patient at high risk for adverse effects; older individuals are three times as likely to show adverse reaction as young patients. The use of a large number of drugs also increases the likelihood of harmful drug interactions. Added to this is the fact that older individuals are less likely to properly adhere to their medication regimen, missing medications or "double-dosing" due to failure to carefully monitor their intake.

The physiological changes that occur with the aging process also contribute to placing the older patient at high risk for adverse drug effects. Changes in drug absorption, distribution, metabolism (biotransformation), and elimination influence the effect of drugs in the elderly. Drug distribution is altered by the increase in relative proportion of body fat and concomitant decrease in lean body mass and water.

As a result, drugs like digoxin, which is distributed in lean body tissue, have higher concentrations in the blood, while substances that are stored in fatty tissue (e.g., barbiturates, phenothiazines, diazepams) have a larger reservoir, effectively prolonging their duration of action.[100] A decrease in some plasma proteins, which bind drugs and thereby "inactivate" some portion of the drug, leads to an increase in the amount of active drug. Drug metabolism rate is only one-half to two-thirds that of younger individuals, decreasing the rate at which the drugs are biotransformed so that they may be excreted. Changes in the function of kidney, which are substantial in aging individuals, retards the elimination of water-soluble drugs. Finally, older individuals appear to be more sensitive to certain drugs, for example the anticholinergics.[100] The problems are made more complex because individuals age at different rates, so there is no easily applied "aging correction factor" by which medication dose may be adjusted for the older patient. All of these factors should be kept in mind as one reviews the material in Table 17-1, which contains a list of some of the more common medications used by older individuals, their indications, and their known or reported visual side effects.

PRESCRIPTION MEDICATIONS
Of their sample of 502 patients, Wilcox and Bartlett provide information about the drug groups and specific drugs used by their patients between the ages of 50 and 90 years.[10] Table 17-1 is an adaptation of data from Wilcox and Bartlett's[10] sample of drug use in 502 of their optometric patients.

The properties and visual side effects of *Dyazide* and *Inderal* are discussed above. Many other diuretics and antihypertensives are used to manage edema and high blood pressure, with different active ingredients and mechanisms. Two others that are common, *HydroDIURIL* and *Lasix*, were described above, as were two often-used beta-blocking agents (*Aldomet, Lopressor*).

Synthroid (levothyroxine sodium) is used as replacement or supplemental therapy in patients with hypothyroidism, and adverse effects of any kind are rare. *Tagamet* (cimetidine), which is a histamine H_2 receptor antagonist that inhibits gastric acid secretion, is used as a short-term treatment of active duodenal ulcer or active benign gastric ulcer, maintenance therapy after healing of duodenal ulcer, and for treatment of other hypersecretory conditions.

	Age			
	50–59	*60–69*	*70–79*	*80–89*
Drug Groups Used Most Frequently	Diuretic Antihypertensive Hormones Antidiabetes	Diuretic Antihypertensive Antidiabetes	Antihypertensive Diuretic Analgesic	Anti-anginal
Specific Drugs Used Most Frequently	Dyazide	Dyazide Synthroid	Inderal Tagamet	

TABLE 17-1
Frequently Used Drugs and Drug Groups in Older Individuals

Hallucinations have been reported as part of reversible confusional states predominantly, though not exclusively, in severely ill patients.

Antiparkinsonians are used to treat paralysis agitans, a common senile condition. *Levodopa* (L-dopa) is widely used to treat parkinsonism, and produces a wide variety of side effects. Blurred vision, miosis, and diplopia have been reported, as well as oculogyric crises. Visual hallucinations are a recognized adverse effect associated with Levodopa therapy that correlates with duration and dose of use.[101]

NONPRESCRIPTION (OVER-THE-COUNTER) PREPARATIONS

Older individuals use a variety of over-the-counter preparations. Most common among these are analgesics, antacids, cough and cold preparations, and laxatives. As many individuals do not consider over-the-counter preparations to be "real" drugs, it is common for them to omit them from drug histories. Nonetheless visual side effects have been associated with some of these products.

ANALGESICS, ANTI-INFLAMMATORY AGENTS, ANTIRHEUMATICS. *Aspirin:* Possible visual side effects include diplopia, nystagmus, field contraction, toxic amblyopia, red-green color defects, chromatopsia, xanthopsia, scintillating scotomas, and optic atrophy. Rarely, transient cortical blindness has been reported. Many analgesic preparations and cold remedies contain aspirin. *Acetaminophen (Tylenol):* Generally considered to be free of adverse effects at therapeutic levels. *Ibuprofen (Motrin, Nuprin, Advil):* Visual disturbances including blurred and/or diminished vision (see, e.g., Nicastro[102]), scotomata, and

changes in color vision have been reported in about 5% of patients using this medication. It is suggested that the drug be discontinued if any of these symptoms occur and that the patient receive an ophthalmic examination including central visual fields and color vision testing. Symptoms of toxic amblyopia and changes in the visual evoked potential have also been reported (see, e.g., Collum and Bowen[103]; Hamburger et al.[104]). Others have reported visual effects to be minimal or absent (cited in Lyle and Hayhoe[7]; Nicastro[102]).

COLD REMEDIES (ANTIHISTAMINES, DECONGESTANTS, COUGH MEDICATIONS). Many different active ingredients are used as antihistamines and decongestants, and the many preparations available contain them in a variety of combinations. Unfortunately little has been documented on the visual side effects of the individual ingredients or the combinations. In general, antihistamines are more likely to cause dizziness, sedation, and hypotension in the elderly. Pseudoephedrine hydrochloride is the active ingredient in many decongestants (e.g., Actifed, Sudafed), and it is contraindicated in high blood pressure, heart disease, or thyroid disease. A similar precaution is offered for dextromethorphan hydrobromide, an effective and common cough suppressant ingredient in cough medicines. Many cold medications (e.g., Dimetapp) carry warnings against use in the presence of glaucoma.

Drugs, both prescription and nonprescription, are widely used in our society. Multiple use is common, and in the elderly it is the rule rather than the exception. Unfortunately the documentation of vision side effects is poor or nonexistent for individual drugs and essentially nonexistent for polydrug use. For the elderly the concern must be not only for the wide and multiple use of prescription drugs by individuals with reduced and varied abilities to accommodate their use, but also the potential for these drugs to interact with their use of nonprescription "over-the-counter" drugs. The ophthalmic practitioner must be particularly alert to these possibilities. Finally, it must be kept in mind that most individuals cannot name the medications that they are currently taking. If the ophthalmic practitioner desires a useful drug history, it is best to ask the patient to bring all of their medications with them when they are seen.

References

1. Davidson SI, Rennie IG. Ocular toxicity from systemic drug therapy—An overview of clinically important adverse reactions. Medical Toxicology 1986; 1:217–224.
2. Amerson SR. Ocular Side Effects of Drugs and Basic Pharmacology. St. Louis, Optometric Development Enterprises, 1972.
3. Fraunfelder FT. Drug-Induced Ocular Side Effects and Drug Interactions. Philadelphia, Lea & Febiger, 1976.
4. Fraunfelder FT. Drug-Induced Ocular Side Effects and Drug Interactions (2nd ed). Philadelphia, Lea & Febiger, 1982.
5. Green H, Spencer J. Drugs with Possible Ocular Side Effects, England, Barrie & Rockliff, 1969.
6. Lyle WM. Drugs and conditions which may affect color vision. J Am Optom Assoc 1974; 45:47–61.
7. Lyle WM, Hayhoe DA. Adverse effects of the drugs most frequently administered to the elderly, Part I. 1976;
8. Lyle WM, Hayhoe DA. Adverse effects of the drugs most frequently administered to the elderly, Part II. J Am Optom Assoc 1976; 47:1132–1139.
9. Koneru PB, Lien EJ, Koda RT. Review: Oculotoxicities of systemically administered drugs. J Ocul Pharmacol 1986; 2:385–404.
10. Wilcox TK, Bartlett JD. Systemic drug profiles in adult optometric outpatients. J Am Optom Assoc 1988; 59:122–126.
11. Silverman HI, Walsh RA. The adverse effects of commonly used drugs on the eye. Am J Optom Arch Am Acad Optom 1971; 48:51–74.
12. Silverman HI. The adverse effects of commonly used systemic drugs on the eye, Part 2. Am J Optom Arch Am Acad Optom 1972; 49:335–362.
13. Silverman HI, Harvie RJ. The adverse effects of commonly used systemic drugs on the human eye, Part 3. Am J Optom Physiol Opt 1975; 52:275–287.
14. Wilson G, Mitchell R. The effects of alcohol on the visual and ocular motor systems. Aust J Ophthalmol 1983; 11:315–319.
15. Ikeda H. The effects of ethyl alcohol on the evoked potentials of the human eye. Vision Res 1963; 3:155–169.
16. Jacobson JH, Hirose T, Stokes PE. Changes in human ERG induced by intravenous alcohol. Ophthalmalogica (Suppl), 1969; 158:669–677.
17. Zrenner E, Reidel KG, Adamczyk T, Gilg T, Leibhart E. Effects of ethyl alcohol on the oculogram and color vision. Doc Ophthalmol 1986; 63:305–312.
18. Russell RE, Carney E, Feiock K, Garette M, Karwoski P. Acute ethanol administration causes transient impairment of blue-yellow color vision. Alcohol: Clinical and Experimental Research 1980; 4:396–399.
19. Hill JC, Toffolon G. Effects of alcohol on sensory and sensorimotor visual functions. J Stud Alcohol 1990; 51:108–113.
20. Adams AJ, Brown B, Flom MC, Jones RT, Jampolsky A. Alcohol and marijuana effects on static visual acuity. Am J Optom Physiol Opt 1975; 52:729–735.
21. Adams AJ, Brown B, Haegerstrom-Portnoy G, Flom MC, Jones R. Marijuana, alcohol, and combined drug effects on the time course of glare recovery. Psychopharmacology 1978; 56:81–86.
22. Krill AE, Fishman GA. Acquired color vision defects. Trans Acad Ophthalmol Otolaryng 1971; 75:1095–1111.
23. Wallgren H, Barry H. Actions of Alcohol, Biochemical, Physiological, and Psychological Aspects, Vol 1. Amsterdam, Elsevier, 1970.
24. Adams AJ, Brown B, Haegerstrom-Portnoy G, Flom MC, Jones R. Evidence for acute effects of alcohol and marijuana on color discrimination. Perception ~ Psychophysics 1976; 20:119–124.
25. Adams AJ. Acute effects of alcohol and marijuana on vision. In Cool SJ, Smith EL, III (eds.): Front in Visual Science. New York, Springer-Verlag, 1978.
26. Birch J, Chisholm IA, Kinnear P. Acquired color vision defects. In Pokorny J, Smith VC, Verriest G, Pinckers AJLG (eds.): Congenital and Acquired Color Vision Defects. New York, Grune & Stratton, 1979.
27. Sekuler R, MacArthur RD. Alcohol retards visual recovery from glare by hampering target acquisition. Nature 1977; 270:428–429.
28. Levett J, Jaeger R. Effects of alcohol on retinal potentials, eye movements, accommodation, and the pupillary light reflex. In Merigan WH, Weiss B (eds): Neurotoxicity of the Visual System. New York, Raven Press, 1980.
29. Raskin NH, Sligar KP, Steinberg RH. Dark adaptation slowed by inhibitors of alcohol dehydrogenase in the albino rat. Brain Res 1973; 50:496–500.
30. Adams AJ, Brown B, Flom MC. Alcohol-induced changes in contrast sensitivity, following high intensity light exposure. Perception ~ Psychophysics 1976; 19:219–225.

31. Adams AJ, Brown B. Alcohol prolongs time course of glare recovery. Nature 1975; 257:481–483.

32. Brown B, Adams AJ, Haegerstrom-Portnoy G, Jones RT, Flom MC. Effects of alcohol and marijuana on dynamic visual acuity, I. Threshold measurements. Perception and Psychophysics 1975; 18:441–446.

33. Jampolsky A, Flom MC, Adams AJ, Jones RT. Objective testing of marijuana-induced vision changes. Final Report to the US Army Medical Research and Development Command. Washington, DC, 1973.

34. Hogan RE, Gilmartin B. The relationship between tonic vergence and oculomotor stress induced by ethanol. Ophthalmic Physiol Opt 1985; 5:4351.

35. Hogan RE, Linfield PB. The effects of moderate doses of ethanol on heterophoria and other aspects of binocular vision. Ophthalmic Physiol Opt 1983; 3:21–31.

36. Wist ER, Hughes FW, Forney RB. Effect of low blood alcohol level on stereoscopic acuity and fixation disparity. Percept Mot Skills 1967; 24:83–87.

37. Levett J, Karras L. Effects of alcohol on human accommodation. Aviat Space Environmen Med 1977; 48:434–437.

38. Stapleton JM, Guthrie S, Linnoila M. Effects of alcohol and other psychotropic drugs on eye movements: Relevance to traffic safety. J Stud Alcohol 1986; 47:426–432.

39. Brown B, Adams AJ, Haegerstrom-Portnoy G, Jones RT, Flom MC. Pupil size after use of alcohol and marijuana. Am J Ophthalmol 1977; 83:350–354.

40. Skoglund CR. On the influence of alcohol in the pupillary light reflex in man. Acta Physiol Scand 1943; 6:94–96.

41. Flom MC, Brown B, Adams AJ, Jones RT. Alcohol and marijuana effects on ocular tracking. Amer J Optom and Physiol Opt 1976; 53:764–773.

42. Mergler D, Blain L, Lemaire J, Lalande F. Colour vision impairment and alcohol consumption. Neurotoxicol Teratol 1988; 10:255–260.

43. Verriest G, Francq P, Pierart P. Results of colorvision tests in alcoholic and mentally disordered subjects. Ophthalmol 1980; 180:247–256.

43b. Verriest E, Francq P, Pierart P. Results of color vision tests in alcoholic and in mentally disordered subjects. Ophthalmol 1980; 180:247–256.

44. Cruz-Coke R. Defective color vision and alcoholism. Modern Problems in Ophthalmology 1976; 11:174–177.

45. Cruz-Coke R, Varela A. Colour blindness and alcohol addiction. Lancet 1965; 2:1348.

46. Cruz-Coke R, Varela A. Inheritance of alcoholism: Its association with colour blindness. Lancet 1966; 2:1282–1284.

47. Sassoon RF, Wise JB, Watson JJ. Alcoholism and color vision: Are there family links? Lancet 1970; 2:367–368.

48. Sakuma Y. Studies on color vision anomalies in subjects with alcoholism. Ann Ophthalmol 1973; 5:1277–1292.

49. deSchweinitz GE. Toxic Amplyopias. Lea Brothers & Co., Philadelphia, 1896.

50. Walsh FB, Hoyt WF. Clinical Neuro-Ophthalmology (3rd ed). Baltimore, Williams & Wilkins, 1969

51. Primo SA. Alcohol amblyopia. J Am Optom Assoc 1988; 59:392–396.

52. Le Dain G. Cannabis: A Report of the Commission of Inquiry into the NonMedical Use of Drugs. Ottawa, Information Canada, 1972.

53. Green K. Marijuana and the eye—A review. Journal of Toxicology, Cutaneous and Ocular Toxicology 1982; 1:3–32.

54. Johnson BA. Psychopharmacological effects of cannabis. Br J Hosp Med 1990; 43:114–121.

55. McClane NJ, Carroll D. Ocular manifestations of drug abuse. Surv Ophthalmol 1986; 30:298–313.

56. Allentuck S, Bowman KM. The psychiatric aspects of marijuana intoxication. Am J Psychiatry 1942; 99:248–251.

57. Julien RM. A Primer of Drug Action (3rd ed.). San Francisco, WH Freeman & Co., 1975.

58. Caldwell DF, Meyers SA, Domino EF, Merriam PE. Auditory and visual threshold effects of marijuana in man. Percept Mot Skills 1969; 29:755–759.

59. Clark LD, Nakashima EN. Experimental studies of marijuana. Am J Psychiatry 1968; 125:379–384.

60. Frank IM, Hepler RS, Stier S, Rickles WH, Ungerleider J. Marijuana, tobacco and functions affecting driving. Presented at the Annual Meeting of the American Psychiatric Association, Washington, DC, May 3–7, 1971.

61. Duckman R. Marihuana—how it affects vision, perception and memory. J Am Optom Assoc 1972; 43:160–163.

62. Halikas JA, Goodman DW, Guze SB. Marihuana effects—a survey of regular users. JAMA 1971; 217:692.

63. Hepler RS, Frank IR, Ungerleider JT. Pupillary constriction after marijuana smoking. Am J Ophthalmol 1972; 7:1185.

64. Weil AT, Zinberg NE, Nelson JM. Clinical and psychological effects of marijuana use in man. Science 1968; 162:1234–1242.

65. Hepler RS, Frank IR. Marihuana smoking and intraocular pressure. JAMA 1971; 217:1392.

66. Purnell WD, Gregg JM. Δ-9 tetrahydrocannabinol, euphoria, and intraocular pressure in man. Ann Ophthalmol 1975; 7:921–924.

67. Shapiro D. Ocular manifestations of the cannabinols. Ophthalmologica 1974; 168:366–369.

68. Flom MC, Adams AJ, Jones RT. Marijuana smoking and reduced intraocular pressure in human eyes: Drug action or epiphenomenon? Invest Ophthalmol Vis Sci 1975; 14:52–55.

69. Thomas R, Chester G. The pharmacology of marijuana. Med J Austr 1973; 2:229–234.

70. Valk L. Hemp in connection with opththalmology. Netherlands Optalmol Soc 1973; 167:413.

71. Dawson WW, Jimenez-Antillon CF, Perez JM, Zeskind JA. Marijuana and vision after ten years' use in Costa Rica. Invest Ophthalmol Vis Sci 1977; 16:689–699.

72. Roberts JD, Adams AJ. The short term effects of smoking on ocular accommodation and pupil size. J Am Optom Assoc 1969; 40:528–530.

73. Sibony PA, Evinger C, Manning KA. Tobacco-induced primary-position upbeat nystagmus. Ann Neurol 1987; 21:53–58.

74. Sibony PA, Evinger C, Manning KA. The effects of tobacco smoking on smooth pursuit eye movements. Ann Neurol 1987; 23:238–241.

75. Fotzsch R, Podemski R, Brzecki A, Bogdanska R. Behavior of visual evoked potentials (pattern reversal VECP) in smokers. Psychiatr Neurol Med Psychol (Leipz) 1986; 38:518–525.

76. Oku H, Fukushimi K, Sako H, Namba T, Wakakura M. Chronic toxicity of tobacco smoke on the visual system. Nippon Ganka Gakkai Zasshi. Acta Societatas Ophthalmologicae Japonicae 1989; 93:617–624.

77. Flaye DE, Sullivan KN, Cullinan TR, Silver JH, Whitelocke RAF. Cataracts and cigarette smoking: the City Eye Study. Eye 1989; 3:379–394.

78. West S, Munoz B, Emmett EA, Taylor HR. Cigarette smoking and the risk of nuclear cataracts. Arch Ophthalmol 1989; 107:1166–1169.

79. Berninger TA, Bird AC, Arden GB. Leber's hereditary optic atrophy. Ophthalmic Paediatr Genet 1989; 10:211–227.

80. Dews PE. Caffeine: Perspectives from Recent Research. New York, Springer-Verlag, 1984.

81. Putz-Anderson V, Setzer JV, Croxton JS. Effects of alcohol and methyl chloride in man. Psychol Rep 1981; 48:715–725.

82. Diamond AL, Cole RE. Visual threshold as a function of test area and caffeine administration. Psychonomic Sci 1970; 20:109–111.

83. Braverman DM, Cassagrande E. Effect of caffeine on performance of a perceptual-restructuring task at different stages of practice. Psychopharmacology 1982; 78:252–255.

84. Lieberman HR, Wurtman RJ, Emde GG, Coviella ILG. The effects of low doses of caffeine on human performance. Psychopharmacology 1987; 92:308–312.

85. Klemen JP, Diamond AL, Smith E. Effects of caffeine on enhancement of foveal simultaneous contrasts. J Exp Psychol 1961; 61:18–22.

86. Lichter PR. Caffeine and other prescriptions for patients with glaucoma (editorial). Ophthalmol 1990; 97:995–996.

87. Adams BA, Brubaker RF. Caffeine has no clinically significant effect on aqueous humor flow in the normal human eye. Ophthalmol 1990; 97:1030–1031.

88. Higginbotham EJ, Kilimanjaro HA, Wilensky JT, Batenhorst RL, Herman D. The effect of caffeine on intraocular pressure in glaucoma patients. Ophthalmol 1989; 96:624–626, 1680–1681.

89. Levine L. Reported ocular side effects of the ten most frequently prescribed drugs. J Am Optom Assn 1979; 50:221–227.

90. Arronson JK, Ford AR. The use of color vision measurement in the diagnosis of digoxin toxicity. Q J Med 1980; 195:273–282.

91. Chaplin S. Benzodiazepine prescribing [letter]. Lancet 1988; 1(8577):120–121.

92. Canon SH. Optometric implications of systemic drug therapy. J Am Optom Assn 1985; 56:843–844.

93. Gengo FM, Fagan SC, dePadova A, Miller JK, Kinkel PR. The effect of β-blockers on mental performance on older hypertensive patients. Arch Intern Med 1988; 148:779–784.

94. Robertson DM, Hollenhorst RW, Callahan JA. Receptor function in digitalis therapy. Arch Ophthalmol 1966; 76:640–645.

95. Applebaum M. Drug toxicity and visual fields. J Am Optom Assn 1980; 51:859–862.

96. Johnson D, Hopf R, Frauendorf A, Woodcock BG, Mujtaba F. The effect of cardiac glycosides on the visual system of man measured with cortical evoked potentials. Arsneimittelforschung 1986; 36:260–262.

97. Ross JVM. Visual disturbances due to the use of digitalis and similar preparations. Am J Ophthalmol 1950; 33:1438–1439.

98. Lanthony P. La xanthopsie de Van Gogh. Bulletin des Societes Ophthalmalogie France 1989; 10:1133–1134.

99. Weleber RG, Denman ST, Hanifin JM, Cunningham WJ. Abnormal retinal function associated with isotretinoin therapy for acne. Arch Ophthalmol 1986; 104:831–837.

100. Braude MC. Drugs and drug interactions in the elderly woman. Women and drugs: A new era for research. Nida Research Monograph Series 1986; 65:58–64.

101. Banerjee AK, Falkai PG, Savidge M. Visual hallucinations in the elderly associated with the use of levodopa. Postgrad Med J 1989; 65:358–361.

102. Nicastro NJ. Visual disturbances associated with over-the-counter ibuprofen in three patients. Ann Ophthalmol 1989; 29:447–450.

103. Collum LMT, Bowen DI. Ocular side-effects of ibuprofen. Br Ophthalmol 1971; 55:472–477.

104. Hamburger HA, Beckman H, Thompson R. Visual evoked potentials and ibuprofen (Motrin) toxicity. Ann Ophthalmol 1984; 16:328–329.

105. Pinckers AJLG, Pokorny J, Smith VC, Verriest G. Classification of abnormal color vision. In Congenital and acquired color vision defects. Pokorny J, Smith VC, Verriest G, Pinckers LG (Eds), Grune & Stratton, New York, 1979.

106. Grant WM. Toxicology of the eye. Springfield IL, Charles C Thomas, 1962.

107. Sanford JP. Guide to antimicrobial therapy. Bethesda, MD, Antimicrobial Therapy Inc., 1990.

Index